DAVID M. WITTEN, M.D., M.S. (Radiology), F.A.C.R.

Professor and Chairman, Department of Diagnostic Radiology,
University of Alabama School of Medicine,
Birmingham, Alabama

GEORGE H. MYERS, Jr., M.D., F.A.C.S.

Clinical Professor of Surgery (Urology),
University of Kansas School of Medicine,
Kansas City, Kansas; Consultant in Surgery (Urology),
Veterans Administration Hospital,
Kansas City, Missouri

DAVID C. UTZ, M.D., M.S. (Urology), F.A.C.S.

Professor of Urology, Mayo Medical School;
Chairman, Department of Urology, Mayo Clinic,
Rochester, Minnesota

1977
W. B. SAUNDERS COMPANY
Philadelphia, London, Toronto

Fourth Edition

Emmett's

CLINICAL
UROGRAPHY

*An Atlas and Textbook
of Roentgenologic Diagnosis*

VOLUME II

W. B. Saunders Company: West Washington Square
                           Philadelphia, PA   19105

                           1 St. Anne's Road
                           Eastbourne, East Sussex BN21 3UN, England

                           833 Oxford Street
                           Toronto, Ontario, M8Z 5T9, Canada

Library of Congress Cataloging in Publication Data

Emmett, John Lester, 1903–1974

Emmett's clinical urography.

First ed. by W. F. Braasch and J. L. Emmett.

First–3d ed. (1951–1971)published under title:
Clinical urography.

Includes bibliographies.

1. Genito-urinary organs — Radiography.   I. Witten,
   David M., 1926–   II. Myers, George Henry, 1935–
   III. Utz, David C., 1923–   IV. Title. [DNLM: 1.
   Urography. WJ141 E54c]

RC874.E45 1977   616.6 ;   76-19614

ISBN 0-7216-9472-1

Emmett's Clinical Urography

                                    Complete Set 0-7216-9471-3
                              Volume I   ISBN   0-7216-9472-1
                              Volume II ISBN   0-7216-9473-X
                              Volume III ISBN   0-7216-9474-8

Last digit is the print number: 9   8   7   6   5   4   3   2   1

CONTENTS

VOLUME II

Chapter 9

ANOMALIES OF THE GENITOURINARY TRACT 565

Clinical Classification of Anomalies 565

The Kidney and Ureter 566

    Embryology of the Kidney and Ureter 566

    Anomalies in Number 569

    Anomalies in Size 577

    Anomalies in Position 579

    Anomalies in Form 604

    Anomalies in Structure 642

The Renal Pelvis and Ureter 642

    Anomalies in Number 642

    Anomalies of Ureteropelvic Juncture; Obstruction at
Ureteropelvic Juncture 672

    Anomalies in Position and Form of Ureter 672

    Anomalies of Origin and Termination of the Ureter 684

The Bladder and Urethra 729

    Embryology of the Bladder 729

    Anomalies of the Urachus 732

    Anomalies of the Bladder 736

    Embryology of the Urethra 751

    Anomalies of the Urethra 755

Deep Pelvic Cysts 765

Congenital Absence of the Abdominal Muscles (Prune
Belly Syndrome) 777

Intersexuality: Genitography in the Intersexual State 779

    by Charles E. Shopfner

    The Nature of Sex 780

    Technique of Genitography 784

    Classification of Anatomy 785

    Comment 790

Urologic Aspects of Ectopic Anus (Imperforate Anus;
Anal Atresia) 791

    by Charles E. Shopfner

    Embryology 792

    Technique of Roentgenographic Examination 793

    Classification of Roentgen Findings 795

    Associated Congenital Anomalies 798

                    Suggested Method of Management................................. 799
                    Comment 800
            References 801

Chapter 10

INFECTIOUS DISEASES OF THE GENITOURINARY TRACT 809
            by Glen W. Hartman, Joseph W. Segura, and Robert R. Hattery

            Acute Pyelonephritis 809
                    Gross Pathologic Appearance in Acute Pyelonephritis...... 809
                    Microscopic Findings in Acute Pyelonephritis................. 809
                    Roentgen Findings in Acute Pyelonephritis 810
            Chronic Pyelonephritis 817
                    Routes of Infection... 818
                    Gross Pathologic Changes in Chronic Pyelonephritis 818
                    Intrarenal Reflux and the Role of Infection 819
                    Roentgen Diagnosis in Chronic Pyelonephritis............... 821
                    Vesicoureteral Reflux in Adults................................... 837
                    Chronic Pyelonephritis in Children............................. 838
            Xanthogranulomatous Pyelonephritis................................... 839
                    Radiographic Findings in Xanthogranulomatous
                            Pyelonephritis 840
            Renal and Perirenal Abscess.. 842
                by H. Peter Jander
                    Etiology of Renal and Perirenal Abscesses..................... 842
                    Pathophysiology of Renal and Perirenal Abscesses.......... 843
                    Clinical Aspects of Renal and Perirenal Abscesses.......... 844
                    Roentgen Findings in Renal and Perirenal Abscesses....... 848
            Responses of the Collecting System to Infection...................... 867
            Pyeloureteritis and Cystitis Cystica...................................... 873
            Malacoplakia 876
            Gas-Producing Infections of the Urinary Tract......................... 878
            Cystitis 883
                    Bacterial Cystitis.. 883
                    Interstitial Cystitis.. 883
                    Cyclophosphamide Cystitis 885
                    Eosinophilic Cystitis 885
                    Cystitis Glandularis... 885
                    Tubercular Cystitis.. 888
            Prostatitis (Acute Bacterial Prostatitis, Chronic
            Bacterial Prostatitis, Chronic Prostatitis
            ["Prostatitis"]); Prostatic Duct Abscess................................ 888
                    Granulomatous Prostatitis.. 891
            Brucellosis of the Urinary Tract... 891
                    Roentgen Findings in Brucellosis 891
            Fungal Infection of the Kidney.. 895
                    Renal Candidiasis and Actinomycosis........................... 895
            Tuberculosis of the Genitourinary Tract 898
                    Pathogenesis of Genitourinary Tuberculosis................... 898
                    Clinical and Laboratory Findings in Genitourinary
                            Tuberculosis... 898
                    Roentgen Findings in Genitourinary Tuberculosis........... 899
                    Genitotuberculosis 918

Genitourinary Bilharziasis (Schistosomiasis)............................ 921
    by Abdel Aziz Zaky Hanna
        Pathogenesis of Genitourinary Bilharziasis...................... 922
        Pathology of Genitourinary Bilharziasis 922
        Genital Involvement in Bilharziasis 927
        Roentgen Diagnosis in Genitourinary Bilharziasis........... 927
Echinococcus Cysts (Renal Hydatidosis)................................ 940
        Epidemiology of Renal Hydatidosis 940
        Pathogenesis of Genitourinary Infestation in
            Renal Hydatidosis.. 941
        Diagnosis of Renal Hydatidosis 942
References 949

Chapter 11
**URINARY STASIS: THE OBSTRUCTIVE UROPATHIES,
ATONY, VESICOURETERAL REFLUX, AND NEUROMUSCULAR
DYSFUNCTION OF THE URINARY TRACT** 955
    Terminology.. 955
    Classification of Stasis.. 955
        Obstructive and Nonobstructive Varieties of Stasis.......... 955
    Pyelectasis (Hydronephrosis).. 955
        Pathophysiologic Changes in the Kidney 955
        Roentgen Findings in Pyelectasis 956
        Renal Radioisotopic Studies in Pyelectasis..................... 971
    Localized Dilatation of Calyx (Hydrocalyx, Calyceal
        Diverticulum, and Pyelogenic Cyst); Hydrocalycosis.............. 974
        Hydrocalycosis.. 983
        Vascular Obstruction of the Infundibulum of the
            Upper Calyx.. 983
    Obstruction at the Ureteropelvic Juncture............................ 986
        Pathogenesis of Ureteropelvic Juncture Obstruction........ 987
        Urographic Diagnosis of Ureteropelvic Juncture
            Obstruction 999
    Ureterectasis and Ureteropyelectasis 1005
        Obstructive Ureterectasis; Obstruction At or Above
            the Ureterovesical Juncture.................................. 1011
    Vesicoureteral Reflux... 1017
        by Panayotis P. Kelalis
        General Considerations.. 1018
        Roentgen Findings in Vesicoureteral Reflux................... 1018
        Etiology of Vesicoureteral Reflux............................. 1038
        Factors Affecting the Course and Prognosis of
            Vesicoureteral Reflux...................................... 1050
        Vesicoureteral Reflux in Adults............................... 1059
        Management of Vesicoureteral Reflux........................... 1062
    Stasis Involving the Lower Part of the Urinary Tract................ 1080
        by David C. Utz and David M. Barrett
        Neurogenic Bladder 1080
        Congenital Obstruction of the Vesical Neck and
            Urethra; Distal Urethral Obstruction; Stenosis of
            the Urethral Meatus 1100
        Congenital Urethral Valves 1106
        Urethral Polyps in Boys....................................... 1119
        Congenital Stenosis of the Urethral Meatus................... 1122

Congenital, Iatrogenic, and Traumatic Strictures
of the Urethra in Infants and Children 1123
Vesical Diverticulum 1129
Obstruction of the Bladder Outlet in the
Adult Male 1135
Urethral Diverticulum in the Male 1149
Urethral Stricture in Adult Males 1150
Postoperative Incontinence in the Male 1162
References 1162

Chapter 12
CALCULOUS DISEASE OF THE GENITOURINARY TRACT 1171
by Reza S. Malek

General Considerations 1171
Classification 1173
Renal Calculi 1176
Clinical Features of Renal Calculi 1176
Roentgen Studies of Renal Calculi 1179
Pathogenesis and Medical Management 1241
Surgical Management of Renal Calculi 1283
Renal Calculi in Childhood 1284
Nephrocalcinosis 1285
Ureteral Calculi 1294
Clinical Features of Ureteral Calculi 1294
Roentgen Studies of Ureteral Calculi 1294
Management of Ureteral Calculi 1331
Vesical Calculi 1338
Endemic Calculi 1338
Clinical Features and Investigations of Vesical
Calculi 1340
Management of Vesical Calculi 1349
Prostatic Calculi 1349
Classification of Prostatic Calculi 1349
Clinical Features of Prostatic Calculi 1352
Roentgen Features of Prostatic Calculi 1352
Management of Prostatic Calculi 1356
Urethral Calculi 1359
Clinical Features of Urethral Calculi 1364
Diagnosis of Uretheral Calculi 1364
Management of Urethral Calculi 1365
References 1365

INDEX i

ANOMALIES OF THE GENITOURINARY TRACT

Campbell (1963) has stated that "anomalous development attains its highest incidence in the urogenital tract . . ." It is estimated that 35 per cent to 40 per cent of all maldevelopments are urogenital and that approximately 10 per cent of all human beings are born with some anomaly of the urogenital tract. Dees found that, in 9.6 per cent of 1,410 cases investigated urologically, urography disclosed some anomaly of the upper part of the urinary tract. This situation is not surprising when one considers the complicated embryologic development of the urinary tract. In the embryologic evolution of the kidney, *three* essential renal organs—the pronephros, the mesonephros, and the metanephros—develop in rapid succession. The pronephros and metanephros degenerate and become important parts of another system, the genital tract. Furthermore, the formation of the definitive kidney requires a delicate union of endodermal and mesodermal structures. Finally, the great number of changes that the fetal kidney normally undergoes both as to form and position are factors responsible for congenital anomalies. Although not every anomaly or congenital malformation constitutes a pathologic lesion or entity, it may be assumed from the clinical data at hand that practically every congenital malformation of the urinary tract is potentially a clinicopathologic entity.

It is apparent that this classification

CLINICAL CLASSIFICATION OF ANOMALIES

(This classification of possible anomalous states of the genitourinary system is by no means complete or all-inclusive and is confined to the anomalous conditions that can be demonstrated urographically.)

I. THE KIDNEY
  A. Anomalies in number
    1. Supernumerary kidney
    2. Agenesis and dysgenesis (unilateral and bilateral)
  B. Anomalies in size
    1. The small kidney (hypoplasia; atrophy)*
    2. Compensatory hypertrophy

  C. Anomalies in position
    1. Malrotation
    2. Ectopia and dystopia
  D. Anomalies in form
    1. Fusion
      a. Crossed renal ectopia with fusion; horseshoe kidneys
  E. Anomalies in structure
    1. Polycystic disease†
    2. Multicystic disease†

---

*Also considered in Chapter 10.   †Considered in Chapter 13.

II. THE RENAL PELVIS AND URETER
  A. Anomalies in number
    1. Bifid, trifid, and multifid pelves
    2. Duplication of pelvis and ureter
  B. Anomalies of the ureteropelvic juncture‡
  C. Anomalies in position and form of ureter
    1. Rudimentary branched ureter
    2. Blind-ending duplication
    3. Ureteral diverticula
    4. Retrocaval ureter
    5. Congenital obstruction of ureter (stricture, valves, and aberrant blood vessels)
    6. Congenital "nonobstructive" ureterectasis (megaureter)‡
    7. Vesicoureteral reflux‡
  D. Anomalies of origin and termination of ureter
    1. Ectopic ureteral orifices
  E. Ureterocele; ectopic ureterocele

‡Considered in Chapter 11.

III. THE BLADDER AND URETHRA
  A. Anomalies of the urachus
  B. Anomalies of the bladder
    1. Exstrophy-epispadias complex
    2. Duplication of bladder
  C. Anomalies of the urethra
    1. Double urethra and accessory urethra
    2. Diverticulum of the male urethra
IV. DEEP PELVIC CYSTS
  A. Cysts of the müllerian duct
  B. Dilatation of prostatic utricle
  C. Cysts of the seminal vesicles
  D. Cysts of the prostate gland
V. CONGENITAL ABSENCE OF ABDOMINAL MUSCLES
VI. INTERSEXUALITY
VII. ECTOPIC ANUS (IMPERFORATE ANUS, ANAL ATRESIA, URETHRORECTAL "FISTULA")

could be enlarged and compounded if one were to list all the possible combinations of the many conditions enumerated. For instance, in the case of the ectopic ureteral orifice many combinations are possible that depend on whether the condition is unilateral or bilateral, is associated with duplication on one or both sides, involves one or more ureters, or is associated with ectopic or crossed ectopic kidneys. It is obviously impossible in a book of this kind to include urograms to demonstrate every type of anomaly of the kidney and ureter that has been described. Illustrations of the more common conditions will be shown which should be sufficient to permit recognition of almost any type of anomaly likely to be encountered.

Also, it should be readily apparent that in the subsequent discussion the outline cannot be followed rigidly because the various conditions often occur together with a myriad of possible combinations which at times may tax one's diagnostic acumen.

THE KIDNEY AND URETER

Embryology of the Kidney and Ureter*

THE KIDNEY: EARLY PHASES

The duct which drains the mesonephros (wolffian body) is called the *mesonephric* or *wolffian* duct. It originates as the pronephric duct which grows caudad, reaching and emptying into the cloaca at about the 4-mm stage. When mesonephric tubules become connected to the pronephric duct, its name is changed to mesonephric duct. The cloaca divides into a ventral segment, forming the bladder and

*Only the embryology pertinent to the anomalies discussed in this chapter is included here.

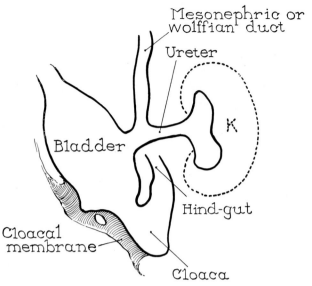

Figure 9–1. Sprouting of ureter from mesonephric or wolffian duct and its division into two branches which are forerunners of two major calyces. Renal mesenchyme, which caps branching ureter, has assumed definite "bean" form. (See text.) (Redrawn from Arey, L. B.)

the urogenital sinus, and a dorsal segment, which becomes the rectum. Even before the cloaca divides, a bud appears on the dorsal surface of the wolffian duct a short distance from the cloacal wall. This is called the *ureteral bud* and is the anlage of the adult ureter. The cranial end of the ureteral bud grows cephalad into a mass of undifferentiated mesoderm which soon becomes specialized to form the renal mesenchyme or anlage of the kidney proper. At approximately the 10-mm stage, the cephalic end of the ureteral bud divides into two branches which are the fore-runners of the two major calyces (Fig. 9–1). At this stage the renal mesenchyme, which caps the branching ureter, has assumed a definite "bean" form. The two kidneys at this stage lie close together (almost in apposition and parallel to each other) and are at the level of the second sacral segment. Their upper poles reach to the brim of the true pelvis. The point of bifurcation of the ureteral bud becomes the future renal pelvis.

Further description of the subsequent branching to the ureter is best left to Arey, who said:

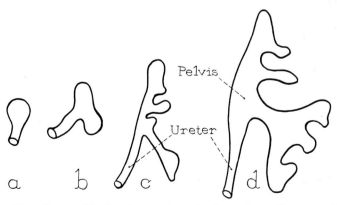

Figure 9–2. Branching of ureteral bud to form major and minor calyces. (See text.) (From Arey, L. B.)

Of the first two [primary divisions of the ureter] one is cranial, the other is caudal in position and between these, two others usually appear [Fig. 9–2]. From an ampullary enlargement at the end of each primary tubule sprout off two, three or four secondary tubules. These in turn give rise to tertiary tubules and the process is repeated until the fifth month of fetal life, when it is estimated that twelve generations of tubules have been developed. The pelvis and the primary and secondary tubules enlarge greatly during development. The two primary expansions become the *major calyces* and the secondary tubules opening into them form the *minor calyces.* The tubules of the third and fourth orders are taken up into the walls of the enlarged secondary tubules so that the tubules of the fifth order, twenty to thirty in number, open into the minor calyces as *papillary ducts.* The remaining orders of tubules constitute the *collecting tubules* which form the greater part of the medulla of the adult kidney.

The renal cortex is formed from the renal mesenchyme, which gives rise to the glomeruli and uriniferous tubules (proximal and distal convoluted tubules and loops of Henle).

Failure of the uriniferous tubules (originating from nephrogenic blastema) to connect with the collecting tubules (derived from the ureteric bud) is the most commonly accepted explanation of *polycystic disease of the kidneys.* However, Mc Kenna and Kampmeier, in 1934, advanced a different explanation based on Kampmeier's original concept of three zones in the developing cortex of the kidney, namely a vestigial zone, a provisional zone, and a growth zone (Fig. 9–3). Kampmeier expressed the belief that the tubules of the vestigial zone are rudimentary and disappear without a trace, those of the provisional zone unite with the collecting ducts only to break away from them again, and those of the growth zone form the definitive renal cortex. McKenna and Kampmeier stated that the uriniferous tubules of the provisional zone usually collapse and disappear after they lose their connections to the collecting tubules, but that some of them may persist and expand to form cysts. They explained all types of renal cysts (solitary, multiple, and polycystic disease) on this basis. [*This explanation of cyst formation has been challenged repeatedly in recent years, and it does not now appear to be correct. The subject is discussed in detail in chapter 13.*]

THE URETER

Returning now to consideration of the lower end of the ureter, it will be recalled that originally the ureter sprouted from the dorsal surface of the wolffian duct just proximal to its junction with the cloaca. The ureter next shifts its position to the lateral aspect of the wolffian duct. The lower end of the duct, from which the ureter arises, expands and through a rather complicated form of growth is absorbed as a part of the bladder in its vesicourethral portion so that the ureter and the mesonephric duct open separately (Fig. 9–4). This change is taking place at about the same time that the kid-

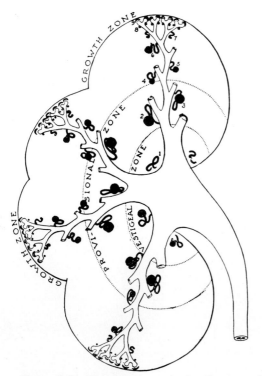

Figure 9–3. The three zones in development of uriniferous tubules. (From Kampmeier, O. F.)

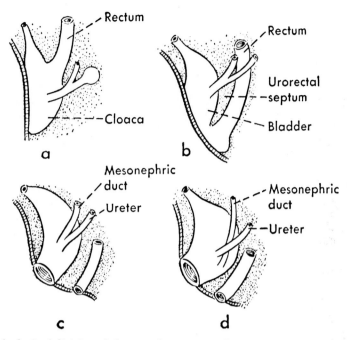

Figure 9-4. Method of subdivision of cloaca and separation of openings of mesonephric duct (vas deferens in male) and ureter. A, Primitive condition. B, Urorectal septum has separated rectum from urinary bladder. C, Common stem of mesonephric duct and ureter has been largely absorbed into wall of bladder. D, Differential growth of wall of bladder is carrying mesonephric duct distally toward urethra. (From Hollingshead, W. H.)

neys are undergoing rotation and ascent. The portion of the bladder that receives the ureters and wolffian ducts grows in an uneven manner so that the ureters migrate laterally and cranially while the distal ends of the wolffian ducts remain close together in the midline and appear to migrate somewhat distally, their orifices eventually being situated in the verumontanum in the distal portion of the floor of the prostatic urethra. Embryologically, therefore, an area bounded by the ureteral orifices and the mesonephric (ejaculatory) ducts is thought to be of mesodermal origin, whereas the remainder of the bladder is of entodermal origin. There is still some difference of opinion concerning this last statement, however. This area of mesonephric tissue in the male includes the trigone and proximal part of the prostatic urethra. In the female it includes the trigone and almost all of the urethra.

Anomalies in Number

"FREE" SUPERNUMERARY KIDNEY

One of the rarest anomalies encountered in the urinary tract is the free supernumerary kidney (Bacon; Carlson; Hanley; Kretschmer; Mills; Stewart; Swick) (Figs. 9-5 through 9-8). Up to five free supernumerary kidneys in one individual have been described. One must be exceedingly careful when making such a diagnosis not to confuse it with a duplicated pelvis or a complete duplication in a segment of a horseshoe kidney (see Figure 9-99).

Embryogenesis

The embryogenesis of the supernumerary kidney is similar to renal duplication. Two ureteric buds arise from different positions on the wolffian duct, reaching the

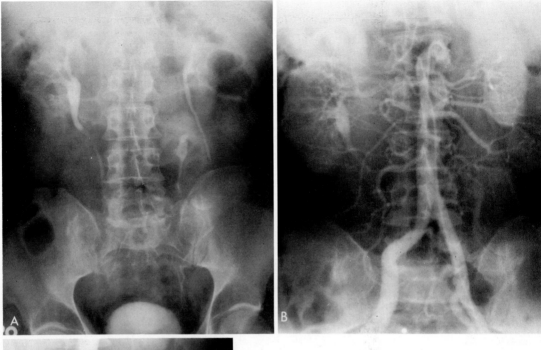

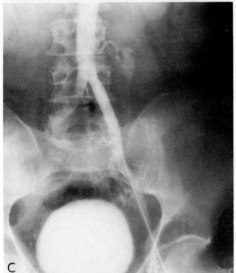

Figure 9–5. Supernumerary kidney with benign cyst. Man aged 49 with crampy abdominal pain. **A,** *Excretory urogram.* Three separate renal units, each having its own separate and complete ureter. The ureter of the left superior kidney is deviated laterally by the supernumerary kidney. **B** and **C,** *Abdominal aortogram.* **B,** normal blood supply to the two normal kidneys but several small arteries entering supernumerary kidney. **C,** One renal artery to supernumerary kidney selectively demonstrated. Surgical exploration and nephrectomy revealed a 4 cm benign cyst arising from the lower pole of the supernumerary kidney. (From Wulfe-kuhler, W. V., and Dube, V. E.)

nephrogenic mesenchyme (nephrogenic blastema) so divergent that two separate renal units develop. Usually the kidney in the inferior position is the supernumerary unit, but it may be superior. The supernumerary kidney is usually smaller and is often hypoplastic and histologically less organized than the normal kidney. For this reason there is often poor function, making the supernumerary kidney difficult to visu-

alize by excretory urography. The ureter of the supernumerary kidney may join the normal ureter or enter the bladder separately. Rarely, the ureter of the upper kidney joins the lower kidney's pelvis (Fig. 9–9), or the ureter of the supernumerary kidney has an ectopic opening (Samuels and associates). Simultaneous anomalies of other parts of the urogenital tract as well as a high incidence of pathologic changes in supernumerary kidneys have been reported (Wulfekuhler and Dube).

RENAL AGENESIS AND DYSGENESIS

Terminology

Ashley and Mostofi, in their comprehensive necropsy study on this subject, have suggested the following terminology: (1) If no vestige of renal tissue is formed, the condition is called *agenesis*. (2) If the kidney is represented by a nodule of tissue that bears no morphologic or histologic resemblance to normal renal parenchyma, it is called *dysgenesis*. (3) If the kidney is

tiny but otherwise similar to a normal organ, it is called *hypoplasia*. Other terms that have been used in the literature for the latter two terms are *aplasia, dysplasia,* and *congenital atrophy.*

Embryogenesis

Renal agenesis and dysgenesis result from a failure of the ureteric bud to make contact with the nephrogenic blastema at the proper time. The reason for this failure may be one of several: (1) failure of the ureteric bud to form, (2) failure of the bud to reach the blastema before it migrates upward, (3) failure of the wolffian duct to

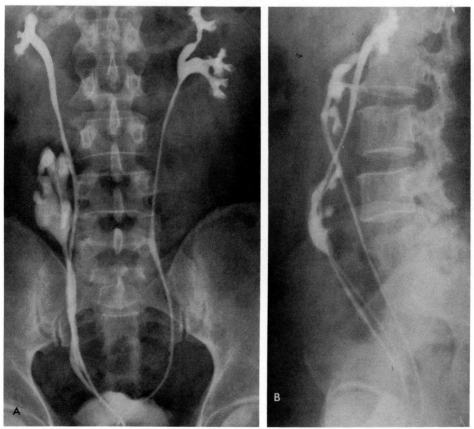

Figure 9–6.   **Supernumerary kidney associated with pyelectasis on right side,** opposite fourth and fifth lumbar vertebrae. This is associated with **complete duplication of right ureter and two ureteral orifices in bladder.** Little if any function remains in right supernumerary kidney. **A,** *Bilateral retrograde pyelogram,* showing three separate kidneys. **B,** *Lateral film.* Exploration revealed supernumerary kidney 6 to 7 cm long on right side, lying in groove between psoas muscle and vertebral bodies in approximate area of right sacroiliac articulation. Upper right kidney and left kidney were palpated and found to be normal except that right kidney was about one third smaller than normal. (From Stewart, C. M.)

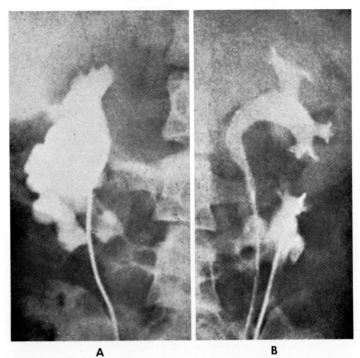

Figure 9–7. **Horseshoe kidney associated with supernumerary kidney. A,** *Right retrograde pyelogram.* Larger half of horseshoe kidney is on right, smaller on left. **Moderate pyelocaliectasis on right. B,** *Left retrograde pyelogram.* Pelvis supplying left half of horseshoe is smaller than right. Above is supernumary kidney which at surgical exploration was freely movable in all directions and separate from horseshoe kidney; separate vascular pedicle could also be palpated. (From Hanley, H. G.)

develop, or (4) the absence of the metanephrogenic mesenchyme. When there is failure of the urogenital ridge to form, there is absence of all internal genital and upper urinary tract structures, including the trigone on the affected side. When the ureteric bud fails to reach or enter the nephrogenic blastema at the proper time, there is either absence or dysgenesis of the kidney. The ureter is absent in most cases of renal agenesis and is usually atretic or absent when dysgenesis is present.

Incidence

Autopsy Material. It is impossible to give any firm data concerning the incidence of renal agenesis. Autopsy studies provide the most significant data. Clinical data are notoriously inaccurate; however, since excretory urography has become so widely used, clinical data are becoming

more significant. Of course, *bilateral agenesis* is extremely rare, incompatible with life, and, therefore, of little clinical importance. Potter described a characteristic facial appearance in infants with bilateral renal agenesis. The face shows an increased space between the eyes and a prominent fold arising at the inner canthus which sweeps downward and laterally below the eyes. In addition, there are a flattened nose, receding chin, and low-set ears. *Unilateral agenesis* appears to be not too uncommon. Most urologists encounter this condition frequently enough to constantly have it in mind.

From a collection of 245,000 autopsy protocols in the files of the Armed Forces Institute of Pathology, Ashley and Mostofi found 364 cases of renal agenesis or dysgenesis as follows: bilateral agenesis—47 cases; unilateral agenesis—240 cases (including 8 cases of crossed ectopia);

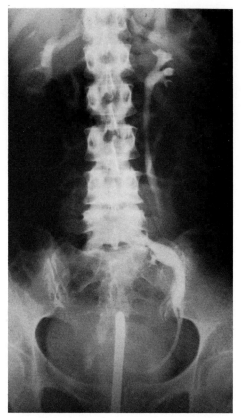

Figure 9–8. *Retrograde pyelogram.* **Supernumerary left kidney** overlies left sacro-iliac synchondrosis. Diagnosis was confirmed at laparotomy. (Courtesy of Dr. W. E. Kittredge.)

cent) were female; the sex was not given in 69 cases.

Braasch and Merricks were able to find 69 cases of unilateral agenesis in the records of the Mayo Clinic from 1909 through 1937. Only 27 of these were verified by operation or autopsy. Longo and Thompson in a later clinical study found an additional 94 cases seen at the Mayo Clinic in a 12-year period, 1938 through 1949. Only five of these cases were verified by operation, but all were exhaustively and carefully studied. The authors stated that unilateral renal agenesis is found in about 1 of every 1,000 autopsies and clinically in about 1 of every 500 urologic patients.

In the past, unilateral agenesis has been considered to occur more commonly in females than in males, but in Longo and Thompson's series 60.6 per cent of the cases involved males and only 39.3 per cent females. It was their opinion that because females have a greater frequency of complications and associated anomalies (especially genital) than males, they are led to seek medical consultation more often.

bilateral dysgenesis—11 cases; unilateral dysgenesis—57 cases; and mixed anomaly (dysgenesis on one side and agenesis on the other)—9 cases.

Because of the military nature of the population from which the study was drawn (high proportion of young men), data concerning sex incidence and age are not significant.

In 19,046 autopsies of children, Campbell (1963) found bilateral agenesis in seven cases (ratio of 1:2,721); whereas, in another series of 51,880 autopsies, there were 94 cases of unilateral agenesis (ratio of 1:552).

Clinical Material. Collins collected 581 cases of unilateral agenesis from the world literature. Of the 581 patients, 281 (48.3 per cent) were male and 231 (39.7 per

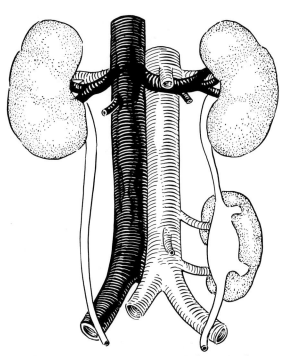

Figure 9–9. Supernumerary kidney. (Redrawn from Kretschmer, H. L. By permission of Surg., Gynec. & Obst.)

Much of the literature on agenesis concerns itself with unusual and special situations—for instance, solitary kidneys in various types of ectopic positions such as pelvic (sacral) (Köhler), crossed ectopia, and so on. In many of these articles the chief interest concerns the associated genital anomalies, such as *absence of the vagina.*

Associated Anatomic Abnormalities

A knowledge of anatomic variations of the genitourinary system that may accompany renal agenesis may be helpful in diagnosis.

Adrenal Glands. There has been much imprecise information in the literature concerning whether or not the adrenal gland is present or absent in cases of unilateral renal agenesis. Ashley and Mostofi reported that in their 240 cases of unilateral agenesis there was homolateral absence of the adrenal gland in 19 (8 per cent). In 22 cases the gland was not mentioned. Both adrenal glands were present in 44 of the 47 cases of bilateral agenesis; in the other 3, the glands were not mentioned. Collins' data agree; of his 581 cases of unilateral agenesis, absence of the homolateral adrenal gland was found in only 66 (11.4 per cent).

The Solitary Kidney. Compensatory hyperplasia of the solitary kidney is commonly seen. It was noted in 308 (53 per cent) of Collins' 581 cases and in 46 (49 per cent) of Campbell's (1963) 94 cases. Anomalies (principally ectopia and malrotation) were noted in 7 (10.1 per cent) of Braasch and Merricks' cases. Malrotation was present in 11 (11.7 per cent) and ectopia in 5 (5.3 per cent) of Longo and Thompson's cases.

Ureters. The homolateral ureter is completely absent in the majority of cases of agenesis, but in some cases portions of the ureter (principally the lower part) may be present. In Collins' series it was reported to be absent in 297 (51.1 per cent) of the 581 cases. Information concerning the ureter was available in 157 of Ashley and Mostofi's cases of unilateral agenesis. They reported the ureter completely absent in 138 (87 per cent). In 19 cases (12 per cent) some of the lower portion of the ureter was present. In no case was a completely formed ureter present. In the 47 cases of *bilateral agenesis* there was complete absence of both ureters in 39, and partial absence in 3. Campbell (1963) mentions one case in which an incomplete atrophic ureter joined the vagina. Saalfeld and associates reported a patient with vaginal atresia, unilateral renal dysgenesis, retroiliac ureter, and anomalies of the abdominal aorta and its branches.

Bladder and Trigone. In their 47 cases of *bilateral renal agenesis,* Ashley and Mostofi encountered complete absence of the bladder in 10 (21 per cent) and a defective urethra in 8 of the 10. In 14 other cases, the bladder was dysplastic, being represented by a vestigial fibrous structure "either without a lumen or with only a minute slit."

In cases of *unilateral renal agenesis,* failure of development of the homolateral half of the trigone is a common finding. This is a finding well known to urologists and is searched for cystoscopically in suspected cases. In 75 of Longo and Thompson's 94 clinical cases of unilateral agenesis, cystoscopy was carried out, and absence of one ureteral orifice and the corresponding half of the trigone and interureteric ridge was noted in 37 cases (49.3 per cent). They also stated that there was an absent ureteral orifice but a normal appearing trigone and interureteric ridge in about one third of the cases. A ureteral orifice appeared to be present in another 13 cases but was apparently a blind ureteral lumen, as the ureteral catheter met obstruction at or near the ureterovesical juncture.

In the necropsy study of Ashley and Mostofi, of the 138 cases of *unilateral agenesis* in which the ureters were completely absent, absence of development of the corresponding side of the trigone was observed in 123 (89 per cent). As these data suggest, absence of the ureteral orifice and corresponding half of the trigone is almost pathognomonic of unilateral renal agenesis.

However, a normally developed trigone does not exclude it. The difficulties and errors associated with cystoscopic diagnosis of a hemitrigone will be discussed later.

Renal Arteries. With the availability and common usage of arteriography, data concerning the status of the renal arteries become of clinical importance. The most significant data come from Ashley and Mostofi's autopsy study. There were only 108 of their cases in which the state of the renal vessels was mentioned, and there was no case in which a major renal vessel was present in conjunction with an absence or gross deficiency (dysplasia) of the kidney. They stated, "in general, the smaller the remnant of kidney tissue, the more likely was the renal vessel to be completely absent."

Associated Anomalies of the Genitalia

Guizzetti estimated that anomalies of the genitalia are present in a third of the cases of renal anomalies. Longo and Thompson state, "It is well established that genital anomalies are associated more frequently with a congenital solitary kidney than they are with any other type of renal malformation."

Associated genital anomalies are nearly always "homolateral" (on the same side as the absent kidney) and are found more frequently in females than males. Fortune, in a study of 381 cases of solitary kidney, noted genital anomalies in 69.9 per cent of 183 females but in only 21.2 per cent of 198 males. In addition to being more frequent in the female, they are also more "traumatic" clinically, resulting in problems that require medical attention; the *well-known syndrome of the absent or hypoplastic vagina and solitary kidney* is a good example.

Although almost every variety of genital anomaly has been encountered in cases of renal agenesis (Ashley and Mostofi; Collins), the most common are as follows.

In the Male. There may be (1) hypo- plasia (atrophy) or absence of all or part of the seminal tract (epididymis, vasa vasorum, seminal vesicle, and ejaculatory ducts); (2) hypoplasia (atrophy) or absence of the testis,* and (3) malformation of the external genitalia such as hypospadias, cleft scrotum, and so on.

In the Female. The most commonly encountered anomalies involve the uterus and vagina.

Uterine Abnormalities. Most often, there is an unicornuate or bicornuate uterus (Shumacker), with or without a rudimentary horn, or a double uterus (uterus didelphys) sometimes associated with a vaginal septum.

Vaginal Abnormalities. Absence or aplasia of the vagina is a well-known anomaly that may send a young woman to the physician (Figs. 9–10 and 9–11). Double vagina is also seen (see Chapter 19, Hematocolpos). In the records of the Mayo Clinic, Phelan, Counsellor, and Greene found 129 cases of congenital absence of the vagina. Excretory urograms, done in 72 cases, revealed unilateral renal agenesis in 10 and renal ectopia in 6. In 1957, this series was increased to 143 cases (Counseller and Flor).

Abnormalities of Ovaries and Fallopian Tubes. Absence and hypoplasia of the ovaries or fallopian tubes, or both, with or without associated anomalies of the uterus and vagina, also occur. Gynecologists are so aware of the association of genital and renal anomalies in the female that an excretory urogram is now almost the first examination requested in such a situation.

The Clinical Problem

The clinical problem obviously is concerned only with *unilateral* renal agenesis (solitary kidney). Special situations arising from anomalies of the solitary kidney such as malrotation, ectopia, duplication of the pelvis and ureter, ectopic ureteral orifices,

---

*Radasch reported absence of the homolateral testis in 15 (7 per cent) of 225 cases of unilateral agenesis.

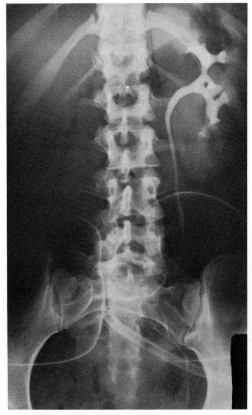 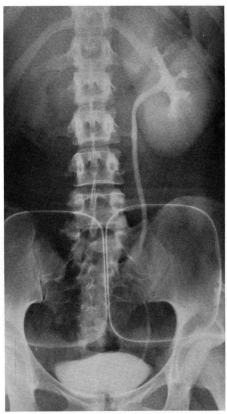

Fig. 9–10   **Fig. 9–11**

Figure 9–10. *Excretory urogram.* Absence of vagina and agenesis of right kidney.
Figure 9–11. *Excretory urogram.* Congenital absence of vagina associated with agenesis of right kidney. Note the compensatory renal hypertrophy.

and so on will be considered subsequently under the proper headings. Only the general problem of recognizing *unilateral agenesis or dysgenesis* concerns us at this point.

In most cases the problem presents itself when, during the course of a urologic investigation, an excretory urogram reveals only one kidney. The question arises, is this a patient with a nonfunctioning kidney secondary to disease (ureteral obstruction, hydronephrosis, and so on), or is it a case of unilateral renal agenesis? Absence of a renal shadow (either parenchyma or renal pelvis) does not necessarily mean an absent kidney. Braasch and Merricks suggested that the outline of the psoas muscles on the side in question may be poor or less definite than on the normal side. Meyers and associates pointed out the frequency of intestinal malposition related to renal agenesis or ectopia. A good tip to remember when reading urograms is: Whenever it appears that one kidney is absent, one should scrutinize the region of the bony pelvis carefully for signs of an ectopic pelvic kidney (see Figs. 9–37 and 9–38). The likelihood that the pelves and calyces of ectopic pelvic kidneys will be incompletely visualized urographically is high. Such spotty areas of contrast medium are easily obscured and overlooked when they overlie bone.

Cystoscopy may provide a relatively easy solution. If a ureteral orifice is present and can be catheterized, the status of the kidney may be settled. If the ureteral orifice and one half of the trigone on the side in question are absent, this is almost pathognomonic of agenesis. But it is not always easy to be sure cystoscopically that one half of the trigone is absent, since often the entire trigone and interureteric bar are indefinite in appearance, and experienced cystoscopists not infrequently have been mistaken; moreover, ureteral orifices are notorious in their being able to "hide" and escape detection. Also, there is always the problem that the ureteral orifice in question is ectopic, located in some obscure position—such as the urethra, urethral meatus, introitus, vagina, or cervix of a female or the seminal tract or prostatic urethra of a male. A ureterocele may also be easily overlooked. Duplication of the pelvis and ureter of the solitary kidney may further compound the diagnostic problem. Arteriography (Kincaid) may be helpful (Fig. 9–12). Absolute diagnosis may require surgical exploration, but fortunately from a clinical standpoint most cases do not demand such unequivocal proof.

The unilateral multicystic or dysplastic kidney (see Chapter 13) is the most common abdominal mass encountered in the newborn infant as well as the most common cystic disorder of the kidney in children (Bearman and associates; Sanders; Stuber and associates). Specialized techniques including sonography (Chapter 5) and high-dose excretory urography are helpful in diagnosis. The characteristic sonographic finding is a cystic structure with or without multiple septa. High-dose excretory urography may reveal opacification of cyst walls (Newman and associates). The retrograde ureterogram will help distinguish between congenital ureteropelvic juncture obstruction with hydronephrosis and renal dysplasia with multiple cysts. In renal dysplasia the ureter ends blindly, is atretic, or is absent.

Anomalies in Size

THE SMALL KIDNEY (CONGENITAL HYPOPLASIA; ATROPHIC PYELONEPHRITIS; RENAL ATROPHY)

Renal atrophy may result from either developmental or acquired factors. Atrophy of embryonic origin usually is referred to as *congenital hypoplasia* or *infantile kidney*. The congenital form of hypoplasia repre-

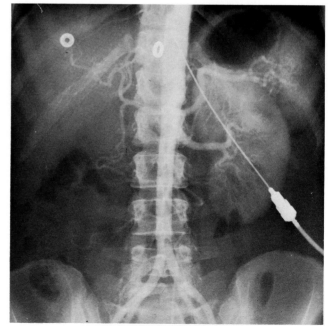

Figure 9–12. *Translumbar aortogram* showing **absence of right renal artery associated with agenesis of right kidney.**

sents an insufficient response of the metanephrogenic mesoderm to the stimulus of the ureteric bud. The reason for this inadequate stimulus is unknown. Gray and Skandalakis believe that the fault lies in the ureteric primordium rather than in the mesenchyme. They base their theory on the fact that the hypoplastic kidney does not have a renal pelvis and calyces of normal size, suggesting, therefore, that the renal substance would be thin if the defect were solely with the mesenchyme. "Acquired" renal atrophy may occur as a result of extensive pyelonephritis or infarction from occlusive vascular disease. Acquired varieties of atrophy have been rather loosely spoken of as *atrophic pyelonephritis*. It is difficult to differentiate between congenital hypoplasia and acquired atrophy on either gross or microscopic examination of the kidney. Urologic and clinical data, however, may occasionally permit such differentiation. (The subject of the atrophic kidney is considered more fully in Chapters 10 and 17.)

COMPENSATORY HYPERTROPHY

Compensatory hypertrophy of a kidney is an acquired condition that occurs when one kidney is called on to perform the function normally carried on by two kidneys. It may follow nephrectomy, atrophy of one kidney, or unilateral renal agenesis. The increase in size of all parts of the kidney is visualized urographically by an enlarged outline of the kidney and to a lesser extent of the pelvis and calyces (Figs. 9–13 and 9–14). (See also Figure 9–11 and Chapter 8.)

The ability of the kidney to undergo compensatory hypertrophy is greatest in childhood and early adult life. Later in adulthood, this response diminishes. This fact has been studied in adult donors for renal transplantation. Functional changes in the remaining kidney occur in a matter of days, but the urographic evidence for compensatory hypertrophy is more subtle and develops more slowly if at all (Donadio and associates; Orecklin, Craven, and

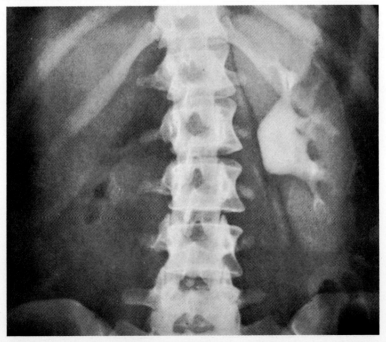

Figure 9–13. *Excretory urogram.* **Compensatory hypertrophy of left kidney secondary to right nephrectomy** for infected right hydronephrosis 8 years before. Note that right renal shadow is absent and right psoas muscle is not as well outlined as left; liver is well visualized.

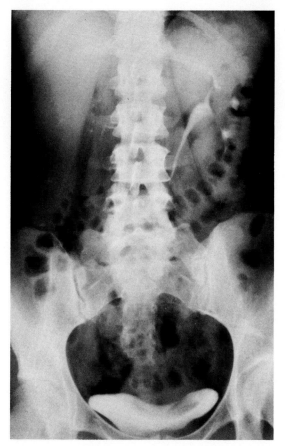

Figure 9–14. Renal hypoplasia with contralateral compensatory hypertrophy. *Excretory urogram.* Right kidney is small and barely visualized, and lies very close to vertebrae. Left kidney shows compensatory hypertrophy.

Lecky). Formation of dilute urine begins about the fourteenth week of fetal life, but the development of compensatory hypertrophy does not occur until after birth because until that time, the excretory function of the kidneys is served by the placenta. (Laufer and Griscom). Thus, the "solitary" kidney of a child born with renal agenesis or dysgenesis will not reveal compensatory hypertrophy until after birth, when the placenta is no longer performing its functions. In the early months of the postnatal period there is already evidence of compensatory hypertrophy when compared to other children (Hodson and associates).

Anomalies in Position

Embryogenesis

At the end of the sixth week of gestation the renal pelvis lies at the level of the second lumbar vertebra. At this stage, the renal pelvis faces ventrally (forward). During the next two weeks the kidneys will rotate outwardly through 90° so that the renal pelvis now faces medially. Should this process fail to proceed normally, resulting in malrotation, the kidney may face ventrally (anteriorly), dorsally (posteriorly), or laterally (Fig. 9–15).

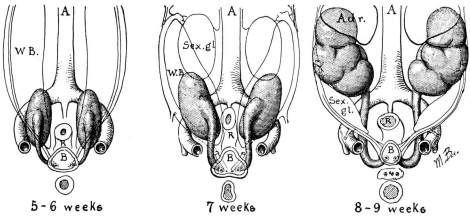

Figure 9–15. Ascent and rotation of kidneys. (See text.) (From Kelly, H. A., and Burnam, C. F.: Diseases of the Kidneys, Ureters, and Bladder, With Special Reference to the Diseases in Women. New York, D. Appleton and Company, 1914.)

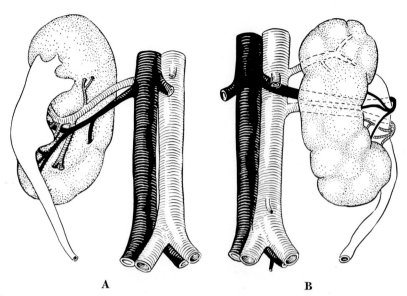

Figure 9–16. Abnormal renal rotation (malrotation). **A,** Reverse rotation. **B,** Hyperrotation (After Weyrauch, H. M., by permission of Surg., Gynec. & Obst.)

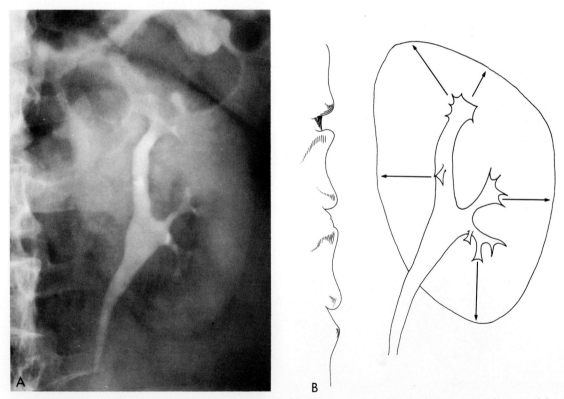

Figure 9–17. **A,** *Excretory urogram.* **Malrotation, left kidney.** No other abnormality present. The tips of the minor calyces are well cupped, the fornices are sharp, and the overlying parenchyma is normal. **B,** *Line drawing, same case* emphasizes that the anatomic relationships of the calyces to the overlying parenchyma are the same in renal anomalies as they are in normal kidneys.

MALROTATION (ABNORMAL ROTATION; INCOMPLETE ROTATION)

Anomalous types of rotation are most frequently associated with ectopia but also may be present in normally placed kidneys. The most common type of malrotation is the persistent anterior position of the renal pelvis or some variation between the fetal anterior and the adult medial positions. Four major types of anomalous rotation have been described (Braasch; Weyrauch), namely, nonrotation, incomplete rotation, reverse rotation, and excessive rotation. The most commonly encountered anomalies are nonrotation (pelvis forward or ventral) and incomplete rotation, in which case the pelvis is between the forward (ventral) and medial positions. Reverse and excessive rotations (Fig. 9–16) are rare. It is obvious from Figure 9–16 that reverse rotations cannot be distinguished from excessive rotations from the uro-

grams alone. In reverse rotation the renal vessels are twisted anteriorly around the kidney; in excessive rotation they are carried posteriorly to the kidney.

Malrotation may be unilateral or bilateral. It may occur in kidneys that are normally located in the renal fossae and in those which are displaced or fused. The incidence of malrotation is much higher in ectopic and fused kidneys than in normally situated kidneys. Malrotation is responsible for more errors in urographic interpretation than almost any other condition. The commonest error is the reporting of the presence of a definite pathologic condition when in reality the kidney is entirely normal except for malrotation. For this reason we are illustrating this condition with a rather large group of films to demonstrate the various urographic appearances that may be encountered.

One must constantly keep in mind that when the kidney is malrotated, the renal

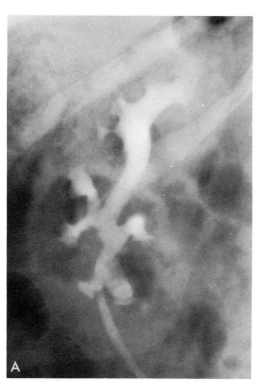
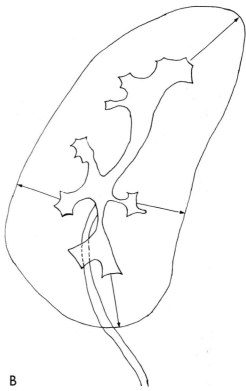

Figure 9–18. *Excretory urogram.* **Malrotation, otherwise normal.** Note normal calyces and corticocalyceal relationships. The ureter is deviated by passing over the lower pole of the kidney. **B,** *Line drawing, same case.*

parenchyma, calyces, and pelvis are often anomalous in shape, giving a bizarre-appearing urogram that is easily misinterpreted as showing disease. This error can be avoided if one carefully examines the appearance of the tips of the calyces and their relation to the overlying renal parenchyma (the individual renal lobes). As pointed out in Chapter 8 in discussion of the normal urogram, the papilla in the normal renal lobe protrudes into the calyx, forming a clearly defined cup-shaped image. The fornices of the minor calyx are sharp, and the renal parenchyma overlying the calyx surrounds it in a symmetrical

fashion. If one carefully examines the individual calyces with their overlying renal parenchyma in an anomalous but otherwise normal kidney, it is apparent that these same anatomic relationships are seen; normal calyceal cupping is present, the fornices of the minor calyces are sharp, and the overlying parenchyma is of the same thickness and bears the same relationship to the individual calyces as it does in a kidney with the usual (normal) morphology (Figs. 9–17 and 9–18). In contrast, mild caliectasis is identified by evidence that the fornices of the calyces are blunted (Fig. 9–19) and not by the bizarre appearance of

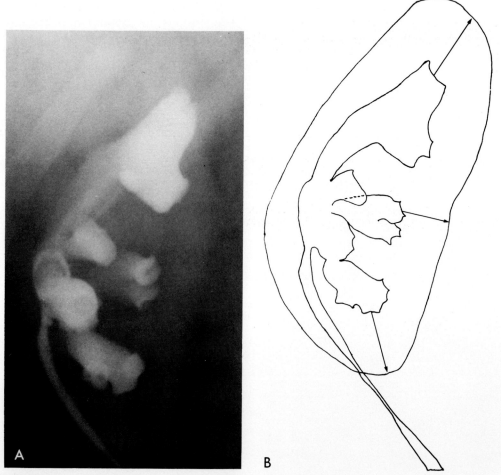

Figure 9–19. *Excretory urogram* (oblique). **Malrotation with mild obstruction.** The pelvis and ureter lie on the anterior and lateral aspect of the kidney. The fornices of the calyces are moderately distended, indicating early caliectasis. The relationship of each calyx to its overlying cortex remains normal. **B,** *Line drawing, same case.* Emphasizes the persistence of normal morphologic relationship of calyces to parenchyma.

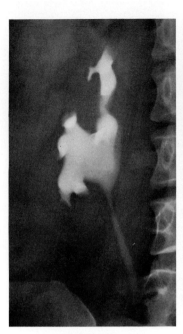 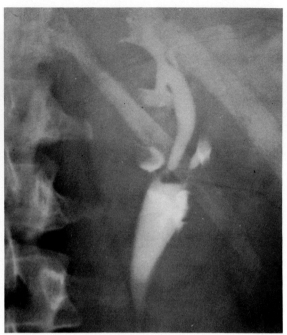

Fig. 9–20   Fig. 9–21

Figure 9–20. *Right retrograde pyelogram.* **Malrotation.**
Figure 9–21. *Left retrograde pyelogram.* **Malrotation with bifid type of pelvis.**

the renal pelvis. More severe changes—for example, cortical atrophy or scarring—are identified by loss of renal parenchymal thickness over one or more minor calyces. Renal masses are identified in the usual manner by an increase in parenchymal thickness and by displacement of calyces.

Because of the anterior or lateral position of the renal pelvis, the upper part of the ureter often appears to be displaced laterally; this should not be misinterpreted as displacement from a pathologic lesion. The pelvis of the malrotated kidney may be elongated, suggesting dilatation when in reality none is present. The arrangement of the calyces may exaggerate this apparent dilatation when their shadows overlie that of the renal pelvis. In some cases, at first glance a calyx may appear to be completely obliterated. The pelvis may lie in any location, varying from its normal medial position to one completely lateral, with the calyces pointing medially. This latter position, however, is not so confusing in urographic interpretation as are the intermediate positions in which the pelvis overlies the calyces and the calyces are projected in more or less of an anteroposterior direction.

At times, oblique or lateral views are necessary to clarify the diagnosis (Figs. 9–20 through 9–23).

In an occasional case the abnormal ro-

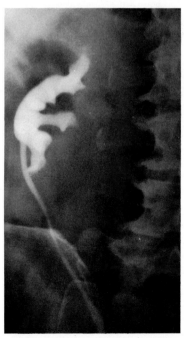

Figure 9–22. *Right retrograde pyelogram.* **Malrotation.**

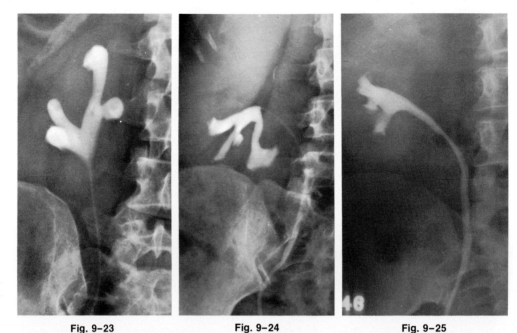

Fig. 9–23   **Fig. 9–24**   **Fig. 9–25**

Figure 9–23. *Right retrograde pyelogram.* Malrotation.

Figure 9–24. *Right retrograde pyelogram.* Malrotation of right kidney around anteroposterior axis, associated with ptosis.

Figure 9–25. *Right retrograde pyelogram.* Acquired (postoperative) malrotation of right kidney around transverse axis. Duplication was excluded at surgical exploration.

tation has been **around the anteroposterior or transverse axis** so that the calyces may point caudal, cephalad, or in some intermediate direction. When this condition is apparent, however, one must make sure that the displacement is not the result of acquired conditions such as retroperitoneal tumor, perinephric abscess, or deformity resulting from previous surgical procedures. To a lesser extent these conditions must be considered and excluded in the ordinary varieties of malrotation or excessive rotation around the **longitudinal axis** of the kidney (Figs. 9–24 and 9–25).

Associated Pathologic Conditions

Stones, tuberculosis, cysts, polycystic disease, tumors, and other lesions also affect malrotated kidneys and at times are responsible for bizarre and interesting urograms (Figs. 9–26 through 9–30).

ECTOPIA

The terms *renal ectopia* and *renal dystopia* describe kidneys that are congenitally located in abnormal anatomic positions (Thompson and Pace). These terms do not apply to acquired renal ptosis. As a result of congenital factors the kidney is firmly fixed near or below the brim of the pelvis (Figs. 9–31, 9–32, and 9–33) and is served by blood vessels that are derived from the regional vascular trunks.

Embryogenesis

Approximately between the 14- and the 30-mm stage of the embryo, ascent of the kidney occurs. The definitive kidney formed by the union of the ureteric bud and nephrogenic blastema at first lies far caudally in the body (Fig. 9–15). To attain the normal position in the adult, the kid-

Text continued on page 588

Fig. 9–26

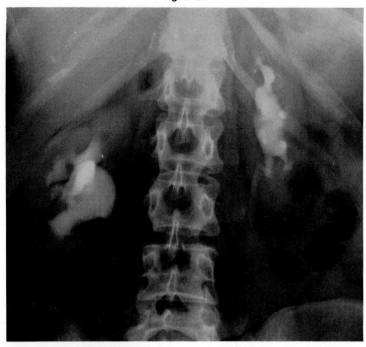

Fig. 9–27   Fig. 9–28

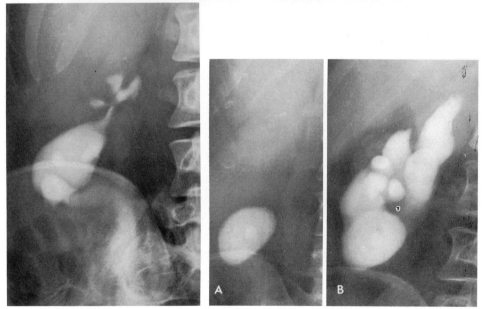

Figure 9–26. *Excretory urogram.* Bilateral malrotation, most marked on left, with associated pyelectasis, greater on right than on left.

Figure 9–27. *Excretory urogram.* Malrotation with associated pyelectasis, grade 2, on right. Also note low-lying kidney which might represent borderline ectopia. Some loss of renal parenchyma is seen in the upper pole.

Figure 9–28. Nephrolithiasis in malrotated kidney. **A,** *Plain film.* Large laminated stone lying just above border of ilium. **B,** *Excretory urogram.* Malrotated right kidney with pyelocaliectasis. Stone included in pelvis.

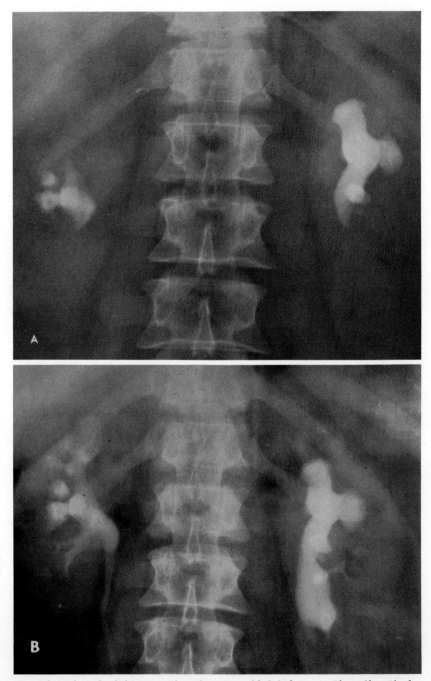

Figure 9–29.   Bilateral nephrolithiasis, with malrotation of left kidney. **A,** *Plain film.* Shadows of branched calculi in both kidneys. **B,** *Excretory urogram.* Malrotation of left kidney, with upper calyces and most of pelvis filled with stone. Normal function of right kidney, with stone filling pelvis and middle calyces.

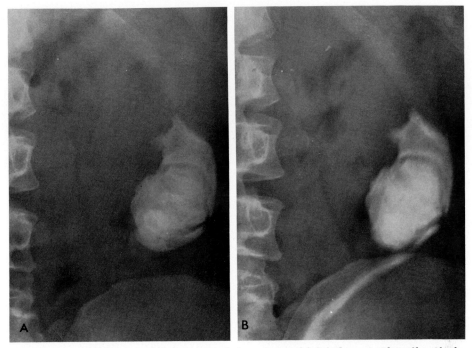

Figure 9–30. Nephrolithiasis and hydronephrosis in malrotated left kidney. **A,** *Plain film.* Shadow of large laminated stone over left renal area. **B,** *Left retrograde pyelogram.* Ureter swings laterally, entering kidney at apparent lateral margin. Stone completely obstructs and no contrast medium enters kidney. Surgical exploration revealed malrotated kidney with hydronephrosis, stone in pelvis, and obstruction at ureteropelvic juncture.

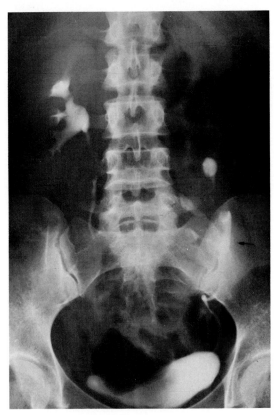

Figure 9–31. *Excretory urogram.* **Ectopic left kidney.** The kidney is malrotated and overlies the sacrum *(arrow).* The ureter is short, its length in keeping with the position of the kidney, a feature that distinguishes ectopia from ptosis.

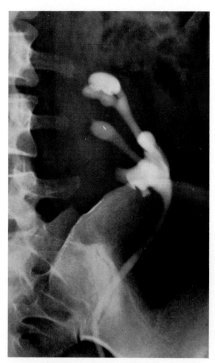

Figure 9–32. *Left retrograde pyelogram.* **Low-lying, malrotated kidney; borderline ectopia.**

neys must migrate upward out of the pelvis and into the abdominal cavity. Whether the kidneys actually ascend or merely remain stationary while the body grows caudally is still a controversial point. During its so-called ascent the kidney is supplied in succession by arteries located higher and higher in the nephrogenic ridge.

In addition to ascent the kidney also undergoes rotation. The renal pelvis, which originally lay on the ventral surface of the kidney (forward), finally comes to face medially in the adult. At about the 25- to 30-mm stage the kidneys have reached their normal adult positions on each side of the second lumbar vertebra. When they have reached this position, permanent vascularization of the kidneys occurs.

Simple Renal Ectopia

Simple renal ectopia (kidney situated on its normal side but below its normal adult level) results from failure of normal ascent. A minimal degree of ectopia may be

difficult to distinguish from secondary ptosis. The length of the ureter may help in differentiation. Also, the presence of some degree of malrotation tends to speak for ectopia rather than ptosis, as does an anomalous type of blood supply, usually from multiple vessels. *It is of interest that in most cases of renal ectopia the adrenal gland is in normal position.*

Ectopia Versus Ptosis

The distinction between ptosis and ectopia may be confusing in cases where the kidney is still above the pelvis. In most patients, ectopia can be distinguished from ptosis by the length of the ureters. In ectopia it is short, with its length in keeping with the position of the ureter (Fig. 9–31),

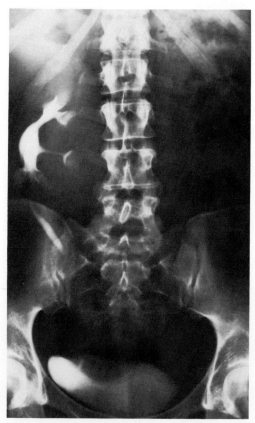

Figure 9–33. *Excretory urogram.* **Solitary ectopic right kidney.** Agenesis of the left kidney was associated with hypoplasia of the left lung in this patient.

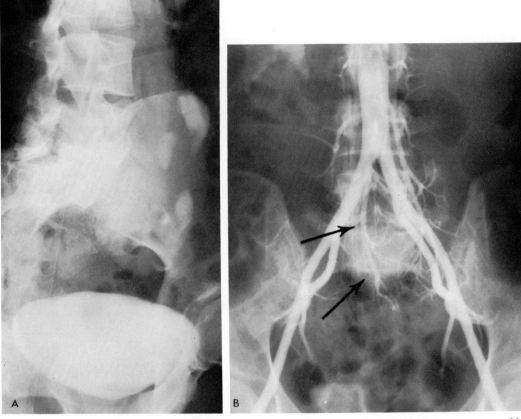

Figure 9–34. Vascular supply of ectopic left kidney overlying left ilium. **A,** *Excretory urogram, oblique view.* **B,** *Arteriogram* showing anomalous ectopic blood supply *(arrows)* arising from near bifurcation of aorta.

whereas the ptotic kidney has a ureter of normal length. Braasch and Merricks stated that to be classified as ectopic, the kidney must be below the level of the second or third lumbar vertebra. Thompson and Pace agreed with this and added that the bizarre position of the renal pelvis (malrotation) tends to support the diagnosis of ectopia. They classified renal ectopia in their 97 cases as follows:

(1) Pelvic: Kidney located in the true pelvis.

(2) Iliac: Kidney located either in the iliac fossa or opposite the crest of the ilium.

(3) Abdominal: The kidney is "fixed" above the crest of the ilium or below the level of L2 and L3.

Of the 97 cases in the series, 88 were diagnosed by means of urography; the other 9 ectopic kidneys were encountered

at autopsy. The distribution of the cases according to their classification was as follows: Pelvic—56 (64 per cent), iliac—7 (8 per cent), and abdominal—25 (28 per cent).

Obviously, demonstration of the renal blood supply by arteriography would clarify the classification in the large majority of cases because a truly ectopic kidney would have an ectopic blood supply (Figs. 9–34, 9–35, and 9–36) (Kincaid). However, there would still be borderline cases in which it would be difficult to state whether the renal vessels were in normal position or were situated "just a little lower" on the aorta and vena cava than normal. In most cases of ptosis the kidneys are freely movable and may be quite easily manipulated manually and restored to their normal position.

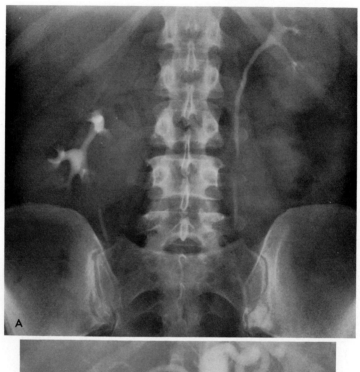

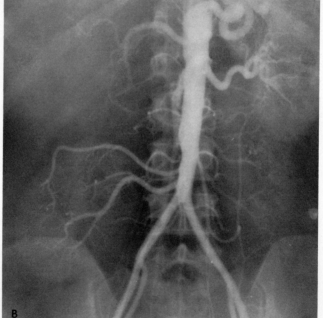

Figure 9–35.   Demonstration of vascular supply of ectopic right kidney with lower pole lying below crest of ilium. **A,** *Excretory urogram.* **B,** *Arteriogram.* This is ectopia rather than ptosis because the renal arteries come off the aorta lower than the normal position (just above the bifurcation), and the ureter is short.

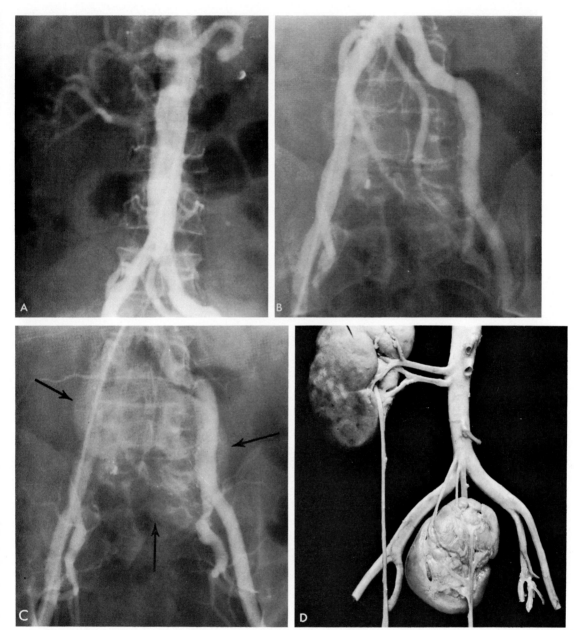

Figure 9–36. *Angiogram* of patient with ectopic midline (left) kidney which overlies lumbosacral area. **A,** Normally placed right renal artery but *no* left renal artery. There are, however, some large arteries arising from distal portion of aorta and from right common iliac artery. **B,** Close-up view of iliac arteries showing these anomalous arteries. **C,** *Nephrographic phase.* Left kidney outline *(arrows)* lies obliquely in midline across lumbosacral spine. (From Kincaid, O. W.) **D,** *Necropsy specimen* from an almost identical case. (From Baggenstoss, A. H.)

PELVIC OR SACRAL KIDNEYS

Inasmuch as most true ectopic kidneys are situated in the bony pelvis, the terms *pelvic kidney* and *sacral kidney* appear in the literature. Many ectopic kidneys, in addition to being misplaced, are malrotated. The combination of ectopia and malrotation presents bizarre urograms. Since such kidneys usually lie against some bony structure such as the sacrum or ischium, they are easily overlooked, especially in an excretory urogram, because the pelvis and calyces are most often only fractionally visualized. The reason for this appears to be the short ureter which drains the kidney so rapidly that complete filling with contrast medium is difficult. It is a good rule to remember in urographic interpretation that *whenever a kidney seems to be either nonfunctioning or absent, one should carefully scrutinize the area adjacent to the bladder in the urogram for evidence of the ureter from an ectopic kidney; the ureter is frequently well-visualized and may be the only clue to the diagnosis of ectopic kidney. In addition the area of the lumbar vertebrae and sacrum should be examined for evidence of isolated spots of contrast medium that would disclose the presence of an ectopic kidney.* Often such kidneys are difficult to visualize properly with the excretory urogram, and retrograde pyelography must be employed for accurate identification (Figs. 9–37 through 9–40).

Although most of the illustrations so far

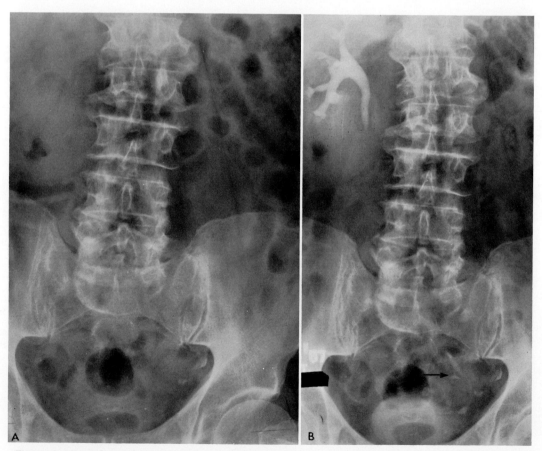

Figure 9–37. **Pelvic (sacral) left kidney.** **A,** *Plain film.* Left kidney area is obscured by gas, and renal outline of neither kidney is clearly demonstrated. **B,** *Excretory urogram.* Right kidney functions normally. On left, presence of well-outlined ureter reveals ectopic but normally functioning kidney. One calyx may be seen pointing medially and distally *(arrow).*

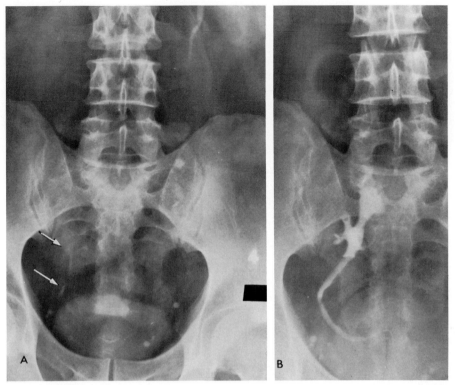

Figure 9–38. **Ectopic (pelvic) kidney. A,** *Excretory urogram.* Characteristic incomplete visualization of pelvic kidney on right, overlying sacrum. Could easily be missed and diagnosed as nonfunctioning right kidney if film were not scrutinized carefully. Fragmentary contrast medium over sacrum. (*Arrows* point to contrast medium in kidney and ureter.) **B,** *Right retrograde pyelogram.* Outline of ectopic (sacral) kidney.

have been concerned with unilateral ectopia, bilateral ectopia does occur (Fig. 9–41). Associated congenital anomalies such as absent or hypoplastic vagina may be encountered (Fig. 9–42). Ectopia may be present in cases of unilateral agenesis (solitary kidney) (Nalle, Crowell, and Lynch) (see Figure 9–33). Thompson and Pace recorded 8 such cases in their series of 97 ectopic kidneys.

INTRATHORACIC KIDNEY

Ectopic kidneys situated above the normal renal level are infrequent, but occasionally a true intrathoracic kidney is encountered (Figs. 9–43 through 9–45). Malter and Stanley found only 36 cases in the literature up to 1971. Although the right and left side have both been affected, it is more common on the left side, with only two cases having occurred bilaterally.

In the congenital form the kidney may rise above the diaphragm before it is completely formed, which does not occur until after two months of gestation. The kidney may also herniate through the foramen of Bochdalek or it may attain an intrathoracic position following traumatic rupture of the diaphragm. At times it may be impossible, without exploration, to determine that a kidney in a high ectopic position is actually beneath the diaphragm (Fig. 9–46).

CROSSED RENAL ECTOPIA

Crossed renal ectopia, because of its relative rarity, is the basis of many case reports in the literature. (Takahashi and Iwashita). *Crossed ectopia with fusion* is not too uncommon. Crossed ectopia *without* fusion is rare, and *crossed ectopia with solitary kidney* is very rare.

Embryogenesis

Several theories have been put forward to explain crossed renal ectopia. The two main theories are: (1) the ureter somehow crosses the midline and induces formation of kidney from the contralateral nephrogenic blastema, and (2) a normally developing kidney becomes attached to the kidney from the opposite side and is dragged across the midline during the ascent. Neither one of these hypotheses explains the variations of fusion and nonfusion, the occasional superior position of the ectopic kidney, the crossed ectopia of a solitary kidney, nor the renal vasculature also crossing with the ectopic kidney.

If, in addition to incomplete ascent, a kidney migrates to the opposite side of the vertebral column, the condition is spoken of as *crossed renal ectopia.* The crossed kidney usually lies below the other, although in rare instances it may lie medial or superior to it. In most cases malrotation

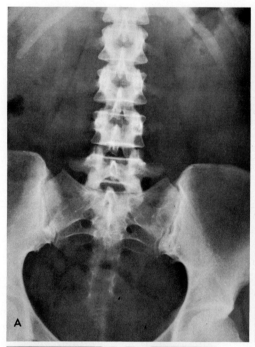
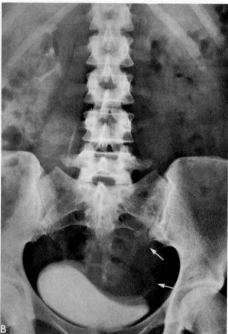
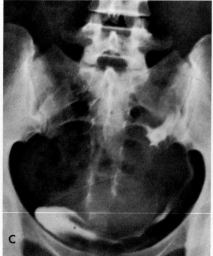

Figure 9–39. Ectopic (pelvic) left kidney, which might easily be missed on excretory urogram. **A,** *Plain film.* Right renal outline can be seen in normal position; left not seen. **B,** *Excretory urogram.* Right kidney in normal position and functioning normally, though incompletely outlined. Lower part of left ureter can be visualized *(lower arrow),* but no medium is seen in normal renal position. On careful examination one can see an area of increased density over left wing of sacrum *(upper arrow).* This is not apparent in plain film and constitutes an incompletely visualized calyx of pelvic kidney, which is more completely outlined in *left retrograde pyelogram* (**C**).

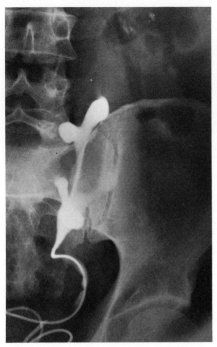

Figure 9–40. *Left retrograde pyelogram.* Ectopic kidney with typical malrotation and bifid pelvis.

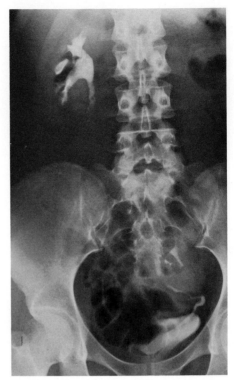

Figure 9–42. *Excretory urogram.* Ectopic (pelvic) left kidney with congenital absence of vagina.

is associated, the commonest condition being an anteriorly (forward) placed pelvis. In some cases the pelvis of the upper, normally situated kidney is projected anteromedially, and that of the lower kidney is projected anterolaterally. The descriptive terms, *sigmoid kidney,* is applied to this condition. In the large majority of cases of crossed ectopia, kidneys are fused and the condition is called *crossed renal ectopia with fusion* or *unilateral fused kidney* (Fig. 9–47). The ureter serving the crossed kidney crosses the midline to enter the bladder on its normal side.

Text continued on page 600

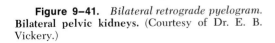

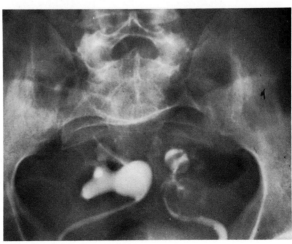

Figure 9–41. *Bilateral retrograde pyelogram.* Bilateral pelvic kidneys. (Courtesy of Dr. E. B. Vickery.)

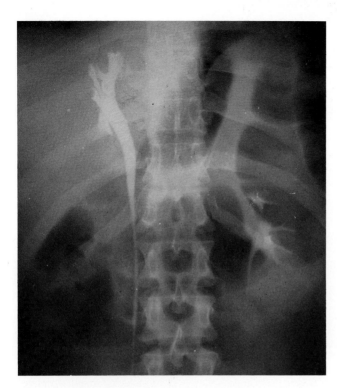

Figure 9–43. Intrathoracic ectopic kidney. *Bilateral retrograde pyelogram.* Surgical exploration showed kidney to be situated in pulmonary ligament. Surgeon stated that part of blood supply to kidney came from pulmonary artery. (Courtesy of Dr. G. W. Strom.)

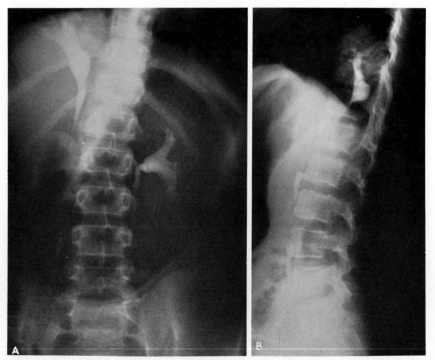

Figure 9–44 Intrathoracic right kidney. **A,** *Excretory urogram.* Anteroposterior view. **B,** *Lateral view.* **C,** Upper pole of right kidney extends well above diaphragm.

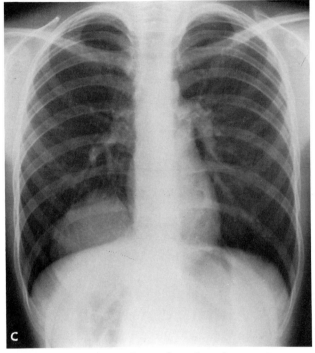

Figure 9–44 *Continued.   See legend on the opposite page.*

Figure 9–45. *Excretory urogram.* Intrathoracic right kidney of 19-year-old boy.

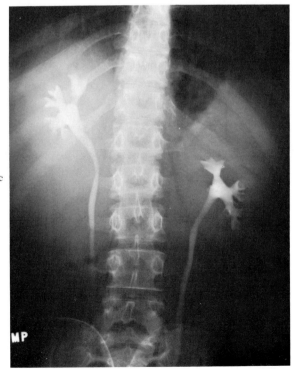

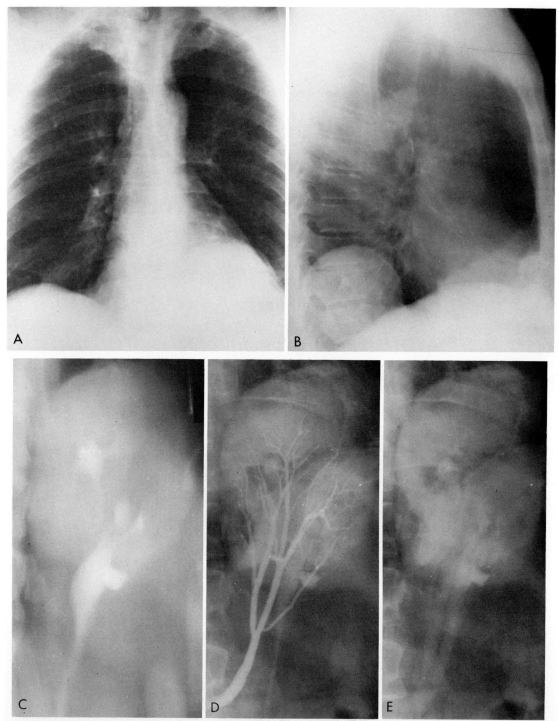

Figure 9–46. **Ectopic kidney having intrathoracic appearance.** Man aged 54. Pain in left upper abdominal quadrant and left lower chest following water skiing injury. **A** and **B,** *Chest x-ray.* **A,** Frontal, homogeneous mass density left base with sharp convex margin. **B,** Lateral, mass noted in posterior location. **C,** *Excretory urogram.* Tomograms reveal the mass to be left kidney. **D** and **E,** *Selective renal arteriogram.* **D,** There is upward stretching of renal artery to unusual renal outline. **E,** Venous phase. Bifid renal vein draining to normal lumbar level. Surgical exploration revealed kidney to lie beneath the diaphragm. (From Malter, I. J., and Stanley, R. J.)

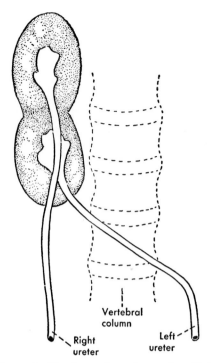

Figure 9–47. Crossed renal ectopia with fusion (unilateral fused kidney). (From Hollinshead, W. H.)

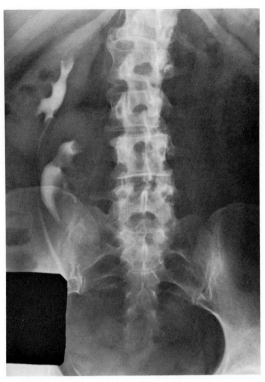

Figure 9–49. *Excretory urogram.* **Crossed renal ectopia.** It is impossible to determine whether fusion exists without surgical exploration.

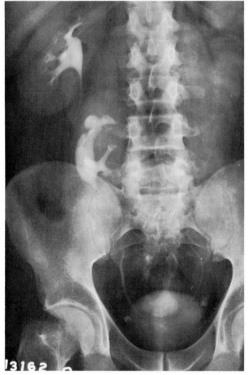

Figure 9–48. *Excretory urogram.* **Crossed renal ectopia without fusion.** (From Arduino, L. J.)

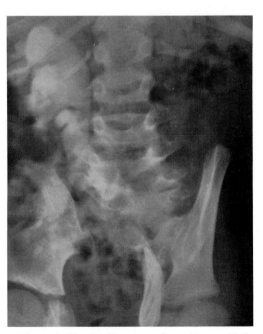

Figure 9–50. *Right retrograde pyelogram.* **Hydronephrosis** in congenital solitary kidney with crossed ectopia.

Crossed Ectopia Without Fusion

Crossed ectopia without fusion (Fig. 9–48) is much less common than ectopia with fusion. In 1965, Arduino collected 59 cases from the literature and added 2 of his own. When the two renal shadows are well separated, diagnosis is not difficult. In the majority of cases, however, some portions of the renal parenchyma overlie one another so that even though the parenchymal outlines are clear and distinct an absolute diagnosis of "no fusion" cannot be made without surgical exploration (Fig. 9–49).

Crossed Ectopia With Solitary Kidney

Crossed renal ectopia with a solitary kidney is extremely rare (Magri) (Fig. 9–50). In 1965, Tabrisky and Bhisitkul were able to find nine cases in the literature and added one of their own, that of a 17-year-old girl who had associated absence of the vagina and of the right half of the trigone. Diagnosis was confirmed by arteriography (Fig. 9–51).

Purpon's case involved a 13-year-old boy and was associated with perineal hypo-

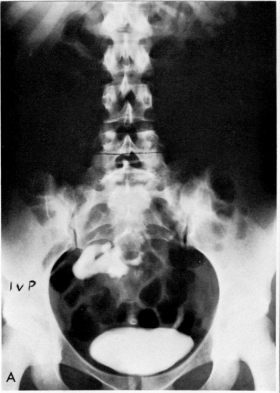
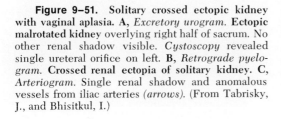
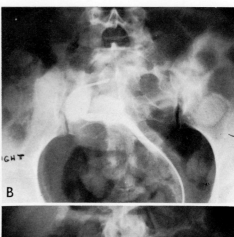
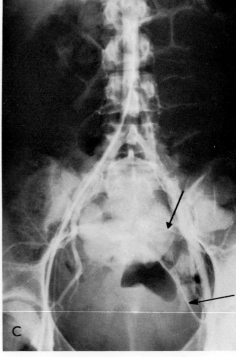

Figure 9–51. Solitary crossed ectopic kidney with vaginal aplasia. **A,** *Excretory urogram.* Ectopic malrotated kidney overlying right half of sacrum. No other renal shadow visible. *Cystoscopy* revealed single ureteral orifice on left. **B,** *Retrograde pyelogram.* **Crossed renal ectopia of solitary kidney. C,** *Arteriogram.* Single renal shadow and anomalous vessels from iliac arteries *(arrows).* (From Tabrisky, J., and Bhisitkul, I.)

the urinary tract there is a high incidence of coexisting anomalies of the anorectal, cardiovascular, skeletal, and gastrointestinal systems (Berdon and associates; Malek, Kelalis, and Burke; Kelalis, Malek, and Segura; Newman, Molthan, and Osborn). These conditions will be discussed subsequently under the subject of anomalies of the renal pelvis and ureter.

Pathologic Conditions Associated With Ectopia

A pelvic ectopic kidney may be suspected because of an abnormal mass palpable in the lower abdomen. Much has been written about ectopic *pelvic kidneys in pregnant women* causing difficulty during labor. Although this has been reported, if the ectopic kidney is otherwise normal it seldom becomes a problem, and a trial of labor can be allowed if the patient's pelvic measurements are adequate (Bergqvist).

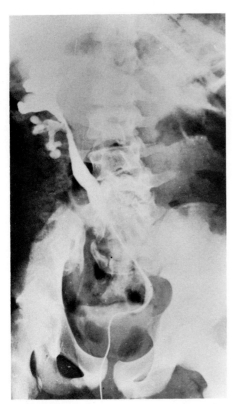

Figure 9–52. *Retrograde pyelogram.* **Crossed renal ectopia of solitary kidney.** Only one ureteral orifice present in bladder, and *excretory urogram* showed no contrast medium on left side or at any other location. Also present were undescended testes, perineal hypospadias, and cleft scrotum. (From Purpon, I.)

spadias and a cleft scrotum (Fig. 9–52). Marshall and Keuhnelian reported the ninth known case of a normotopic kidney with the ureter crossing the midline and entering the contralateral side of the trigone (Fig. 9–53).

Crossed Ectopia With Fusion

This condition will be discussed below under the heading of "Fusion."

Miscellaneous Associated Congenital Conditions

It is apparent that many combinations of ectopy with other congenital malformations such as agenesis, dysgenesis, pelvic and ureteral duplication, and so on are possible. In addition to coexisting anomalies of

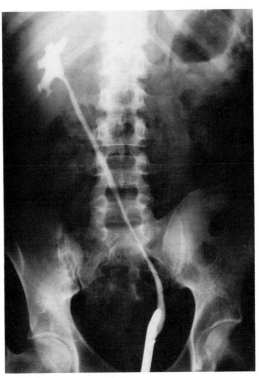

Figure 9–53. **Crossed ureteral ectopia with solitary normotropic kidney.** Man aged 37. Evaluation of azoospermia. *Retrograde pyelogram.* Normal position of right kidney with ureter crossing to left side of trigone. (From Marshall, V. F., and Keuhnelian, J. G.)

Figure 9–54. Ectopic (pelvic) kidney displaced during pregnancy. A, *Left retrograde pyelogram before pregnancy.* B, *Excretory urogram during pregnancy.* This is extremely unusual in that kidney has been displaced well out of pelvis and above innominate bone. (Courtesy of Dr. George Prather.)

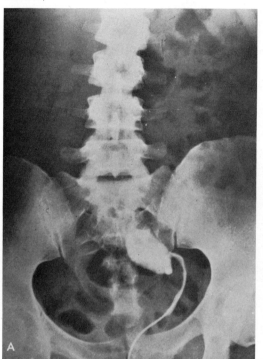

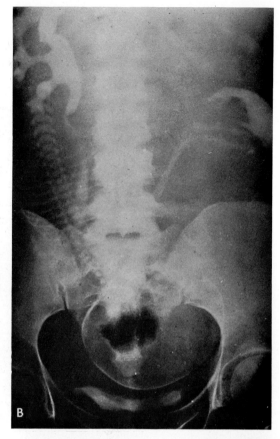

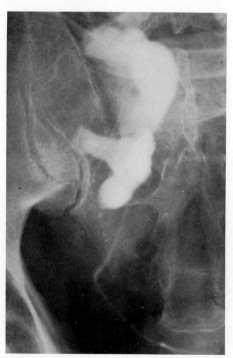

Figure 9–55. *Right retrograde pyelogram.* Pyelocaliectasis in ectopic (pelvic) right kidney.

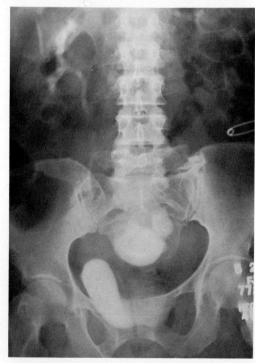

Figure 9–56. *Excretory urogram.* Left ectopic (pelvic) kidney with hydronephrosis displacing bladder. Right kidney in normal position. (From Thompson, G. J., and Pace, J. M.) (By permission of Surg., Gynec. & Obst.)

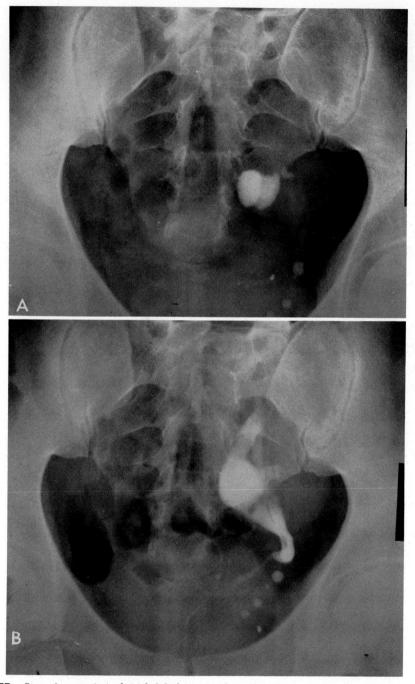

Figure 9–57. Stone in ectopic (pelvic) left kidney. **A,** *Plain film.* Large calcific shadow overlying left half of midsacrum. **B,** *Left retrograde pyelogram.* Pelvic kidney with malrotation and dilated pelvis which contains stone.

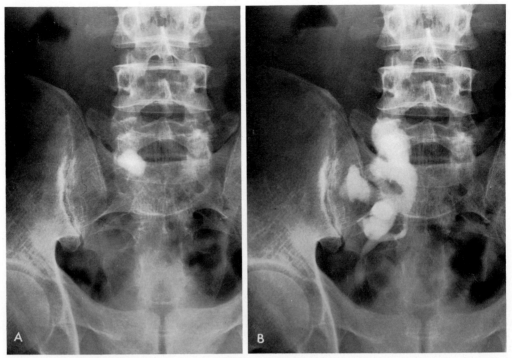

Figure 9–58. Right ectopic (pelvic) kidney with stone in upper group of calyces. **A,** *Plain film.* **B,** *Retrograde pyelogram.* (From Thompson, G. J., and Pace, J. M. By permission of Surg., Gynecol., Obstet.)

Prather encountered an unusual case in which a pelvic kidney was displaced well up into the abdomen during pregnancy (Fig. 9–54).

Occasionally, ectopic kidneys are discovered during an episode of acute infection or stone, the symptoms simulating appendicitis or salpingitis. Many abdominal and pelvic explorations have been done for such conditions only to encounter an acutely infected or obstructed ectopic kidney. Such errors are becoming infrequent since excretory urography has become such a routine diagnostic procedure before abdominal and pelvic operations.

Hydronephrosis, stone, cyst, tuberculosis, and tumor have all been encountered in ectopic kidneys and may cause considerable confusion and difficulty in diagnosis (Figs. 9–55 through 9–66).

Anomalies in Form

Minor anomalies such as *fetal lobulation* and variations in the shape of the kid-

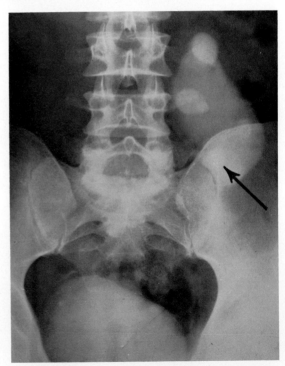

Figure 9–59. *Excretory urogram.* **Left ectopic kidney with malrotation, pyelectasis, and stone** (*arrow*). (Right kidney is also ectopic, overlying right side of sacrum, but is too fractionally visualized in this film to be seen.) (From Thompson, G. J., and Pace, J. M.) (By permission of Surg., Gynecol., Obstet.)

Text continued on page 608

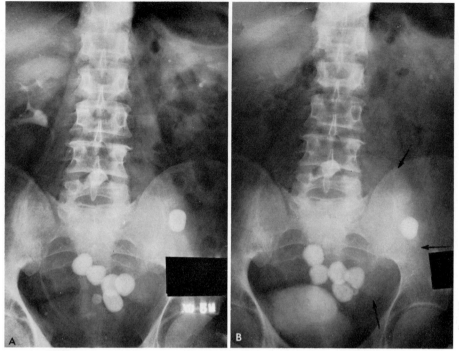

Figure 9–60. Nephrolithiasis in hydronephrotic ectopic (pelvic) left kidney. **A,** *Excretory urogram,* 5-minute film. Right kidney and ureter normal. Bladder not outlined. Multiple calcific shadows suggesting vesical calculi overlying midportion of pelvis and one lying high over left ilium. Indefinite shadow of contrast medium over this same area. **B,** *Forty-five minute film.* Bladder outlined. Shadows excluded from bladder and are seen to be multiple stones in large hydronephrotic pelvic kidney *(arrows).*

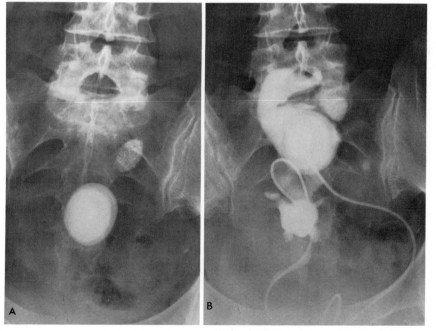

Figure 9–61. Bilateral ectopic (pelvic) kidneys with left nephrolithiasis. **A,** *Plain film.* Large laminated calcific shadow over midsacrum. Smaller mottled calcific shadow above and to left. **B,** *Bilateral retrograde pyelogram.* Bilateral pelvic kidneys; left lies above right, over sacrum, and laminated shadow apparently is included in pelvis, which is moderately dilated. Upper shadow apparently is stone in dilated calyx. Typical malrotation of both kidneys.

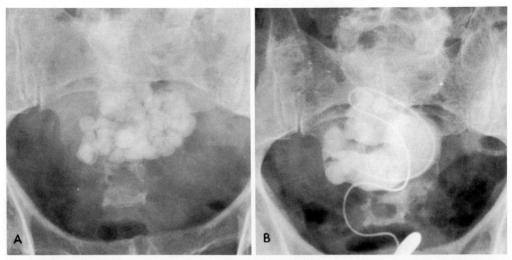

Figure 9–62. Calculi in pelvic kidney simulating vesical calculi. **A,** *Plain film.* Numerous calculi overlying bladder region. **B,** *Retrograde pyelogram.* All of calculi apparently are situated in pelvis of ectopic right kidney. (Courtesy of Dr. H. B. Simon.)

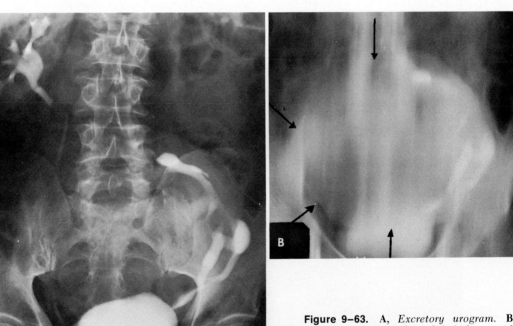

Figure 9–63. **A,** *Excretory urogram.* **B,** *Tomogram.* Ectopic (pelvic) left kidney with large solitary cyst *(arrows).*

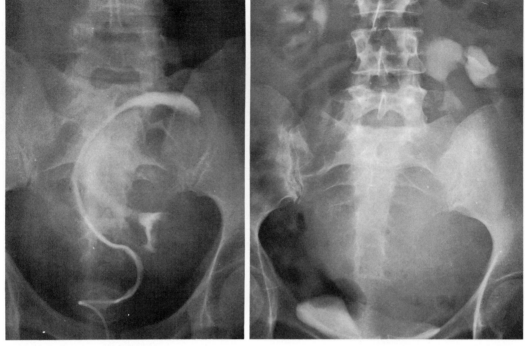

Fig. 9–64   Fig. 9–65

Figure 9–64. *Left retrograde pyelogram.* **Simple (solitary) cyst of renal cortex and papillary epithelioma of lower calyx in ectopic (pelvic) left kidney.** Typical crescentic deformity from cyst and moth-eaten appearance of lower group of calyces from papillary tumor.

Figure 9–65. *Left retrograde pyelogram.* **Hypernephroma in ectopic left kidney.**

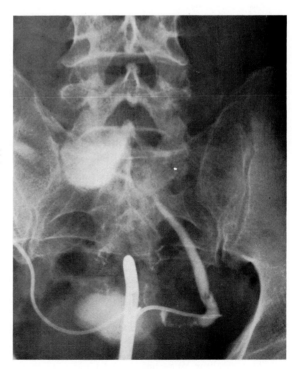

Figure 9–66. **Primary ureteral tumor involving ureter of a crossed ectopic (pelvic) left kidney.** *Left retrograde pyelogram.* Lead catheter in each ureter. Pelvic kidney with typical filling defect of terminal portion of ureter due to primary ureteral tumor. (Courtesy of Dr. S. J. Arnold, Dr. S. Immergut, and Dr. Z. R. Cottler.)

ney have been considered in Chapter 8 as variations of normal.

FUSION

The term *fusion* indicates that two (or more) kidneys are anatomically joined in some manner. As one might surmise, there are endless possibilities for the types and configurations that can occur. Bizarre types of fusion can be most confusing, and they account for a generous percentage of errors in urologic diagnosis. It is apparent that one kidney must cross the midline to be joined to its mate (*unilateral fused kidney*), or the kidneys may approach each other

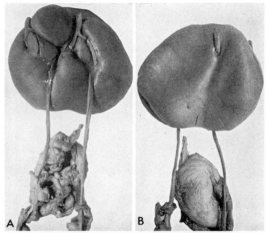

Figure 9–67.   A and B, "Cake," "disk," or "lump" kidney. (From Campbell, M. F.)

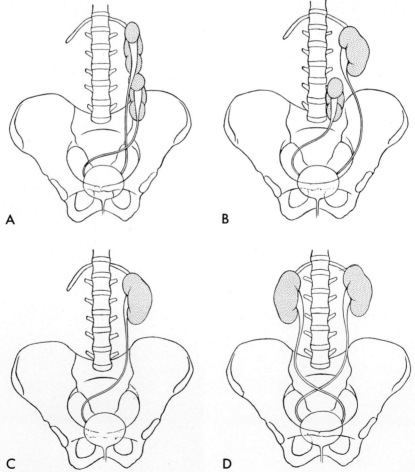

Figure 9–68.   Four varieties of **crossed renal ectopia. A, With fusion. B, Without fusion. C, Solitary. D, Bilateral.** (Redrawn from McDonald, J. H., and McClellan, D. S., as reproduced by Abeshouse, B. S., and Bhisitkul, I.)

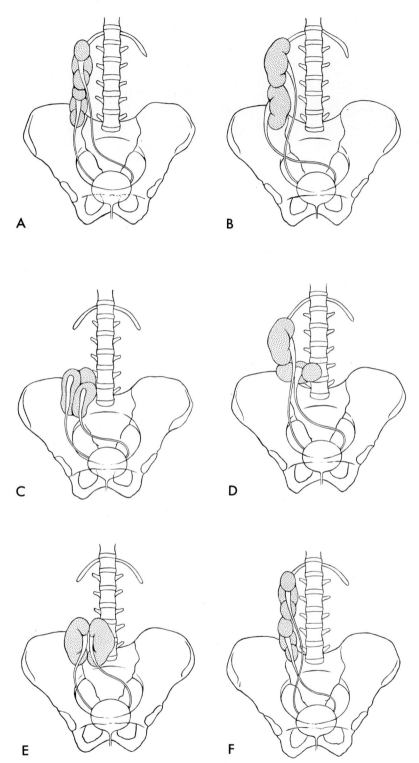

Figure 9–69. Six varieties of crossed renal ectopia with fusion. A, Unilateral fused kidney, superior ectopia. B, Sigmoid or S-shaped kidney. C, "Lump" kidney. D, L-shaped kidney. E, "Disk" kidney. F, Unilateral fused kidney, inferior ectopia. (Redrawn from McDonald, J. H., and McClellan, D. S., as reproduced by Abeshouse, B. S., and Bhisitkul, I.)

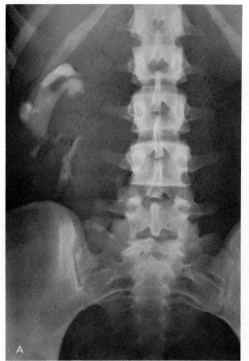
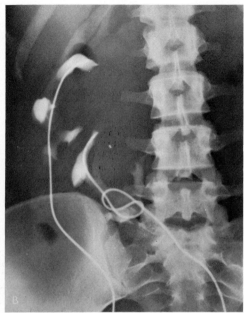

Figure 9–70. Unilateral fused kidney (crossed ectopia with fusion). **A,** *Excretory urogram.* Incomplete filling of lower (left) kidney. **B,** *Bilateral retrograde pyelogram.*

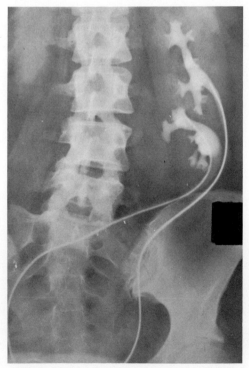

Figure 9–71. *Bilateral retrograde pyelogram.* Unilateral fused kidney (crossed ectopia with fusion).

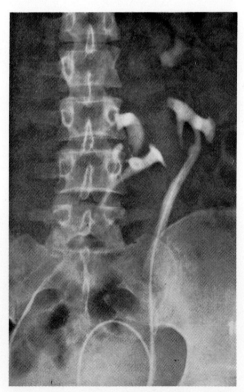

Figure 9–72. *Bilateral retrograde pyelogram.* Unilateral fused kidney (crossed ectopia with fusion).

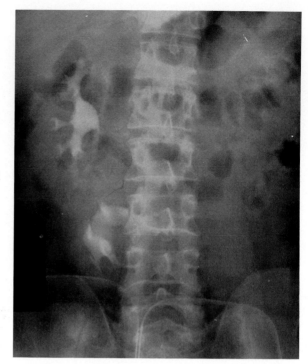

Figure 9–73. *Excretory urogram.* **Crossed renal ectopia with fusion.**

and be joined in the midline (*horseshoe kidney*). Between these two definite situations myriad conformities may occur which defy conventional classification. In nearly all cases of fusion, malrotation around the vertical axis of the kidney is present with the pelvis lying in some type of anterior position. Also some degree of "vertical" ectopia is usually present when the kidney lies below the normal renal level.

Embryogenesis

It has generally been postulated that renal fusion occurs if the nephrogenic blastema is pressed together by the umbilical arteries as the developing kidneys ascend out of the pelvis. The association of renal ectopia and fusion with other anomalies of genitourinary, anorectal, cardiovascular, skeletal, and gastrointestinal systems implies the influence of more than mere mechanical factors (Kelalis, Malek, and Segura). Friedland and DeVries hypothesized that renal ectopia and fusion result

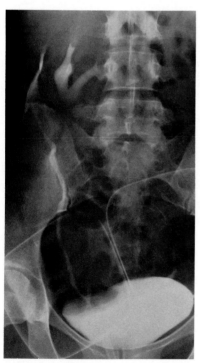

Figure 9–74. *Excretory urogram.* **Crossed renal ectopia with fusion.** Rather unusual variant, as both kidneys are at same level.

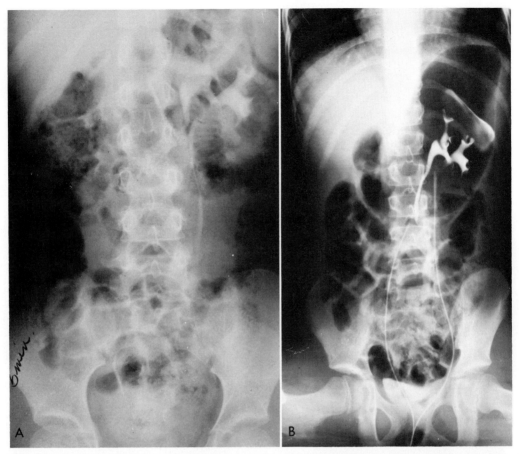

Figure 9–75. **Crossed renal ectopia with fusion.** Girl aged 7. Recurrent urinary tract infections. **A,** *Excretory urogram.* The ectopic kidney assumes a slight superior position. Collecting system appears normal, without malrotation, in both kidneys. **B,** *Retrograde pyelogram.* Confirms slight superior position of ectopic kidney. (From Schwartz, S. J., and Shaheen, D. J.).

from an inhibition of growth at specific developmental stages. They therefore reasoned that renal fusion occurs at a time when the kidneys are already nearly fused anyway, which is before they ascend between the umbilical arteries.

The commonest type of fusion is *horseshoe kidney.* In more than 90 per cent of cases fusion is at the lower poles, and the area of fusion (isthmus) across the midline corresponds to the toe of a horseshoe. The isthmus may be composed of renal parenchyma or rather seldom simply of a band of fibrous tissue. Horseshoe kidneys usually lie rather low in the abdomen, the isthmus lying in the region of the aortic bifurcation.

This isthmus almost always lies in front of the great vessels, but rare cases have been reported in which it lay either behind both the great vessels or behind the vena cava but in front of the aorta. In most cases the superior hypogastric sympathetic plexuses lie in front of the isthmus. The pelves are situated ventrally and usually lie anterior to the renal vessels. The renal vessels vary considerably in position, size, and number. In almost all cases the course of the ureters is downward, anterior to the renal substance and isthmus.

A less common type of fusion is the single disk, sometimes called a *cake, disk,* or *lump kidney* (Fig. 9–67). It is usually situated lower than the horseshoe kidney and lies over the sacrum. This condition has also been called *fused pelvic kidneys.*

Crossed Renal Ectopia With Fusion (Unilateral Fused Kidney)

Crossed renal ectopia without fusion has been considered previously in this chapter. It was pointed out that crossed ectopia is much more common *with fusion* than *without fusion* (378 to 40 in McDonald and McClellan's series of cases). This condition has been most commonly spoken of as *unilateral fused kidney.* Abeshouse and Bhisitkul have graphically described the difficulties that may be encountered in diagnosis of crossed ectopia with fusion as follows:

When the crossed ectopic kidney fuses with its opposite mate, many variations may occur in the extent of the fusion, the location of the fused renal mass, the axial deviation of the fused renal components, the direction and position of the pyelocalycal [sic] system and the

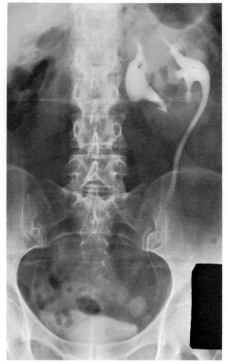

Figure 9–76. *Excretory urogram.* **Crossed renal ectopia**—"disk" kidney? Unusual in that kidneys are at normal level. **Congenital absence of vagina.**

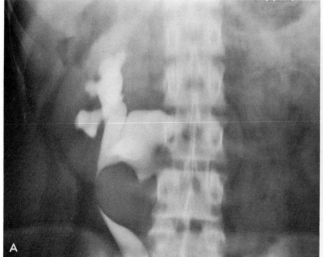

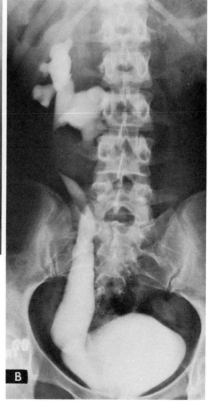

Figure 9–77. Unusual variety of crossed renal ectopia with fusion. Only one ureter and one ureteral orifice are visualized. **A,** *Excretory urogram with tomogram.* Renal mass is well outlined. **B,** *Excretory urogram.* Single right ureter with progressive increase in dilatation from above downward. Note compression of upper part of ureter by renal mass. (Courtesy of Dr. Richard Lyons.)

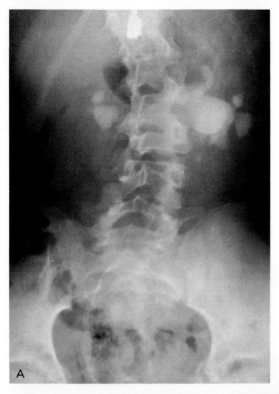

Figure 9–78. Crossed renal ectopia with fusion. A single crossed ureter drains the fused renal mass. Boy aged 13. Evaluation for congenital scoliosis. **A,** *Excretory urogram.* Fused kidney which looks as though it might be an atypical horseshoe kidney. "Right" ureter outlined. **B,** *Infusion excretory urogram with tomogram.* Solitary ureter attached to kidney on the left side of spine. Ureter crosses midline to enter right side of bladder at the site of normal right ureteral orifice. **C,** Ureter is dilated from **vesicoureteral reflux** which was demonstrated by *retrograde cystogram.* Child underwent right ureteroneocystostomy. (From Cass, A. S., and Vitko, R. J.)

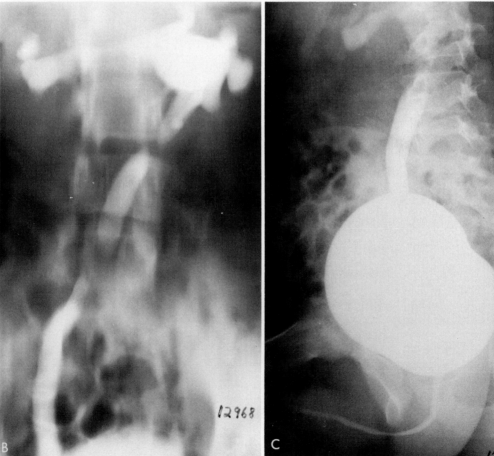

ureters, and the origin and course of the vascular supply of each renal component. The anatomical variations may be so bizarre and confusing that the examining physician may have great difficulty in determining the exact type of crossed ectopia with fusion not only after careful scrutiny of the excretory and retrograde pyelograms but even after a detailed examination of the operative or necropsy findings.

In spite of the complicated problem, attempts at classification of crossed ectopia with fusion have been made. Probably the best has been devised by McDonald and McClellan. In Figure 9–68 these authors illustrate four varieties of crossed renal ectopia as follows: (**A**) crossed ectopia with fusion and (**B**) without fusion, (**C**) crossed ectopia with solitary kidney, and (**D**) bilateral crossed ectopia. In Figure 9–69 they illustrate their classification of six types of *crossed ectopia with fusion*. In the *unilateral fused type (inferior ectopia)*, which is by far the most common, the crossed ectopic kidney is always inferior, with its upper pole fused to the lower pole of the other normally situated kidney. The other five types are much more uncommon. The *sigmoid* or "*S-shaped*" kidney is the second most common type and differs from the previous type only in the degree of axial rotation of the two kidneys. The "lump" kidney (other terms include *clump, cake, renfungiformis,* and so on) and the "disk" kidney are somewhat similar types in that there is extensive fusion of the two kidneys over a wide area to form an irregular mass. They differ in that in the "disk" kidney the fusion occurs along the entire length of the medial concave borders of each kidney. The "*L-shaped*" *kidney* and the *unilateral fused kidney (superior ectopia)* in which the crossed ectopic kidney lies above the normally placed kidney are both extremely rare.

It does not require much stretch of the imagination to appreciate that these six types are quite arbitrary attempts to bring some order out of confusion. Attempts to place each case in one of these categories will often result in failure, as can be seen from Figures 9–70 through 9–81.

With the current widespread use of ar-teriography, the anomalous vascular supply to these kidneys has generated much interest. Thus, arteriography often helps make some form of intelligent classification possible, and it can be very helpful to the surgeon if operation is required.

Differential Diagnosis. Urographically crossed ectopia with fusion may be confused with *crossed ectopia without fusion* (see Figures 9–48 and 9–49) or with an extremely mobile kidney that lies close to the midline or barely crosses it. Surgical exploration is necessary in some cases to verify the fusion. An ectopic kidney with a completely duplicated pelvis and a functionless kidney on the other side also might be confused with crossed renal ectopia with fusion.

Associated Pathologic Conditions. Crossed renal ectopia with fusion with essentially normal kidneys is usually found accidentally during routine excretory urography. If pathologic changes such as infec-

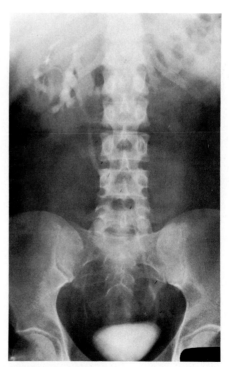

Figure 9–79. *Excretory urogram.* **Crossed renal ectopia (probably with fusion).** Left kidney appears to be superimposed over right. No surgical exploration. (Courtesy of Dr. John I. Mandler.)

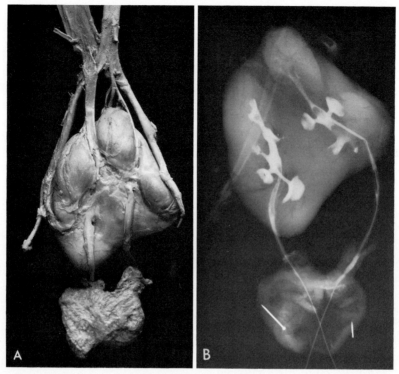

Figure 9–80. A, *Necropsy specimen.* Bilateral ectopic kidneys fused together to form "shield" or "cake" kidney that lay in pelvis between iliac vessels. Note vascular supply from aorta near bifurcation. **B,** *Bilateral retrograde pyelogram* of removed specimen. (From Thompson, G. J., and Pace, J. M.) (By permission of Surg., Gynec. & Obst.)

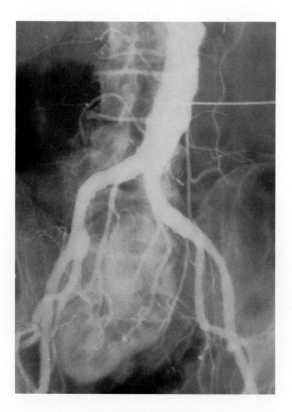

Figure 9–81. Fused "cake" kidney lying in pelvis over the sacrum. *Arteriogram.* Fused kidney lying between iliac arteries. Blood supply coming from the iliac arteries. (No normally located renal arteries were present.)

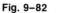

Fig. 9–82

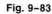

Fig. 9–83

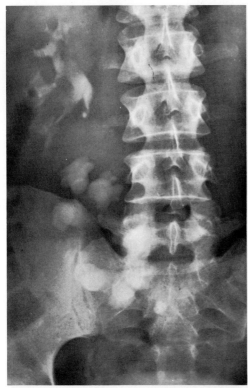

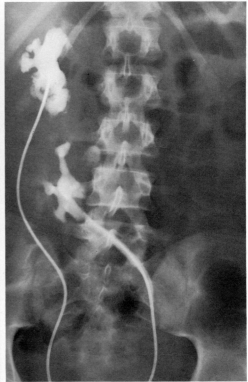

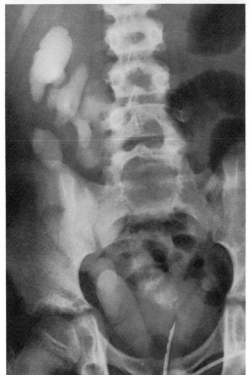

Fig. 9–84

Figure 9–82. *Excretory urogram.* Unilateral fused kidney (crossed ectopia with fusion). Lower (left) kidney is site of pyelocaliectasis. Caliectasis is no doubt exaggerated because of malrotation of calyces in anteroposterior position.

Figure 9–83. *Bilateral retrograde pyelogram.* Unilateral fused kidney (crossed ectopia with fusion) with pyelectasis and multiple cortical abscess of upper (right) kidney. Surgical removal of upper segment was necessary.

Figure 9–84. *Excretory urogram.* Unilateral fused kidney (crossed ectopia with fusion) and **pyeloureterectasis of both kidneys.** Anomalous ureteral orifices, both of which were situated just inside small, shallow pocket immediately proximal to vesical neck at 6 o'clock position.

Fig. 9–85   Fig. 9–86

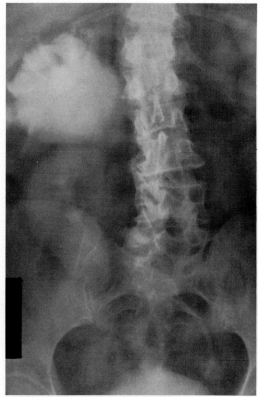 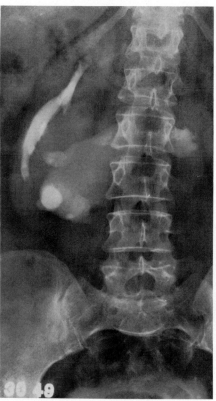

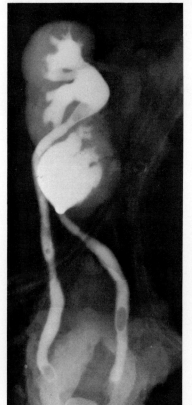

Figure 9–85. *Excretory urogram.* **Unilateral fused kidney (crossed ectopia with fusion).** Marked by hydronephrosis and hydroureter of upper (right) kidney. No evidence of dilatation of lower (left) kidney, calyces of which can be incompletely visualized through shadow cast by dilated upper ureter, which overlies lower kidney.

Figure 9–86. *Excretory urogram.* **Unusual type of unilateral fused kidney which simulates horseshoe kidney.** Hydronephrosis of lower (left) kidney. Ureters not outlined.

Figure 9–87. **Unilateral fused kidney (crossed ectopia with fusion).** Autopsy specimen with both segments filled with contrast medium.

Fig. 9–87

tion, pyelectasis, calculi, and so on are present, however, the symptoms and signs may point to a painful lower abdominal mass, and the patient may be subjected to abdominal surgery for "appendicitis" or "salpingitis." In the past, before excretory urography became a more-or-less routine diagnostic procedure preceding abdominal surgery, surgeons encountered these crossed ectopic kidneys and erroneously thought that they were dealing with some type of tumor.

This anomaly, like other types of fusion, is prone to cause stasis of urine, pyelectasis, caliectasis, and cortical infection with necrosis and stone. The anomalous position of the kidneys and pelves, which necessitates abnormal insertion of the ureters into the pelves as well as an abnormal course as they cross the renal parenchyma, predisposes to poor drainage and may result in extensive hydronephrosis. Kelalis, Malik and Segura point out an increased incidence of vesicoureteral reflux with ectopia and suggest that this abnormality rather than obstruction may account for the increased incidences of infection associated with this anomaly. Other patho-

logic conditions, such as tuberculosis, cyst, polycystic disease, and tumor, may be present and may produce unusual urographic deformities (Figs. 9–82 through 9–87).

HORSESHOE KIDNEY

Embryogenesis $4^{th} - 8^{th}$ wk.

The horseshoe kidney is the most common type of fusion anomaly. It is characterized by fusion of either the upper or the lower poles of the kidneys (almost invariably the latter). The mechanism of fusion is unknown, but it is generally agreed that the developmental defect takes place between the fourth and eighth weeks of embryogenesis. As the kidneys ascend out of the pelvis their blood supply changes from the iliac arteries to segmental aortic branches and finally to the normal position of the renal arteries. During their ascent the kidneys undergo a 90° lateral rotation with the renal hilus changing from a ventral to a medial position. If fusion and improper ascent takes place, as in the horseshoe kidney, then the renal blood supply will arise from multiple sources, the pelves

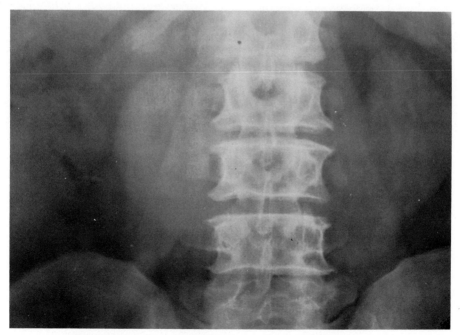

Figure 9–88. *Plain film.* Soft-tissue outline of **horseshoe kidney.**

ventral → medial position hilus
Ascent → 90% lateral rotation

and ureters will assume a ventral position owing to malrotation, and the kidneys will lie in a lower position, thus accounting for the typical urographic findings with this anomaly.

Urographic Findings

It is often possible to surmise that renal fusion exists from examination of the *plain film,* which may show the renal shadows situated nearer the vertebral column and lower than usual and the renal axes somewhat changed so that the lower poles lie closer together than the upper poles. At times it is possible to see the soft tissue outline of the isthmus which connects the two segments across the vertebral column (Fig. 9–88). Accurate diagnosis, however, can be made only from a urogram, arteriogram, or radionuclide renal scan (Figs. 9–89 and 9–90).

Urographically one is impressed by the malrotation of the renal pelves, which usually lie anteriorly. The position of the calyces varies from incomplete lateral projection to anteroposterior or even medial projection. Because of the location of the pelves, they may appear to be dilated and bizarre in outline and may give the erroneous impression of pyelectasis. The pelves usually lie close to the midline (the right often is more medial than the left) and also somewhat lower than in normal kidneys. Probably most diagnostic of all urographic findings is the characteristic appearance of the lower calyces, which in nearly all cases point toward the midline and seem to be reaching out in an effort to join each other. The lower calyces are commonly projected in such a manner that their tips overlie the vertebral column. In occasional cases the tips of the lower calyces actually communicate with each other so that contrast medium injected into one pelvis will outline both segments of the horseshoe kidney. This may present surgical difficulties if removal of one segment becomes necessary. It is rather uncommon to encounter a case in which the upper rather than the lower poles of the kidneys are fused.

It naturally follows that the *course of the ureters* in patients with horseshoe kidney varies considerably. The ureters must

Text continued on page 625

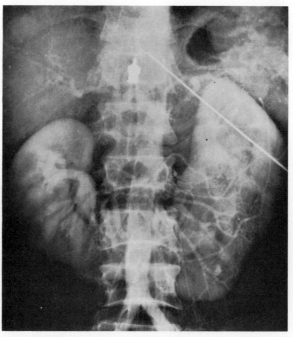

Figure 9–89. *Translumbar aortogram* demonstrating **horseshoe kidney** during nephrographic phase. (Courtesy of Dr. R. S. Hagstrom and Dr. J. R. Robison.)

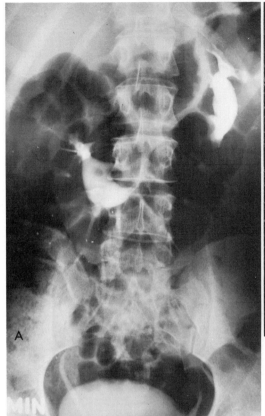
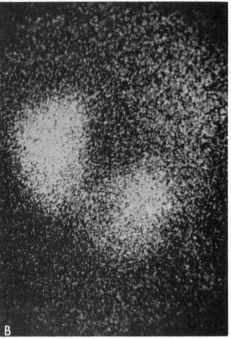

Figure 9–90. *Excretory urogram.* Horse-shoe **kidney** with right side partially displaced over spine. **B,** *Radionuclide renal scan* (kidneys viewed from back). The relative position of the two kidneys and fusion of the lower poles at the isthmus is well shown.

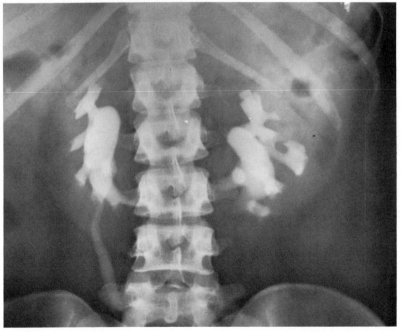

Figure 9–91. *Excretory urogram.* **Horseshoe kidney.** Both segments lie close to spinal column, with medial projection of lower calyces and malrotation; pelves lie anteriorly. Right ureter is lying on lower pole of kidney and isthmus, which illustrates one reason for frequent occurrence of pyelectasis in this condition.

Fig. 9–92

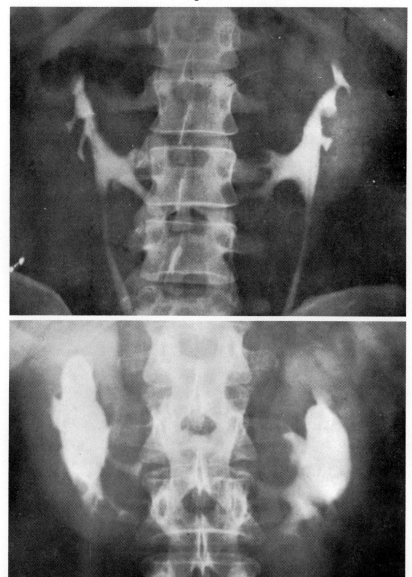

Fig. 9–93

Figure 9–92. *Bilateral retrograde pyelogram.* **Horseshoe kidney** with typical urogram. Lower calyces point downward and medially; those on right overlie vertebral column.

Figure 9–93. *Excretory urogram.* **Horseshoe kidney.** Typical malrotation, with anterior position of pelves and lower calyces projected medially. Position of pelves gives erroneous impression of pyelectasis, which probably is not present, as may be surmised from tips of calyces, which retain their normal terminations.

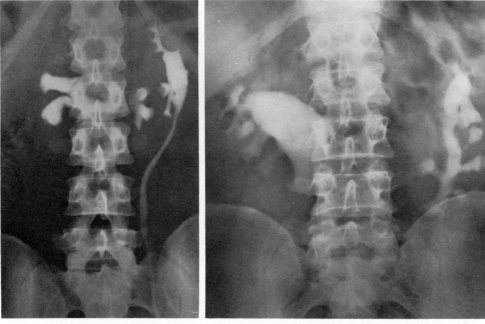

Fig. 9–94   Fig. 9–95

Figure 9–94. *Bilateral retrograde pyelogram.* **Horseshoe kidney.** Right kidney overlies spinal column; left is situated close to midline.

Figure 9–95. *Excretory urogram.* **Horseshoe kidney.** Large elongated extrarenal type of pelvis on right, which probably represents definite early pyelectasis.

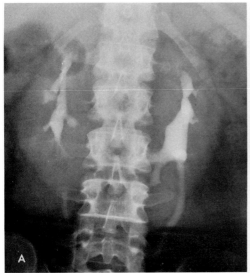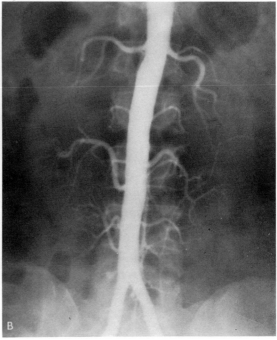

Figure 9–96. Horseshoe kidney. **A,** *Excretory urogram.* **B,** *Arteriogram.* Note two sets of renal arteries supplying renal mass.

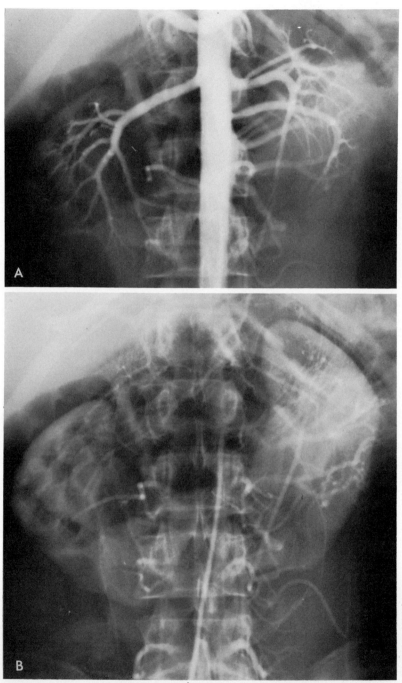

Figure 9–97. *Arteriogram* in case of **horseshoe kidney. A,** *Arterial phase.* Normal-appearing renal artery on right; multiple arteries on left. **B,** *Late nephrographic phase.* Isthmus and both renal segments opacified. (From Kincaid, O. W.)

necessarily lie anterior to the pelves as well as to the substance of the isthmus or lower poles of the kidneys. This gives rise to odd curvatures, which may be one of the factors responsible for the high incidence of obstruction, infection, and calculi in cases of renal fusion (Figs. 9–91 through 9–95). If surgical intervention is required, arteriograms may be helpful in identifying the number and location of renal vessels before operation (Figs. 9–96 and 9–97).

Associated Congenital Anomalies

Horseshoe kidney is not an unusual autopsy finding in severe congenital disorders. However, the cause of death is nearly always related to the other coexisting anomalies and not to the horseshoe kidney (Pitts and Muecke; Segura, Kelalis, and Burke). Although several congenital anomalies of the urinary tract have been associated with horseshoe kidney, the most common is obstruction of the ureteropelvic juncture. Other anomalous conditions of the urinary tract, such as the bifid pelvis or *complete* or *incomplete duplication in one or both pelves*, may be associated with

horseshoe kidneys as well (Figs. 9–98 through 9–101). The urogram in such circumstances might easily be confused with that presented by the supernumerary kidney. In some cases the fusion may be so bizarre in appearance that one cannot be sure of its classification (Fig. 9–102. See also Figure 9–78). *Differential diagnosis* must take into consideration the possibility of bilateral malrotation without fusion (Fig. 9–103). If one kidney is lying in a transverse position across the spine with the other kidney in an almost normal position, it may be impossible to decide if it should be classified as an L-shaped crossed ectopia with fusion or as a horseshoe kidney (see Fig. 9–94). The possibility of a normal kidney associated with an ectopic, incompletely rotated a kidney lying close to the spinal column also must be considered. Nonurinary anomalies are not as commonly associated with horseshoe kidney as urinary anomalies; however, a variety including anomalies of the skeleton, cardiovascular system, gastrointestinal system, anorectal region (imperforate anus), and the genital systems are found. *Horseshoe kidneys that have been separated surgically* may present bizarre urographic outlines, de-

Text continued on page 631

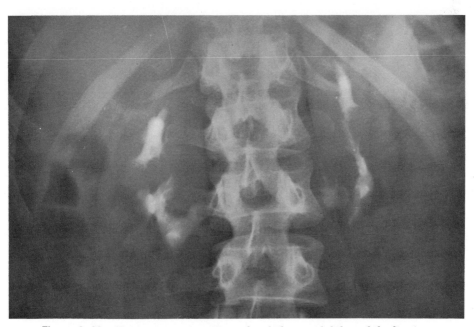

Figure 9–98. *Excretory urogram.* Horseshoe kidney with bilateral duplication.

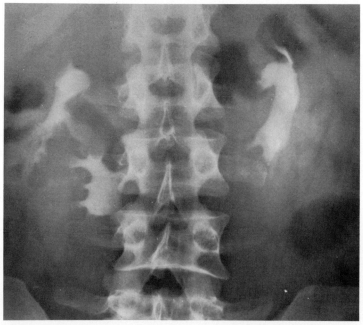

Figure 9–99. *Excretory urogram.* Horseshoe kidney with unilateral duplication (right).

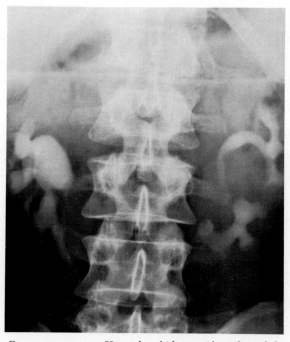

Figure 9–100. *Excretory urogram.* Horseshoe kidney with unilateral duplication on left.

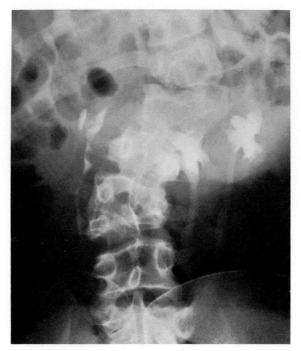

Figure 9–101. *Excretory urogram.* Bizarre type of renal fusion. Horseshoe kidney? Duplication of left half of kidney? Atrophy of right segment?

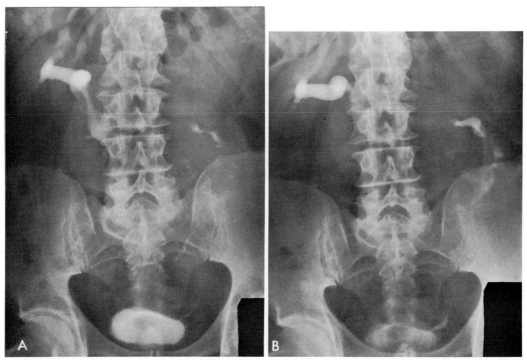

Figure 9–102. *Excretory urograms.* **A,** *Ten-minute film.* **B,** *Twenty-minute film.* Peculiar type of renal fusion. Horseshoe kidney? Duplication of right kidney?

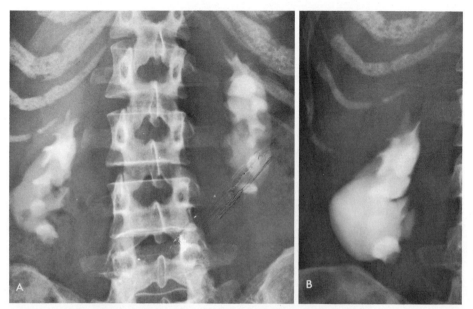

Figure 9–103. Horseshoe kidney simulating bilateral malrotation without fusion. **A,** *Excretory urogram.* Bilateral malrotation. Lower poles of kidneys widely separated. Does not suggest fusion. Moderate pyelocaliectasis is present. **B,** *Right retrograde pyelogram.* More pyelectasis than was suspected from excretory urogram. Surgical exploration revealed horseshoe kidney. Lower poles were joined only by long, narrow, fibrous isthmus.

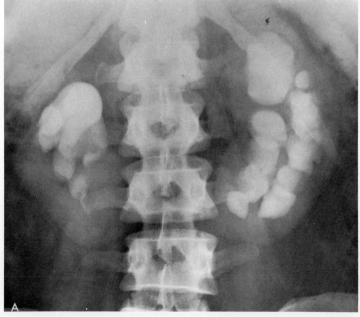

Figure 9–104. *Excretory urograms.* **A,** Typical **horseshoe kidney with rather marked caliectasis, and left nephrolithiasis.** **B,** Three years after surgical separation and left calycectomy, pyeloplasty, and nephropexy.

Illustration continued on following page

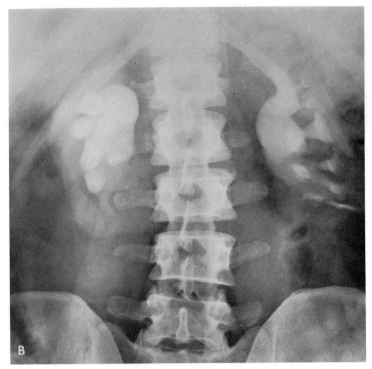

Figure 9–104. *Continued.*

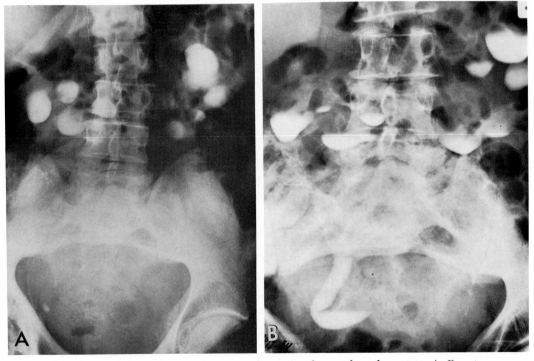

Figure 9–105. Horseshoe kidney and urinary obstruction from enlarged prostate. **A,** *Excretory urogram.* Hydronephrosis, grade 3, bilaterally. Note faint convex outline of hugely distended bladder overlying iliac bones and fourth lumbar vertebra. **B,** *In 60-minute film,* fluid levels were visible in most calyces, indicating relative heaviness of contrast medium compared with urine. Note Paget's disease of sacro-iliac bones. *Excretory urogram* (not shown here) 6 months after transurethral prostatic resection demonstrated the bizarre calyceal pattern in both **A** and **B** to be from horseshoe kidney, which resumed normal function and near-normal configuration. (Courtesy of Dr. H. W. ten Cate.)

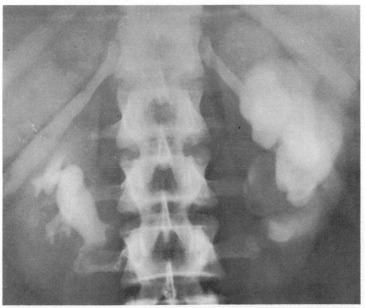

Figure 9–106. *Excretory urogram.* **Horseshoe kidney with pyelocaliectasis involving left half.** No pyelectasis on right.

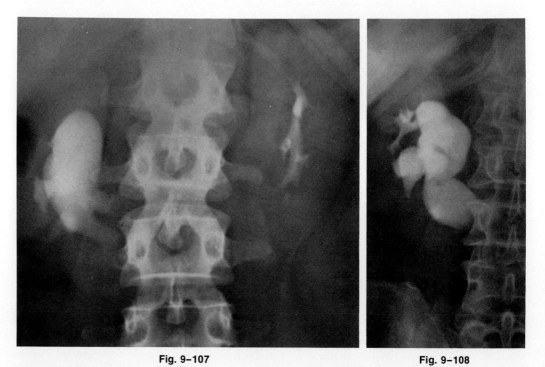

Fig. 9–107   **Fig. 9–108**

Figure 9–107. *Excretory urogram.* **Horseshoe kidney with pyelocaliectasis on right.** No pyelectasis on left.
Figure 9–108. *Right retrograde pyelogram.* **Large anomalous extrarenal pelvis on right in horseshoe kidney** simulates obstruction. Note that the intrarenal portions of the pelvis and the calyceal tips are normal.

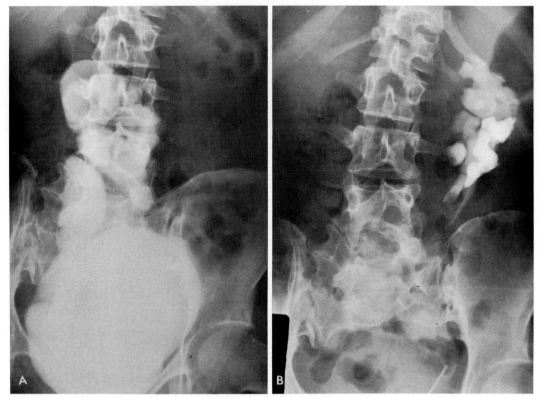

Figure 9–109.   Renal fusion. Horseshoe kidney. **A,** *Retrograde cystogram.* **Vesicoureteral reflux into right segment with advanced hydronephrosis.** Right kidney lies almost in midline. **B,** *Left retrograde pyelogram* after right hydronephrotic segment had been removed. **Malrotation of left segment with moderate caliectasis. Probable atrophy of renal parenchyma.**

pending on the position in which the kidney was fixed at operation (Fig. 9–104).

Associated Pathologic Conditions. It is not surprising that in such an anomalous condition pathologic changes such as *pyelectasis, caliectasis, and urinary calculi* are likely to occur. One must remember that the pelves in a horseshoe kidney may present unusual and bizarre outlines suggesting pyelectasis when in reality no dilatation is present. On the other hand, definite obstruction of the pelves and calyces is not uncommon (Figs. 9–105 through 9–109). At times the anomalous extrarenal pelvis seen with horseshoe kidney and other anomalies of fusion and rotation may simulate obstruction, but close examination of the calyces reveals no calyceal blunting or other evidence of increased intrarenal pressure (see Figure 9–108). When *stone* is present in a fused kidney, the pos-

sibility of fusion may be inferred from the plain film in some cases, because of the characteristic renal shape or position (Figs. 9–110 through 9–117). More often, however, a urogram is necessary before fusion is suspected. Because of the anterior position of the pelves and the unusual position of the calyces, exact localization of the shadows may be difficult even with the urogram.

Any disease that involves ordinary kidneys may be found in anomalous kidneys. Tuberculosis has been encountered (Figs. 9–118 and 9–119). A recent review of the world literature (Blackard and Mellinger) disclosed that cancer in a horseshoe kidney (either of the parenchyma or renal pelvis) has been reported seventy times (Figs. 9–120 through 9–124). Renal cysts and polycystic kidneys have also been encountered (see Chapter 13).

Text continued on page 642.

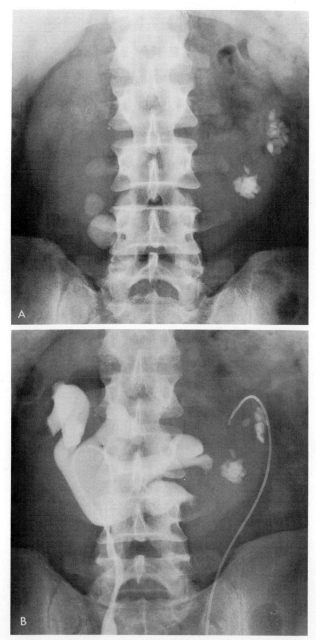

Figure 9–110. A, *Plain film.* Multiple small calculi in left half of horseshoe kidney and two large calculi in pelvis of right half. B, *Retrograde pyelogram* of right segment. Calculi are included in pelvis. Calyces extend across midline and illustrate reason for difficulties sometimes encountered when surgical separation is attempted.

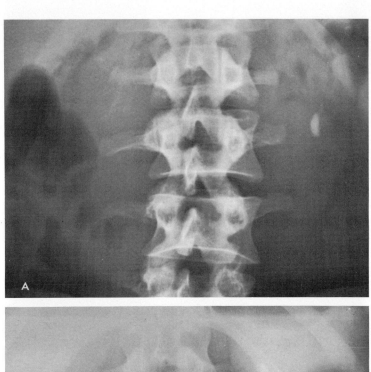

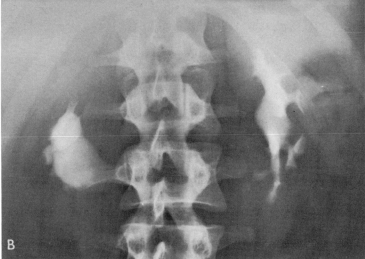

Figure 9–111. **Stone in left half of horseshoe kidney. A,** *Plain film.* Elongated calcific shadow over left renal area, opposite third transverse process. Soft-tissue outline is not pathognomonic of horseshoe kidney. **B,** *Excretory urogram.* Shadow represents stone, apparently included in one of lower calyces of left segment, which overlies upper part of ureter. Little if any pyelocaliectasis on left, but definite **pyelectasis on right.**

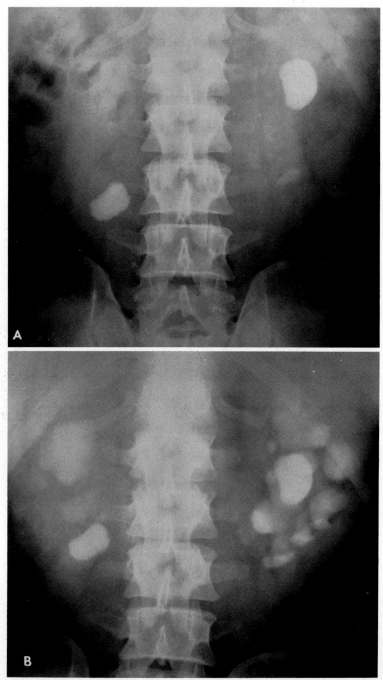

Figure 9–112. **Bilateral nephrolithiasis in horseshoe kidney. A,** *Plain film.* Large calcific shadow opposite right third lumbar transverse process. Multiple shadows over left renal area. **B,** *Excretory urogram.* **Bilateral pyelocaliectasis.** Shadow on right in plain film represents large stone, apparently in one of lower calyces. Larger shadow on left apparently represents stone in pelvis. Smaller shadows above and below this indicate stones in dilated calyces.

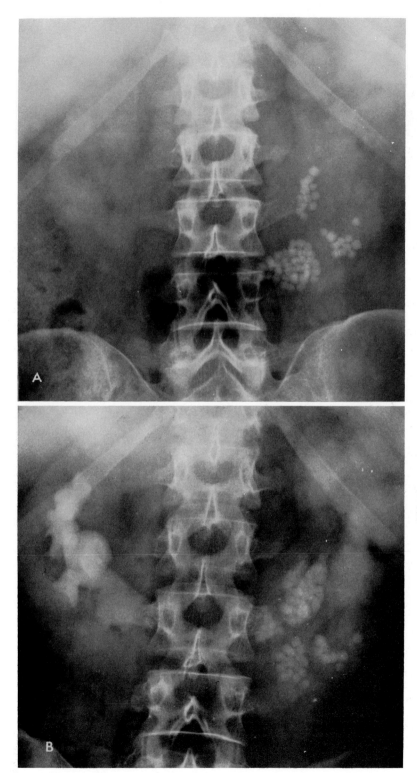

Figure 9–113.   Multiple stones in left half of horseshoe kidney. **A,** *Plain film.* Multiple calcific shadows overlying lower pole of left half of horseshoe kidney. Soft-tissue mass shows definite horseshoe kidney. **B,** *Excretory urogram.* **Marked pyelocaliectasis of left segment.** Stones apparently included in calyces, which are projected downward and medially. Right segment shows little if any pyelectasis. Lower calyx extends over spinal column.

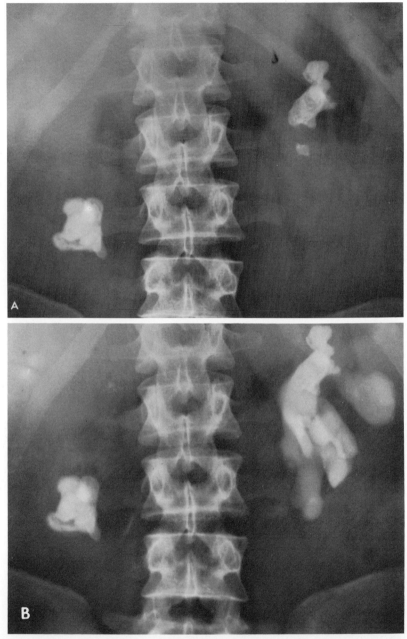

Figure 9–114. **Bilateral nephrolithiasis in horseshoe kidney. A,** *Plain film.* Large calcific shadow of branched variety overlying both renal areas. **B,** *Excretory urogram.* Typical horseshoe kidney; on left, stone fills pelvis, upper and part of lower calyx, producing dilatation of all calyces. *Little if any function remains on right,* although there seems to be slight amount of medium in ureter adjacent to pelvic stone.

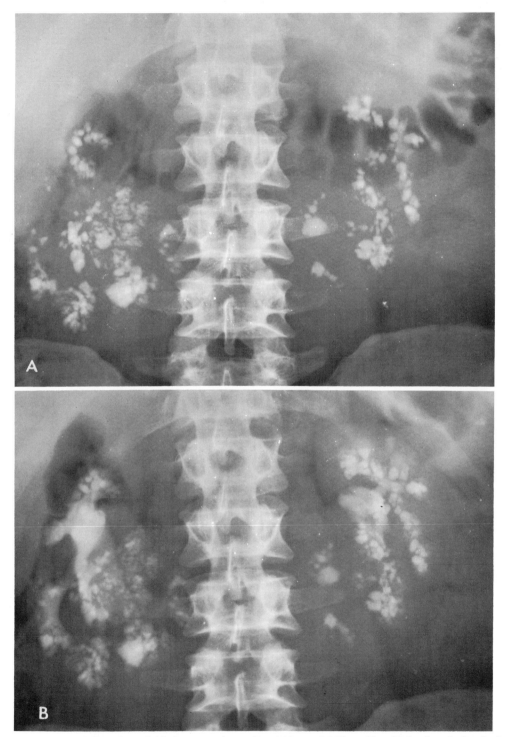

Figure 9–115. Bilateral nephrolithiasis in horseshoe kidney. **A,** *Plain film.* Multiple calcific shodows of various sizes overlying area suggest contour of horseshoe kidney. **B,** *Excretory urogram.* Definite horseshoe kidney. Shadows apparently are included in calyces. Could easily be confused with nephrocalcinosis or medullary sponge kidney.

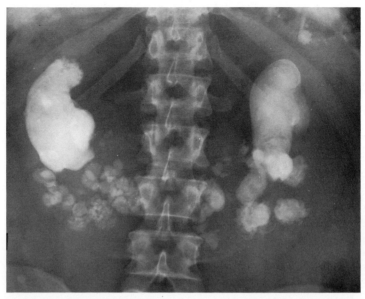

Figure 9–116. *Plain film.* **Advanced nephrolithiasis in horseshoe kidney. Branched calculus** filling pelves and calyces.

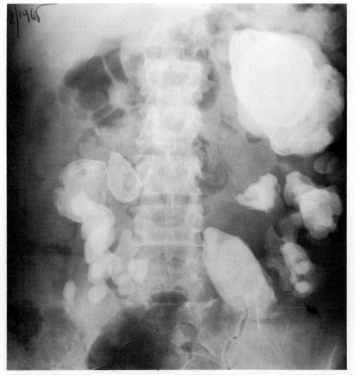

Figure 9–117. *Plain film.* **Extensive calculi in horseshoe kidney.** (Courtesy of Dr. George Marngos, Nicosia General Hospital, Cyprus.)

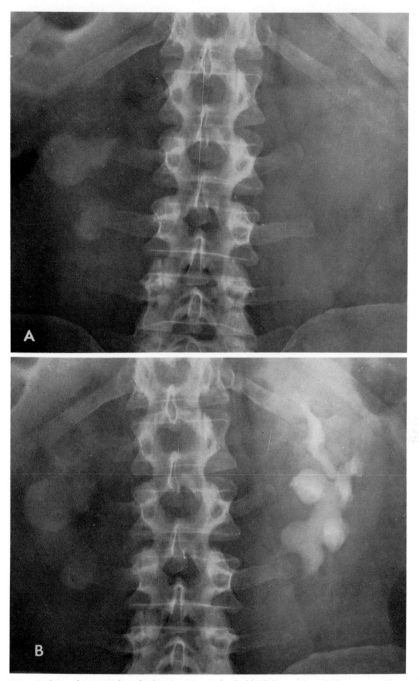

Figure 9–118.   Tuberculosis with calcification in right half of horseshoe kidney. **A,** *Plain film.* Irregular, mottled, calcific shadow overlying right renal area. Soft-tissue shadow on left suggests horseshoe kidney. **B,** *Excretory urogram.* Only left half of horseshoe kidney visualized. Typical projection of lower calyces toward midline, with irregular dilatation of pelvis and middle and lower calyces. No function on right.

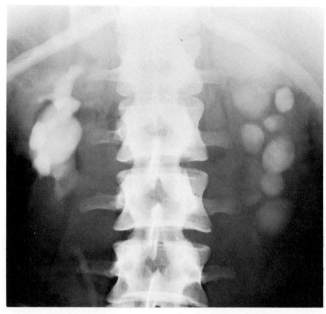

Figure 9–119.   *Excretory urogram.* Horseshoe kidney with marked caliectasis of left segment secondary to tuberculosis.

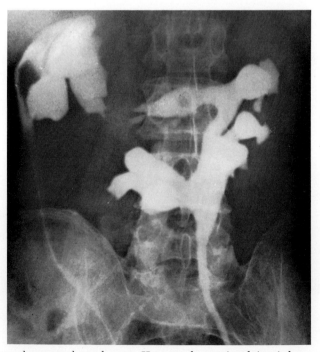

Figure 9–120.   *Bilateral retrograde pyelogram.* Hypernephroma involving isthmus and right half of horseshoe kidney. (Courtesy of Dr. M. Pesqueira.)

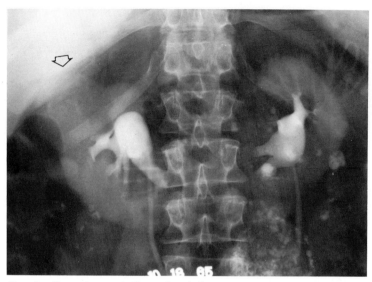

Figure 9–121. **Renal cell carcinoma in horseshoe kidney.** *Excretory urogram.* Typical horseshoe kidney with malrotated renal pelvis. Mass *(arrow)* (renal cell carcinoma) upper pole right. Abdominal calcification from old granulomatous peritonitis.

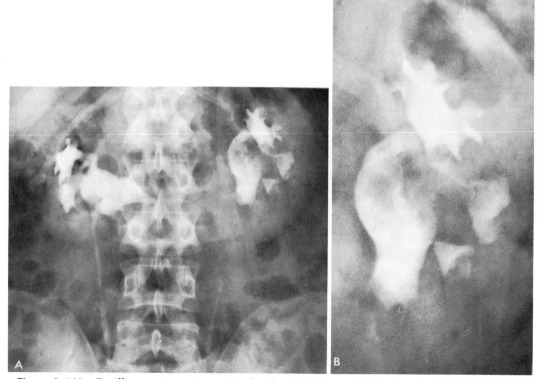

Figure 9–122. **Papillary carcinoma (transitional cell epithelioma grade 2) of renal pelvis (left) of horseshoe kidney. A,** *Excretory urogram.* Horseshoe kidney with filling defect in left renal pelvis from papillary tumor. **B,** Close-up view of left renal pelvis. (From Blackard, C. E., and Mellinger, G. T.)

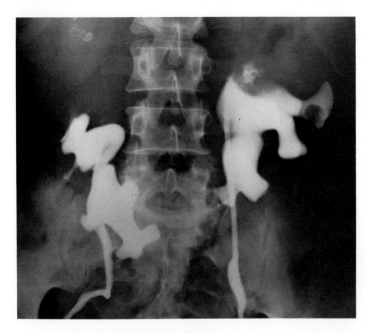

Figure 9–123. *Bilateral retrograde pyelogram.* **Horseshoe kidneys with epithelioma involving pelvis and upper calyces of left kidney.** (Courtesy of Dr. C. L. Deming.)

Anomalies in Structure

POLYCYSTIC AND MULTICYSTIC KIDNEYS

Polycystic disease probably should be included in this chapter, since it is the result of anomalous development. Nevertheless, we have considered it in Chapter 13 because polycystic disease is so often confused clinically and urographically with renal cysts. Multicystic disease is discussed in the same chapter.

THE RENAL PELVIS AND URETER

Anomalies in Number

INCOMPLETE URETERAL DUPLICATIONS (BIFID URETER)

Abnormal bifurcation or splitting of the ureteral bud is thought to account for incomplete ureteral duplication, in which case the two ureters join to form a common ureter with only one ureteral orifice (Fig. 9–125). If the branching is high so that the point of juncture is at or just below the ure-

teropelvic juncture, the condition is called a *bifid pelvis. Trifid pelvis* and triplicated ureter are encountered occasionally.

COMPLETE URETERAL DUPLICATION

Complete duplication of the ureter (double ureter) with each ureter having its own orifice is the result of two ureteral buds sprouting separately from the wolffian duct (Fig. 9–126). Logically, the ureteral bud sprouting from the higher level on the wolffian duct should serve the upper renal pelvis; the lower, the lower renal pelvis. Clinically, however, the *lower*, more medially situated ureteral orifice almost always serves the upper renal pelvis, whereas the upper, more cranially and laterally situated orifice serves the lower pelvis. This situation comes about in the following manner: As mentioned previously, the portion of the bladder that contains the wolffian duct and ureter grows in an uneven manner so that the ureter migrates laterally and cranially. As shown again, in Figure 9–126, the lower ureter is first absorbed into the bladder, while the upper ureter is carried caudally by the

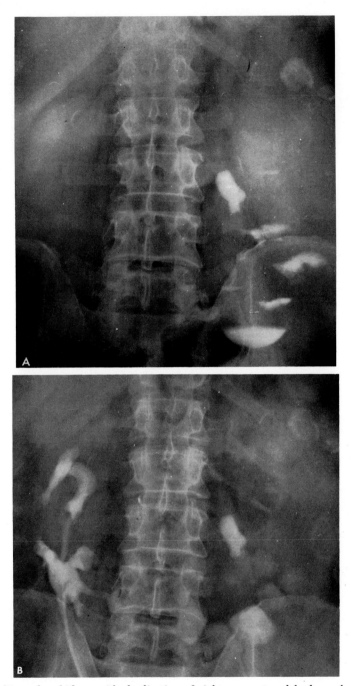

Figure 9–124. Horseshoe kidney with duplication of right segment and hydronephrosis, nephrolithiasis, "milk of calcium" stones, and rhabdomyosarcoma of left segment. **A,** *Plain film* (standing position). Multiple areas of calcific material over left kidney. Lowermost shadow, opposite second sacral segment, is crescentic in outline, with definite fluid level, and suggests contrast medium, although none had been injected. **B,** *Right retrograde pyelogram* (impossible to catheterize left ureteral orifice). **Horseshoe kidney with duplication on right.** Calcific shadows persist on left. Layering of calcific substance over lower pole of left kidney not seen in this film, as this was made with patient in dorsal position. Surgical exploration showed **horseshoe kidney, perinephritis, hydronephrosis, and rhabdomyosarcoma.** The layering of medium over lower pole was caused by thick suspension of calcium crystals and pus in dilated lower calyces of left segment of horseshoe kidney. (Courtesy of Dr. J. H. Kiefer and Dr. R. D. Herrold.)

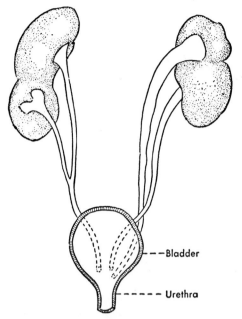

Figure 9–125. Bifid, double, or duplicated ureter. Incomplete duplication of right ureter, complete duplication of left ureter. (From Hollinshead, W. H.)

they fuse to become one ureter is not clear (Fig. 9–127).

BIFID, TRIFID, AND MULTIFID PELVIS

Double formation of the renal pelves and ureters is the most common form of malformation of the urinary organs (Nordmark; Thompson and Amar). It is more common in females than in males. Bifid renal pelvis is said to occur in 10 per cent of the population. It does not require much imagination to visualize the many variations that could occur during the branching of the cranial end of the ureter. Probably the most minor variation that occurs is the partial division of the renal pelvis to form a *bifid, trifid,* or *multifid* pelvis (Fig. 9–128), depending on the number of divisions that

migrating mesonephric duct, and only as still more of the duct is absorbed into the bladder or urethra does this ureter attain its independent opening. Because of this, the orifice serving the lower renal pelvis is always situated cranial and lateral to the orifice serving the *upper* ureter and renal pelvis. This is known as the *Weigert-Meyers rule.* Only rare instances have been reported in which this rule did not hold. The two ureters course downward side by side to the pelvis, and just before the bladder is reached, the ureter from the lower pelvis crosses the other to enter the bladder, while the other ureter continues on to enter at a lower and more medial position. As will be discussed subsequently, in the completely duplicated ureter, whenever one ureteral orifice is in an ectopic (extravesical) location the lower or ectopic orifice always serves the upper renal pelvis.

A rare type of ureteral duplication is the inverted Y in which two ureteral orifices are present but the duplicated ureters join to form a common ureter before reaching the single renal pelvis. This condition is thought to result from two ureteral buds sprouting from the wolffian duct. Just how

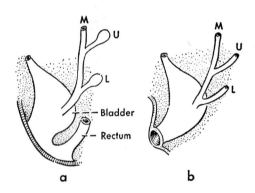

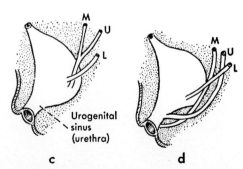

Figure 9–126. A to D, Development of complete ureteral duplication demonstrating reason why lower, most medial ureteral orifice connects with ureter which serves upper renal pelvis. M = mesonephric (wolffian duct); U = upper ureter (serving lower renal pelvis); L = lower ureter (serving upper renal pelvis). (From Hollinshead, W. H.)

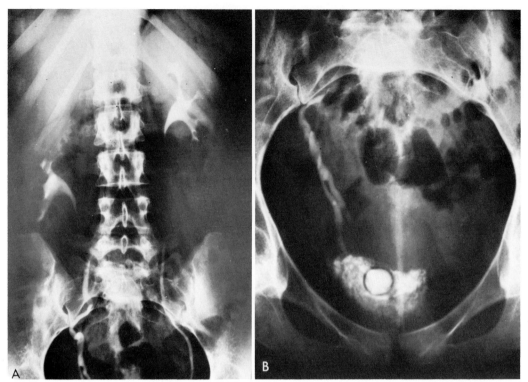

Figure 9–127.   Inverted Y ureteral duplication. Woman aged 25. Recurrent urinary tract infections and right lower quadrant pain. **A** and **B,** *Excretory urogram.* **A,** Lower right ureter divides into two branches. **B,** *Postvoiding film.* Inverted Y ureteral duplication with ureterocele. Cystoscopic examination revealed two right ureteral orifices with ureterocele involving most distal and medial orifice (From Klauber, G. T., and Reid, E. C.).

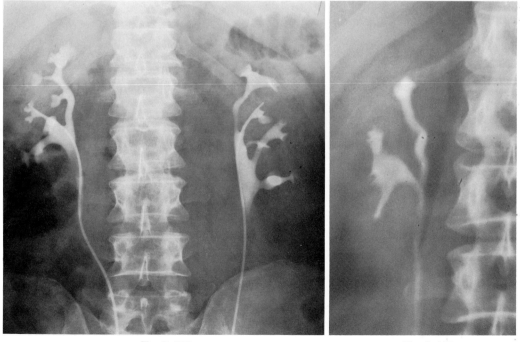

Fig. 9–128   Fig. 9–129

Figure 9–128.   *Bilateral retrograde pyelogram* illustrating **multifid pelves.**
Figure 9–129.   *Right retrograde pyelogram.* **Incomplete duplication;** point of junction just below normal site of ureteropelvic juncture. Note small upper pelvis.

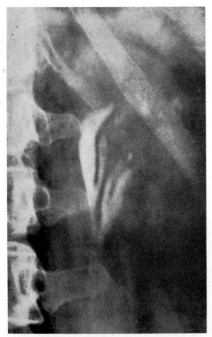

Figure 9–130. *Excretory urogram.* **Incomplete duplication** with both pelves of bifid type.

are created. This abnormal condition has been considered in detail in the chapter devoted to the normal renal pelvis, as it occurs frequently enough to be considered as an almost normal finding (see discussion of normal renal pelvis, Chapter 8). It may be difficult at times to distinguish partial duplication from complete duplication of the renal pelvis because no fixed anatomic landmarks separate the two. In most instances, when the juncture of the divisions of the pelvis is distal to the point at which the normal ureteropelvic juncture should be, the condition generally should be regarded as duplication (Goyanna and Greene; Greene) (Figs. 9–130).

DUPLICATION OF THE PELVIS AND URETER

Terminology

Duplication of the renal pelvis may be unilateral or bilateral, incomplete or complete. The term *incomplete duplication*

signifies that the ureters from the two pelves unite before emptying into the bladder. The term *complete duplication* signifies that the two ureters enter the bladder (or other structures) through separate orifices. In rare instances, triplication and even quadruplication is seen (Fig. 9–131). A kidney in which duplicated pelves are present is spoken of as a *duplex kidney.* Other terms used in the ensuing discussion include the following: *upper pole* and *lower pole,* applied to the renal pelvis, ureter, and ureteral orifice, to indicate the association of those structures with drainage of the upper or lower part of the kidney, respectively; *ectopic ureteral orifice,* to signify that the orifice occurs in other than the normal position—it may be classified as (1) intravesical, (2) extravesical, or (3) extraurinary; and *ectopic ureter,* to designate a ureter that serves an ectopic orifice in case of duplication.

In the case of incomplete duplication, the ureters may join at any level. An incomplete duplication in which the ureters join above the level of the bladder has been spoken of as a *Y-type ureter* (Lenaghan) (Figs. 9–132, 9–133, and 9–134); a malformation in which the junction is in the intramural portion of the ureter, has been termed a *V-type ureter* (Hartman and Hodson).

Comparative Size of Duplicated Pelves

In the vast majority of cases of duplication, the upper-pole pelvis is much smaller than the pelvis of the lower pole, often consisting of only a single minor calyx (Figs. 9–135, 9–136, and 9–137; also, see Fig. 9–129). It must not be forgotten, however, that cases are encountered in which the upper-pole pelvis is as large as or larger than the lower-pole pelvis (Figs. 9–138 through 9–142).

The two ureters usually cross each other just below the renal pelvis; if the juncture is low enough, they usually recross just above the bladder (see Figs. 9–135 and 9–136). The upper-pole ureter is usually situated anterior to the lower-pole

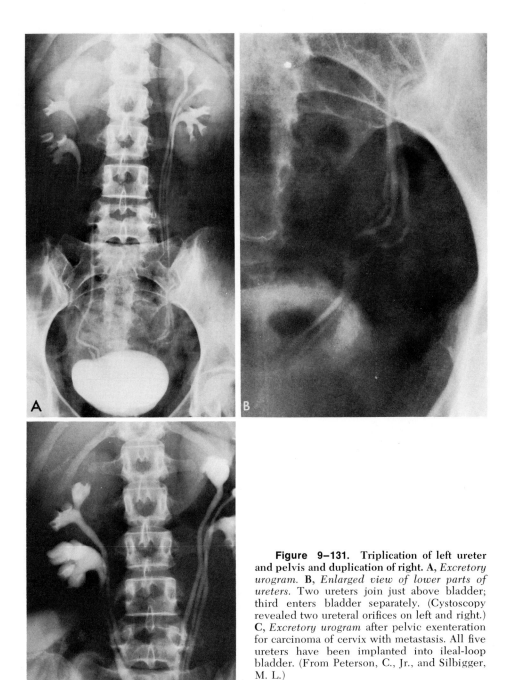

Figure 9–131. Triplication of left ureter and pelvis and duplication of right. **A,** *Excretory urogram.* **B,** *Enlarged view of lower parts of ureters.* Two ureters join just above bladder; third enters bladder separately. (Cystoscopy revealed two ureteral orifices on left and right.) **C,** *Excretory urogram* after pelvic exenteration for carcinoma of cervix with metastasis. All five ureters have been implanted into ileal-loop bladder. (From Peterson, C., Jr., and Silbigger, M. L.)

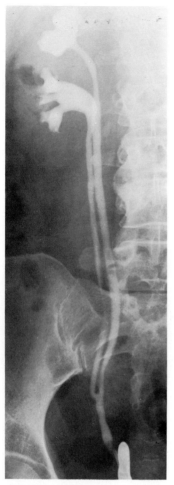

Figure 9–132. *Bulb pyeloureterogram.* Junction of **incompletely duplicated ureters** is well shown to be just above bladder.

ureter (Stephens, 1958). In some cases there is no crossing (see Figure 9–137). A most important rule to remember is that the upper-pole ureter is always drained by the most distal (caudad) and medial orifice; the lower-pole ureter, by the most proximal (cephalad) and lateral orifice. Exceptions to this rule have been encountered only very rarely (Lund) (Fig. 9–143).

Retrograde Peristalsis in One Limb of Incompletely Duplicated Ureter

For many years it has been appreciated that children with duplicated ureters have a higher incidence of urinary infection than do those without duplication. Partial obstruction at the juncture of the two ureters has been considered as a possible factor (Stephens, 1956), as not infrequently (in 41 per cent of cases) some dilatation of the two forks above the Y is observed (Fig. 9–144) (Kaplan and Elkin). The more recent demonstration of reverse peristalsis of one limb of the Y (Campbell, 1967; Kaplan and Elkin; Lenaghan) has been most illuminating with respect to this problem. The phenomenon, also described as a to-and-fro movement of urine from one arm of the forked ureter to the other, is said to occur in approximately 84 per cent of cases of incomplete duplication. The peristaltic wave begins in one limb as *antegrade peristalsis*, and when it reaches the Y juncture, it proceeds up the other limb of the Y as *retrograde peristalsis*. The limbs of the Y tend to alternate in the direction of the peristaltic flow (see Fig. 9–134).

THE DUPLEX KIDNEY

A duplex kidney is usually from 1 to 3 cm longer than its contralateral normal nonduplex mate (see Figures 9–141, 9–142, and 9–143). Rarely, it is of the same size, but it is never smaller. In the case of bilateral duplex kidneys, the length of each is increased. It has been pointed out (Hodson) that calyceal distribution of two kidneys in the same individual tends to be symmetric in approximately 85 per cent of individuals (see Chapter 8). This is associated with essentially equal thickness of the renal parenchyma (including that of all four poles). Duplication results in asymmetry in this regard; the parenchymal thicknesses of the two poles of a duplex (but otherwise normal) kidney may differ by as much as 1 cm, and frequently the combined thickness of the two poles is less than the combined thickness of the two poles of the contralateral (normal nonduplex) mate (Hartman and Hodson).

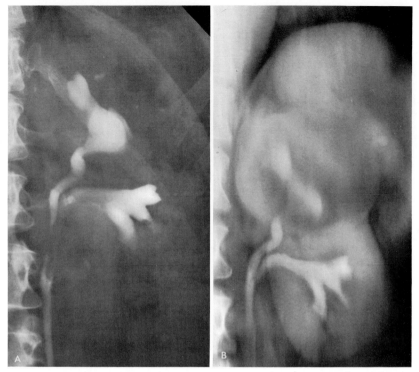

Figure 9–133. Cyst in upper segment of duplex kidney with duplication of pelvis and incomplete duplication of ureter. **A,** *Retrograde pyelogram.* **B,** *Nephrotomogram.*

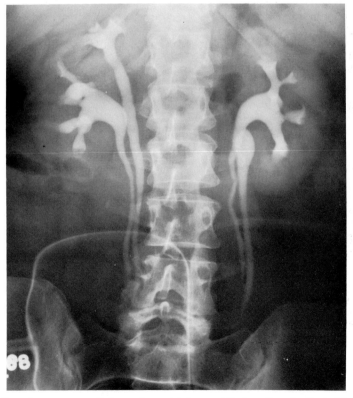

Figure 9–134. *Excretory urogram.* **Retrograde peristalsis up blind-ending duplicated left ureter.** Junction of ureters is at left of transverse process of L-5. The blind-ending segment has been filled by retrograde flow of urine.

649

Pseudotumor (Lobar Dysmorphism)

In the duplex kidney, an enlarged and somewhat irregular septum of Bertin that may form a tumor-like mass of tissue is often seen. This abnormality apparently represents a type of anomalous fusion of adjacent lobes in the upper and lower segment. The overgrowth of parenchymal tissue in this area may produce a "mass," which may be large enough to cause compression of the adjacent pelvis or pelves. This "mass" may appear sufficiently dense in an excretory urogram, nephrotomogram, or arteriogram to suggest a tumor (hypernephroma) (Hartman and Hodson; King, Friedenberg, and Tena). Such pseudotumors have been encountered when surgical exploration has been carried out on the basis of an incorrect diagnosis. Being alert to the possibility, plus the use of an arteriogram or a radioisotopic scan of the kidney, should clarify the diagnosis (Figs. 9–145, 9–146, and 9–147) (Charghi and associates).

Text continued on page 654.

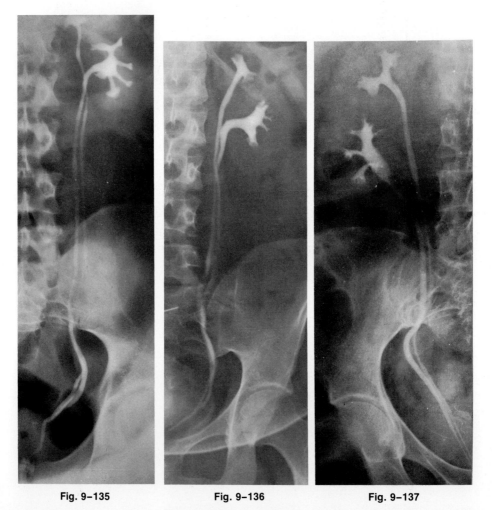

Fig. 9–135   Fig. 9–136   Fig. 9–137

Figure 9–135. *Left retrograde pyelogram.* **Complete duplication on left.** Note typical crossing of ureters as they descend into pelvis. Small upper pelvis also is typical.

Figure 9–136. *Left retrograde pyelogram.* **Complete duplication** with typical crossing of ureters before reaching bladder.

Figure 9–137. *Right retrograde pyelogram.* Note typical small upper pelvis. **Complete duplication** with no crossing of ureters.

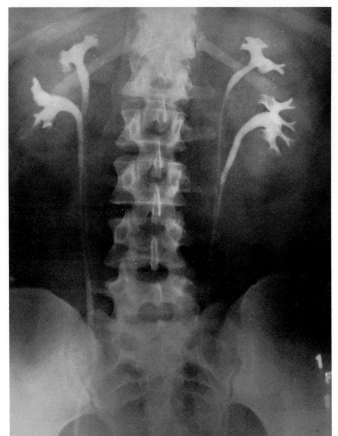

Figure 9–138. *Bilateral retrograde pyelogram.* **Bilateral complete duplication.** Upper pelves and calyces are larger than in average case.

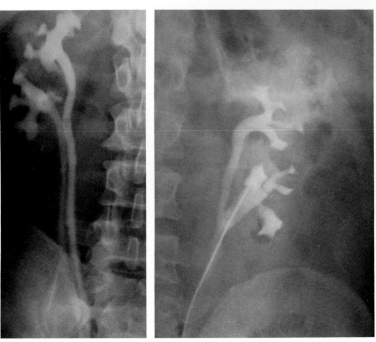

Fig. 9–139   Fig. 9–140

Figure 9–139. *Right retrograde pyelogram.* **Incomplete duplication.** Unusual in that upper and lower pelves are almost equal in size.

Figure 9–140. *Left retrograde pyelogram.* **Incomplete duplication.** Unusual type of case in which upper and lower pelves are almost equal in size.

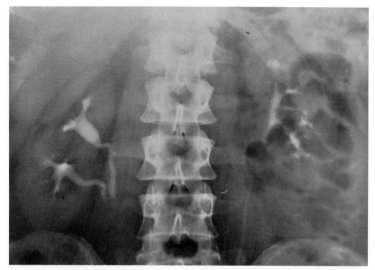

Figure 9–141. *Excretory urogram.* **Duplication on right.** Unusual because upper pelvis is larger than lower.

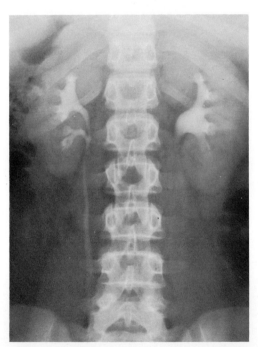

Figure 9–142. *Excretory urogram.* **Duplication of right renal pelvis.** Unusual because upper-pole pelvis is much larger than lower.

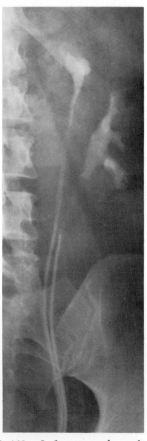

Figure 9–143. *Left retrograde pyelogram.* **Complete duplication.** Unusual in that the ureters do not cross, and extremely rare in that the most lateral and proximal ureteral orifice serves the upper rather than the lower pelvis. Note typical small upper pelvis. (From Lund, A. J.)

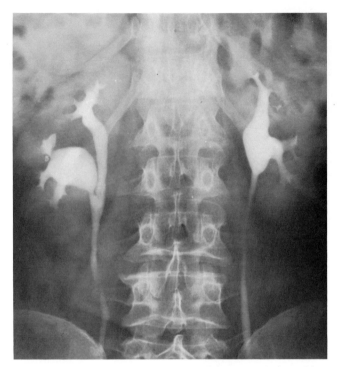

Figure 9–144.   *Excretory urogram.* **Y-type duplication of right ureter.** There is dilatation of both forks above stem.

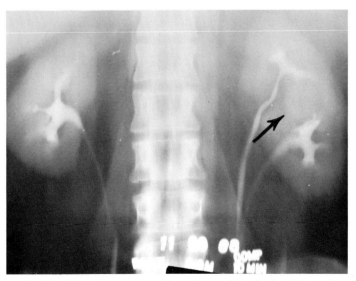

Figure 9–145.   *Nephrotomogram.* "Pseudotumor" in duplex kidney *(arrow).*

Associated Anomalies

Duplication of the pelvis and ureter may be associated with almost any other type of anomaly such as malrotation, unilateral agenesis, fusion, and ectopia. In the case of malrotation either one or both of the pelves may be involved (Figs. 9–148 through 9–152).

Obstruction and Reflux

The incidence of reflux and obstruction is increased in duplication. *Reflux* is more common from the orifice of the lower-pole ureterovesical juncture (Fig. 9–153), which is thought to be the result of a developmental fault; the intramural portion of this ureter tends to come through the bladder in a perpendicular rather than in the normally oblique manner. In a study of 27 cases of duplication of the ureter, Ambrose and Nicolson found lower-pole reflux in only 2. Lower-pole reflux occurred three times as frequently as upper-pole reflux in Stephens' (1956) cases. Reflux may be suspected from the excretory urogram when

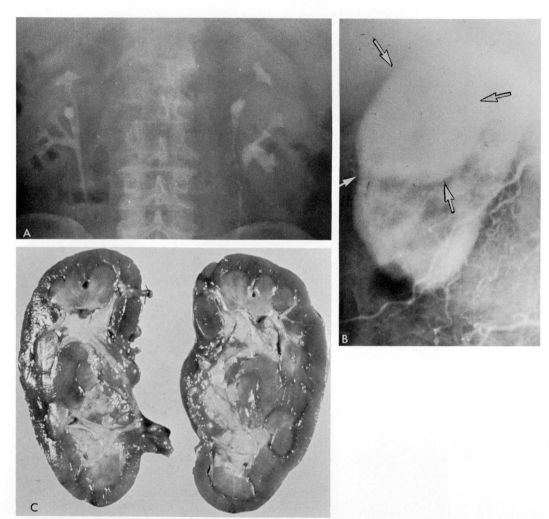

Figure 9–146. "Lobar dysmorphism" (misplaced renal lobe or "pseudotumor") in bifid, duplex type, right kidney, simulating tumor. **A,** *Excretory urogram.* Bifid type pelvis on right. Duplex kidney on left, with incomplete duplication of ureter. **B,** *Aortogram, nephrographic phase.* Large mass with "blush" in midrenal area, near upper pole. (Surgical exploration and nephrectomy were done.) **C,** *Gross specimen.* Mass turned out to be deep-seated renal lobe composed of normal parenchyma. (From Charghi, A., Dessureault, P., Drouin, G., Gauthier, G. E., Perras, P., Roy, P., and Charbonneau, J.)

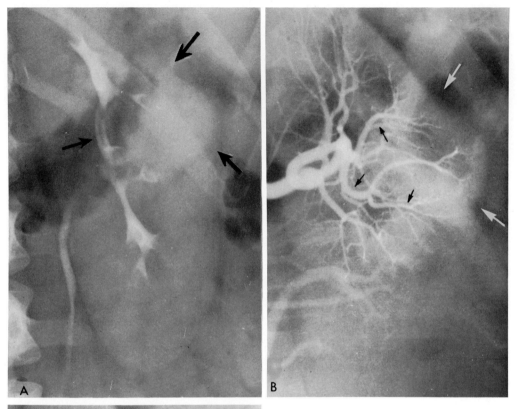

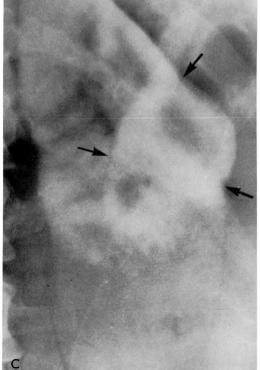

Figure 9–147. Duplex kidney with "mass" of normal parenchyma simulating tumor ("lobar dysmorphism"; "pseudotumor"). **A,** *Excretory urogram.* Circular form of renal mass causes spreading and crescentic deformity of upper calyces. **B,** *Selective arteriogram, arterial phase.* No evidence of pathologic vascularization, tumor stain, or puddling. **C,** Selective arteriogram, nephrographic phase. "Mass" is well outlined and is shown to have greater density than does rest of kidney. (Surgical exploration revealed mass to be composed of normal parenchyma.) (From Charghi, A., Dessureault, P., Drouin, G., Gauthier, G. E., Perras, P., Roy, P., and Charbonneau, J.)

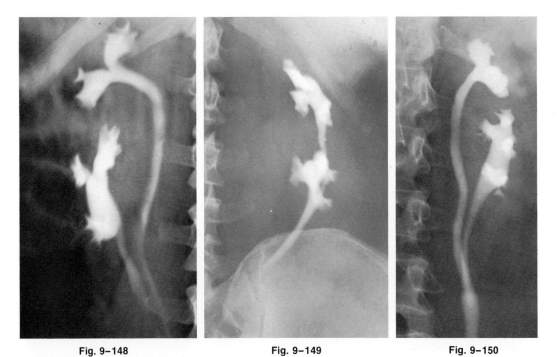

Fig. 9–148 Fig. 9–149 Fig. 9–150

Figure 9–148. *Right retrograde pyelogram.* Duplication, with malrotation of lower pelvis.
Figure 9–149. *Left retrograde pyelogram.* Duplication, incomplete, with malrotation of both pelves.
Figure 9–150. *Left retrograde pyelogram.* Duplication, incomplete, with malrotation of lower pelvis.

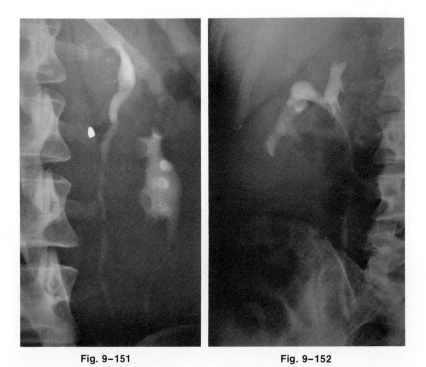

Fig. 9–151 Fig. 9–152

Figure 9–151. *Excretory urogram.* Duplication, with malrotation of lower pelvis.
Figure 9–152. *Right retrograde pyelogram.* Incomplete duplication with unusual contour, apparently resulting from malrotation of lower pelvis around both vertical and anteroposterior axes.

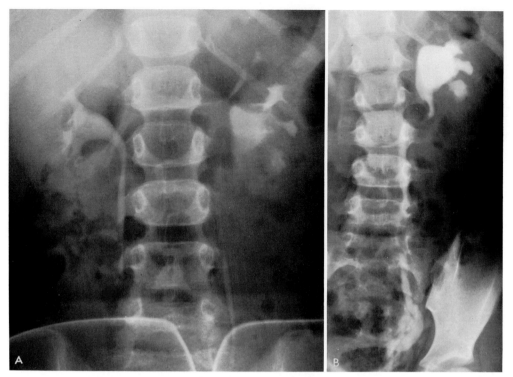

Figure 9–153. Reflux up lower-pole ureter of duplex left kidney with dilatation of the lower pelvis. **A,** *Excretory urogram.* Duplication (complete) with moderate pyelectasis of lower-pole pelvis. **B,** *Retrograde cystogram.* Reflux up lower-pole ureter filling pelvis.

it indicates such findings as pyeloureterectasis, undue distensibility of the upper urinary tract when ureteral compression is applied, and the sudden appearance of contrast medium in a previously nonopacified part of the upper urinary tract (Hartman and Hodson). Atrophy and pyelonephritic scarring or a small kidney with associated caliectasis may be the tip-off (see Chapter 10).

Obstruction, on the other hand, more commonly affects the upper-pole ureter because so often its orifice is ectopic, being located in the vesical neck, the urethra, or even in an extraurinary position. Various degrees of dilatation of the upper-pole pelvis and ureter may result, as may various degrees of reduction of function of the upper-pole segment. This situation produces some of the most difficult diagnostic problems encountered in urology, particularly in pediatric urology. The upper-pole pelvis too often is not visualized, even with delayed films (several hours after injection of contrast medium); thus, the diagnosis must be made on the basis of indirect findings and clinical data, requiring considerable deduction and "sleuthing" on the part of an alert examiner.

Extreme hydronephrosis involving upper-pole pelves may result in bizarre urograms (Fig. 9–154). Obstruction reaches its greatest incidence and degree in malformations in which the ureters terminate in an ectopic position (including ectopic ureterocele). These conditions are considered later under appropriate headings.

Recognition of Lower-Pole Renal Pelvis (When the Upper-Pole Pelvis Is Not Visualized).

It is most important that the student learn to recognize the lower-pole pelvis of a duplication (Fig. 9–155), because a high incidence of obstruction is associated with nonfunction and nonvisualization of the upper-pole pelvis, especially if the upper-

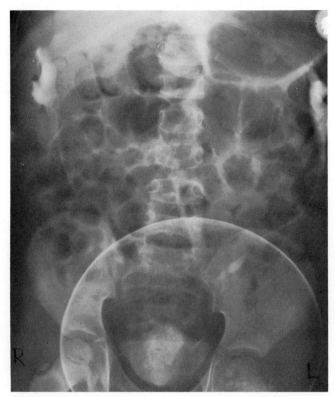

Figure 9–154. Bilateral ureteropelvic duplication with ectopic upper-pole ureters in 6-year-old boy. Obstruction of both upper-pole ureters was associated with **tremendous hydronephrotic dilatation of both upper-pole pelves,** causing marked lateral displacement of both kidneys suggesting a retroperitoneal tumor. Presenting complaint was that of enlarging abdomen. *Excretory urogram* shows marked lateral displacement of kidneys (only lower pelves are visualized) with some malrotation. It would be difficult, with only these films, to state that bilateral duplication exists. (Bilateral heminephrectomy was performed.) (Courtesy of Dr. A. J. Palubinskas.)

pole ureter terminates ectopically. The characteristics which may suggest that a renal pelvis drains only the lower pole of the kidney include the following:

(1) The calyces may be fewer in number than normal; for instance, there may be two major calyces instead of three.

(2) The upper calyx appears shortened and does not reach into the upper pole of the kidney (Figs. 9–155 *A, C,* and *D* and 9–156 through 9–160; also, see Fig. 9–154). Obviously, the parenchymal outline of the upper pole of the kidney must be visualized or mistakes easily can be made. If the outline is poor, a tomogram will clarify it. *The alert examiner will always insist that the parenchyma of the upper pole of the kidney be adequately outlined before he will commit himself to a diagnosis.*

(3) The lower pole of the kidney may be displaced downward by a dilated upper pelvis; this may be indistinguishable from other space-occupying lesions (Fig. 9–161).

(4) The upper pole of the kidney may appear to be rotated laterally and downward on its anteroposterior axis (counterclockwise on the left side, clockwise on the right) causing the pelvis and calyces to be so rotated, producing a "drooping flower" appearance (Fig. 9–155 *B* and 9–156). Williams and Woodard have spoken of this as the "down and out" displacement of the lower-pole pyelogram.

(5) The renal pelvis may be displaced laterally; and the ureter, instead of proceeding directly medially toward the vertebral column and then downward (a right-angle course), takes instead a direct course

Text continued on page 662

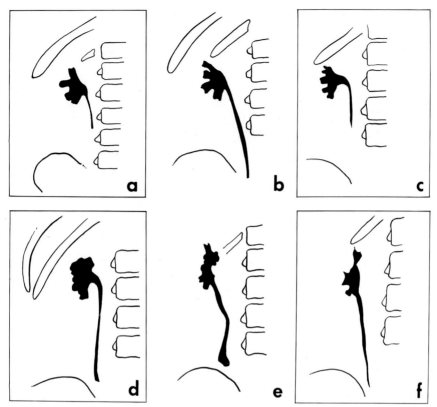

Figure 9–155. Varieties of lower renal pelves associated with duplication. (Redrawn from Williams, D. I., 1958b.)

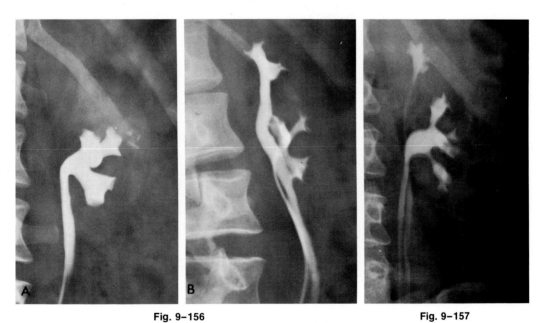

Fig. 9–156   Fig. 9–157

Figure 9–156. **A,** *Left retrograde pyelogram.* **Lower pelvis of duplication** visualized. Although there are three major calyces, elongated renal outline furnishes evidence that there must be duplication, since upper half is not served by visualized pelvis. Note "drooping flower" appearance of renal pelvis. **B,** *Left retrograde pyelogram* (lateral view). **Complete duplication** visualized since there is catheter in each ureter. Upper and lower pelves visualized.

Figure 9–157. *Left retrograde pyelogram.* **Complete duplication.** Typical small upper pelvis with larger lower pelvis. If upper pelvis were not visualized, one might mistake lower pelvis for only one supplying kidney, as there are three definite major calyces.

Fig. 9–158

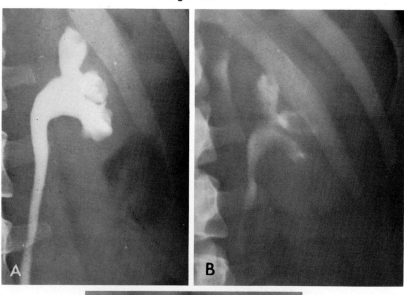

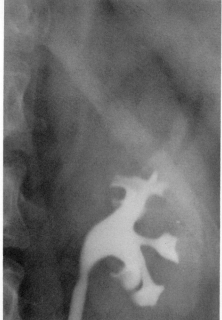

Fig. 9–159

Figure 9–158. **Duplication** which could easily be missed. **A,** *Left retrograde pyelogram.* Fairly normal-sized pelvis with three major calyces. Soft-tissue outline of kidney is indistinct. **B,** *Extretory urogram.* Duplication. Diminutive upper pelvis can be seen in region of upper pole near spinal column.

Figure 9–159. *Excretory urogram.* **Lower half of duplication.** Interesting because pelvis seems to be almost normal in size and has three major calyces. However, soft-tissue outline of kidney is well delineated, and it can be seen that upper half is not served by pelviocalyceal system. Further examination showed upper pelvis to be present.

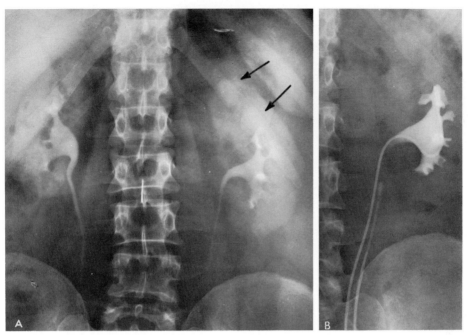

Figure 9–160. **Poorly functioning, hydronephrotic upper segment of duplicated left kidney** from obstruction in upper third of upper-pole ureter. **A,** *Excretory urogram.* Right: normal. Left: pelvis and calyces of lower segment appear normal, with three major calyces that in themselves would not suggest duplication. However, soft-tissue outline of kidney reveals that upper pole is not served by upper calyx. Also, there are two indistinct circular areas of apparent contrast medium over upper pole of left kidney, apparently dilated calyces *(arrows).* **B,** *Left retrograde pyelogram.* **Duplicated ureters** found on cystoscopy. Ureter serving upper pelvis is occluded opposite third lumbar transverse process.

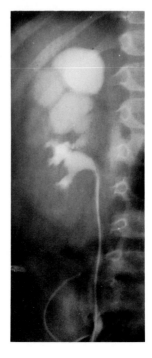

Figure 9–161. Duplication of pelvis and ureter, with upper-pole ureter terminating in the urethra, and hydronephrosis of upper segment of kidney. *Retrograde pyelogram* of lower-pole pelvis. Typical lateral and downward rotation of lower-pole pelvis, with some compression of upper calyces by dilated upper-pole pelvis.

toward the spinal column at the lumbosacral level ("cutting across" the hypotenuse of the triangle) and then downward to the bladder (Figs. 9–155 *B* and *F* and 9–160).

(6) The ureter may be displaced or compressed by the dilated upper-pole pelvis (Fig. 9–162).

(7) The upper calyx of the lower pole may be deformed by pressure of the dilated upper-pole pelvis; this may suggest cyst or tumor. A good nephrogram may help clarify such a situation.

In order to become proficient in recognizing the lower-pole pelvis of a duplication of the renal pelvis, the student should study all duplex kidney illustrations in this section as well as those in the section on ectopic ureteral orifices and ectopic ureteroceles.

Associated Pathologic Conditions

Pyelectasis; Pyeloureterectasis. Dilatation of the pelvis and ureter from either reflux or obstruction incident to the duplicated state of the ureteral orifices has already been discussed. Obstruction may also occur at a higher level in the ureters or at either ureteropelvic juncture (Figs. 9–163 through 9–166).

Renal and Ureteral Calculi. Renal and ureteral calculi are not uncommon in cases of duplication of the ureter. *In the case of ureteral calculi,* if satisfactory visualization of both ureters is not obtained with the excretory urogram, it may be most difficult to decide in which ureter the stone is located; also, if the upper-pole pelvis is not visualized, the presence of a second ureter

Text continued on page 666.

Figure 9–162. **Duplication with lateral ureteral displacement.** Boy aged 5. Acute right epididymitis and urinary tract infection. **A,** *Excretory urogram.* Lateral displacement and dilatation of upper right ureter. **B,** *Voiding cystogram.* Delayed film shows marked dilatation and tortuosity of ureter to duplicated upper segment.

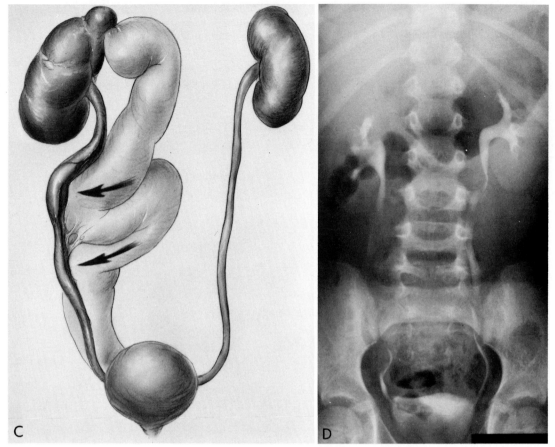

Figure 9–162 *Continued.*   **C,** Diagrammatic representation of situation. **D,** *Excretory urogram.* Nearly normal ureter after excision of upper renal segment and its ureter. (From Amar, A. D.)

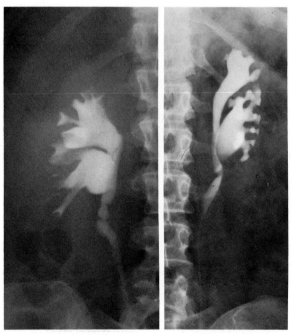

Fig. 9–163   Fig. 9–164

Figure 9–163.   *Right retrograde pyelogram.* Incomplete duplication with mild pyelectasis of both pelves.
Figure 9–164.   *Left retrograde pyelogram.* Moderate pyelectasis of both segments of duplicated left kidney.

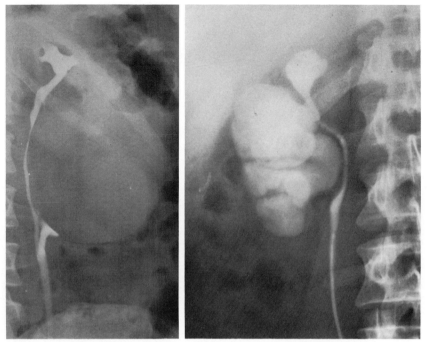

Fig. 9–165   **Fig. 9–166**

Figure 9–165. *Left retrograde pyelogram.* Nonfunctioning, hydronephrotic lower segment of incomplete duplication on left. Complete obstruction at ureteropelvic juncture of lower segment.

Figure 9–166. *Right retrograde pyelogram.* Incomplete duplication, with hydronephrosis of lower segment (which showed no function on excretory urogram).

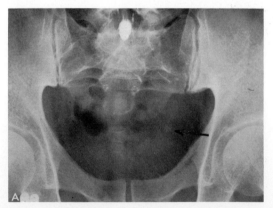

Figure 9–167. **Unrecognized ureteral duplication on left with calculi in dilated upper-pole ureter** causing flank pain, infection, and fever. **Incomplete duplication of ureter;** ureters, joined in intramural portion, had only one ureteral orifice. **A,** *Plain film.* Small shadows suggesting calculi in region of lower part of left ureter *(arrow).* There are questionable minute calculi in lower pole of each kidney. **B,** *Excretory urogram.* Malrotated pelvis without evidence of obstruction. Upper calyx is long, but outline of upper pole is indistinct. Duplication not suspected. At operation on lower part of left ureter, surgeon encountered hugely dilated duplicated upper-pole ureter containing calculi. Heminephrectomy and ureterectomy were performed.

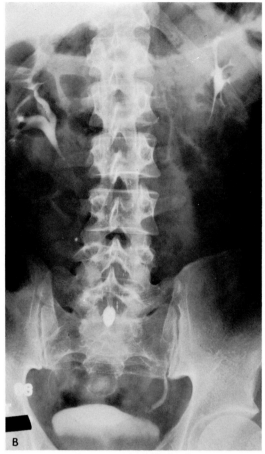

Fig. 9–167 *Continued.*

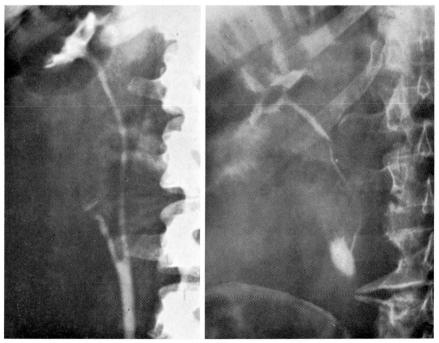

Fig. 9–168   **Fig. 9–169**

Figure 9–168. Ureteral calculus in duplicated ureter. *Right retrograde pyelogram.* Incomplete duplication. Upper pelvis normal. Lower pelvis not outlined. Complete obstruction of ureter serving lower pelvis, caused by stone about 3 cm above point of junction of ureters. No medium enters lower pelvis. (Courtesy of Dr. M. Pesqueira.)

Figure 9–169. *Right retrograde pyelogram.* **Nonopaque ureteral stone in duplicated ureter.**

may not be suspected (Figs. 9–167, 9–168, and 9–169). *In the case of renal calculi,* either one or both pelves of the kidney may be involved (Figs. 9–170 through 9–174).

Other Pathologic Lesions. Tuberculosis, tumor, cortical abscess, cyst, and polycystic disease, when associated with duplication of the pelvis and ureter, may produce

Text continued on page 672.

A

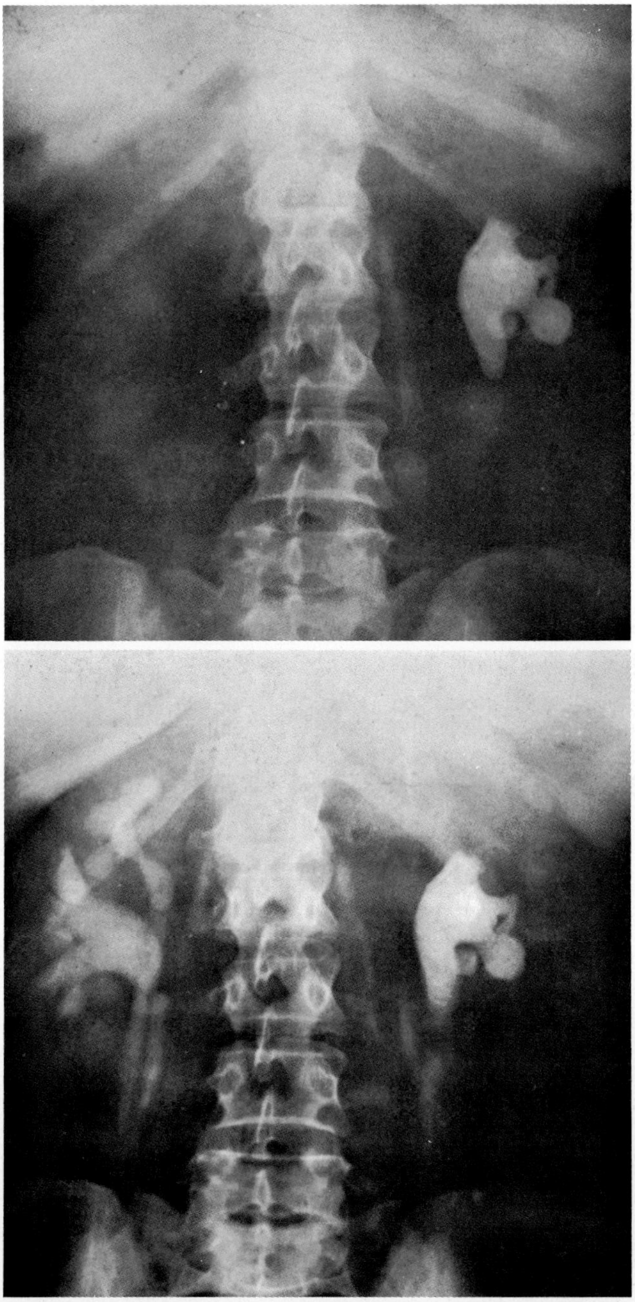

B

Figure 9–170. Left nephrolithiasis in duplicated left kidney. **A,** *Plain film.* Branched calculus filling pelvis and calyces of lower segment. **B,** *Excretory urogram.* Bilateral duplication. Branched calculus fills lower segment of duplicated left kidney.

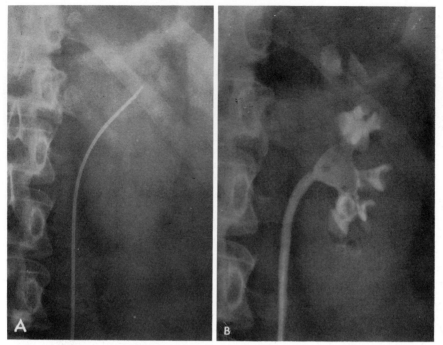

Figure 9–171. Slightly opaque calculi in duplicated left kidney. **A,** *Plain film.* Opaque catheter in left ureter; shadow of poor density at level of transverse process of L1. **B,** *Left retrograde pyelogram.* Incomplete duplication. Ureter to upper segments not completely outlined, but calyces of upper segment are shown. Negative filling defect of lower pelvis and lower calyces from calculi of poor density.

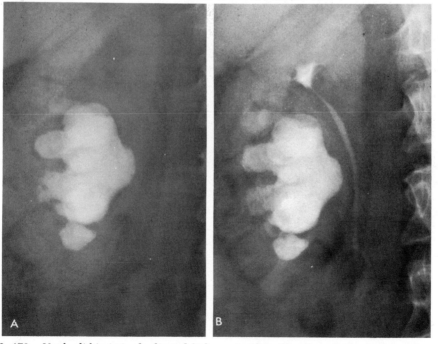

Figure 9–172. Nephrolithiasis in duplicated kidney. **A,** *Plain film.* Branched calculus outling pelvis and calyces of lower two thirds of right kidney. **B,** *Excretory urogram.* Duplication. Normal upper segment and ureter. Branched calculus filling dilated pelvis and calyces of lower segment. There is function remaining in lower segment, as indicated by contrast medium around periphery of stone.

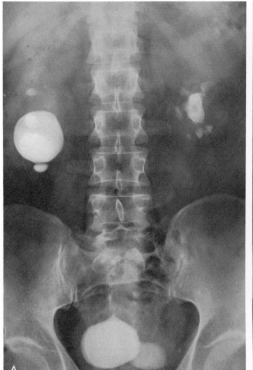

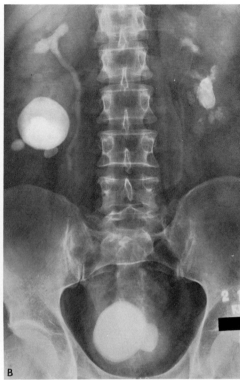

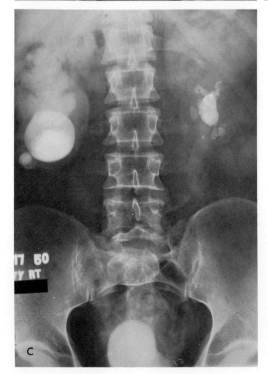

Figure 9–173. Bilateral nephrolithiasis in lower pelves of bilateral duplicated kidneys. Marked hydronephrosis of lower pelvis of right kidney. Multiple large vesical calculi. **A,** *Plain film.* Multiple large calculi overlying lower pole of both kidneys. Two large vesical calculi. **B,** *Excretory urogram, 35-minute film.* Upper pelves of bilateral duplication only are visualized. No apparent function in either lower pelvis, both of which contain calculi. **C,** *Excretory urogram, 5-hour film.* Both lower pelves are now visualized in this delayed film. Lower segment of duplicated right kidney shows marked hydronephrosis, with **apparent obstruction at ureteropelvic juncture.** Ureter incompletely visualized but also suggests dilatation. Ureter serving lower pelvis of left kidney is outlined with medium and is dilated. There is no apparent hydronephrosis on this side. Pelvis seems to be contracted around largest stone.

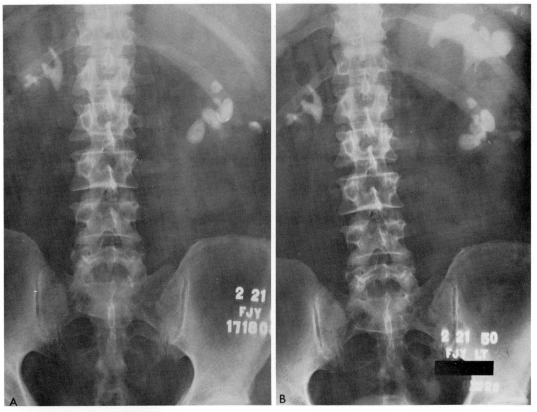

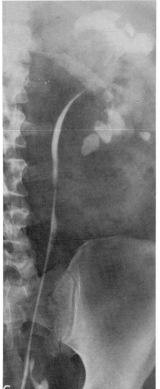

Figure 9–174. Calculi in pyonephrotic lower segment of duplicated left kidney, associated with perinephric abscess and draining sinus. Staghorn calculus in right kidney. **A,** *Plain film.* Staghorn calculus in small atrophic right kidney. Large renal outline on left, with multiple calculi over midportion and lower pole. **B,** *Excretory urogram.* Function is best on right, as medium can be seen in ureter. Upper pelvis on left is functioning. Calyces dilated. Apparently no function in lower segment. **C,** *Left retrograde pyelogram.* Ureteral catheter inserted in lowermost ureteral orifice, which was in edge of small vesical diverticulum. Upper pelvis and ureter serving it are outlined. Some medium has run around catheter into diverticulum and has run retrograde up lower 3 cm of duplicated left ureter (orifice of which is in bottom of diverticulum).

Fig. 9–175   Fig. 9–176

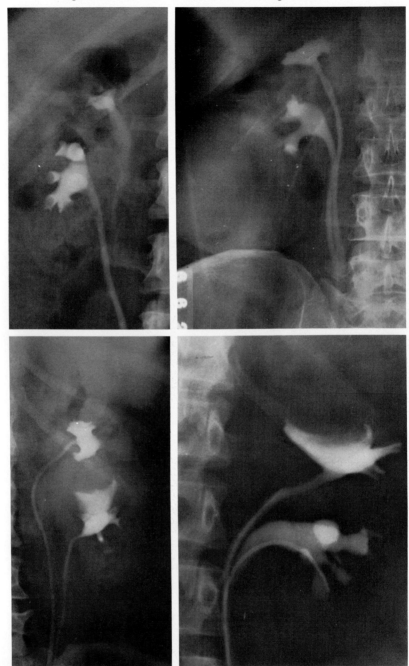

Fig. 9–177   Fig. 9–178

Figure 9–175. *Right retrograde pyelogram.* **Tuberculosis in duplicated right kidney.** Evidence of cortical necrosis in upper segment, which is partially obscured by gas in bowel. Lower segment appears to be urographically normal. At operation entire kidney was found to be seat of caseous tuberculosis.

Figure 9–176. *Right retrograde pyelogram.* **Simple (solitary) cyst involving lower pole of completely duplicated right kidney.**

Figure 9–177. *Left retrograde pyelogram.* **Simple (solitary) cyst in midportion of left kidney, which is site** of complete duplication. Cyst is deforming upper calyces of lower pelvis. Irregularity of calyces, which surround cyst, could easily be confused with tumor.

Figure 9–178. *Left retrograde pyelogram.* **Multilocular cyst associated with complete duplication of left kidney. Cyst involves upper pole of kidney** and is producing deformity of upper pelvis. Loss of normal terminal irregularities of upper calyces could suggest tumor. At operation multilocular cyst found. (Heminephrectomy done.)

670

Fig. 9–179

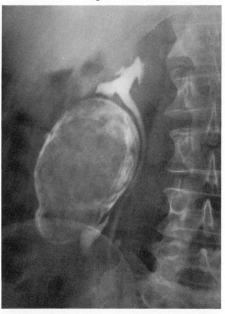

Fig. 9–180

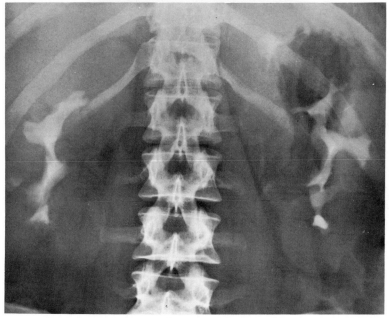

Figure 9–179. *Right retrograde pyelogram.* Calcified simple (solitary) cyst involving lower half of duplicated right kidney. Complete obstruction of ureter serving lower segment at ureteropelvic juncture.
Figure 9–180. *Excretory urogram.* Bilateral polycystic disease associated with duplication on left.

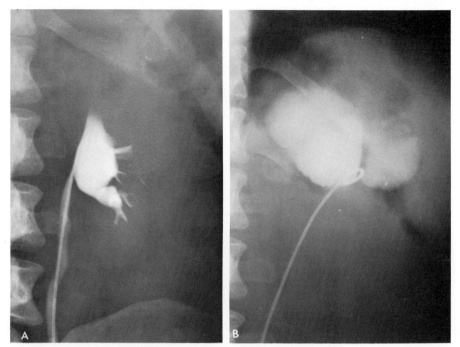

Figure 9–181. Cortical abscess involving upper pole of duplicated left kidney. *Retrograde pyelograms.* **A,** Only lower pelvis is visualized; mass obliterates upper calyx, suggesting possible **tumor of upper pole. B,** Catheter is in ureter serving upper pelvis and has perforated the **cortical abscess,** now filled with contrast medium.

an endless variety of urographic deformities (Figs. 9–175 through 9–183; also, see Fig. 9–133).

Anomalies of Ureteropelvic Juncture; Obstruction at Ureteropelvic Juncture

These subjects are considered in Chapter 11.

Anomalies in Position and Form of Ureter

RUDIMENTARY BRANCHED URETER

A rudimentary branched ureter with a blind "ending" or pouch (Figs. 9–184 through 9–187) is a fairly uncommon anomaly. About 50 cases have been reported (Haber). It is considered to be the result of multiple budding from the wolffian duct or of premature cleavage of a single ureteral bud. Essentially the same situation may be present in which the blind ureter arises not

from the ureter but adjacent to it and has a separate ureteral orifice similar to a complete ureteral duplication. Such an anomaly may be difficult to distinguish from a vesical diverticulum, especially if it becomes dilated. It probably represents an abortive attempt at complete ureteral duplication. Haber has been successful in demonstrating the branched ureter by utilizing both the prone and supine Trendelenburg positions during excretory urography (Figs. 9–188 and 9–189).

SINGLE URETERAL DIVERTICULUM

The single ureteral diverticulum is considered here because at present some authors (Rank and associates) who have considered this subject now think a true diverticulum is simply a rudimentary branched ureter which has become dilated and assumed an ovoid or round shape (Figs. 9–190 and 9–191). Richardson found 30 cases in the literature in 1942 and added

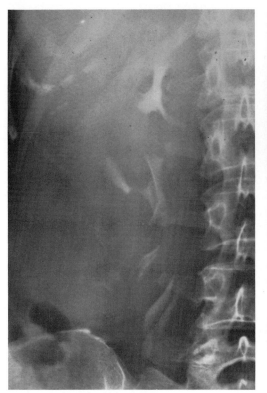

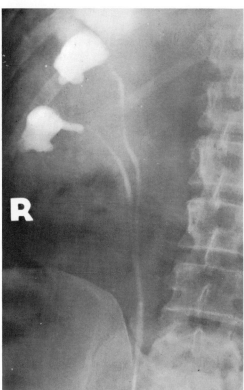

Fig. 9–182   Fig. 9–183

Figure 9–182. *Excretory urogram.* **Hypernephroma involving lower half of duplicated right kidney.**

Figure 9–183. *Right retrograde pyelogram.* **Renal sarcoma in duplicated kidney.** Incomplete duplication of ureters. Mass in right renal area, with bizarre deformity of calyces. Surgical exploration revealed huge tumor of right kidney. Kidney removed. **Pathologic diagnosis was round cell sarcoma** with complete destruction of renal substance.

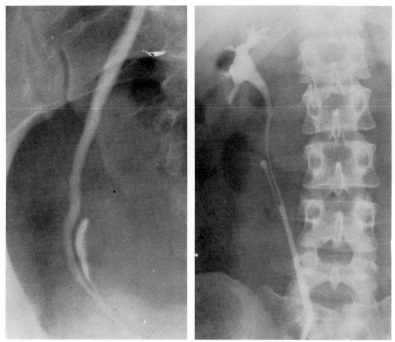

Fig. 9–184   Fig. 9–185

Figure 9–184. *Right retrograde pyelogram.* Rudimentary branched ureter with blind ending.

Figure 9–185. *Retrograde pyelogram.* Ureteral diverticulum or abortive attempt at duplication of ureter.

673

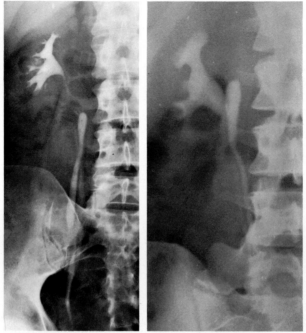

Fig. 9–186   Fig. 9–187

Figure 9–186. *Retrograde pyelogram.* **Abortive blind-ending ureter or ureteral diverticulum** (Courtesy of Dr. Hugh Robinson.)

Figure 9–187. *Right retrograde pyelogram.* **Rudimentary branched ureter with blind ending.**

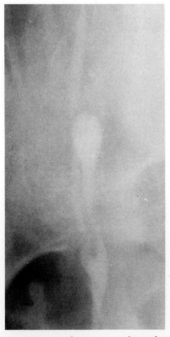

Figure 9–188. **Rudimentary branched ureter with blind ending.** Man aged 64 with right flank pain. *Excretory urogram.* Prone Trendelenburg position used to fill blind-ending branch. (From Haber, K.)

1 case of his own, that of a huge diverticulum containing 3,500 ml of urine.

In 1947, Culp studied the subject in depth. He found 52 cases in the literature and added 1 of his own, in which a huge diverticulum (1,600 ml in capacity) arose from the upper part of the ureter (Fig. 9–192). Of the 52 cases studied, Culp found that 13 had been confused with such conditions as hydronephrosis, ureteroceles, and vesical diverticula; 10 were hydroureters, and 14 were rudimentary branched ureters with a blind pouch. Only 15 met the criteria he laid down for a true diverticulum, namely, having ovoid or round shape, containing all of the ureteral coats, and communicating through a distinct stoma. Since then, several more cases have been reported (Gettel and associates). Most of the cases seem to be acquired rather than congenital diverticula. Although the mechanism of acquired diverticula has not been elucidated, there seems to be a strong correlation with infection.

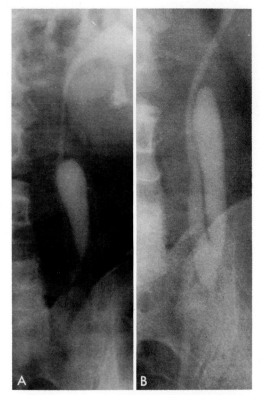

Figure 9–189. Rudimentary branched ureter with blind ending. **A** and **B,** *Excretory urogram.* Prone and supine Trendelenburg positions demonstrate differences in filling of blind-ending branch. (Courtesy of Dr. K. Haber.)

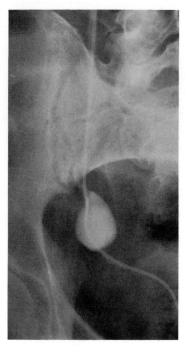

Figure 9–190. *Right   retrograde   pyelogram.* Right ureteral diverticulum.

MULTIPLE URETERAL DIVERTICULA
(Fig. 9–193)

Multiple ureteral diverticula were first described by Holly and Sumcad in 1957. Since that time, several other reports of this condition have appeared (Dolan and Kirkpatrick; Mims; Norman and Dubowy; Williams and Goodwin). At present, neither the etiology nor the microscopic anatomy is too well worked out because there has been very little material available for study. Infection has been present in most cases. In the surgical specimen studied by Williams and Goodwin, the diverticula contained all the muscle layers of the normal ureter.

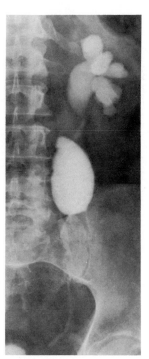

Figure 9–191. *Retrograde   pyelogram.* Large ureteral diverticulum with moderate pyelectasis.

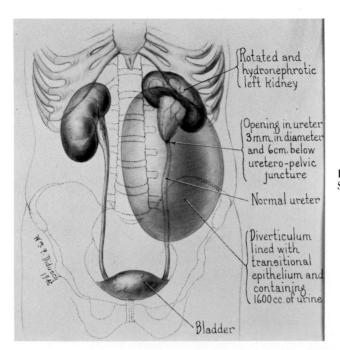

Figure 9–192. Artist's conception of large ureteral diverticulum. (From Culp, O. S., 1947.)

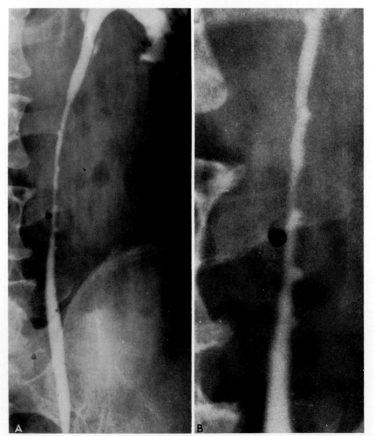

Figure 9–193. Multiple diverticula of left ureter. **A,** *Retrograde pyeloureterogram.* **Multiple diverticula** in midureter. **B,** *Close-up view* of involved area. (From Norman, C. H., Jr., and Dubowy, J.)

RETROCAVAL URETER (POSTCAVAL AND CIRCUMCAVAL URETER)

Retrocaval ureter is the only anomaly of the genitourinary tract that is essentially limited to the right side. An instance of left-sided retrocaval ureter associated with situs inversus has been reported (Brooks) (see Figure 9–202). Apparently the first case in which an accurate preoperative diagnosis was made was reported by Harrill in 1940. The second case was reported by Greene and Kearns in 1946. Cases have been reported with increasing frequency as urologists have become more cognizant of the lesion (Considine; Duff; Laughlin; Pitt).

Embryogenesis

In this anomalous condition the ureter turns abruptly medial from a normal position in its upper third and passes behind the vena cava, then passes forward between the vena cava and aorta, then passes across the front of the vena cava to reach its normal position lateral to the vena cava. In its course it makes a "hook" around the vena cava (Fig. 9–194). The embryologic error here is probably one of the vena cava rather than the ureter. In all reported cases except one, the condition has been on the right side. Hollinshead described the origin of this anomaly as follows:

Without going into details, it can be stated that most of the infrarenal segment of the inferior vena cava is usually formed from a persistent venous channel (supracardinal vein) which lies dorsal to the ureter, but that during the development of the inferior vena cava there is also a subcardinal vein which lies ventral to the ureter [Fig. 9–195]; if the subcardinal vein persists as the infrarenal segment of the vena cava then the ureter passes behind the definitive vein, but in front of the dorsally formed iliac vein, and necessarily makes a hook around this anomalously formed vena cava as the vessel is shifted toward the midline. The majority of retrocaval ureters occur, then, because of the persistence of a ventral venous element and the disappearance of a dorsal element; occasionally, as in the case reported by Gruenwald and Surks, both dorsal

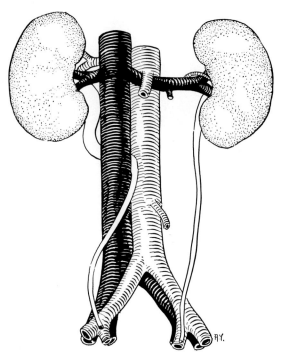

Figure 9–194. Retrocaval ureter. (From Hollinshead, W. H.)

and ventral elements persist simultaneously, so that the retrocaval ureter actually passes between two portions of the vena cava, an anterior and posterior. Again, however, it is the persistence of the ventral portion that causes the anomaly.

Clinical Features

This condition has no pathognomonic signs or symptoms. It becomes a clinical problem only because the hydronephrosis may result from obstruction of the ureter as it passes behind and around the vena cava. Any patient who has pyelectasis on the right side and dilatation involving only the upper part of the ureter may be suspected of having retrocaval ureter.

Urographic diagnosis may be rather difficult, as it is often impossible to fill the ureter adequately with contrast medium. An opaque catheter inserted into the ureter may establish the diagnosis, since it may be seen to pass toward the midline, so that it overlies the vertebral column in the region of the third and fourth lumbar ver-

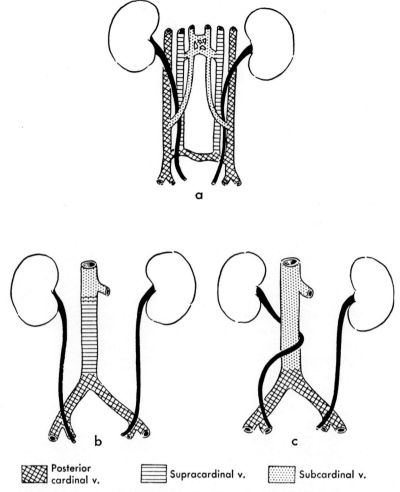

Figure 9–195. Relation between **development of infrarenal portion of inferior vena cava and retrocaval ureter. A,** Primitive condition, with ureter winding between three cardinal veins. **B,** Usual method of formation of vena cava from right supracardinal vein (dorsal to ureter) has left ureter free. **C,** Subcardinal vein, ventral to ureter, has formed main portion of vena cava. (From Hollinshead, W. H.)

tebrae. In this manner a sickle-shaped curve is imparted to the catheter. A satisfactory ureterogram will disclose a gentle curving of the midportion of the ureter, which is close to the vena cava, and with the convexity directed superiorly and medially. Rowland, Bunts, and Iwano have demonstrated the relationship between the ureter and vena cava by securing a roentgenogram after an opaque catheter had been passed into the ureter and the vena cava simultaneously had been visualized with opaque medium (Figs. 9–196 through 9–202).

RETROILIAC URETER (POSTARTERIAL URETER AND PREURETERAL ILIAC ARTERY)

Retroiliac ureter was first reported by Dees in 1940. Since then there have been only a few cases of this rare anomaly reported (Corbus and associates; Hock and associates; Seitzman and Patton). Like the retrocaval ureter, this is primarily a vascular malformation. It results from a failure of the dorsal intersegmental branch, which joins the aorta to umbilical arteries, to replace the ventral branch. The persistence of the ventral root places the common iliac

Fig. 9–196

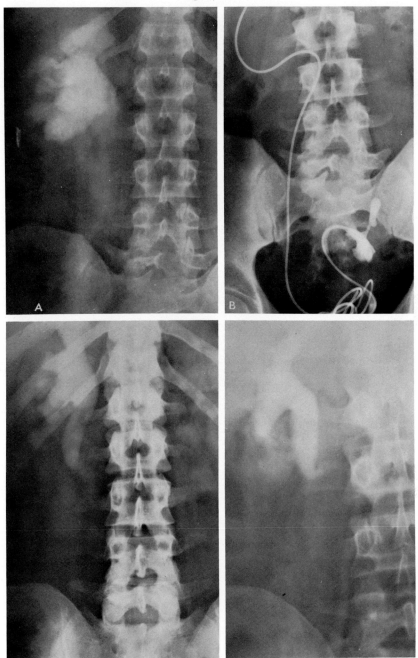

Fig. 9–197   Fig. 9–198

Figure 9–196. Retrocaval ureter. A, *Excretory urogram.* **Pyelocaliectasis on right;** ureter not outlined. Point of obstruction not apparent. **B,** *Lead catheter in ureter* demonstrates typical sickle-shaped curve of ureter as it passes around vena cava at level of third and fourth lumbar vertebrae. Proved at operation. Note **ectopic left kidney.**

Figure 9–197. *Excretory urogram.* **Retrocaval ureter with moderate pyelectasis.** Note gentle curve of upper part of ureter toward midline, which suggests but does not prove diagnosis. Proved at operation. (From Greene, L. F. and Kearns, W. M.)

Figure 9–198. *Excretory urogram.* **Retrocaval ureter.** Excellent demonstration of ureter as it bends abruptly toward spinal column to encircle vena cava. (Courtesy of Dr. R. P. Middleton and Dr. A. W. Middleton.)

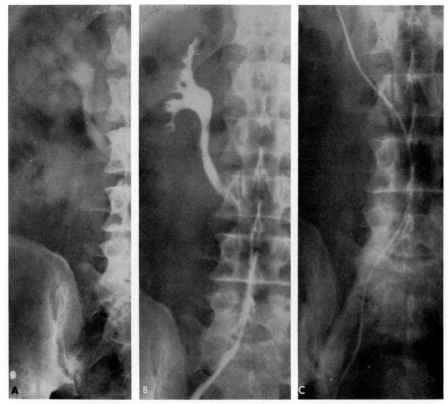

Figure 9–199. Retrocaval ureter. **A,** *Excretory urogram.* **Moderate pyelectasis of right kidney** with dilatation of upper part of ureter. Ureter directed toward spinal colum suggests but does not prove retrocaval ureter. **B,** *Right retrograde pyelogram.* Complete ureter outlined showing that ureter makes abrupt swing over spinal column to encircle vena cava. **C,** *Lead catheter in ureter.* Iliac vein and vena cava have been faintly outlined with contrast medium by femoral venipuncture. (From Duff, P. A.)

artery in front of the ureter. Although this is a rare congenital anomaly, it is occasionally seen following aortoiliac replacement when the graft is placed in front of the ureter, resulting in ureteral obstruction (Fig. 9–203).

CONGENITAL OBSTRUCTION OF URETER

Stricture

Much has been written about *congenital ureteral stricture,* and the literature suggests that it is a fairly common condition, especially in infants and children (Campbell, 1963). The lesions are said to occur most frequently at the ureterovesical juncture, with a lesser number involving the ureteropelvic juncture.

Nearly all of the illustrative cases show markedly dilated ureters which taper down as they pass into the bladder, and the diagnosis is usually "confirmed" either by encountering "tightness" to a ureteral catheter as it passes through the intramural ureter or by inability to pass the catheter. "Dilation" of the terminal part of the ureter has been advised as proper treatment.

In our experience almost none of such cases are bona fide strictures, the real problem being ureterectasis of indeterminate etiology associated with a normal intramural ureter. "Tightness" or resistance to a ureteral catheter as it passes through the ureter is a normal phenomenon which we think has no diagnostic importance. This poorly understood problem is considered fully in Chapter 11, as is also the problem of the ureteropelvic juncture. There is no

Fig. 9–200

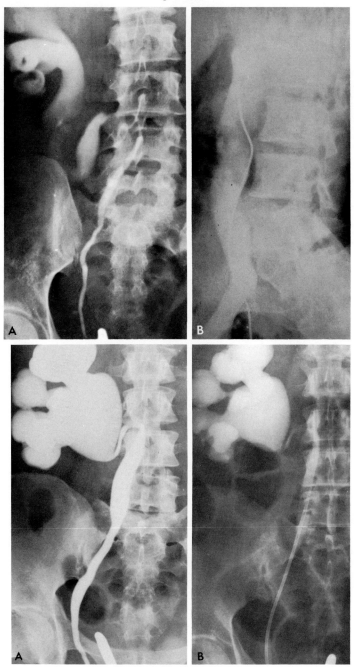

Fig. 9–201

Figure 9–200. Retrocaval ureter. A, *Retrograde pyelogram* demonstrates abnormal course of right ureter. **B,** *Inferior vena cavagram,* with lead catheter in ureter, lateral view. Relationship between ureter and vena cava is demonstrated. (From Rowland, H. S., Jr., Bunts, R. C., and Iwano, J. H.)

Figure 9–201. Retrocaval ureter with solitary kidney. A, *Retrograde pyelogram* of woman, 36 years of age, with right renal pain and anuria, who was 7 months pregnant. **Advanced pyelectasis and retrocaval ureter** demonstrated. Ureteral catheter was passed to renal pelvis and left for several days. Obstruction relieved. Normal delivery 2 months later. Operation refused. **B,** *Retrograde pyelogram 10 years later.* **Less pyelectasis** than present 10 years before when pregnant (From Laughlin, V. C.)

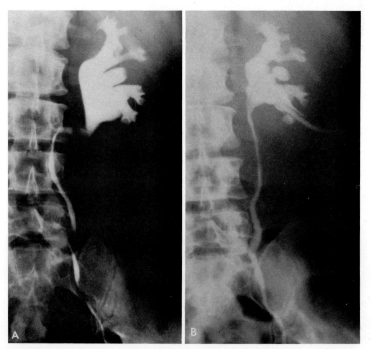

Figure 9–202. Left retrocaval ureter with complete situs inversus in 43-year-old man. **A,** *Left retrograde pyelogram.* **Pyelectasis.** At operation ureter was divided obliquely, brought out from under vena cava, and re-anastomosed. **B,** *Postoperative film.* (From Brooks, R. E., Jr.)

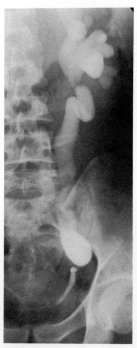

Figure 9–203. *Left retrograde pyeloureterogram.* Marked dilatation of renal pelvis and upper two thirds of ureter secondary to **congenital obstruction caused by aberrant blood vessels.** Diagnosis proved surgically.

doubt that a congenital stricture of the midureter is encountered in rare instances, but it is difficult to be sure that such strictures are not inflammatory. This problem also is discussed in Chapter 11.

Valves

Ureteral valves are rare. They consist of transverse folds of redundant mucosa, are commonly found in the fetus, and usually disappear during the first few months of life. Occasionally one may persist and cause obstruction. Wall and Wachter proposed the following criteria for "bona fide" ureteral valves: (1) anatomically demonstrable transverse folds of ureteral mucosa which contain bands of smooth muscle, (2) changes of obstructive uropathy above the valve with a normal urinary tract below, and (3) no other evidence of mechanical or functional obstruction. In 1955, Simon, Culp, and Parkhill reported two cases and included illustrations of both the gross and microscopic

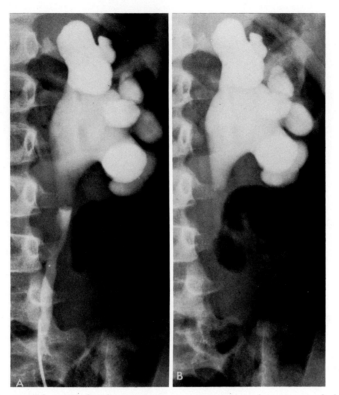

Figure 9–204. **Congenital ureteral valve.** *Excretory urogram* (not shown) revealed left hydronephrosis. Point of obstruction appeared high. Right kidney appeared normal. **A** and **B,** *Retrograde pyelograms.* **A,** Note valve below ureteropelvic juncture. No obstruction is present in distal ureter as evident by free flow of dye into bladder at ureterovesical juncture. **B,** Valve again is clearly delineated. Note retention of dye proximally. Normal-appearing ureter is seen distal to valve. (From Passaro, E., Jr., and Smith, J. P.)

findings. In each case the valve consisted of a transverse mucosal fold containing muscularis and covered with transitional epithelium.

In 1959, Foroughi and Turner found nine cases in the literature, two of these being in children. In 1960, Passaro and Smith reported a case involving a 5-year-old girl, which they stated was the third case affecting a child to be reported. The excretory urogram and retrograde pyelogram (Fig. 9–204) demonstrate pyelectasis with retention of contrast medium above the valve which is outlined almost as a "meniscus" about 2 cm below the ureteropelvic juncture. In 1972, Mering and associates found only 14 cases reported, and they added 2 of their own. In one of their patients a calculus had become impacted by the valve in the midureter (Figs. 9–205 and 9–206).

Aberrant Blood Vessels

Aberrant blood vessels may be factors in ureteral obstruction. They are rare but when seen are commonly encountered at the ureteropelvic juncture (Chapter 11). Occasionally, they are seen in other locations also (see Figure 9–203). See also Chapter 17 on renal vascular diseases.

CONGENITAL NONOBSTRUCTIVE URETERECTASIS (MEGAURETER)

This subject is discussed in Chapter 11.

VESICOURETERAL REFLUX

This subject is discussed in Chapter 11.

Anomalies of Origin and Termination of the Ureter

ECTOPIC (ABNORMALLY PLACED) URETERAL ORIFICES

It is customary to limit application of the term *ectopic ureter* to a ureter that has an opening in some location other than the bladder. Although abnormally located ureteral orifices within the bladder are anatomically ectopic, they are not considered ectopic from a clinical standpoint (Mackie and Stephens).

Ureteral orifices in ectopic locations are of great clinical importance because (1) if the orifice is outside the vesical and urethral sphincters, urinary incontinence may result; and (2) ureters that open into abnormal locations are prone to become obstructed, resulting in pyeloureterectasis, with or without reflux, infection, and impairment of renal function. As a matter of fact, this general category of anomalies accounts for a generous proportion of all urinary problems encountered in infants and children. They are of course also encountered in adults, but in the majority of cases they require medical attention before the individual reaches adulthood.

Embryogenesis

In order to understand the embryogenesis of the ectopic ureter, one must first ap-

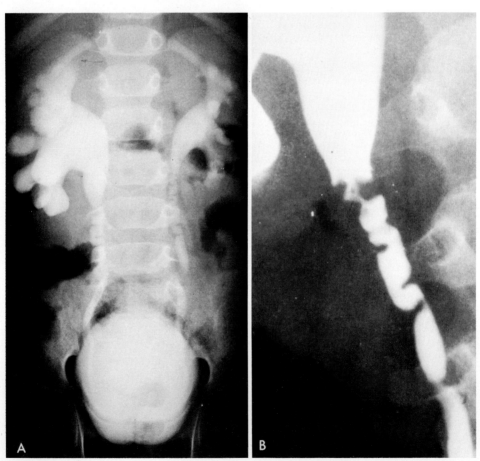

Figure 9–205. Congenital ureteral valves. Boy aged 3. Acute renal failure and oliguria. **A,** *Excretory urogram.* Serpiginous tortuosity of both upper ureters, and right pyelocaliectasis. **B,** *Retrograde pyelogram.* Multiple ureteral folds with marked narrowing in upper ureter which has appearance of stricture. Ureterotomy revealed the presence of valves. A ureteropyeloplasty was performed on the right. (From Mering, J. H., Steel, J. F., and Gittes, R. F.)

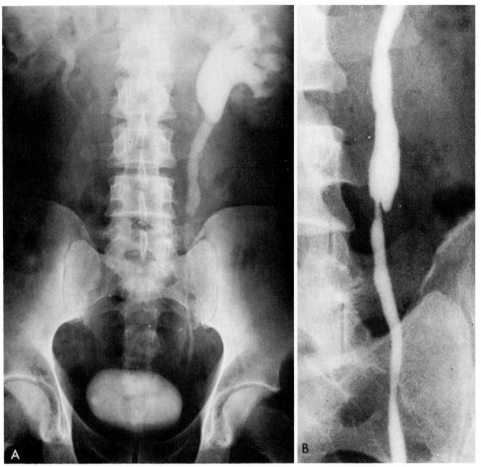

Figure 9–206. Ureteral valve with impacted calculus. Man aged 54. Left ureteral colic. **A,** *Excretory urogram.* Left-sided ureterectasis and pyelocaliectasis. Calculus not seen but is adjacent to transverse process of L_4 vertebra. **B,** *Retrograde pyelogram.* Ureteral valve demonstrated with proximal ureterectasis. Ureterotomy revealed calculus impacted at ureteral valve. Valves were excised and calculus was removed. (From Mering, J. H., Steel, J. F., and Gittes, R. F.)

preciate the relationship of the developing ureter with the mesonephric or wolffian duct. The ureter first begins as a cephalad growing bud from the lower end of the wolffian duct. As the caudad portion of the wolffian duct is incorporated into the posterior wall of the cloaca, the developing ureter is separated from the wolffian duct by the downward growth of the urogenital septum. This results in a separate orifice for both ureter and wolffian duct in the posterior wall of the primitive bladder. Additional growth of the urogenital sinus further separates the two orifices. In the female, the wolffian duct system degenerates, and its remnants are known as

Gartner's ducts. In the male, the wolffian duct orifices become the openings of the ejaculatory ducts.

Ectopic ureteral orifices result when the ureteric bud arises from the wolffian duct more cephalad than usual. It may be the only bud, but more often it is a second outgrowth. When the ureteral outgrowth originates in an unusually high position, incorporation of the ureteral orifice into the urogenital sinus is delayed. The ureter, therefore, remains attached to the wolffian duct during the latter's downward growth, resulting in a lower than normal ureteral orifice. In ureteral duplication one bud usually originates in a normal position

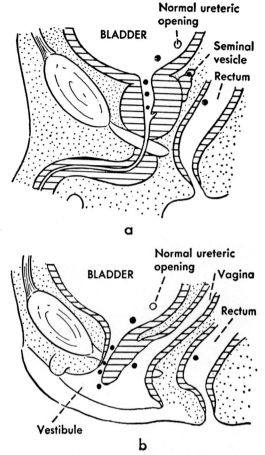

a

b

Figure 9–207. Possible abnormal sites of ureteral orifices. **A,** Male. **B,** Female. (From Hollinshead, W. H.)

(draining the lower renal pole); the other grows from a high position (draining the upper renal pole). For this reason, it is the ureter to the upper renal pole that ends up in a more distal or ectopic position (Fig. 9–207). In the male, ectopic ureters always open at some site cephalad to the external urethral sphincter so that incontinence is rarely, if ever, a symptom. In the female, on the other hand, the ectopic orifice is frequently situated distal to or beyond the jurisdiction of the external sphincter so that incontinence of urine is a common complaint.

If the ureteral bud arises even more cephalad, there is failure of separation from the wolffian duct. In the male, this may cause the ureter to open into the ejaculatory duct, the seminal vesicles, or the vas deferens. In the female, this may cause the ureter to open into the wolffian duct remnant, or Gartner's duct.

When ectopic ureters are found in the fallopian tubes, uterus, cervix, or vagina, the explanation is more difficult, as those structures are formed from the paired müllerian ducts. In such a situation the most common explanation centers around Gartner's ducts, which are the remnants of the wolffian ducts in the female. It has been demonstrated that vestigial remnants

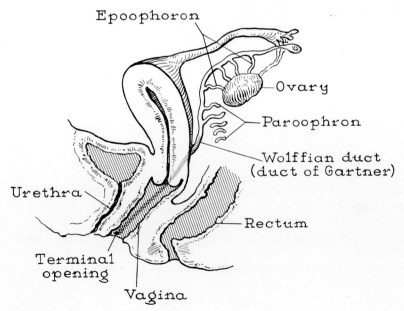

Figure 9–208. Remnants of wolffian duct in female. (Redrawn from Keith, A.)

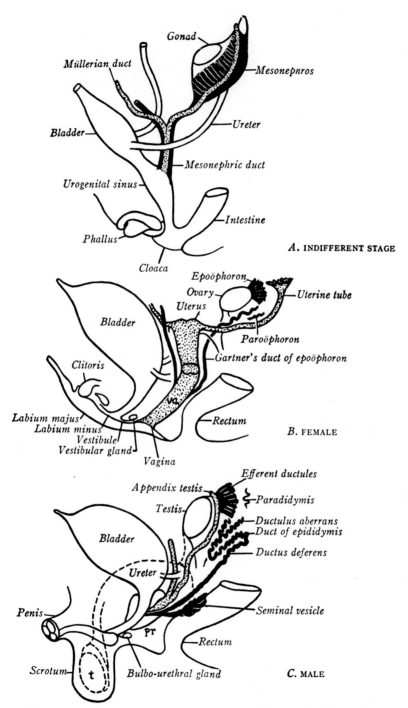

Figure 9–209. Diagrams illustrating transformation of an indifferent, primitive genital system into definitive male and female types (Thompson). (From Arey, L. B.)

of the wolffian ducts in the female may be found along a line running from the hymen (homologue of the verumontanum) through the anterior and lateral walls of the vagina, through the cervix, the wall of the uterus, and between the layers of the broad ligament to the epoophoron (Figs. 9–208 and 9–209). Inasmuch as the ureters arise from the wolffian duct, it seems reasonable to assume that their openings could be found anywhere along its course.

Another explanation, favored by Kjellberg, Ericsson, and Rudhe, calls attention to the intimate relationship of the wolffian and müllerian ducts during their embryologic development. Kjellberg and associates cited the work of Gruenwald, who demonstrated that the müllerian duct actually grows *inside* the basal membrane of the wolffian duct and may be derived from the cells of the wolffian duct. Such a common origin and close association, therefore, could explain the presence of a wolffian duct structure (ureter) terminating in some organ formed by the müllerian ducts (vagina, cervix, uterus, or fallopian tubes).

As mentioned previously, in rare instances ectopic ureteral openings in the rectum have been reported. The best explanation advanced for this error of development is faulty division of the cloaca by the urorectal septum.

Pertinent Statistical Data

Sex. The problem of ectopic ureteral orifices is far more common in females than males (Grossman and associates, 45 of 50 cases; Wiggishoff and Kiefer, 20 of 21 cases).

Duplication or No Duplication. Most cases are associated with ureteral duplication. Figures commonly quoted state that ureteral duplication is present in more than two thirds of cases (Moore), whereas cases with no duplication constitute 10 per cent to 20 per cent. Grossman and coworkers, reporting on a 5-year experience at New York Hospital, found 50 cases of ectopic ureter; in 45 (90 per cent), there was associated duplication and in 5, the ureters

were nonduplicated ("single" or "solitary") (Figs. 9–210 through 9–214). They stated, "Rarely, however, an unduplicated ureter draining an entire kidney terminates ectopically," Wiggishoff and Kiefer's figures were similar, that is, 19 of 21 ectopic ureters were associated with duplication. Cox and Hutch reviewed the subject of *bilateral* ectopic ureteral orifices *without duplication* and found only 19 cases; they added 2 of their own. Each of their patients was a little girl with urinary leakage, and *both* ectopic orifices were located in the urethra in each instance. Johnston, in 1969, added 2 more cases, while Williams and Lightwood added 10 more in 1972. It has been pointed out that patients with bilateral single ec-

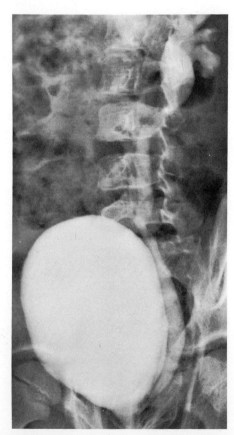

Figure 9–210. Ectopic (nonduplicated) left ureter which opened into bladder neck of 5-year-old girl. *Voiding cystourethrogram.* Reflux up dilated ureter. **Right side of trigone was absent. Moderately atrophic kidney with pyelectasis.** (From Grossman, H. L., Winchester, Patricia H., and Muecke, E. C.)

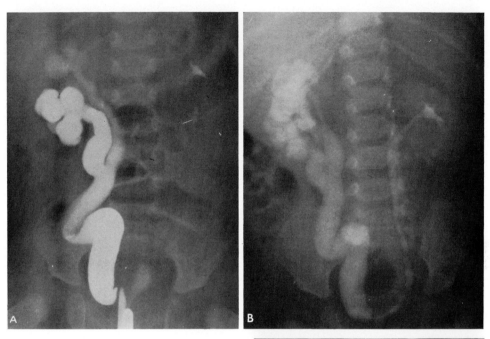

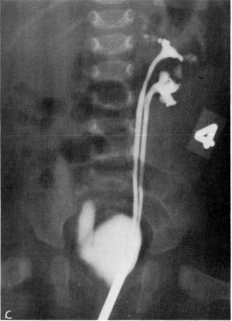

Figure 9–211. Ectopic ureteral orifice serving nonduplicated (single) ureter of 8½-pound female infant, age 3½ months. Clinical diagnosis was **urinary sepsis associated with failure to thrive.** Only one orifice of hemitrigone was visible on left side. Dilated right ureteral orifice was found in midurethra. **A,** *Right retrograde pyeloureterogram* made with Braasch bulb catheter through panendoscope. **Incomplete duplication** with point of juncture in upper third of ureter. **Marked pyeloureterectasis;** residual medium in duplex left kidney. **B,** Film exposed 1 hour later. Contrast medium still present in right ureter, but it now shows, in addition, **triplication of pelvis. C,** *Left retrograde pyelogram* made with catheter inserted just inside meatus. **Incomplete ureteral duplication** with point of juncture located in intramural portion of ureter. In previous cystogram (not shown here) reflux into upper pole of pelvis was demonstrated. (Courtesy of Dr. Jerry D. Giesy.)

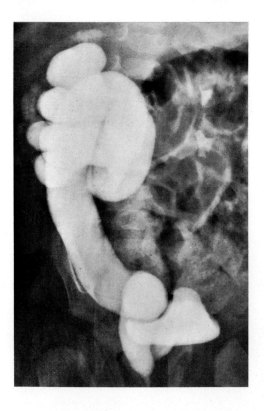

Figure 9–212. Ectopic (nonduplicated) markedly dilated right ureter, opened into posterior wall of urethra of 1-month-old girl. *Retrograde pyelogram* through ectopic orifice. **Advanced pyeloureterectasis.** (From Grossman, H. L., Winchester, Patricia H., and Muecke, E. C.)

topic ureters also have incomplete formation of the bladder neck.

Unilateral Versus Bilateral Ectopic Orifices; Associated Contralateral Duplication

In a small percentage of cases, bilateral ectopic orifices are present (Figs. 9–215 through 9–219). Grossman and coworkers found 8 instances in their series of 50 cases of ectopic ureter; in 2 of these 8 there was no ureteral duplication. It is a relatively common experience to see *duplication without ectopia* on one side and *duplication with ectopia* on the other side.

Sites of Ectopic Orifices

After a survey of the literature, Kjellberg, Ericsson, and Rudhe found the relative incidence of the sites of ectopic ureteral orifices to be as follows:

Males:

Posterior urethra	54 per cent
Seminal vesicles	28 per cent
Vas deferens	10 per cent
Ejaculatory ducts	8 per cent

Females:

Vestibule	38 per cent
Urethra	32 per cent
Vagina	27 per cent
Uterus	3 per cent

In Wiggishoff and Kiefer's 21 cases (20 females), the ectopic orifice was located in the urethra in 8 cases, in the vestibule adjacent to the urethral meatus in 4, and in the vagina in 5; in 4 cases, the orifice was never found.

In Grossman and coworkers' five cases without duplication, in two of which the anomaly was bilateral, four ectopic orifices were located in the bladder neck and three in the posterior urethra.

Double Ectopic Orifices

In the case of duplication, if only one orifice is ectopic it is always the most distal (caudad) one that serves the ureter to the upper-pole pelvis. If both orifices are ectopic, the proximal orifice serving the

THE RENAL PELVIS AND URETER

lower-pole pelvis is always nearer to the normal position.

Obstruction Versus Reflux

In complete ureteral duplication (with two separate orifices), whether or not either is ectopic, the general rule still applies—namely, that *obstruction* more commonly involves the upper-pole orifice and *reflux,* the lower-pole orifice.

An ectopic position of a ureteral orifice predisposes to obstruction, reflux, infection, and impaired renal function. Inasmuch as the majority of cases are associated with duplication, this means that the upper renal segment is most often involved, frequently to the point where it is unable to excrete contrast medium in sufficient concentration to be visualized on the excretory urogram. For this reason, it is most important to recognize radiographic changes (often very minor) in the appearance of the "normal" lower-pole pelvis that will alert the examiner to the possibility of duplication. The fact that, in the presence of complete duplication with ectopia, the upper renal pelvis may be diminutive and serve a tiny amount of upper-pole parenchyma compounds the problem, as the lower

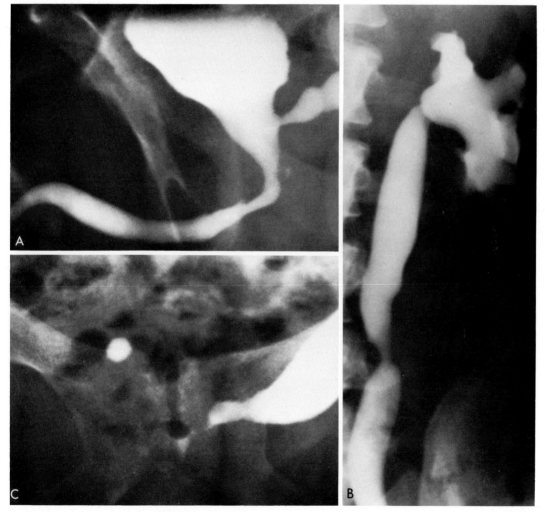

Figure 9–213. Ectopic (nonduplicated) solitary ureter. Man aged 31. Incontinence noted since birth. **A** through **C,** *Voiding cystourethrogram.* **A,** Reflux up dilated left ureter entering urethra. Bladder neck is wide open. **B,** Reflux up solitary dilated ureter is total, revealing pyelocaliectasis. **C,** Postvoiding film demonstrates markedly dilated lower ureter. (From Mogg, R. A.)

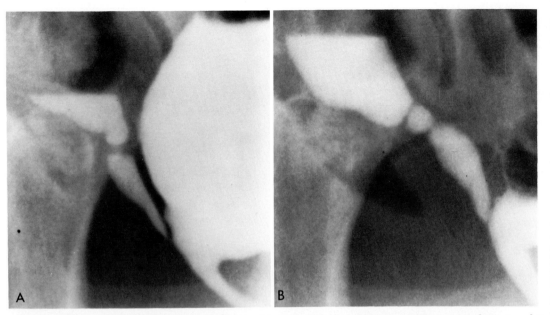

Figure 9–214. Ectopic (nonduplicated) ureter with contralateral renal agenesis. Woman aged 26. **A** and **B**, *Voiding cystourethrogram.* **A**, Reflux up dilated ureter entering proximal urethra. **B**, Postvoiding film shows marked ureterectasis. (From Mogg, R. A.)

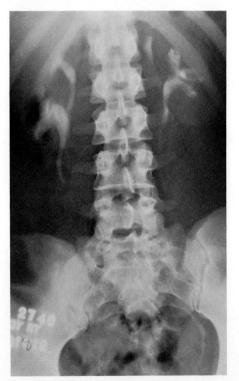

Figure 9–215. *Excretory urogram* of girl aged 21. **Urinary incontinence. Bilateral duplication with bilateral ectopic orifices.** Right ectopic orifice located in vesical neck; left could not be found, but was most likely in urethra. (Left heminephrectomy eliminated urinary leakage.)

pelvis tends to be large enough to simulate a normal single kidney without duplication. (This subject is thoroughly discussed under the heading of "Duplication of the Pelvis and Ureter".)

Ectopic Ureteral Orifices in the Female; Urinary "Incontinence"

Inasmuch as the overwhelming majority of ectopic ureteral orifices are found in females and most are located distal to the urinary sphincter, it is not surprising that the most common presenting symptoms are those of dribbling urinary incontinence, which may or may not be associated with symptoms of infection from the accompanying ureteropyelectasis.

Little girls have urinary leakage from an ectopic ureteral orifice not uncommonly, yet it is surprising how many of these patients reach adult life before the diagnosis is made. For instance, of Wiggishoff and Kiefer's 20 female patients, only 10 were less than 10 years old, while 6 were more than 30. The pathognomonic presenting symptoms is *continuous leakage of urine associated with normal micturition.*

Figure 9–216. Bilateral complete duplication with ectopia and **ureteropyelectasis of upper segment on both sides** in 6-month-old boy. **A,** *Excretory urogram.* Lower pelves of both kidneys visualized—**slight pyelectasis. B,** *Right retrograde pyelogram.* Lower pelvis and ureter visualized, showing only slight dilatation. (Pyelogram of left lower segment was similar to that on right.) **C,** *Right retrograde pyeloureterogram of ureter and upper pelvis.* (Urethral catheter inadvertently entered right ectopic upper-pole orifice.) Ureteral orifice was never visualized cystoscopically. **Marked hydroureter.** At operation bilateral duplication with pyeloureterectasis of both upper segments was found. (Bilateral heminephrectomy relieved patient's recurring chills and fever.)

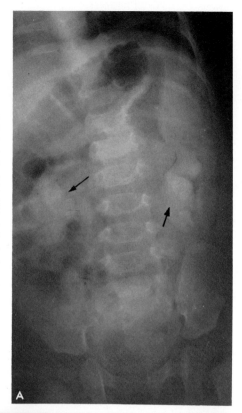

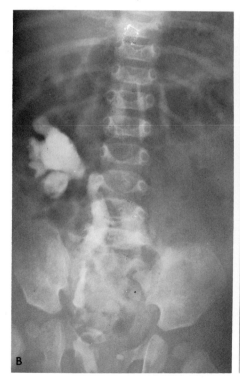

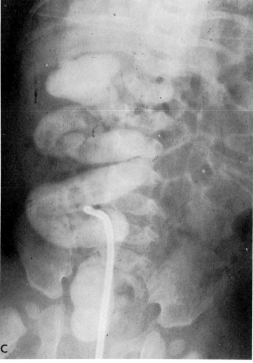

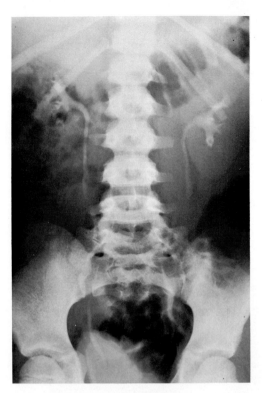

Figure 9–217. Girl with incontinence from bilateral duplication and bilateral ectopic orifices opening into urethra. (Ectopic orifices could never be found.) *Excretory urogram.* Typical "drooping flower" type of lower pelvis of duplication on left. No function in upper segment. Right pelvis also suggestive of duplication but not as typical. Left heminephrectomy reduced amount of leakage but some persisted. Right kidney then was explored, duplication was found, and heminephrectomy was done, eliminating leakage completely.

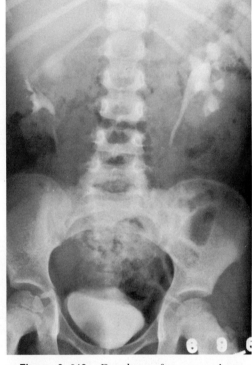

Figure 9–218. Daughter of woman whose excretory urogram taken 22 years earlier is illustrated in Figure 9–217. Was brought to Mayo Clinic by her mother because of **urinary incontinence.** *Excretory urogram.* **Duplication on right with pyelectasis of upper pelvis.** Left lower pelvis is typical of **duplication with some malrotation; no function of upper segment.** Both ectopic orifices eventually were found in vestibule adjacent to urethral meatus.

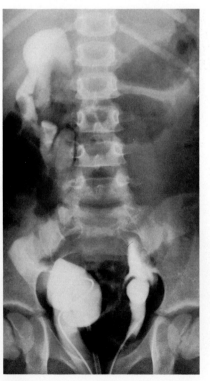

Figure 9–219. (Same case as in Figure 9–218). *Retrograde pyelogram.* Catheters in both ectopic ureters show them to be dilated and tortuous. (Bilateral heminephrectomy eliminated leakage.)

Diagnostic Methods

Radiographic Diagnosis. Diagnosis may be made on the basis of an excretory urogram only if there is sufficient function remaining in the upper-pole pelvis. Too often, however, because of the associated obstruction, there either is no function or the function is reduced sufficiently that the upper pole pelvis and ureter are visualized poorly. In such a case the upper-pole ureter and pelvis may be entirely overlooked by the examiner, unless late films (after 1 to 6 hours) are taken. Also, for some unexplained reasons, occasionally the upper-pole pelvis may not be visualized (or at least so poorly visualized that it is over-looked) at one examination, yet at another time it may be well seen. If visualization is poor, the pelvis may be mistaken for a bowel shadow (Figs. 9–220 and 9–221). It is imperative that the physician think of the condition so that he will carefully evaluate the films for signs typical of a *lower-pole pelvis* with no visualization of the upper pelvis. A voiding or cine cystourethrogram may occasionally prove helpful, if the ectopic meatus is located in the urethra and is sufficiently dilated to permit reflux.

Cystoscopy, Urethroscopy, and Examination of Vestibule and Vagina. A careful search of the vestibule should be made for ectopic orifices. They are frequently located near the urethral meatus. If there is

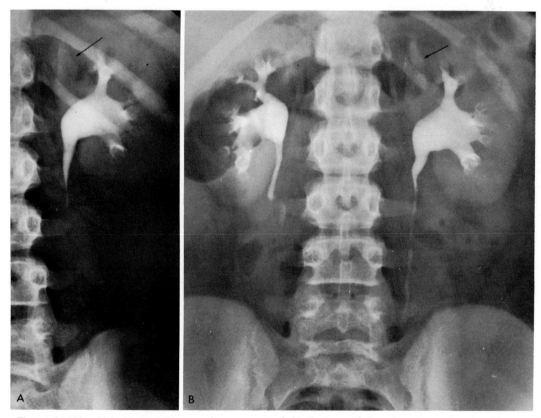

Figure 9–220. Urinary incontinence from ectopic (left) "upper-pole" orifice situated in vestibule at 5 o'clock position adjacent to urethral meatus. **A,** *Excretory urogram* (made in home community 1 year before registration at Mayo Clinic). Duplication missed because lower pelvis is large with reasonably long upper calyx. Upper pole of kidney, however, is not well outlined. Contrast medium is present in dilated upper pelvis *(arrow),* but was of such poor density that it was considered to be part of bowel shadows. **B,** *Excretory urogram* made at Mayo Clinic. Shadow of upper pelvis is of better density, and there is less overlying gas, permitting easier recognition. (Cystoscopically, drops of urine could be seen coming from 5 o'clock position at urethral meatus, but it was impossible to catheterize ectopic orifice. Left heminephrectomy relieved incontinence.)

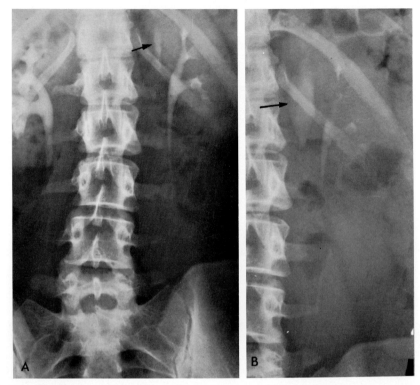

Figure 9–221. **Duplication with ectopic orifice** in woman aged 22 with life-long incontinence. **A,** *Excretory urogram, 5-minute film.* Faint narrow streak of contrast medium *(arrow)* medial to upper pole of left kidney might easily be overlooked. **B,** *Excretory urogram, 45-minute film.* Shadow now more dense and of greater width, outlining dilated upper pelvis *(arrow)*. Ectopic orifice was probably in urethra, but we were unable to find it. (Left heminephrectomy eliminated the leakage.)

reasonably good function of the upper-pole pelvis, drops of urine may be seen effluxing from the orifice. Too often, however, this is not the case. Locating an orifice within the vagina may be most difficult. In examining little girls the panendoscope is preferable to a vaginal speculum. Wiggishoff and Kiefer advise using a binocular loupe for examination of the vestibule and vagina.

Unless the ectopic orifice is dilated, it is usually difficult to visualize if it is located inside the urethra. A urethroscope or panendoscope is necessary for adequate examination. If the urine in the ectopic ureter is cloudy or purulent, stripping of the anterior vaginal wall during urethroscopy may express the urine from the orifice. If the ectopic ureter is located in the vestibule, compression of the inguinal region on the suspected side may accomplish the same result (Wiggishoff and Kiefer).

Chromoscopy. Chromoscopy may be of help and may be used in several ways. Probably the first procedure should be to introduce an indigo carmine solution into the bladder through a urethral catheter, remove the catheter, and then observe the vestibule and urethral meatus for signs of leakage. If leakage continues and the leaking urine is uncolored, urethral incompetence has been excluded; this is almost pathognomonic of an ectopic ureteral orifice.

The intravenous injection of a solution of indigo carmine may be helpful. If reasonably good function remains in the upper-pole segment, the efflux of blue urine may demonstrate the orifice either in the urethra (during urethroscopy) or in the vestibule or vagina. Even though the function of the upper-pole segment is poor, the examination may still prove to be of value; several hours after the injection, when the patient again is voiding clear uncolored urine from the bladder, a delayed oozing of faint blue urine from the ectopic orifice may clinch the diagnosis. Amar has suggested introducing a blue solution into the bladder, asking the patient to void and empty the bladder, and then performing cystoscopy. If there is reflux up the ectopic ureter, the blue that refluxed up during voiding may now run back down and be observed effluxing from the "hidden" orifice. In difficult cases, he also suggested *percutaneous needle injection* (see discussion of percutaneous antegrade pyelography, Chapter 3) of the dilated renal pelvis with contrast medium mixed with blue solution; this may both outline the ectopic ureter radiographically and permit the orifice to be located cystoscopically (or by careful examination of the vestibule). *Arteriography* might be considered as a last resort.

Despite all these modalities of examination, however, the ectopic orifices sometimes are never found. This was the case in 4 (20 per cent) of Wiggishoff and Kiefer's 20 cases. Urograms from more or less typical cases are shown in Figures 9–222 through 9–226).

Atypical Cases

Unusual cases may be encountered in which the symptoms are not typical. It has been mentioned that in probably half of the cases the diagnosis is not made until the patient is an adult. This may be because either the physician has been unable to make the diagnosis or the patient has been embarrassed by her problem and has hesitated to seek medical advice. In some cases, however, leakage may have been either not present, so minimal that it was not detected, or not apparent until the patient reached adulthood. In some recorded cases it has not appeared until after childbirth (Idbohrn and Sjöstedt) or pelvic operation. If the ectopic orifice is located in the proximal part of the urethra or near the vesical neck, this might be explained on the basis of weakening of the pelvic muscles or

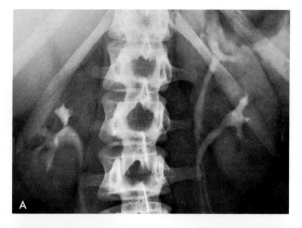
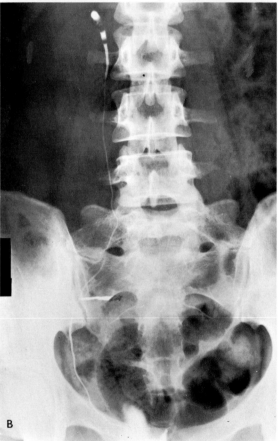

Figure 9–222. Ectopic ureteral orifice in woman 23 years of age, with **bilateral duplication** which could easily be missed urographically. **A,** *Excretory urogram.* Right kidney appears normal and one would not suspect duplication from this film. Duplication on left. **B,** *Right retrograde pyelogram,* made by catheterizing ectopic ureteral orifice situated in vestibule, shows **atrophic duplicated ureter serving small upper segment of right kidney.** (At operation [heminephrectomy] upper pelvis was minute and lay just under renal capsule.)

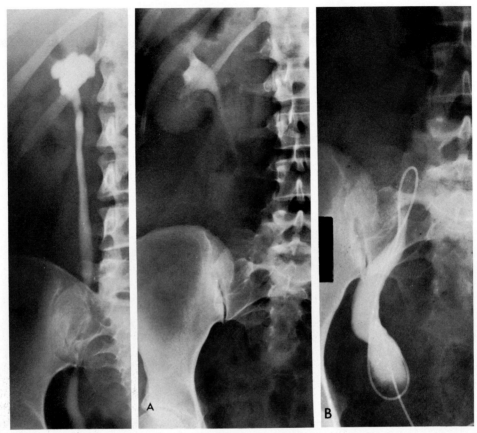

Fig. 9–223   **Fig. 9–224**

Figure 9–223. Ectopic ureteral orifice associated with duplication of right kidney in woman, 22 years of age. *Excretory urogram* (not shown) showed normal lower pelvis and nonfunctioning upper pelvis. **Ectopic ureter** situated in floor of midurethra. *Right retrograde pyelogram* of ectopic ureter and upper pelvis shows **moderate pyeloureterectasis.**

Figure 9–224. Ectopic ureteral orifice in woman, 34 years of age, associated with **complete duplication on right.** Ectopic orifice situated at vesical neck in 6 o'clock position. **A,** *Excretory urogram.* Pelvis and ureter of lower segment normal. No function of upper segment. Duplication might not be suspected here because three major calyces are presented and pelvis appears quite normal. However, it is obvious that upper pole of kidney is not adequately served by pelvis. **B,** *Right retrograde ureterogram,* made with catheter introduced into ectopic ureteral orifice, shows **dilated lower part of ureter that serves upper pelvis.** Upper pelvis and adjacent ureter not outlined.

urethral musculature; but, if the orifice is located in the vestibule or vagina, explanation is more difficult. DeWeerd and Litin reported a case in which the ectopic orifice, located in the vestibule, had caused no incontinence; the patient, a 19-year-old girl, had an attack of left flank pain associated with chills and fever that led to the diagnosis (Fig. 9–227). They stated that they had been able to find reports of five other similar cases in the literature.

A 33-year-old woman, para 4, was sent to the Mayo Clinic for repair of a "vesico-vaginal fistula." During her first delivery she had been badly torn and afterward noted some mild "stress incontinence" which required her to wear a pad for protection when she was away from home. There had been three subsequent deliveries which were uneventful. Four months before admission, a vaginal hysterectomy and repair had been done, after which urinary leakage was greatly increased and was constant. A vesicovaginal fistula secondary to operation had been suspected. Our excretory urogram showed

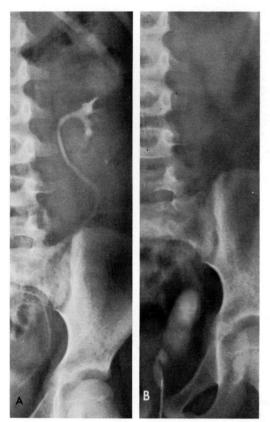

Figure 9–225. Ectopic ureteral orifice, in a girl 6 years of age, associated with **duplicated left kidney.** **A,** *Excretory urogram.* Lower pelvis and ureter of duplicated left kidney. Functionless upper segment. **B,** *Retrograde ureterogram,* with catheter inserted into **ectopic ureteral orifice, which was located in floor of midurethra. Marked ureterectasis** of ureter to upper segment; upper pelvis not filled.

duplication of the left kidney with a dilated upper-pole pelvis (Fig. 9–228). An ectopic orifice in the vestibule near the urethral meatus was found and could be catheterized. A dilated upper-pole ureter was visualized by means of retrograde urography. Heminephrectomy eliminated the patient's leakage.

Wesson discussed the problem of the patient with both urethral leakage and an ectopic (vaginal) ureteral orifice.

Not uncommonly, the patient complains of a "vaginal discharge." This may be more-or-less constant or may be intermittent with exacerbations of a "vaginal infection" that in reality is an acute infection

involving the ectopic ureter, emptying into the vagina (Fig. 9–229). Wiggishoff and Kiefer described a patient who complained of leakage only at night when she was in bed.

Ectopic Orifice Simulating Urethral Diverticulum

If an ectopic orifice is located in the urethra and the attached ureter is dilated,

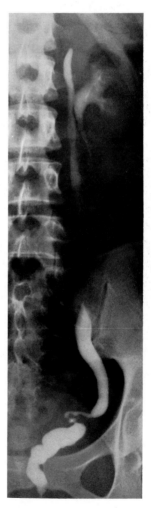

Figure 9–226. Bilateral duplication with ectopic ureteral orifice in woman, 26 years of age. *Simultaneous excretory urogram and left retrograde pyelogram.* Duplication with ureter serving upper segment of left kidney opening in **ectopic position at introitus, just lateral to urethral meatus.** (Lifetime history of incontinence, cured by heminephrectomy.) (Courtesy of Dr. E. Burns.)

the condition may be mistaken for a urethral diverticulum. This has been described as an "ectopic orifice within a diverticulum" (Willmarth), but most likely it simply represents a dilated ectopic orifice and the dilated terminal portion of the ectopic ureter (Vanhoutte). The dilatation in such instances may result from infection. A case in which this condition was encountered and a "diverticulectomy" was done because of a mistaken diagnosis is illustrated in Figure 9–230. To exclude an ectopic ureter and thus avoid this pitfall, all urethral diverticula should be examined by means of cystourethrograms and urethroscopy, and an attempt should be made to pass a urethral catheter.

Familial Tendency

Although no recognized hereditary tendency to duplication and ectopic orifice has been demonstrated, the occasional situation in which the condition occurs in more than one member of a family is of interest. DeWeerd and Feeney reported a case of bilateral ureteral ectopia occurring in a mother and daughter. The mother, when a child, had been brought to the Mayo Clinic in 1938 with constant urinary leakage associated with normal micturition. An excretory urogram (see Figure 9–217) suggested duplication on the left with a typical "drooping flower" type of lower pelvis and no function of the upper segment. A similar

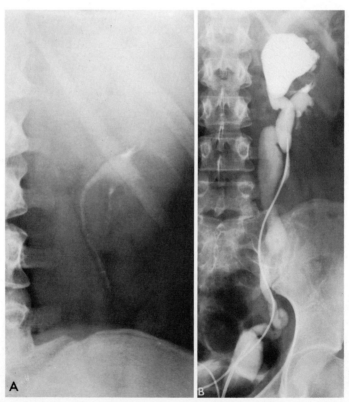

Figure 9–227. Ectopic left ureteral orifice located in vestibule near urethral meatus of 19-year-old girl. (No history of incontinence. Patient sought medical help because of chills, fever, and left flank pain.) **A,** *Excretory urogram.* Typical "drooping flower" appearance of lower pelvis of duplication. (See Fig. 9–155). No function in upper segment. **B,** *Retrograde pyelogram.* Lower part of ectopic ureter was catheterized. Injected contrast medium shows hydronephrotic upper pelvis and connecting ureter. Normal lower pelvis also is visualized with catheter passed well up into it.

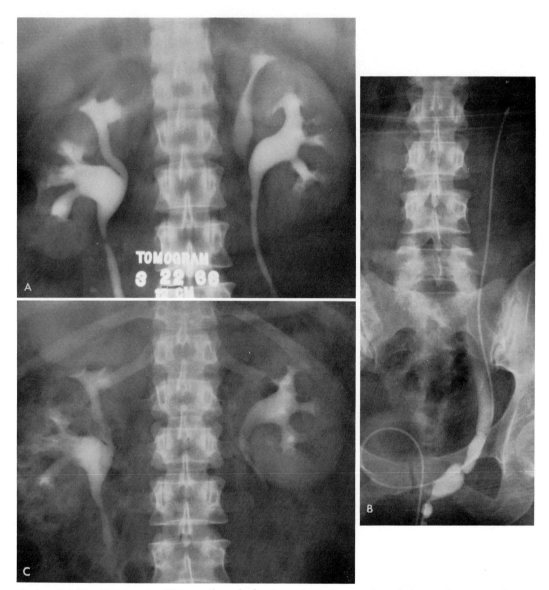

Figure 9–228. Woman age 33, para four, had **urinary incontinence from left ectopic upper-pole ureter** which did not appear until after first delivery. Severity increased after vaginal hysterectomy and perineal repair 4 months before urograms were made. Postoperative vesicovaginal fistula was suspected. **A,** *Excretory urogram with tomogram.* Duplication on left with mild dilatation of upper pelvis. **B,** *Retrograde pyelogram* (ectopic orifice in vestibule near urethral meatus). Dilated upper-pole ureter. Acorn catheter is in lower-pole ureter, but contrast medium has not been injected. (Left heminephrectomy eliminated incontinence.) **C,** *Postoperative excretory urogram.*

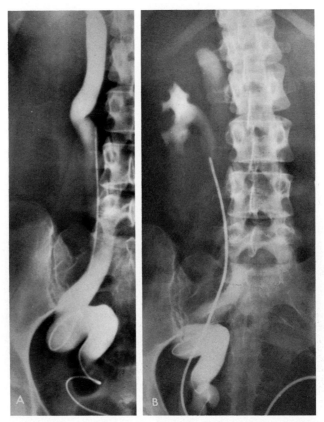

Figure 9–229. Duplicated ureter in woman, 34 years of age, with **ectopic opening in deep vaginal vault** just to left of cervix. *Right retrograde pyelograms.* **A,** Catheter inserted into ureteral orifice in edge of cervix outlines tortuous dilated ureter with practically no renal pelvis. **B,** Catheter inserted into ureteral orifice in normal position in bladder outlines normal lower segment of right kidney. (Patient complained of recurring attacks of fever, with severe "vaginal discharge." Examination disclosed *Trichomonas* infection of ectopic ureter and upper pelvis. Ureteral orifice was on posterior lip of cervix and difficult to find.) (Courtesy of Dr. R. M. Bobbitt.)

situation appeared to be possible on the right side also, but the appearance of the pelvis was not as characteristic. It was believed that the ectopic ureteral orifices were probably located in the urethra, but they could never be found. Left heminephrectomy reduced the amount of leakage substantially, but some persisted. The right kidney was then explored, duplication with a dilated upper pelvis found, and heminephrectomy performed, eliminating the leakage completely.

In 1962, this girl (now a married woman) returned to the Clinic with her 5-year-old daughter, who also had incontinence. The mother recognized the symptoms as identical to those she had had as a

child in 1938. An excretory urogram demonstrated duplication on the right with a dilated poorly functioning upper pelvis; on the left, the pelvis had the typical characteristics of a duplicated lower pelvis and a nonfunctioning upper renal segment. An ectopic orifice with efflux of urine could be seen in the vestibule just to the left of the urethral meatus. It was successfully catheterized, and injection of contrast medium outlined the lower part of a dilated ectopic ureter. Left heminephrectomy was performed, which eliminated about half the leakage. The patient returned 3 months later, at which time the right ectopic orifice was found in the vestibule just to the right of the urethral meatus; both ectopic ureters were then catheterized and injected, demonstrating both the dilated ectopic ureters (see Figs. 9–218 and 9–219). After a right heminephrectomy the leakage ceased entirely.

Unusual Cases of Ectopic Ureteral Orifice

It does not require much stretch of the imagination to contemplate the innumerable possibilities, if ectopic termination of single or duplicated ureters is combined with other congenital anomalies. These situations may require clever deduction and diagnostic improvisation on the part of the examiner. They form the basis of interesting single case reports, many of which read like detective stories as the urologist unfolds the details of his examination in a baffling, obscure situation.

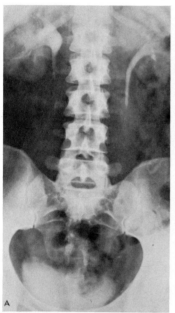
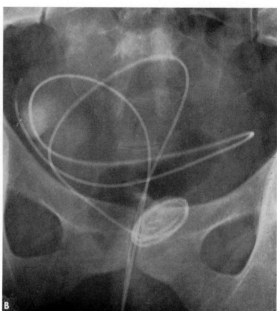
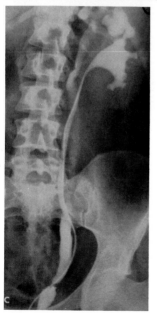

Figure 9–230. Ectopic ureteral orifice simulating urethral diverticulum in female patient. **A,** *Excretory urogram,* which was erroneously interpreted as "grossly normal." However, appearance of left renal pelvis suggests it to be lower pelvis of duplication. **B,** *Ureteral catheters coiled in pocket* in floor of urethra which was considered to be urethral diverticulum. **C,** *Injection of contrast medium through catheters* to outline "diverticulum" demonstrated it to be terminal portion of dilated ectopic ureter which served upper segment of duplicated left kidney. Opening in floor of urethra was ectopic ureteral orifice. Urethral catheter has been passed up normally situated ureter and pyelogram made of lower pelvis.

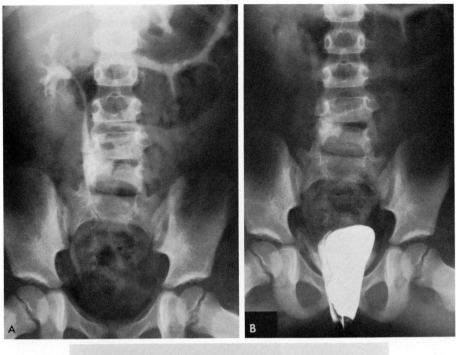

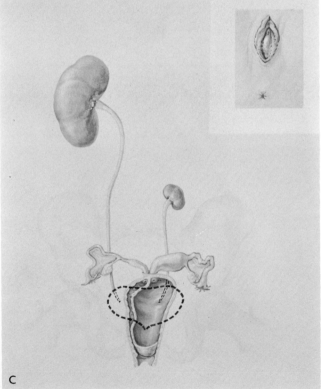

Figure 9–231.   Ectopic ureter, hydrocolpos, double vagina, and uterus didelphys. **A**, *Excretory urogram.* No visualization of left kidney. **Compensatory hypertrophy of right kidney. B**, *Vaginogram.* (Contrast medium injected through needle in cystic mass bulging from vagina.) **Double vagina with hydrocolpos on left.** Right half of vagina is partially outlined by leakage of contrast medium from left. **C**, Relationship of anomalous anatomic structures. (From Constantin, H. M.:)

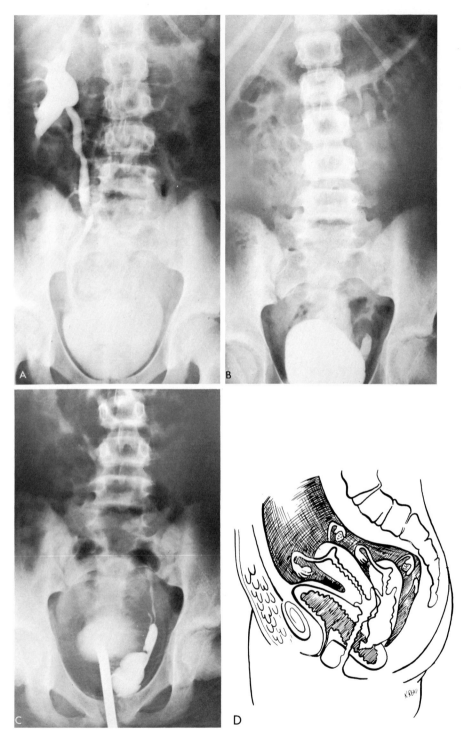

Figure 9–232. Ectopic atretic left ureter serving a dysplastic kidney terminating into occluded double vagina which communicates with bladder; uterus didelphys. **A,** *Excretory urogram.* Only right kidney is visible. **No function on left. B,** *Voiding cystogram* reveals 3-cm tubular structure resembling lower part of ureter. **C,** *Left bulb ureterogram.* Bizarre structure suggests ectopic pelvic kidney. **D,** Appearance of anomaly at operation. Double uterus and vagina. Left vagina was stenotic, filled with blood (hematocolpos); it connected with and drained into bladder. Small atretic left ureter (coming from minute dysplastic kidney) entered hematocolpos laterally. (From Weiss, J. M., and Dykhuizen, R. F. Official U.S. Navy Photograph.)

Constantian reported the case of a 6-year-old girl who experienced dribbling after voiding and had a "bulging membrane" at the introitus. She finally proved to have a hypoplastic left kidney with a single (unduplicated) ureter which emptied ectopically into the occluded half of a double vagina (unilateral vaginal atresia) which was distended with fluid (hydrocolpos). A double uterus (uterus didelphys) was also present (Fig. 9–231).

Weiss and Dykhuizen reported the case of an 11-year-old girl complaining of grossly bloody urine. The final diagnoses in this case were uterus didelphys and double vagina, the left half of which was occluded (unilateral vaginal atresia), dysplasia of a single (unduplicated) left ureter consisting of only a strand of tissue without a lumen and terminating ectopically in the occluded left vagina, and hypoplasia (dysplasia) of the left kidney. There was also an anomalous communication between the occluded vagina and the bladder, the opening being situated where the left ureteral orifice normally should be located (Fig. 9–232).

Ectopic Ureteral Orifices in the Male

As has been mentioned previously, most ectopic ureteral orifices are found in females. Because of this, few data are available relative to males.

In the male, the ectopic ureteral orifice is found in the vesical neck, prostatic urethra, or seminal tract (chiefly the seminal vesicles). *In contrast to the situation in the female, ureteral duplication is less common than is single ectopic ureter; this is especially true when the ureter empties into one of the seminal vesicles.*

Ectopic Ureteral Orifice in Vesical Neck and Prostatic Urethra. Whereas the chief symptom of females with ectopic orifices is dribbling incontinence, symptoms experienced by males having ectopic orifices in the vesical neck and prostatic urethra consist primarily of urinary infection, dysuria, obstruction, and in some

cases sexual dysfunction and infertility. Abdominal or flank pain caused by hydronephrosis and hydroureter may be present. The diagnostic problem is essentially the same as that described for the female, special attention being given to the possibility of duplication with the upper-pole pelvis not visualized on the excretory urogram.

Generally speaking, *cystoscopy* and *cystourethroscopy* are more rewarding than in examination of the female because of the larger lumen of the prostatic urethra and the greater ease with which it may be examined. Also, if an ectopic orifice is visible, its catheterization may be more easily accomplished. Cine or voiding cystourethrograms may outline the ectopic ureter, if reflux is present (Fig. 9–233).

Ectopic Ureteral Orifices Terminating in the Seminal Vesicle. This is a rare anomaly. In 1946, Riba, Schmidlapp, and Bosworth collected only 36 cases from the world literature (since 1852): 32 of these were autopsy cases, only 4 having been diagnosed clinically. They added one clinical case, making a total of five. Allansmith reviewed the literature in 1958 and found a total of 15 "clinical cases" to which he added one autopsy report of a stillborn infant. In 1965, the literature was again reviewed by Schnitzer, who found an additional 4 clinical cases and added 4 of his own, making a total of 23 clinical cases. Since then there have been several additional cases reported (Brannan and Henry; Malek and associates; Mulholland and associates; Orquiza and associates; Sargent and associates). In addition, several cases of ectopic ureter entering the seminal vesicle have been noted to be associated with renal dysplasia or agenesis (Figs. 9–234 and 9–235).

From an analysis of these cases, it is at once apparent that the condition is more commonly encountered on the left side and that *duplication of the involved ureter is rare.* Riba and associates' case (Fig. 9–236) is a notable exception. Uson, Lattimer, and Melicow reported one case; also one case was reported by Mogg. In most reported cases, the kidney is rudimentary (dys-

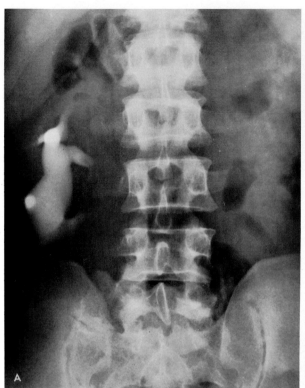

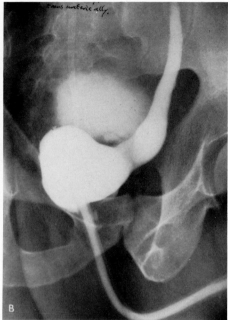

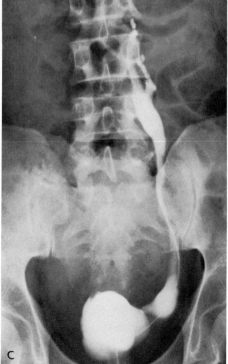

Figure 9–233. Dysplastic left kidney with ureter terminating ectopically into prostatic urethra near verumontanum of 29-year-old man. Patient had never ejaculated and was infertile. **A,** *Excretory urogram.* Ectopic malrotated right kidney. **No function on left. B,** *Cystourethrogram.* Reflux outlines dilated left ureter terminating in large subtrigonal cavity or cyst which in turn communicates with prostatic urethra. **C,** *Retrograde pyelogram.* Rudimentary dysplastic kidney. (From Mogg, R. A.)

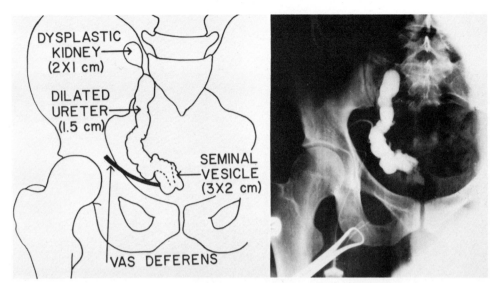

Figure 9–234. Ectopic ureter entering seminal vesicle with renal dysplasia. Man aged 23. Right testalgia, especially following ejaculation, and perineal pain. **A,** *Diagrammatic representation* of anomalous structures. **B,** *Vasoseminal vesiculography.* Reflux up dilated ectopic right ureter. Surgical exploration confirmed ectopic ureter plus presence of dysplastic kidney. (From Gordon, H. L., and Kessler, R.)

plastic), and in many cases, the ureter is also dysplastic and atretic.

Symptoms include pain in the testis (epididymis), groin, or both, which may or may not be aggravated by sexual intercourse and ejaculation. Pain on defecation, pain in the flank and lower quadrant of the abdomen, dysuria, and pyuria may all be present.

A cystic mass may be palpable above the prostate gland on digital rectal examination, and putting pressure on this mass with the examining finger may reproduce the pain. An *excretory urogram* will show no function on the side involved. Cystoscopy will show absence of the ureteral orifice on the side in question, and there may be an elevation, mass, or cystic swelling of the side of the trigone on the involved side. Occasionally a dilated ejaculatory duct is seen which may be so large as to simulate the opening of a prostatic abscess and lend itself to catheterization and injection of contrast medium (Figs. 9–237 and 9–238).

Diagnosis is accomplished by the following: (1) demonstration of a nonfunctioning kidney on the involved side; (2) injec-

tion of contrast medium into the vesicle through a catheter in the ejaculatory duct or through a vasotomy incision; (3) transvesical needle injection of the cystic mass either (a) cystoscopically with a needle attached to a ureteral catheter (Schnitzer), the needle being plunged directly into the trigonal mass, or (b) through a suprapubic cystostomy incision; (4) needle injection of the dilated seminal vesicle through the rectum (Schnitzer); or (5) injection of the ureter during surgical exploration, if the ureter has a patent lumen (Figs. 9–239 and 9–240).

A much rarer form of ureteral ectopia is for the ureter to enter the vas deferens (Fig. 9–241).

URETEROCELE

Simple Ureterocele

Simple ureterocele is described as a congenital cystic dilatation of the lower end of the ureter. It is usually relatively small, of the "cobra head" or "spring onion" type, situated completely within

Text continued on page 713

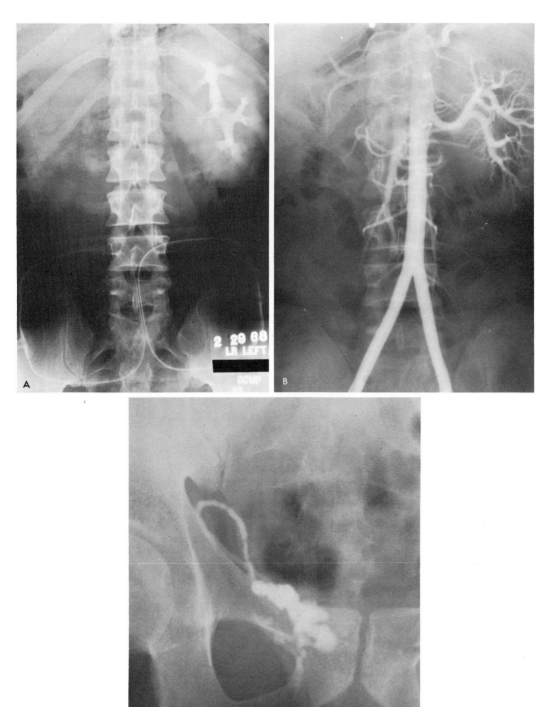

Figure 9–235. **Unduplicated right ureter terminating in seminal vesicle.** Patient complained of pain in right testis and right inguinal region, aggravated by sexual intercourse. **A,** *Excretory urogram.* **Solitary left kidney with malrotation. B,** *Arteriogram.* **Absence of right renal artery. C,** *Seminal vesiculogram* (made through vasotomy incision). **Irregularity and dilatation of ampulla;** incomplete visualization of seminal vesicle. Operation revealed **congenitally atrophic (atretic) ureter** attached below to right seminal vesicle and above to small nubbin of tissue (**dysplastic kidney**). (Ureterectomy and seminal vesiculectomy relieved pain.)

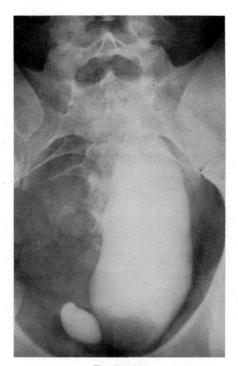

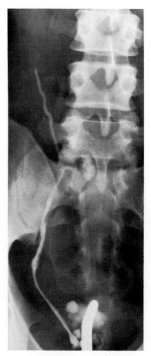

Fig. 9–236   **Fig. 9–237**

Figure 9–236. *Retrograde vesiculogram.* Complete duplication on left, with upper-pole ureter emptying into left seminal vesicle. *Excretory urogram* showed **marked hydronephrosis** of upper pelvis. Lower pelvis normal. Catheter inserted into left ejaculatory duct outlines slightly dilated right vesicle and hugely dilated left vesicle, into which ectopic left ureter drains. Proved on surgical exploration. (From Riba, L. W., Schmidlapp, C. J. and Bosworth, N. L. By permission of the Williams & Wilkins Company.)

Figure 9–237. *Right retrograde ureterogram.* Ectopic ureteral orifice in man, which apparently opens into seminal vesicle. Catheter introduced into opening in prostatic urethra (**dilated ejaculatory duct?**) outlines ectopic ureter and right seminal vesicle. Excretory urogram made prior to this showed no function on right. Exploration revealed small aplastic kidney with practically no function remaining. (Courtesy of Dr. Gordon Strom.)

Figure 9–238. **Ectopic ureter opening into seminal vesicle.** *Excretory urogram* showed absence of function in left kidney and compensatory enlargement of right kidney. *Retrograde pyelogram.* On cystoscopy, no left ureteral orifice could be demonstrated. There was cavernous type of opening in left floor of prostatic urethra which proved to be dilated ejaculatory duct. Ureteral catheter was passed into it and contrast medium injected, which outlined dilated left seminal vesicle, ureter, and renal pelvis of left kidney. Kidney is hypoplastic. Proved surgically. (From Engle, W. J.: Ureteral Ectopic Opening Into the Seminal Vesicle. J. Urol. *60*:46–49 [July] 1948.)

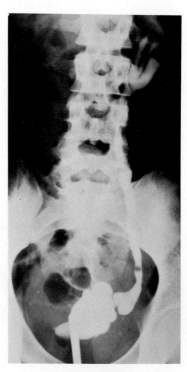

Fig. 9–238

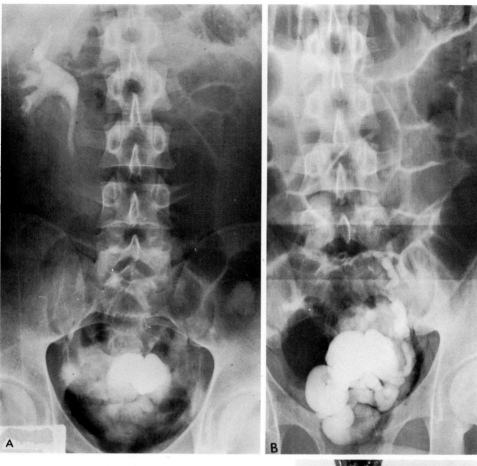

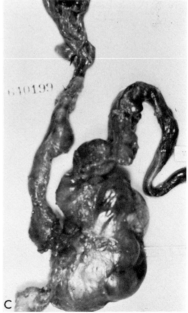

Figure 9–239.   Nonduplicated left ureter with ectopic termination into seminal vesicle; dysplastic left kidney. **A,** *Excretory urogram plus cystoscopic transvesical injection of left seminal vesicle.* **No evidence of function of left kidney; dilated seminal vesicle. B,** *Ureterogram of left ureter during operation.* Ureter connects with seminal vesicle. **C,** *Surgical specimen.* **Dysplastic kidney (with ureter attached to dilated seminal vesicle),** vas deferens, and prostate gland. (From Schnitzer, B.)

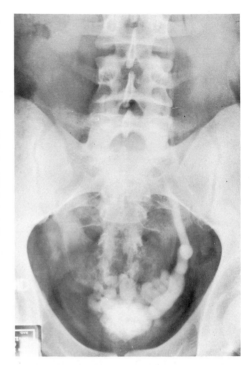

Figure 9–240. Nonduplicated left ureter with ectopic termination into seminal vesicle. Excretory urogram (not shown) showed no function of left kidney and compensatory hypertrophy of right kidney. Cystoscopy showed large cystic mass elevating left side of trigone. When mass was incised (cystoscopically), pus and sperm emptied into bladder. *Retrograde cystogram after incision.* Dilated seminal vesicle and lower third of dilated ectopic ureter are visible. (From Schnitzer, B.)

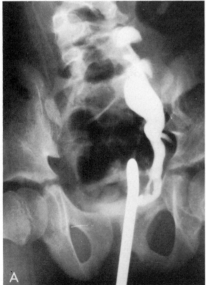

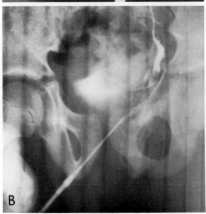

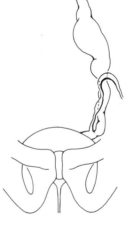

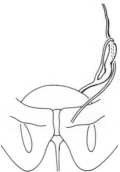

Figure 9–241. Ectopic vas deferens communicating with ureter. Boy aged 7. Bilateral undescended testes, perineal hypospadias, and pelvic kidney. **A,** *Retrograde pyelogram.* Pelvic kidney with dilated ureter and reflux into vas deferens. **B,** *Vasogram.* Reflux up ureter and efflux into bladder. Communication between vas deferens and ureter seen. (From Alfert, H. J., and Gillenwater, J. Y.)

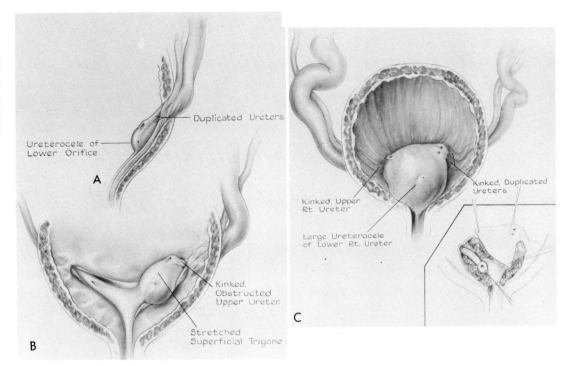

Figure 9–242. Ureterocele in duplicated ureter. A and **B,** Small ureterocele. Note relationship of upper ureteral orifice to expanding ureterocele underneath. **C,** Giant ureterocele in duplicated system compressing ipsilateral and contralateral ureters and encroaching on bladder neck. Insert shows effect of complete excision of ureterocele. (From Tanagho, E. A.)

the bladder, and located where the normal ureteral orifice should be. Simple ureteroceles are encountered most commonly in adults and more frequently in females than in males. They may be associated with ureteral duplication, but this is not often the case—in contrast to the high incidence of ureteral duplication in cases of ectopic ureterocele in infancy.

The degree of ureterectasis complicat-

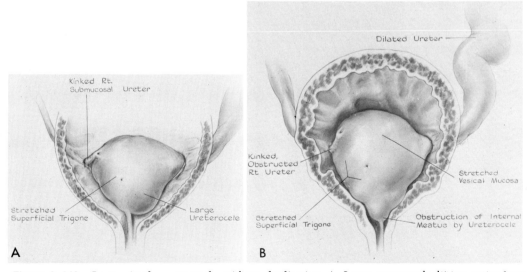

Figure 9–243. Large simple ureterocele without duplication. A, Large ureterocele lifting entire base of bladder and compressing contralateral ureter. **B,** Further enlargement causes bladder neck obstruction. (From Tanagho, E. A.)

ing simple ureterocele usually is minimal and limited to the lower third of the ureter, but in some cases it may be marked and may involve the entire ureter and renal pelvis. In the absence of marked ureterectasis and pyelectasis—if the urine in uninfected and there are no calculi or symptoms—simple ureteroceles should be considered only as incidental findings and left alone. Only rarely do they become large enough to cause vesical neck obstruction (Figs. 9–242 and 9–243). Incision of the ureterocele cystoscopically may result in reflux and persistent infection which later could require either ureteroneocystostomy or nephrectomy for relief. To avoid this complication, Hutch and Chisholm advise open operation if treatment is neces-

sary, combining the excision of the ureterocele with an antireflux type of ureteroneocystostomy.

Urographic findings usually are pathognomonic of the condition, but in some cases cystoscopy is necessary for confirmation. Thompson and Greene in 1942 found that diagnosis was made by means of excretory urography only (without cystoscopy) in only 4 of their 37 cases. The advances in excretory urography since that time, however, including the development of better contrast media and the use of higher concentrations and larger doses of media, provide a much higher incidence of good ureteral and bladder filling; thus, urographic diagnosis should be possible in most cases.

When the ureterocele is well demon-

Fig. 9–244

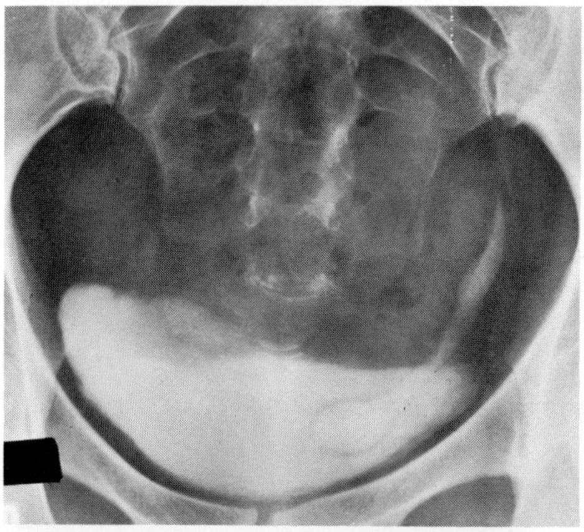

Fig. 9–245

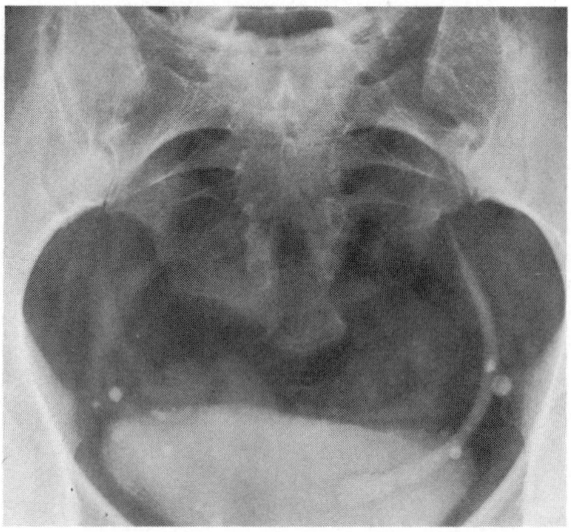

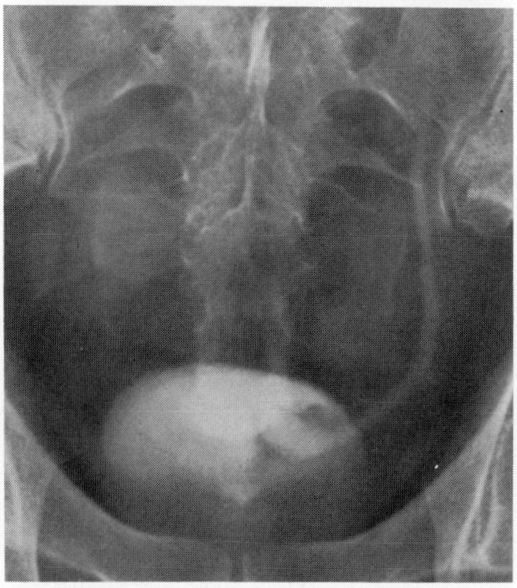

Fig. 9–246

Figure 9–244. *Excretory urogram.* **Ureterocele** on left, with cobra-head filling defect in vesical outline.

Figure 9–245. *Excretory urogram.* **Ureterocele** on left, with cobra-head filling defect.

Figure 9–246. *Excretory urogram.* **Ureterocele** on left, with more-advanced cobrahead filling defect in vesical outline.

strated, the resulting urogram is quite dramatic in appearance. In the classic situation, the dilated, cystic, terminal portion of the ureter projects into the bladder to produce a characteristic urographic deformity. One of the most common findings is the *cobra head* or *spring onion* filling defect in the bladder (Figs. 9–244 through 9–248). This shadow is produced by the intravesical projection of the dilated terminal portion of the ureter. A thin negative shadow or "halo" surrounds and outlines the rounded ureterocele filled with contrast medium (Figs. 9–249, 9–250, and 9–251). In some cases the ureterocele is not filled well with contrast medium, so that it casts only a negative shadow that may easily be confused with a nonopaque vesical calculus, a vesical tumor, or gas in the rectum (Figs. 9–252 through 9–255). The lodging of calculi within a ureterocele is occasionally seen (Figs. 9–256, 9–257, and 9–258).

Ectopic Ureterocele

The term *ectopic ureterocele* was first introduced by Ericsson in his classic mono-

Text continued on page 719

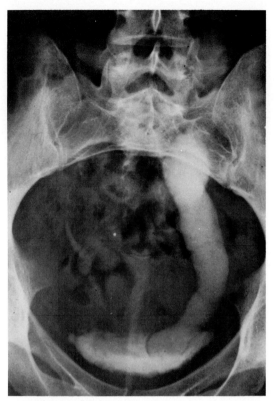

Figure 9–247. *Excretory cystogram.* **Ureterocele on left** with cobra-head filling defect. (From Wines, R. D., and O'Flynn, J. D.)

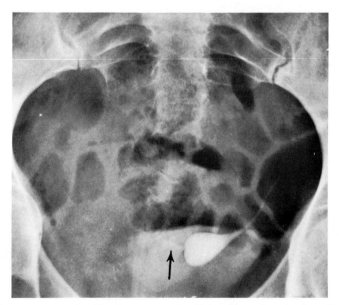

Figure 9–248. *Excretory urogram.* **Simple ureterocele.** Note efflux of contrast medium from orifice in its mid-distal aspect *(arrow).* (Courtesy of Dr. E. W. Phillips.)

Fig. 9-249

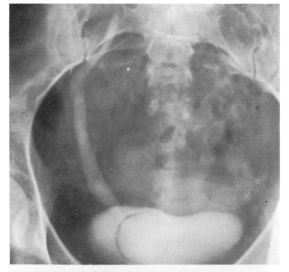

Fig. 9-250

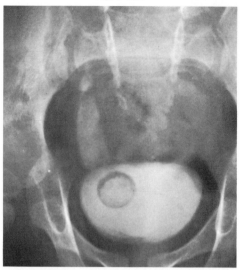

Fig. 9-251

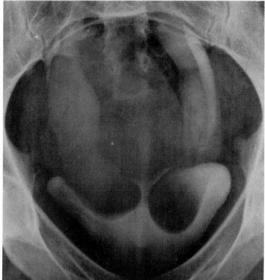

Figure 9-249. *Excretory urogram.* **Ureterocele** on right, with negative halo surrounding cystic outline of ureterocele.

Figure 9-250. *Excretory urogram.* **Right ureterocele** with typical negative halo surrounding rounded, cystic outline of ureterocele. **Obstruction indicated by dilated ureter.**

Figure 9-251. *Excretory cystogram.* Bilateral oval negative filling defects caused by **bilateral ureteroceles in duplicated systems.** (From Wines, R. D., and O'Flynn, J. D.)

Figure 9-252. *Excretory urogram.* Oval negative filling defect situated in left side of bladder, caused by **ureterocele,** which is not filled with contrast medium. Could be confused with negative shadow of nonopaque vesical calculus or tumor.

Figure 9-253. *Excretory urogram.* Filling defect in left half of bladder from **huge ureterocele** (which does not fill with contrast medium). Could be confused with filling defect from vesical tumor or from vesical diverticulum which does not fill with contrast medium.

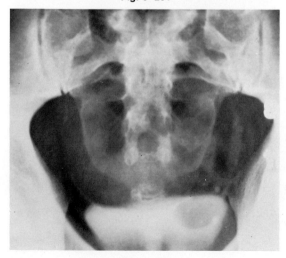

Fig. 9-252

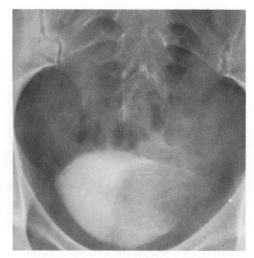

Fig. 9-253

Fig. 9–254

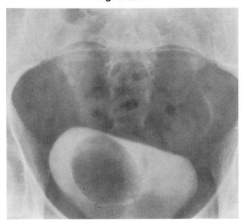

Figure 9–254. *Excretory urogram.* Filling defect in right half of bladder from large ureterocele which is not filled with contrast medium. Could be confused with gas bubble in rectum.

Fig. 9–255

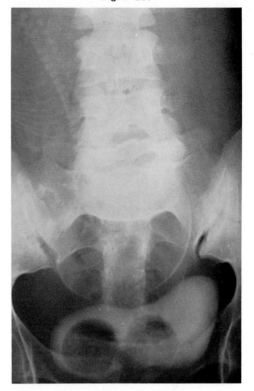

Figure 9–255. *Retrograde cystogram.* Filling defects from **bilateral ureteroceles** in pregnant woman. Fetus visible. (Courtesy of Dr. J. G. Olson.)

Figure 9–256. **A,** *Plain film.* Three calcific shadows overlying lower portion of right ureter. **B,** *Excretory urogram.* **Right ureterocele** with typical halo deformity, **containing three stones** with relation to each other different from that in **A.**

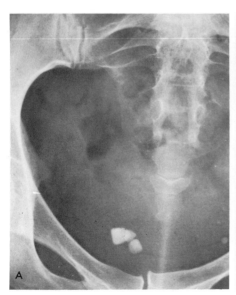

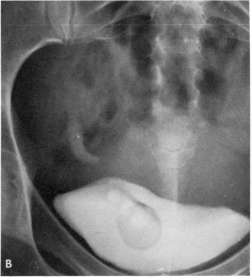

Fig. 9–256

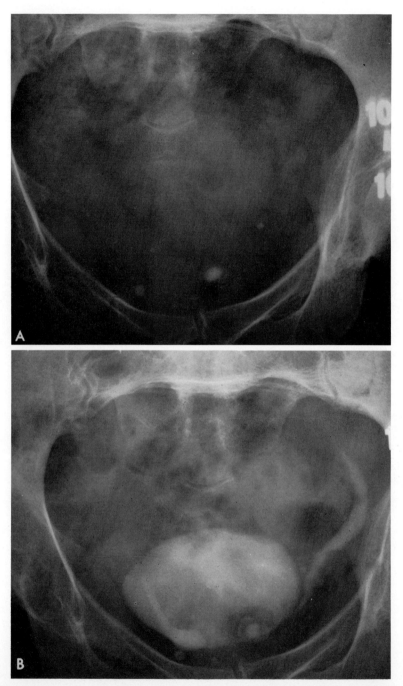

Figure 9–257. Ureterocele containing stone. **A,** *Plain film.* Multiple shadows in bony pelvis. Largest shadow is to left of midline, irregular in outline, and surrounded by ring of less-dense calcific substance. **B,** *Excretory urogram.* **Bilateral ureterocele,** with typical cobra-head deformity on right. On left there is halo deformity surrounding shadow seen in **A.**

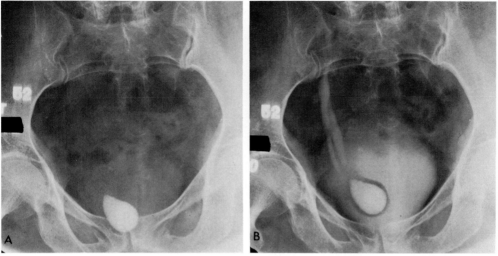

Figure 9–258   Duplicated ureter with ureterocele containing stone. **A,** *Plain film.* Calcific shadow suggesting ureteral calculus or vesical calculus on right side of bony pelvis. **B,** *Excretory urogram.* Typical halo deformity surrounding shadow of stone.

graph on that subject in 1954. This work has been a contribution of major importance and has done much to clarify a difficult subject. His first report dealt with a series of 14 cases. In 1957 (Kjellberg, Ericsson, and Rudhe), the series was enlarged to 28 cases. Since then Williams (1958a) has contributed substantially to the understanding of the subject and has brought it to the attention of the entire profession. In 1964, he reported 68 cases (Williams and Woodard), which is the largest series yet presented. Previous to this clarification such terms as "cystic ureterovesical protrusion" had been used (Mertz and associates).

This lesion is encountered principally in children, in contrast to simple ureterocele, which is found most commonly in adults. Although there initially was considerable resistance to the concept of ectopic ureterocele, it has now become quite generally accepted. Ericsson defined the lesion as involving a ureter with an ectopic termination, either at or distal to the bladder neck. He stated that an ectopic ureterocele "invariably reaches down into the urethra. It is a *ureterocele* in that it is an intravesical cystic ballooning of the lower part of the ureter, lying between the bladder mucosa and the detrusor muscle; it is

ectopic in the ´sense that it arises from a ureter whose orifice is located either at the vesical neck (on its distal "slope") or immediately distal to this in the adjacent urethra. Ureteral duplication is almost always present, the ectopic ureterocele being connected to the upper-pole ureter (Fig. 9–259). Mogg, however, states that it can also be encountered with a single (unduplicated) ureter and reports one such case. Reflux into the ureterocele and attached ureter is present in some cases—3 of 18 (Kjellberg and associates) and 3 of 25 (Williams and Woodard).

Terminology.   Because reflux into the ureterocele can and does occur, some workers have objected to the term *ectopic ureterocele.* They feel that the term *ureterocele* has been used for such a long time to describe *simple ureterocele* (which is never involved in reflux) that it is a misnomer here. They have advocated that the condition be called simply *ureterectasis associated with an ectopic orifice.* At present, however, the term seems to have been quite generally accepted, and it fills a definite need.

Embryogenesis.   Several theories have been put forth to explain the ureterocele. The obstructive theory is based on the frequent finding of a pin-point ureteral

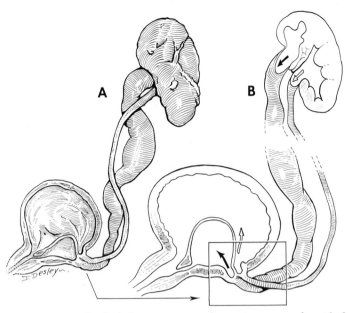

Figure 9–259. Ectopic ureterocele. Pathologic anatomy of ectopic ureterocele with duplication. (Modified from Williams, D. I., 1958a; and Williams, D. I., and Woodard, J. R.)

orifice associated with the ureterocele. This theory fails to explain many instances of ureterocele, especially the frequent absence of ureterectasis above the ureterocele. The most commonly accepted theory postulates the persistence of Chwalle's membrane, an epithelial sheet separating the lumen of the terminal portion of the wolffian duct from the urogenital sinus. This membrane covers the ureteral orifice until about 60 days, when it begins to desquamate to unveil the ureteral orifice. Ericsson's theory proposes that the membrane between the wolffian duct and the vesicourethral canal is not reabsorbed: a caudal opening forms in the membrane for the wolffian duct. The ectopic ureteral orifice is buried beneath this membrane. Both Chwalle's and Ericsson's theories can explain the formation of stenotic ectopic ureteroceles but cannot adequately explain the sphincteric types. Stephen has postulated that the ureterocele forms by a failure of the ureteral orifice to expand and not by membrane occlusion. He believes that the stimulus that causes the bladder to expand does not affect the normally positioned ureter. In the ectopic ureter, however, the distal end expands like the bladder, to form a ureterocele. This theory explains why an ectopic ureterocele can form even though the ureteral orifice is normal or larger than normal.

Anatomic Description. As has been mentioned, ectopic ureteroceles are found almost exclusively in infants and children and *are almost always associated with ureteral duplication.* They are usually large (much larger than simple ureteroceles) and poorly demarcated from the rest of the bladder, in contrast to simple ureteroceles, which are sharply defined. The cystic swelling may appear as a huge subtrigonal mass projecting into and at times almost filling the bladder lumen, or it may appear only as a mild elevation of one side of the trigone. The size of the cystic swelling may vary from one moment to another because of compression from either intravesical pressure or an examining cystoscope. The compression can reduce the size of the intravesical protrusion and may even be sufficient to evert the sac and make it appear as a bladder diverticulum.

The distal (upper-pole) ectopic orifice may not be macroscopically visible, but it usually is located just distal to the vesical neck. The proximal (lower-pole) orifice is on the proximal edge of the ureterocele and may be displaced upward by it. It is believed that this displacement and distortion can reduce the length of the intramural ureter and thus account for the high incidence of reflux up the "normal" lower-pole ureter. Anatomically the ectopic orifice of the ureterocele is always located either on the distal slope of the vesical neck or on the adjacent part of the urethra (prostatic urethra in the male). Clinically, however, this may be hard to demonstrate. Cystoscopy in infants and small children can be difficult; and, in the presence of distortion and deformity of the bladder neck from the ureterocele, it may be impossible to be sure if the orifice is located proximal to, at, or distal to the vesical neck. This may be the case even at operation with the bladder open; it is especially true when the ureterocele is large or bilateral and causing marked distortion of the entire trigone and base of the bladder. The best cystoscopic view is obtained from the posterior urethra with a urethroscope or Foroblique panendoscope, looking forward into the bladder. If a right-angle telescope is used, it may be most difficult to keep the lens at a sufficient distance from the ureterocele to view it properly. Not uncommonly it is impossible to decide on the basis of cystoscopy on which side the ureterocele is situated.

Associated Involvement of the Upper Urinary Tract. In the case of unilateral involvement, marked dilatation of the upper-pole ureter and pelvis served by the ectopic ureterocele is the rule. Ipsilateral involvement of the duplicated lower-pole ureter and pelvis is frequent, consisting of either reflux, obstruction, or both. Reflux up the ipsilateral lower-pole ureter occurs in approximately 50 per cent of cases (Kjellberg and associates; Williams and Woodard). If the ureterocele becomes large

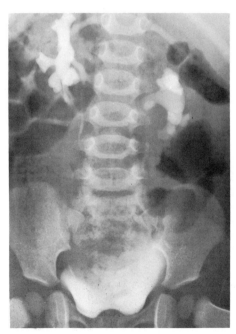

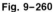
Fig. 9–260

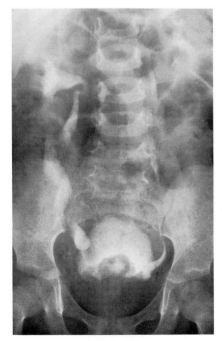
Fig. 9–261

Figure 9–260. Ectopic ureterocele with minimal filling defect at bladder neck. *Excretory urogram.* Ureterocele serves ureter leading from nonfunctioning upper segment of right half of **horseshoe kidney.** (Proved by operation.)

Figure 9–261. Ectopic ureterocele with intermittent prolapse through urethra. *Excretory urogram.* Characteristic negative shadow in base of bladder. Ureterocele serves nonfunctioning upper segment of right kidney.

enough, the contralateral ureter (or ureters if bilateral duplication is present) may also become involved with obstruction or reflux. Mogg has stated:

It is important to appreciate the burrowing characteristic of the ectopic ureterocele, as it can readily dilate and extend in an alarming manner in the subtrigonal and submucosal planes of the bladder, and can thereby obstruct the orifice of the contralateral ureter.

If bilateral ectopic ureteroceles are present, of course, the possible combinations are myriad.

Prolapse of Ureterocele Through Urethra; Obstruction of Vesical Outlet. Most reported cases of prolapses of ureteroceles in little girls concern ectopic ureteroceles that have extruded through the urethra. Obstruction of the bladder outlet from a large ectopic ureterocele pressing against the vesical neck is occasionally encountered.

Symptoms. In most cases, patients with ectopic ureterocele are first brought to medical attention because of urinary infection. Renal insufficiency, with its associated anemia, gastrointestinal symptoms, and so on, may also be present. An enlarged abdomen or palpable abdominal masses representing hydronephrotic kidneys or hugely dilated tortuous ureters may be the presenting complaint. A vaginal "swelling" or "cyst" from a prolapsed ureterocele also may bring the child to the doctor. Symptoms of bladder-neck obstruction from the ureterocele may be present.

Urographic Diagnosis. (Figs. 9–260 through 9–267). A good excretory urogram is the most rewarding urographic modality. The presence of a typical "negative" filling defect in the bladder shadow plus either an ipsilateral nonfunctioning kidney or evidence that only the lower pelvis of a duplication is visualized (with no function in the upper segment) would be quite diagnostic. Unfortunately, the situation often is not this simple and clear-cut, and further inves-

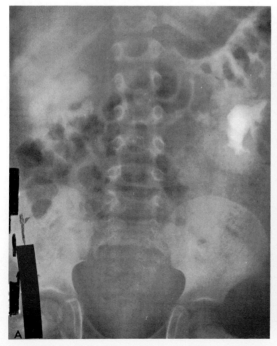 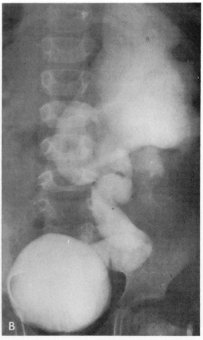

Figure 9–262. **Bilateral ectopic ureteroceles** in boy 3 years old. **A,** *Excretory urogram.* Poor function on right; only hugely dilated calyces dimly outlined. Only lower pelvis of left kidney visualized showing lateral and downward displacement from dilated upper pelvis. Insufficient contrast medium in bladder to outline ureteroceles. **B,** *Retrograde cystogram,* after excision of ureteroceles. Reflux up markedly dilated ureter and pelvis of upper segment of left kidney.

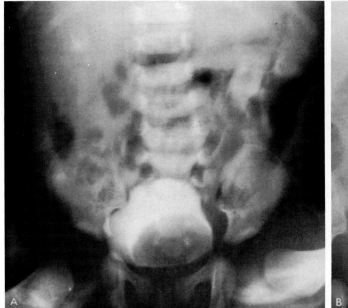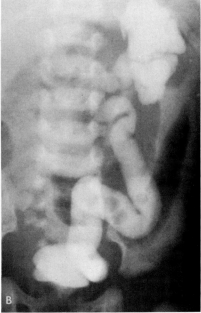

Figure 9–263. Ectopic left ureterocele with prolapse through urethra of 2-week-old girl. **A,** *Excretory urogram.* Characteristic filling defect in lower half of bladder. Rotation and lateral displacement of left kidney suggest lower pelvis of possible duplication with no function of upper segment. **B,** *Retrograde cystogram.* Reflux outlines hydronephrosis and hydroureter of upper-pole ureter and pelvis. *Operative findings:* Thin-walled ureterocele involved left side of trigone. Ectopic orifice of upper-pole ureter was slit-like in appearance and located on distal aspect of ureterocele in region of vesical neck. Orifice of lower-pole ureter could not be located until ureter was dissected out and catheter was passed down into bladder. Single (unduplicated) right ureteral orifice was pulled up high on ureterocele near midline. Left heminephrectomy and ureterectomy. Lower-pole orifice could not be dissected from ectopic ureterocele; it was excised and ureter was reimplanted into bladder.

tigation by means of cystourethrography, cystoscopy, and even surgical exploration may be required. A retrograde or voiding cystourethrogram may be inferior to the cystogram obtained with an excretory urogram because the contrast medium may be so dense that it obscures the ureterocele, or the pressure of the injected medium may reduce the size of the ureterocele.

On the other hand, if reflux into the ureterocele is present, the ureterocele and the dilated ureter to a nonfunctioning upper renal segment may be outlined, clarifying the diagnosis.

The typical bladder defect of an ectopic ureterocele appears as a large, oval, smooth "negative" (lucent) defect which sits "off center" in the lower half or base of the bladder. The defect is larger than that of most *simple ureteroceles*. Its contact with the floor of the bladder is broad, and it

appears to involve the bladder outlet. (The shadow is a little reminiscent of that of benign prostatic hypertrophy with some intravesical protrusion.) At times, however, the shadow may be almost completely surrounded by a thin rim of contrast medium, suggesting only a very narrow contact, if any, with the bladder base and possibly resembling the shadow of a large simple ureterocele. Asymmetry is the rule, but sometimes it is difficult to be sure which side is involved. Bilateral ureteroceles usually appear as double lucent shadows but may appear as a confluent single shadow. Williams and Woodard reported an atypical case involving a 31-year-old woman in whom a large "flabby" ectopic ureterocele (attached to the upper-pole ureter on the left) appeared as a negative shadow lying high in the bladder in the midline and completely surrounded by

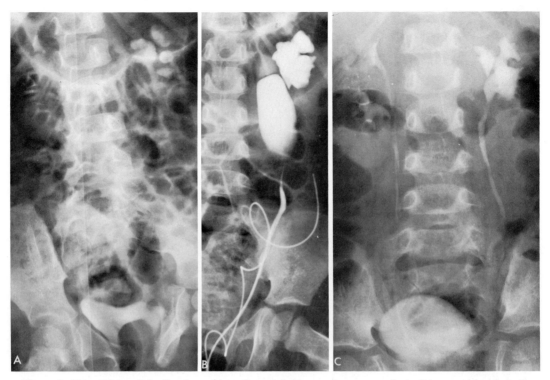

Figure 9–264. Bilateral duplication with unilateral (left) ectopic ureterocele in 3½-year-old girl. **A,** *Excretory urogram.* Filling defect, left base of bladder. **Pyelectasis on left** showing some aspects of lower pelvis of duplication. (*Cystoscopic examination* revealed ureterocele on left with distal orifice just to left of midline in region of vesical neck. Lower-pole orifice was on proximal edge of ureterocele. On right side there were two normal-appearing ureteral orifices in normal location.) **B,** *Left retrograde pyelogram,* both left orifices catheterized. Huge dilatation of upper-pole ureter; pelvis not outlined. Lower-pole pelvis dilated, grade 1. (*Operation* included left heminephrectomy and partial ureterectomy down to level about 4 cm above bladder.) **C,** *Excretory urogram* (1 year postoperatively). Pyelectasis of remaining lower left pelvis. Some flattening at left base of bladder, apparently from remaining uncapped ureterocele.

Figure 9–265. Unilateral duplication (right) with ectopic ureterocele in 6-year-old girl. **A,** *Excretory urogram.* Large filling defect at base of bladder, slightly more on right than left. Thin rim of contrast medium surrounds it entirely, which would suggest possible simple ureterocele. Lower pelvis of duplication is visible on right; good parenchymal shadow shows that upper pelvis is not supplied by upper calyx of lower pelvis. (On cystoscopy, ureterocele was not recognized, apparently because it was compressed by cystoscope. Only some "mild elevation" of right half of trigone was described. Two right orifices were identified; more distal was gaping and was situated at bladder neck. Ureteral catheter was passed into it and contrast medium injected.) **B,** *Right retrograde pyelogram.* Catheter is coiled in ectopic ureterocele, and lower part of ureter is dilated and tortuous. (After heminephrectomy and partial ureterectomy, urinary infection persisted.) **C,** *Excretory urogram* made 4 months postoperatively. "Flabby" type of defect from incompletely filled ureterocele persists. There is reflux up stump of ectopic ureter (*arrow*). (Stump of ureter and ureterocele were removed.) **D,** *Excretory urogram* made 6 months postoperatively.

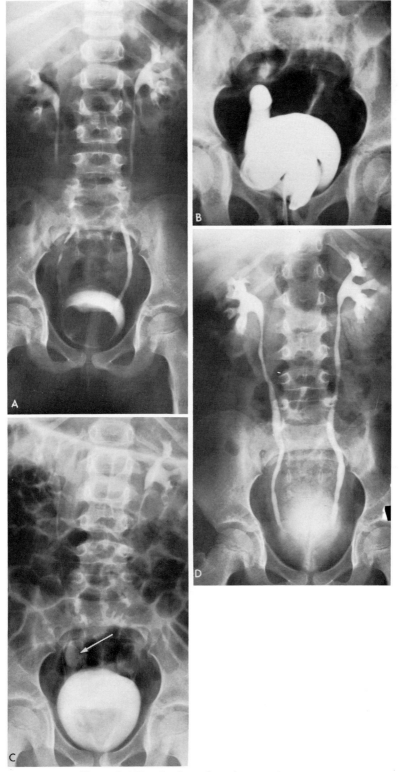

Figure 9–265. *See legend on the opposite page.*

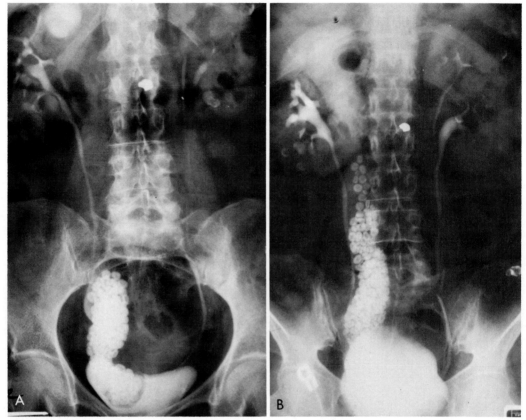

Figure 9–266. *Excretory urogram.* **Duplication on right with ectopic ureterocele containing multiple ureteral calculi** in a 40-year-old woman asymptomatic so far as urinary tract concerned. **A,** and **B,** Stones move freely in the ureter. Stone formation is an uncommon complication of ectopic ureterocele. (Courtesy of Dr. M. L. Duggan.)

contrast medium; there was nothing to suggest contact with the base of the bladder.

It should be pointed out here that the absence of a bladder defect does not entirely exclude an ectopic ureterocele; intravesical pressure may collapse or evert the ureterocele during the radiographic examination so that an erroneous diagnosis of a simple ureteral reflux or even of a vesical diverticulum may be made.

As is true in all cases involving duplication and ectopia, bizarre situations are encountered that may tax the ingenuity and acuity of the examiner. At times, indeed, accurate diagnosis is impossible without surgical exploration. Certainly, one easily may make diagnostic errors, unless he is alert to the various possibilities. It is well to remember that huge hydronephrotic

upper pelves can cause extreme renal displacement (see Fig. 9–154) and that greatly dilated ureters in the infant also may cause marked displacement of the kidneys and even of the bladder (Mogg). Williams and Woodard reported a case of ectopic ureterocele in which the "contralateral" kidney had been removed elsewhere for hydronephrosis because the surgeon had not recognized that an ectopic ureterocele involving the upper-pole ureter of a duplication on the opposite side was the child's basic difficulty. To truly appreciate the many difficult diagnostic problems that may be encountered, the student is urged to read individual case abstracts that appear in the literature from time to time. Selected illustrative groups of case abstracts have been published by Williams and Woodard and also by Mogg.

GENERAL PRINCIPLES IN TREATMENT OF URETERS THAT TERMINATE ECTOPICALLY

The subject of treatment is not in the province of a book of this kind. Nevertheless, stating a few general principles may be in order. The overall problem is that of the duplicated ureter which, because of its ectopic location, is subjected to obstruction, reflux, or both. This, of course, is almost always the upper-pole ureter. Generally speaking, attempts at conservative operations on the upper-pole ectopic ureter have not been good. Such procedures usually consist of an attempt to reimplant the upper-pole ureter into the bladder (Fig. 9–268). Segmental resection of the upper pole (heminephrectomy) is the treatment of choice, but the difficult and controversial

problem is what should be done with the ureter. We have come to some general conclusions as follows:

1. In females, where the ectopic ureteral orifices are distal to the urinary sphincters, ureterectomy is rarely necessary.

2. When the ectopic orifice is located in the vesical neck or in the proximal urethra, the problem is not so straightforward and simple. It is obvious that a dilated stump of a ureter may contain an infected pool of urine or (if reflux is present) may act as an infected vesical diverticulum. On the other hand, it may contract, shrink down, and cause no trouble.

Each case of course must be individualized, but in general our practice has been to proceed with heminephrectomy and par-

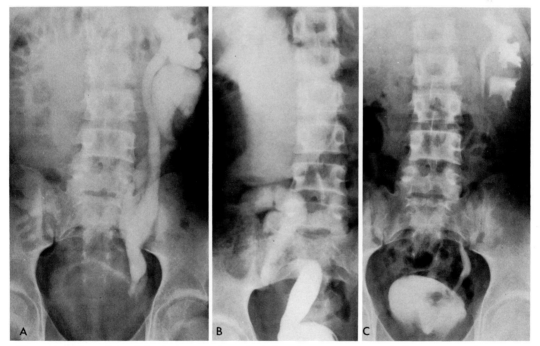

Figure 9–267. **Bilateral duplication with unilateral (right) ectopic ureterocele** in boy aged 15 years. **A,** *Excretory urogram.* Large filling defect occupying most of bladder. Appears to be completely surrounded with contrast medium. No function on right. Duplication on left with moderate dilatation of both ureters and pelves. *Cystoscopic examination.* **Large cystic mass** in right trigone which disappears as bladder is distended with fluid. Two dilated orifices on right—one on proximal lateral margin and the other on distal aspect of cystic mass at vesical neck at 6 o'clock position. Distal orifice catheterized and injected with contrast medium. **B,** *Right retrograde pyelogram* with catheter coiled in upper pole of ureter. Tremendous dilatation of upper-pole pelvis. Catheter then withdrawn and lower-pole orifice catheterized, which showed dilatation of lower pole of pelvis marked but not as great as that of upper pelvis. *Operation.* Complete right nephrectomy and ureterectomy (removing both segments and both ureters). **C,** *Excretory urogram* 2 months postoperatively. Shows duplex left kidney has returned almost to normal. Dilatation was apparently due to pressure on terminal left ureter from huge right ectopic ureterocele.

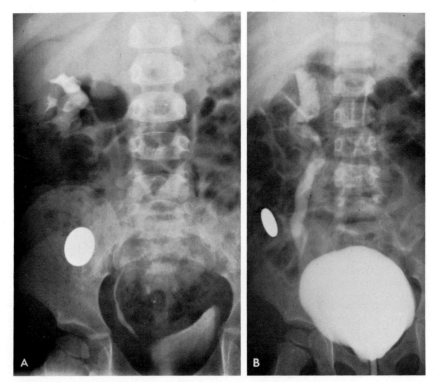

Figure 9–268. Example of poor results which frequently follow conservative operations on duplicated ureters. At age 3 months, this 3½-year-old-girl had had left nephrectomy—apparently because of hydronephrosis, duplication, and ectopic ureteral orifice. One year later duplication on right had also been found with upper-pole orifice in (?) ectopic location. This ureter was reimplanted into bladder, but urinary infection persisted. **A,** *Excretory urogram.* Lower pelvis of duplicated right kidney with **mild pyelectasis. No function of upper segment. B,** *Retrograde cystogram.* Reflux up dilated upper-pole ureter. (Right heminephrectomy and ureterectomy were done.)

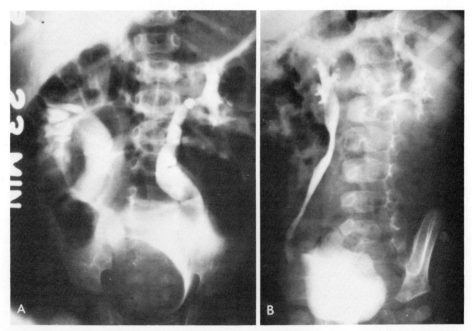

Figure 9–269. Large ureterocele in duplicated collecting system. Boy aged 4. **A** and **B,** *Excretory urogram.* **A,** Duplicated right collecting system with radiolucent bladder defect produced by large right ureterocele. Note ipsilateral and contralateral ureterectasis. **B,** Eight weeks after right upper-pole heminephroureterotomy and complete excision of the ureterocele with bilateral ureteral reimplantation and trigonal reconstruction. (From Tanagho, E. A.)

728

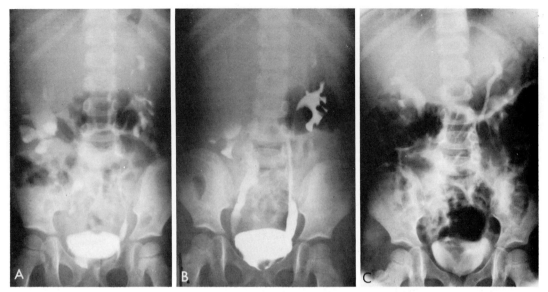

Figure 9–270. Large ureterocele in bilateral duplication. Child aged 4. **A,** *Excretory urogram.* Nonfunctioning right upper pole with ureterectasis and pyelocaliectasis of right lower-pole renal unit. **B,** *Cystogram.* Reflux into all three units but not up the right upper segment. **C,** *Excretory urogram.* Four months after right upper pole heminephroureterotomy, ureterocelectomy, bilateral reimplantation, and trigonal reconstruction. (From Tanagho, E. A.)

tial ureterectomy and then to observe the patient for a few months. If trouble and infection continue, a complete ureterectomy is done as a second-stage procedure.

If an ectopic ureterocele is present, complete ureterectomy and excision (uncapping, unroofing) of the ureterocele are imperative in most cases. Williams (1958a), who has had by far the most experience in these cases, advises it in all cases, although he states that it may be necessary to do the operation in two stages if the infant is in poor general condition. In this case, he advises that the first stage should be the "uncapping" of the ureterocele, the end of the ureter being brought out through the skin as a ureterostomy. Then, at a later elective date, the upper pole of the kidney and the ureter can be removed through a single incision.

Tanagho advocates dissection of the ureterocele sac from under the trigone and complete excision of its inner mucosal lining, followed by reimplantation of the ureter if the kidney is salvageable. If the kidney is seriously damaged, nephroure-terectomy with complete excision of the ureterocele is performed. In the case of a large ureterocele he advises preservation of the superficial trigone to allow for reconstruction and advancement of the contralateral ureter if it has been markedly displaced (Figs. 9–269 and 9–270; see also Figure 9–242C).

THE BLADDER AND URETHRA

Embryology of the Bladder

THE CLOACA

The primitive cloaca (Fig. 9–271) is formed by the distal part of the digestive tract, the hindgut. It receives the allantois (allantoic stalk) and the paired wolffian ducts (with their ureteral buds). It is separated from the outside by the *cloacal membrane.* The *urorectal septum* (urogenital septum, urogenital fold, or mesoderm) grows toward the cloacal membrane, separating the cloaca into the *rectum* (posterior) and the *urogenital sinus**** (Fig. 9–272A through D). The site of the fusion of the urorectal septum with the cloacal membrane becomes the *perineal body.* The part of the cloacal membrane anterior to the point of fusion is called the *urogenital membrane;* the part posterior, the *anal membrane.†* The connection between the rectum and urogenital sinus (just before they are completely divided from each other by the urorectal septum) is called the *cloacal duct.*

---

*Another explanation suggests that the urogenital septum is formed by urogenital folds growing from either side of the cloaca toward the midline and then fusing from above downward. Ladd and Gross stated that failure of fusion of these folds at various levels best explains the occurrence of multiple fistulae between the rectum and the urinary tract.

†This concept has been challenged by Tench, who concluded that the cloacal membrane ruptures before the urorectal septum reaches it so that there is really no separate anal membrane.

THE UROGENITAL SINUS

The urogenital sinus may be subdivided into two parts: (1) The proximal portion above the opening of the wolffian ducts (Müller's tubercle in the undifferentiated embryo, the seminal colliculus or verumontanum in the adult male, or the hymen in the female) develops into the bladder and prostatic urethra in the male and the bladder and entire urethra in the female. (2) The distal portion (the *urogenital sinus proper* or *definitive urogenital sinus*) becomes the remainder of the *urethra* (the cavernous urethra extending to the glans penis) in the male and is represented by the introitus or vestibule in the female.

The narrowed apex of the bladder continuous with the allantoic stalk at the umbilicus is called the *urachus.* In an early de-

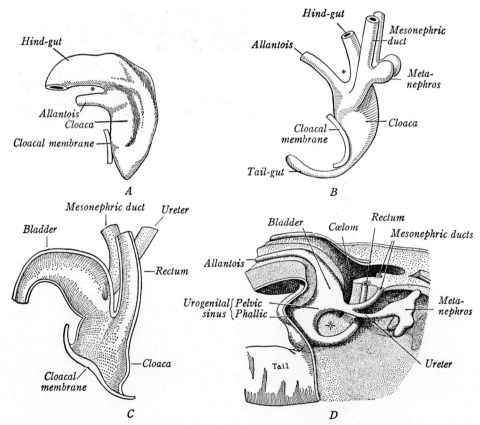

Figure 9–271. **Partial division of human cloaca,** illustrated by models viewed from left side. **A** and **B**, At 3.5 and 4 mm, respectively (after Pohlman; ×50). **C**, At 8 mm (×50). **D**, At 11 mm (after Keibel; ×25). Asterisk indicates position of cloacal septum in **A** and **B**. (From Arey, L. B.)

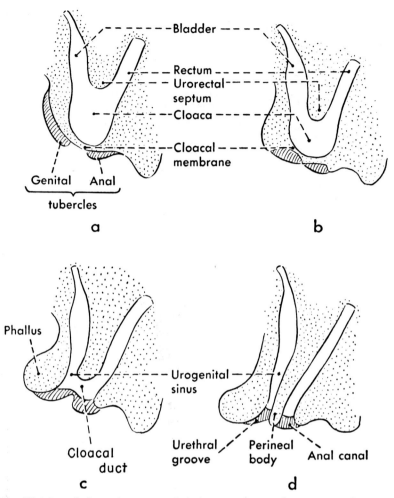

Figure 9–272. Division of cloaca into urogenital sinus, rectum, and anus. Note that paired genital tubercles (in **A**) have fused with each other (in **B** and **C**) to form phallus. (From Hollinshead, W. H.)

velopmental stage this structure undergoes regression that normally results in complete obliteration. Failure to obliterate results in a *patent urachus (urachal fistula)* or *urachal cysts* (Fig. 9–273).

There is some difference of opinion concerning the origin of the bladder. The most widely accepted view (Arey) is that in man the bladder is entirely cloacal in origin; that is, it originates from the urogenital sinus. Another view (Krasa and Paschkis) is that part of the bladder is derived from the allantois. Kjellberg, Ericsson, and Rudhe propose that the part of the bladder lying above the trigone is of allantoic origin, whereas the part below is of cloacal origin. They present urographic and clinical evidence to support the thesis that the level of

the trigone, which they stipulated as being at the first and second sacral vertebrae, is also the level of the juncture of the rectum (which is of cloacal origin) and the colon, which arises from the hindgut. They state that in the adult, this junction is marked by the transverse folds (plica transversalis) of the upper part of the rectum. They emphasize the close relationship between the rectum (below the transverse folds) and the trigone and prostatic urethra and call attention to the fact that in cases of rectal atresia (imperforate anus) in which fistulous communications between the rectum and bladder or urethra are common, the literature contains no report in which the site of fistulous communication was at a higher level than the trigone. In most cases, of

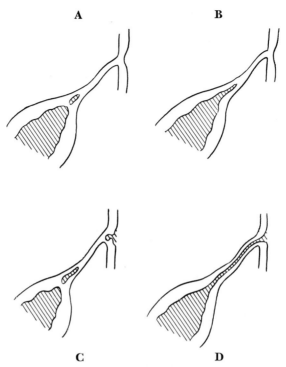

Figure 9–273. Variations in the urachus. **A,** Cavity of urachus not continuous with that of bladder (most common variety; 66 per cent according to Begg). **B,** Lumen of urachus opens into bladder (approximately one third of cases). **C,** Persistent remains of urachus at umbilicus; it may or may not be cystically dilated and may or may not open at umbilicus. **D,** Patent urachus (rare). (From Hollinshead, W. H.)

course, it involves the prostatic or membranous urethra in the region of the seminal colliculus (verumontanum) or an area just distal to it.

Anomalies of the Urachus

In the early embryo, the bladder vertex reaches the umbilicus by its communication with the allantoic duct (Begg, 1927). This umbilical attachment is retained even after complete obliteration and regression of the allantois. As development progresses, the apical portion of the bladder begins to narrow and the urachus begins to form. The bladder, at first an abdominal organ, descends as the pelvis develops, and as this occurs the narrowed urachus elongates (Hammond and associates). The umbilical attachment becomes attenuated as the superior portion of the urachus undergoes various degrees of atrophy. In the adult, the urachus becomes a fibromuscular appendage, about 5 cm long, attached to the bladder apex; however, it retains a minute lumen (less than 1 mm in diameter) lined by a modified transitional epithelium and filled with desquamated debris. In one third to one half of dissections, a minute communication between the urachus and bladder can be demonstrated (Begg, 1927; Hammond and associates; Luschka).

Hinman (1961b) proposed the following classification of urachal abnormalities based on Vaughan's older description: (1) congenital patent urachus ("completely open")—the urachus remains patent or fails to form from the apex of the bladder; (2) vesicourachal diverticulum—the urachus is patent only at its vesical termination ("open internal"); (3) umbilical cyst and sinus—the subumbilical portion of the urachus remains patent ("open external"); and (4) alternating urachal sinus—the vesical and umbilical ends are potentially patent, thereby allowing infection to spread centrally to the bladder, peripherally to the umbilicus, or to both areas simultaneously.

The term *patent urachus* should not be applied to cysts, sinuses, and diverticula, nor to the mere presence of a normal lumen (Steck and Helwig). It should only be applied when there is passage of urine by way of the urachal lumen through an orifice at the umbilicus. This rare condition more commonly affects males than females, the male-female ratio being 3:1 (Mahoney and Ennis; McCauley and Lichtenheld; Nix and associates). The diagnosis is made readily by observing leakage of urine from the umbilicus.

Three types of patent urachus have been described (Nix and associates): (1) persistence of the fetal bladder without descent, resulting in a widely patent urachus; (2) persistence of fetal bladder with descent, producing a double funnel that is narrow in the middle segment; and (3) arrested urachal closure, in which the bladder has a normal position and shape and the urachus is a narrow tube of fairly uniform diameter.

Several diagnostic procedures may be employed to prove the patency of the urachus: (1) passing catheters via the fistula into the bladder; (2) analyzing the draining fluid that identifies it as urine; (3) injecting the fistula with methylene blue and observing the dye in the voided specimen; and (4) intravenously injecting indigo carmine and observing the discoloration of the umbilical fluid (Marshall and Muecke, 1968). An excretory urogram and a voiding cystourethrogram should be obtained before treatment, since this anomaly is often associated with urinary tract obstruction and other anomalies (Herbst). The fistulous tract can be outlined by cystography and is best demonstrated in the lateral position (Fig. 9–274). Cystoscopic examination is helpful in determining the type and size of the patent urachus and in evaluating the lower urinary tract for obstruction. Sanders and associates have utilized B-scan ultrasonography in conjunction with the roentgenologic use of negative and positive contrast material in the evaluation of urachal anomalies.

Vesicourachal diverticulum is usually associated with lower urinary tract obstruction and is most often found in adults. Despite the late appearance, it should be considered a congenital defect that remains asymptomatic until there is superimposed

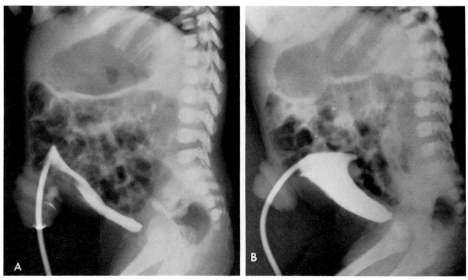

Figure 9–274. **Patent urachus** in newborn infant girl. **A,** Catheter has been inserted into protruding redundant umbilicus, and contrast medium fills urachus and bladder. **B,** Bladder more completely filled; it appears to be attached to umbilicus. (Courtesy of Dr. R. W. Nichols and Dr. R. M. Lowman.)

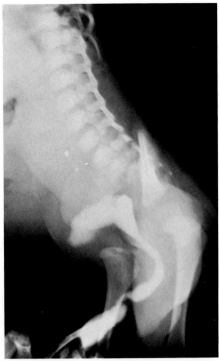

Figure 9–275. Vesicourachal diverticulum in 2-month-old boy with absent abdominal musculature.

obstruction and infection. Calculi have frequently been found within vesicourachal diverticula (Campbell; Siddall; Ward). The diagnosis is made by means of cystoscopy and voiding cystourethrography, the lateral or oblique view best demonstrating the lesion (Felderman and Fetter) (Figs. 9–275 and 9–276).

Umbilical cyst or *sinus*, although more common in adults, originates from a remnant of the urachal duct, which communicates externally in the region of the umbilicus. Symptoms only occur when local infection ensues. A sinogram to demonstrate the extent of the tract before treatment is undertaken may be of value (Hinman, 1961b) (Fig. 9–277).

Alternating urachal sinus, described by Hinman (1961a), causes periumbilical symptoms followed sooner or later by evidence of vesical irritation. It is thought that the path of infection is the patent urachal canal and that the infection arises in the canal and from there spreads both exter-

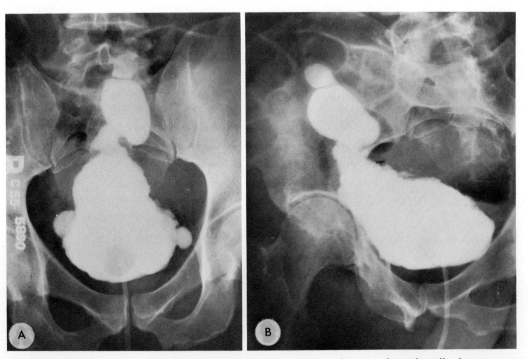

Figure 9–276. *Retrograde cystogram.* **Vesicourachal diverticulum** discovered accidentally during examination of 55-year-old man for urinary obstruction caused by hypertrophy of prostate. Diverticulum per se was asymptomatic and emptied completely with catheter. **A,** *Anteroposterior view.* **B,** *Oblique view.* (Successful excision was followed 8 days later by transurethral prostatic resection.) (From Felderman, E. S., and Fetter, T. R.)

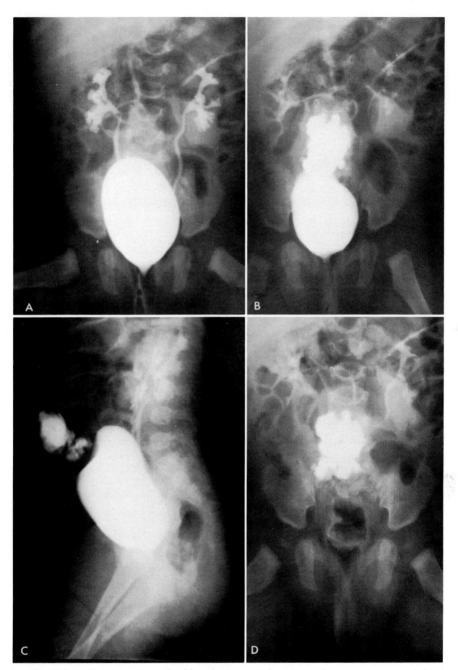

Figure 9–277. Urachal cyst in 4-month-old girl. Presented with tender mass in subumbilical region and high fever. No drainage from umbilicus and no communication with bladder cavity could be demonstrated. *Excretory urograms.* **A,** *Anteroposterior view.* Normal. Smooth bladder outline. Needle introduced into mass and fluid aspirated as contrast medium was injected. Culture of fluid showed *Staphylococcus aureus*. **B,** *Anteroposterior view.* Irregular outline of cyst lying adjacent to and above vesical outline. **C,** *Lateral view* shows relation of cysts to bladder. **D,** *Anteroposterior view after contrast medium evacuated from bladder* shows contrast medium remaining in cyst. Cyst was successfully removed surgically. Specimen measured approximately 3.5 by 6.5 cm. No patent communication with umbilicus or bladder could be demonstrated. (From Constantian, H. M., and Amaral, E. L.)

nally to the umbilicus and internally to involve the bladder. The diagnosis is made by inserting a probe into the sinus, by making a sinogram, and by visualizing a lesion on the dome of the bladder at cystoscopy. Cystography has not been beneficial since no communication exists.

The urachus may also be the site of carcinoma or sarcoma (Begg, 1931; Butler and Rosenberg; Mostofi and associates; Whittle and associates).

Urachal lesions must be distinguished from other disorders of the umbilicus such as omphalitis and patent omphalomesenteric duct, and at times a radiographic study of the upper part of the intestinal tract is essential (Trimingham and McDonald).

Anomalies of the Bladder

EXSTROPHY-EPISPADIAS COMPLEX

Exstrophy of the bladder is a rare congenital anomaly occurring approximately once in every 40,000 to 50,000 live births, with a male-female ratio of 2:1 (Harvard and Thompson). The abnormality involves the musculoskeletal structures of the lower part of the abdomen in addition to the genitourinary tract, and not infrequently it affects the lower part of the gastrointestinal tract. Marshall and Muecke (1962) have listed the variations encountered in the exstrophy-epispadias complex, as follows:

Spade penis only
Epispadias with continence
    Balanic only
    Penile
Epispadias with incontinence
    Subsymphyseal
    Penopubic
Classical exstrophy
Cloacal exstrophy
Superior vesical fissure
Duplicate exstrophy
Pseudoexstrophy

Although the embryogenesis of bladder exstrophy is unknown, several theories have been proposed (Muecke; Patten and

Barry). Unlike most congenital defects, exstrophy cannot be explained as an arrested developmental stage, since it never appears in the normal embryo. If the causative process were one of a mere fusion defect, one would expect the lesser degrees to be the more prevalent, but just the opposite is actually the case.

Classical exstrophy is the most frequently encountered malformation of this anomalous complex, and penopubic epispadias, sometimes referred to as *inferior vesical fissure,* is the next most common (Marshall and Muecke, 1962). In classical exstrophy, the bladder lies open and everted on the surface of the lower part of the abdomen. The trigone and ureteral orifices are easily recognized as urine spurts onto the abdominal wall. The pubic bones are separated, and, on palpation, a fibrous structure can be felt just below the bladder neck. The umbilicus is low and elongated, and a thin fibrous sheet lies between the two divergent rectus muscles, occasionally

Text continued on page 742

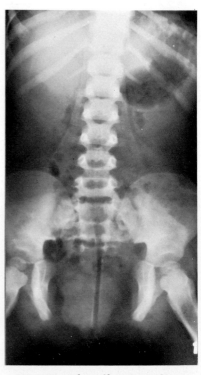

Figure 9–278. *Plain film.* Typical separation of pubic bones of exstrophy-epispadias complex.

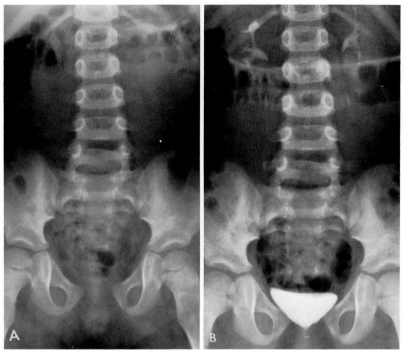

Figure 9–279.   **Epispadias without exstrophy** in 3½-year-old boy. **A,** *Plain film.* Minimal widening of pubic symphysis. **B,** *Excretory urogram.* **Normal upper urinary tracts.** Widened pubis gives appearance of descended bladder.

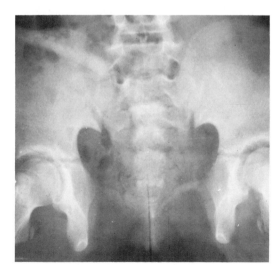

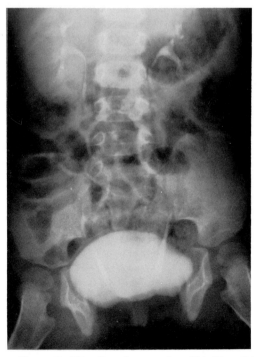

Figure 9–280. **Exstrophy of bladder.** *Plain film* shows typical wide distance between pubic bones with outward rotation of the innominate bones so that they lie parallel to the coronal plane. There is also outward rotation of the ischium and pubis. (Courtesy of Dr. P. R. White and Dr. R. L. Lebowitz).

Figure 9–281. **Pseudoexstrophy of bladder** of 6-month-old girl. *Excretory urogram.* Separation of pubic symphysis is characteristic of exstrophy-epispadias complex. Upper urinary tracts appear normal. Bladder is elevated, and both ureters enter with more medial and direct approach than is normal.

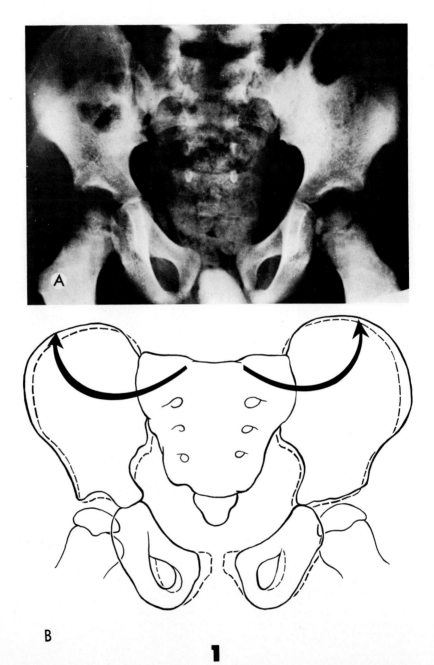

Figure 9–282. Exstrophy-epispadias complex. **A** and **B**, Primary feature (1) in symphyseal widening is outward rotation of innominate bones, relative to sagittal plane of body, along sacro-iliac joints. (From Muecke, E. C., and Currarino, G.)

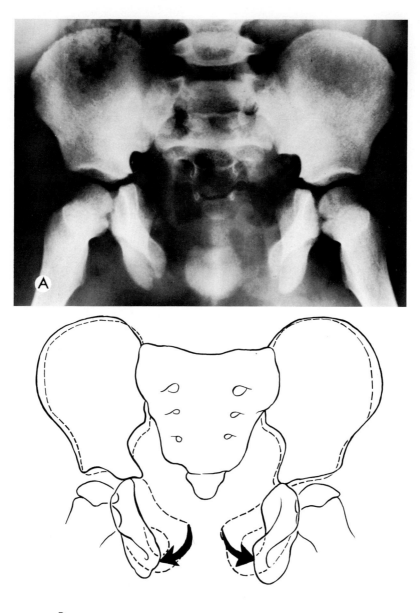

1 + 2

Figure 9–283. **Exstrophy-epispadias complex. A** and **B,** Second feature (1 + 2) in symphyseal widening is eversion or outward rotation of pubic bone at its junction with ischium and ilium. (From Muecke, E. C., and Currarino, G.)

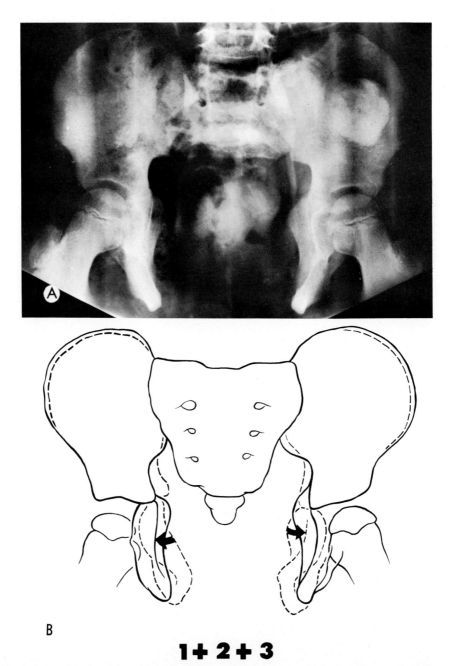

1+ 2+ 3

Figure 9–284.   Exstrophy-epispadias complex. A and **B,** Third component $(1+2+3)$ of congenital symphyseal widening, present in most severe cases, is lateral displacement of innominate bones inferiorly with fulcrum at sacro-iliac joint. (From Muecke, E. C., and Currarino, G.)

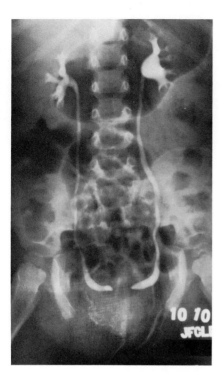

Figure 9–285. Exstrophy of bladder of 3-year-old boy. *Excretory urogram.* Characteristic separation of pubic symphysis. Upper part of urinary tract is normal, except for minimal dilatation of terminal portions of ureters and slight dilatation of left renal pelvis.

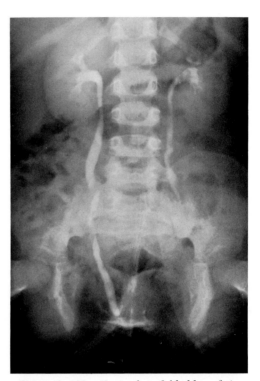

Figure 9–286. Exstrophy of bladder of 4-year-old girl. *Excretory urogram.* Characteristic separation of pubis. **Bilateral ureterectasis** is evident, but renal pelvis and calyces are normal.

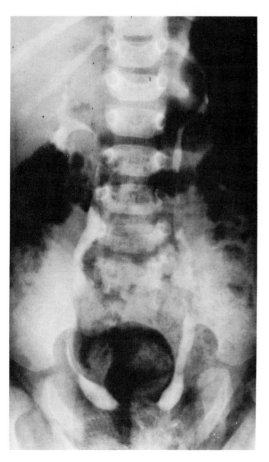

Figure 9–287. Exstrophy of bladder. *Excretory urogram.* Bilateral bulbous dilatation of terminal ureters. Only minimal ureterectasis of upper ureter. (Courtesy of Dr. P. R. White and Dr. R. L. Lebowitz.)

bulging outward as an umbilical hernia. Bilateral inguinal hernias are frequently present, and the testes may be undescended. In the male, the penis is short and upturned, with the epispadiac urethral mucosa covering the dorsal surface. The scrotum is often flattened and may be hypoplastic. In the female, the urethral strip is short and nearly indistinguishable from the bladder mucosa. The clitoris is bifid, and the vaginal orifice is readily recognized, since the labia minora are widely separated.

An anteroposterior roentgenogram of the pelvis shows the separation of the pubic bones that is so characteristic of the exstrophy-epispadias complex (Fig. 9–278). In the normal individual, the distance between the pubic bones does not exceed 10 mm at any age (Abramson and associates;

Heyman and Lundqvist). In patients with the exstrophy-epispadias complex this distance has ranged from 12 to 170 mm, with the amount of separation correlating fairly well with the severity of the complex (Fig. 9–279 and 9–280). Muecke and Currarino studied 89 instances of congenital widening of the pubic symphysis; 66 per cent occurred with classical exstrophy or its variants and 24 per cent occurred in epispadias without exstrophy. The remaining 10 per cent occurred with other unusual entities — namely, anorectal anomalies, urethral duplication, duplicated phallus, congenital hydrocolpos, and pseudoexstrophy (Fig. 9–281). On the basis of their study of pelvic roentgenograms, Muecke and Currarino described three anatomic features related to the pubic separation. First, there is an outward rotation of the in-

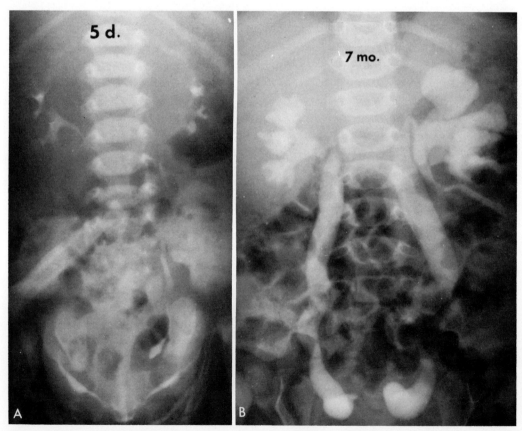

Figure 9–288.   Exstrophy of bladder. **A** and **B,** *Excretory urogram.* **A,** At 5 days of age upper tracts look essentially normal. **B,** At 7 months of age marked ureterectasis and pyelocaliectasis have occurred despite treatment. (Courtesy of Dr. P. R. White and Dr. R. L. Lebowitz.)

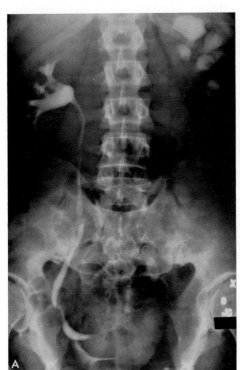

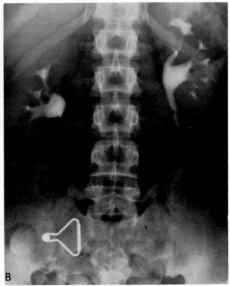

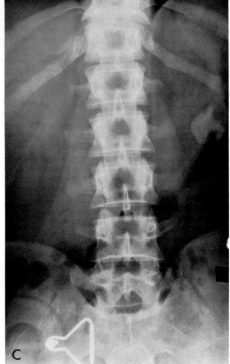

Figure 9–289. Exstrophy of bladder of 31-year-old man. **A,** *Excretory urogram.* Characteristic separation of pubic symphysis. **Mild right ureterectasis and pyelectasis and more severe left pyelocaliectasis** are evident. **B,** *Excretory urogram* 1 month after ileal-conduit diversion. Both kidneys have resumed nearly normal appearance. **C,** *Plain film.* **Staghorn calculus of left kidney** 2 years after diversion.

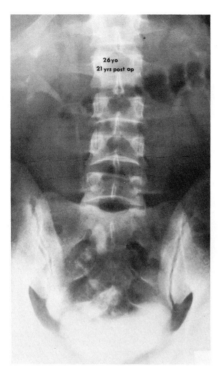

Figure 9-290. Exstrophy of bladder with ureterosigmoidostomy. Man aged 26. *Excretory urogram.* Normal-appearing upper urinary tracts 21 years after ureterosigmoid urinary diversion using antireflux type ureterosigmoid anastomoses. (Courtesy of Dr. P. R. White and Dr. R. L. Lebowitz.)

nominate bones, relative to the sagittal plane of the body, along the sacro-iliac joints (Fig. 9–282). Second, there is an eversion or outward rotation of the pubic bone at its junction with the ischium and ilium (Fig. 9–283). Third, there is, in most of the severe cases, some degree of lateral separation of the innominate bones inferiorly, with the fulcrum at the iliosacral joint (Fig. 9–284).

The excretory urogram may show normal kidneys and ureters, or as so often occurs it may show signs of obstruction (Figs. 9–285 through 9–289). In 17 of 50 cases reported by Maloney and associates, there was unilateral or bilateral ureteropyelocaliectasis when the patients were first seen. Although the ureteral orifices lie exposed, the point of obstruction is the ureterovesical juncture, partly because of the

partial ureteral prolapse and partly because of fibrosis and metaplasia of the bladder mucosa.

Treatment of exstrophy consists of either urinary diversion or primary anatomic closure. The standard method of treatment since 1894 has been ureterosigmoidostomy (Harvard and Thompson). This form of treatment has alleviated suffering and social ostracism for many, yet none have achieved normal life expectancy (Boyce and Vest). The majority of postoperative deaths are of renal origin, usually from pyelonephritis (Harvard and Thompson; Higgins). The creation of competent ureterosigmoid anastomoses by the formation of submucosal "antireflux" tunnels will re-

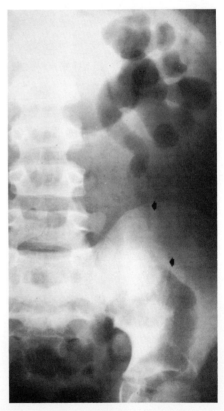

Figure 9-291. Exstrophy of bladder with ureterosigmoid urinary diversion. *Plain film.* Note left "gas" pyelogram due to reflux up dilated ureter. No antireflux ureteral intestinal anastomosis was performed. (Courtesy of Dr. P. R. White and Dr. R. L. Lebowitz.)

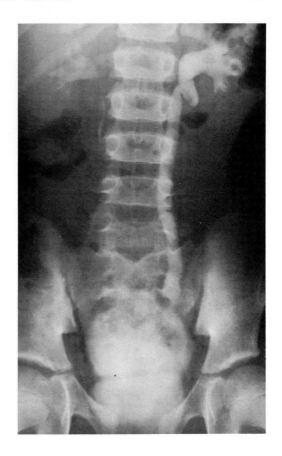

Figure 9–292. Exstrophy of bladder with ureterosigmoid urinary diversion. *Excretory urogram.* Right side is normal. Left reveals **ureterectasis** and **pyelocaliectasis.** Surgical exploration revealed colonic polyps at the site of left ureterosigmoid anastomosis. (Courtesy of Dr. P. R. White and Dr. R. L. Lebowitz.)

duce the incidence of pyelonephritis (Fig. 9–290). If no antireflux tunnel is created, one may observe "gas" refluxing into the ureters and upper collecting system (Fig. 9–291). Hydronephrosis following ureterosigmoidostomy may also result from adenomatous polyp formation (Fig. 9–292) or carcinoma (Fig. 9–293) at the ureterosigmoid anastomosis. Occasionally, calculi form in an obstructed ureter following ureterosigmoidostomy (Fig. 9–294). Urinary diversion by means of the ileal conduit theoretically will offer a longer life expectancy, but this remains to be demonstrated (De-Weerd).

In recent years, there has been a resurgence of interest in primary anatomic closure of the exstrophied bladder (Lattimer and Smith). The overall results have been poor since the majority of these patients remain incontinent and have vesicoureteral reflux and persistent urinary

tract infection (Lattimer and Smith; Marshall and Muecke, 1968; Swenson and associates (Figs. 9–295, 9–296, and 9–297).

DUPLICATION OF THE BLADDER

Duplication of the bladder is uncommon and rarely occurs as an isolated anomaly (Ravitch). Many of the earlier case reports were based on autopsy findings and may actually represent other anomalies, such as vesical diverticulum and ectopic ureterocele (Abrahamson). Several patterns of bladder duplication have been observed, and these have been classified by Burns and coworkers. More recently, Abrahamson modified the classification to include the following: (1) complete duplication, (2) incomplete duplication, (3) complete sagittal septum, (4) incomplete sagittal septum, (5) incomplete frontal septum, (6) multiseptate

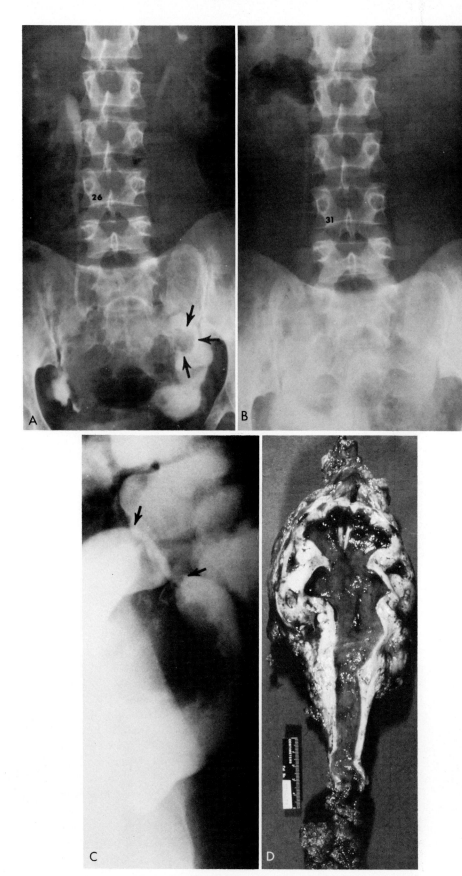

Figure 9–293. *See legend on the opposite page.*

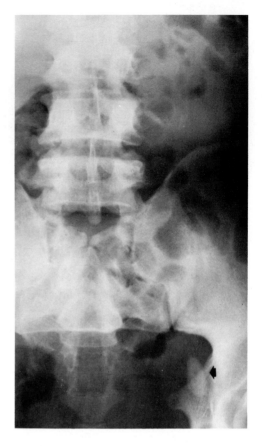

Figure 9–294. Exstrophy of bladder with calculus obstructing ureter following ureterosigmoid urinary diversion. *Plain film.* Calculus overlying left side of pelvis *(arrow).*

bladder, and (7) hourglass bladder. Although these variations have been grouped together on the basis of their clinical descriptions, this does not necessarily mean that they share a common embryogenesis (Marshall and Muecke, 1968; Robson and Ruth).

In cases of complete duplication, the bladders lie side by side, separated by a peritoneal fold (Figs. 9–298, 9–299, and 9–300). Each chamber represents a complete unit formed by normal muscular layers lined by transitional epithelium and receiving a ureter from the ipsilateral kidney (Nesbit and Bromme; Satter and Mossman;

Swenson and Oeconomopoulos). Although each bladder empties through a separate urethra, there may or may not be duplication of the external genitalia. Other anomalies, especially of the lower parts of the gastrointestinal system, are commonly associated with complete duplication of the bladder (Ravitch).

Incomplete duplication occurs less often and is associated with fewer other anomalies than the complete form. The two bladder compartments of the incompletely duplicated bladder share a common vesical outlet and urethra.

Text continued on page 751

Figure 9–293. Exstrophy of bladder with carcinoma developing at ureterosigmoid anastomosis. A and B, *Excretory urogram.* A, Normal-appearing upper urinary tract in 26-year-old woman, 20 years after ureterosigmoidostomy. Filling defect in colon *(arrows)* was not recognized at this time. B, Five years later there is nonfunction on the left side. C, *Barium enema.* Large polyp *(arrows)* at left ureteral orifice. D, *Surgical specimen* following left nephroureterectomy and en bloc resection of colon reveals **villous adenoma with adenocarcinomatous elements** adjacent to ureteral orifice. (Courtesy of Dr. P. R. White and Dr. R. L. Lebowitz.)

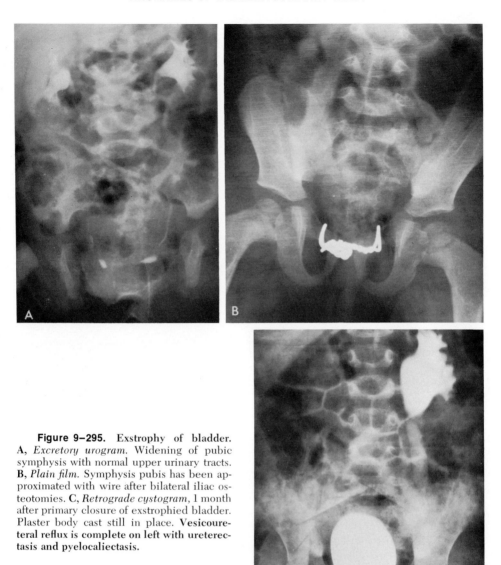

Figure 9–295. Exstrophy of bladder.
A, *Excretory urogram.* Widening of pubic
symphysis with normal upper urinary tracts.
B, *Plain film.* Symphysis pubis has been ap-
proximated with wire after bilateral iliac osteotomies. **C,** *Retrograde cystogram,* 1 month
after primary closure of exstrophied bladder.
Plaster body cast still in place. **Vesicoureteral reflux is complete on left with ureterectasis and pyelocaliectasis.**

Figure 9–296. **Exstrophy of bladder with primary closure. A,** *Excretory urogram.* Untreated girl aged 5.
Normal-appearing upper collecting system with typical separation of pubis. **B,** *Voiding cystourethrogram.* Pubic
bones have been wired together after bilateral iliac osteotomies. There is **bilateral vesicoureteral reflux. C,** *Excretory urogram.* Same patient 4 years after bladder closure and 3½ years after antireflux surgery. (Courtesy of Dr. P.
R. White and Dr. R. L. Lebowitz.)

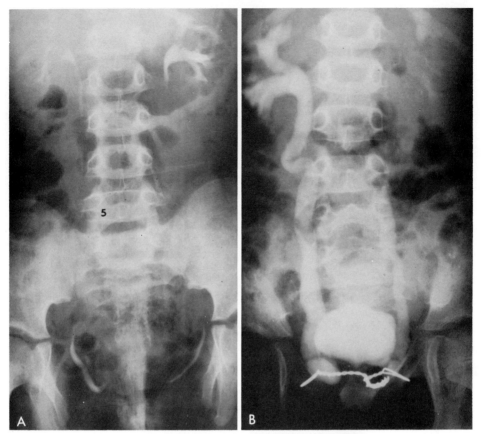

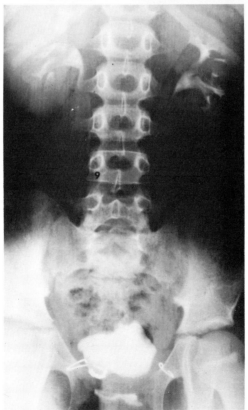

Figure 9–296. *See legend on the opposite page.*

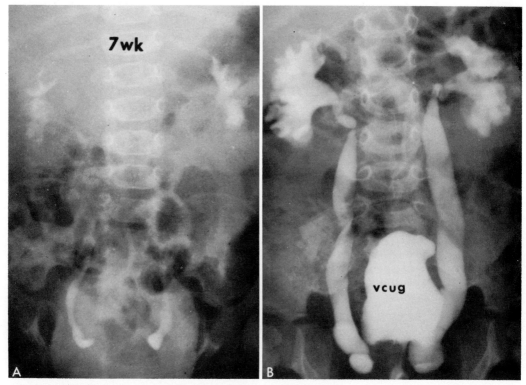

Figure 9–297. Exstrophy of bladder with primary closure. **A,** *Excretory urogram.* Untreated girl aged 7 weeks. Essentially normal upper urinary tract. **B,** *Voiding cystourethrogram.* Same patient at age 1 year, eleven months after bilateral iliac osteotomies and bladder closure. No antireflux surgery has been performed. (Courtesy of Dr. P. R. White and Dr. R. L. Lebowitz.)

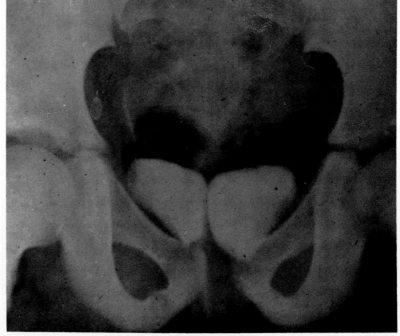

Figure 9–298. *Excretory urogram.* Patient had **double bladder, double penis, and double urethra.** Right ureter empties into right bladder and left ureter into left bladder. (From Nesbit, R. M., and Bromme, W.)

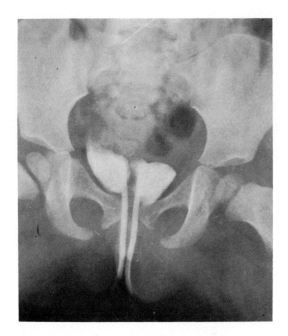

Figure 9–299. *Bilateral retrograde cystogram.* **Duplication of bladder and urethra** in female. (From Satter, E. J., and Mossman, H. W.)

Bladders divided by complete or incomplete septa into chambers of equal or unequal size are also classified with bladder duplication. The septum may be thick and muscular or may consist of little more than two layers of mucosa. Each chamber receives a ureter, and if the septum is complete the obstructed kidney is usually aplastic or hypoplastic (Abrahamson).

Hourglass bladder is a descriptive term used when the bladder is constricted in the horizontal plane, resulting in two equal or unequal chambers (Swenson and Oeconomopoulos). The bladder wall is normal except at the fibromuscular constriction. Although commonly included with bladder duplication, the hourglass deformity is not actually a duplication. The two ureters enter only one chamber—nearly always the lower one (Zellermayer and Carlson). This condition may simulate vesical diverticulum, vesicourachal diverticulum, or a deformity associated with neurogenic dysfunction (Fig. 9–301).

AGENESIS OF THE BLADDER

Agenesis of the bladder is a rare congenital anomaly, usually associated with stillbirth or other defects that are not compatible with life. Campbell reported six autopsy cases, in all of which there were additional severe anomalies. Palmer and Russi reviewed the literature up to 1968 and found 34 collected cases of bladder agenesis. In 29 of these cases, the agenesis was associated with stillbirth. Four of the five patients who survived long enough for a clinical diagnosis to be made were females. If the etiology of this rare anomaly stems from failure of mesonephric duct structures to form the trigone, one can understand why the anomaly is more serious in the male. Without a rudimentary posterior urethra there would be complete obstruction to the outflow of urine, resulting in renal failure. Palmer and Russi added a case of vesical agenesis in a 23-year-old woman with absent urethra. The case reported by Graham in 1972 was the first instance of vesical agenesis in which the urethra was present (Fig. 9–302). The case reported by Vakili was also associated with urethral agenesis (Fig. 9–303).

EMBRYOLOGY OF THE URETHRA

In the male, the *definitive urogenital sinus* below the openings of the wolffian ducts (seminal colliculus) becomes the

Text continued on page 755

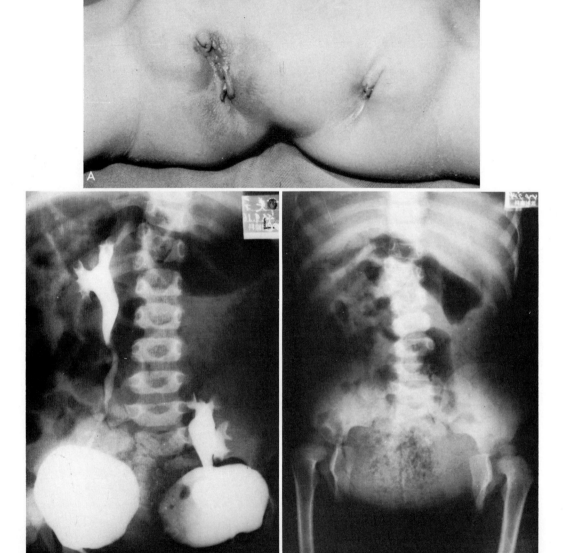

Figure 9–300. **Duplication of bladder and urethra with pelvic kidney.** Girl aged 26 months. Multiple anomalies of genitourinary system. **A,** Two external genitalia, composed of the clitoris and labia majora, are 10 cm apart. On the right, external genitalia, urethral meatus, vaginal opening, and imperforate anus with rectoperineal fistula are observed. On the left side, the urethral meatus exits at the dorsal wall of the vagina (female hypospadias) and the imperforate anus is below the labia. **B,** *Plain film.* Pubic rami are farther apart than is usually seen in exstrophy. **C,** *Retrograde cystograms.* Complete separation of bladders with vesicoureteral reflux. Right kidney is in normal position, whereas left kidney is in pelvis. (From Takaha, M., Nakaarai, K., and Ikoma, F.)

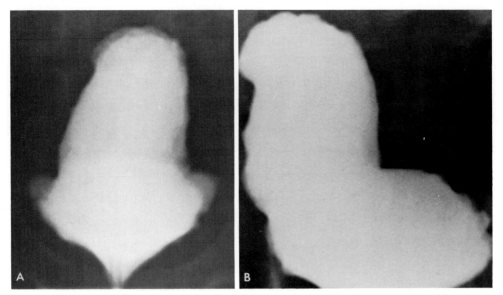

Figure 9–301. *Retrograde cystogram* of girl aged 7 years. **A,** *Anteroposterior view.* **B,** *Oblique view.* **Bladder with saccular compartment,** simulating hourglass bladder. Both portions of bladder emptied completely on voiding.

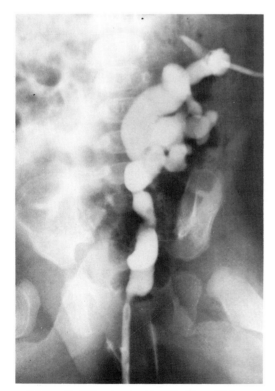

Figure 9–302. Agenesis of bladder. Girl aged 6 weeks. Failure to gain weight. *Antegrade pyeloureterogram.* Tortuous dilated ureter entering the urethra. Catheter is in distal portion of urethra. Surgical exploration revealed solitary left kidney. Nephrostomy tube inserted into upper pole of solitary kidney. (From Graham, S. D.)

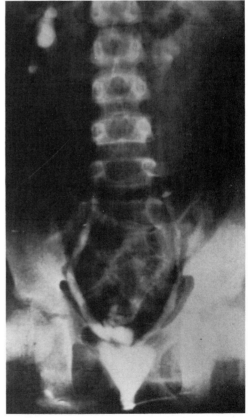

Figure 9–303. Agenesis of bladder and urethra. Girl aged 10 years. Urinary incontinence since birth. *Retrograde study.* Ureters joining near midline and draining into vagina. (From Vakili, B. F.)

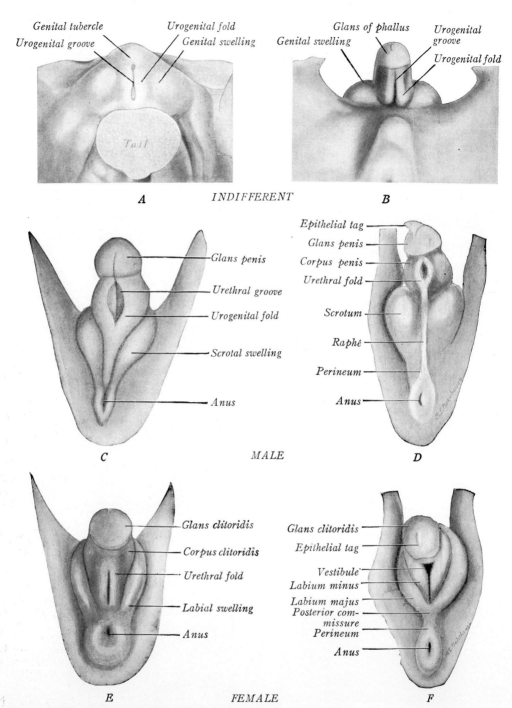

Figure 9–304. **Differentiation of human external genitalia** (after Spaulding). **A** and **B**, Indifferent period, at nearly 7 and nearly 8 weeks (×15). **C** and **D**, Male, at 10 and 12 weeks (×8). **E** and **F**, Female, at 10 and 12 weeks (×8). (From Arey, L. B.)

cavernous urethra, which extends from the membranous urethra to the glans penis.

At the 8-mm stage, the urogenital membrane (anterior half of the cloacal membrane) becomes surrounded by a mound of tissue known as the *genital tubercle.* This tissue assumes the form of folds (urogenital folds) on each side of a groove called the *urogenital groove* or *urogenital sulcus.* The floor of this sulcus is formed by the unruptured *urogenital membrane* (Fig. 9–304). The genital tubercle gradually elongates into a more or less cylindrical phallus (penis in male, clitoris in female) while the urogenital sinus grows with it to form the lining of the future cavernous urethra (Fig. 9–305). At about the 15-mm stage, the urogenital membrane in the floor of the sulcus breaks down, providing the urogenital sinus with an opening to the outside; its external orifice is now the urethral sulcus.

In the male, the edges of the urethral sulcus (the urogenital folds) progressively

fold together and fuse in the midline from behind forward until the entire sulcus to the glans penis is completely enclosed to form the cavernous urethra. The fused edges of the urogenital folds constitute the median raphe. Failure of closure results in varying degrees of *hypospadias.*

In the female, the phallus remains rather small and becomes the clitoris. The urethral sulcus remains shorter and never extends on to the glans, as in the male, but remains open as the *vestibule,* the urethral folds becoming the *labia minora.*

Anomalies of the Urethra

DOUBLE URETHRA AND ACCESSORY URETHRA

Complete duplication of the bladder is often associated with urethral and genital duplication (Wojewski and Kossowski) (see Figure 9–299). The congenital anomaly of

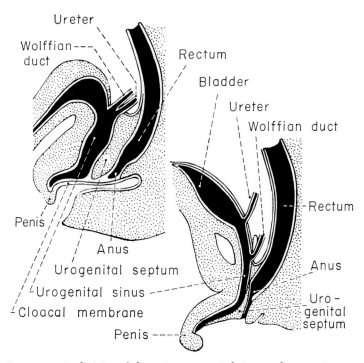

Figure 9–305. Late stages in division of cloaca into urogenital sinus and rectum in anus. Diagrams illustrate manner in which urogenital sinus grows into phallus (penis) to form lining of future cavernous urethra. (Adapted from Keith, A.)

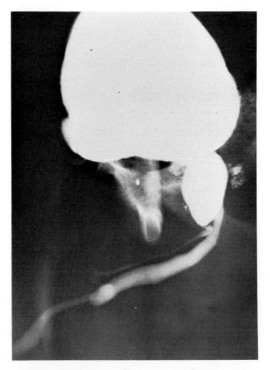

Figure 9–306. *Voiding cystourethrogram.* **Complete urethral duplication.** Major urethra was hypospadic. (From Waterhouse, K.)

double urethra is less common, and the term refers, in the male, only to those cases in which there is complete duplication of the urethra in a single penis. In both sexes, the two channels emerge independently from a single bladder and extend distally without intercommunication (Arnold and Kaylor; Boissonnat; Gross and Moore; Wrenn and Michie). Gross and Moore, after an extensive review of the literature, classified the accessory urethra in urethral duplication in the male as follows:

> Accessory urethra
> Complete—dorsal (22 per cent)
> Incomplete
>   Ventral (4 per cent)
>   Dorsal
>   Ending blindly (59 per cent)
>   Joining main urethra internally
>   (15 per cent)

There have now been over forty reported cases of complete duplication of the male urethra, all but one belonging to the epispadiac type with the upper opening in a groove on the glans or on the dorsum of

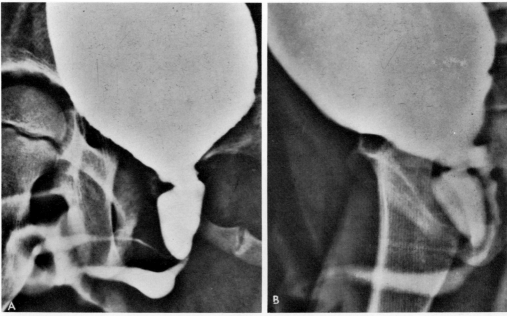

Figure 9–307. *Voiding cystourethrograms.* **Complete duplication of urethra** in male. **A,** *Oblique view* shows complete duplication of all of anterior urethra. **B,** *Lateral view* shows two independent vesical necks and duplication of posterior as well as anterior urethra. (From Boissonnat, P.)

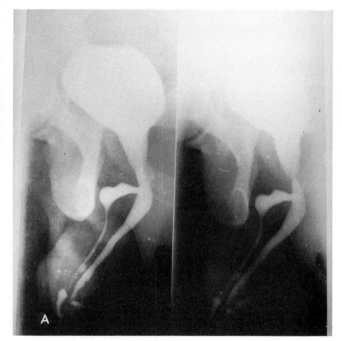
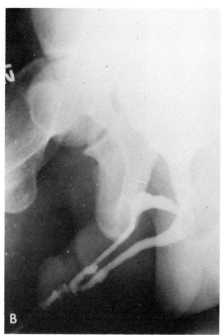

Figure 9–308. Duplication of urethra. Man aged 19. Imperforate anus at birth plus two urethral openings, one at the tip of the glans, the other 2 cm proximal to the corona on ventral surface of penis. **A** and **B,** *Voiding cystourethrograms.* **A,** Preoperative film shows "complete" duplication with accessory urethra opening on the glans. A small calculus was present in the distal dorsal urethra. **B,** Postoperative film after ventral urethra has been joined to dorsal urethra. (From Durrani, K. M., Shah, P. I., and Kakalia, G. R.)

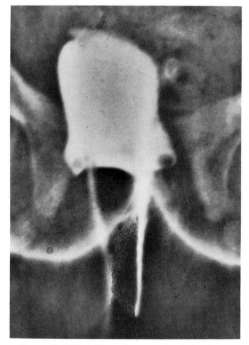

Figure 9–309. Complete urethral duplication in female. *Retrograde cystogram* with contrast medium injected through ureteral catheters inserted in each urethra. Two urethras are entirely independent, run parallel in same frontal plain, and end in two independent bladder necks in widely separated lateral positions. (From Boissonnat, P.)

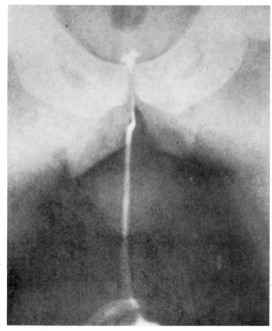

Figure 9–310. *Urethrogram.* **Accessory urethra,** dorsal to true urethra, terminates proximally with blind end just behind symphysis pubis. No communication with true urethra or bladder. (From Irmisch, G. W. and Cook, E. N.)

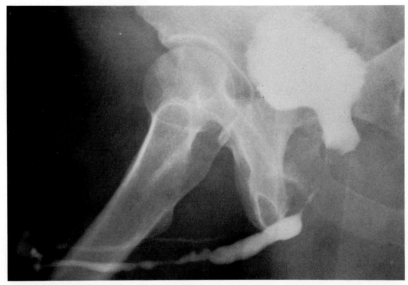

Figure 9–311. *Retrograde urethrogram.* **Accessory urethra** in 62-year-old man. Note multiple urethral strictures, with proximal dilatation, and postoperative changes in prostatic urethra from previous transurethral prostatic resection.

the penis (Arnold and Kaylor; Boissonnat; Gross and Moore; Thevathasan; Waterhouse; Wrenn and Michie). The presenting symptoms associated with complete duplication have included a double urinary stream, incontinence, urethritis, urinary tract infection, and dorsal chordee. The diagnosis can best be confirmed by voiding cystourethrography or retrograde urethrography (Figs. 9–306, 9–307, and 9–308). Complete duplication of the female urethra, with a single bladder, has been

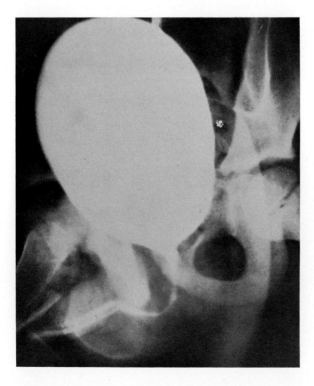

Figure 9–312. *Voiding cystourethrogram.* **Accessory urethra, incomplete, dorsal.** (From Waterhouse, K.)

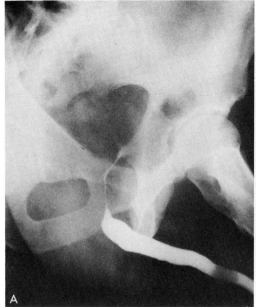

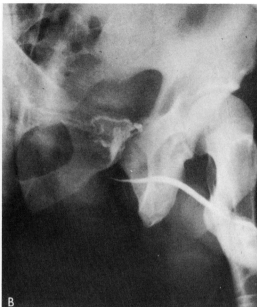

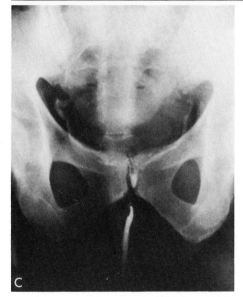

Figure 9–313. Accessory urethra. Man aged 34, father of five children. Purulent drainage from accessory penile opening. **A** through **C**, *Retrograde urethrograms*. **A,** Normal ventral urethra. **B** and **C,** Dorsal accessory urethra with reflux into prostate and ejaculatory ducts, seminal vesicles, and vasa deferentia. No reflux into bladder or normal urethra. (From Schmidt, J. D.)

Figure 9–314. Accessory perineal urethra. Male aged 17. Since birth patient had voided through perineal opening with only few drops from normally located urethral meatus. *Retrograde penile urethrogram.* Small, thin penile urethra with small duct communicating with posterior portion of perineal urethra. (From Selvaggi, F. P., and Goodwin, W. E.)

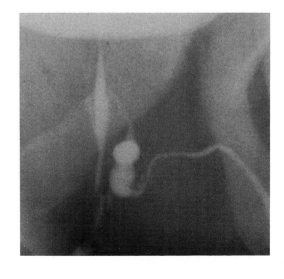

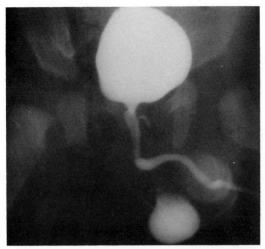

Figure 9–315. Congenital urethroperineal fistula. Newborn male with cystic perineal mass. *Retrograde cystourethrogram.* Fistulous channel arises from posterior urethra and ends in dilated cavity with midline perineal opening. (From Gehring, G. G., Vitenson, J. H., and Woodhead, D. M.)

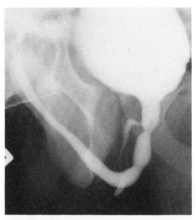

Figure 9–316. Congenital urethroperineal fistula. *Voiding cystourethrogram.* Fistulous channel arising from posterior urethra has its external opening in the median raphe of the scrotum. (Courtesy of Dr. R. Olson.)

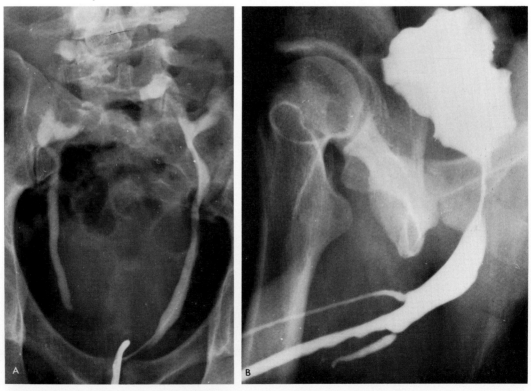

Figure 9–317. Trifurcation of anterior urethra in 22-year-old man. **A,** *Bilateral retrograde pyelogram. Note bilateral pelvic kidneys.* **B,** *Retrograde urethrogram.* (From Forgaard, D. M., and Ansell, J. S.)

reported less than a half dozen times (Bois-sonnat; Brown) (Fig. 9–309).

Most of the reported cases of double urethra are no more than accessory urethral canals or partially duplicated urethral segments that either communicate with the main urethra or, more often, end blindly after a few centimeters (Irmisch and Cook; Lowsley) (Figs. 9–310 through 9–313). A much rarer form of accessory urethra is the one which comes off the posterior urethra and opens onto the perineum as a urethro-perineal fistula (Figs. 9–314, 9–315, and 9–316). Trifurcation of the urethra is a rarity among accessory urethral canals and has been associated with an anomalous appearing upper urinary tract (Forgaard and Ansell (Fig. 9–317).

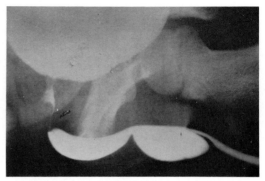

Figure 9–318. Elongated urethral diverticulum opening in bulb of urethra and compressing normal channel in boy 2 years of age. (From Williams, D. I.: Discussion on Lower Urinary Obstruction. Arch. Dis. Childhood 37:132–137 [Apr.] 1962.)

DIVERTICULUM OF THE MALE URETHRA

Diverticulum of the urethra distal to the external sphincter is an uncommon but important cause of urinary obstruction in the male child. These diverticula occur in two forms: saccular and diffuse. Their loca-tion is variable, but they are found mainly in the penile and bulbous portions of the urethra (Abeshouse; Stephens).

Saccular Form. In the saccular form, the orifice is comparatively narrow, and the sac is elongated and lies beside the normal urethral channel, which it compresses when it is distended with urine (Fig. 9–318). Visualization of the opening on

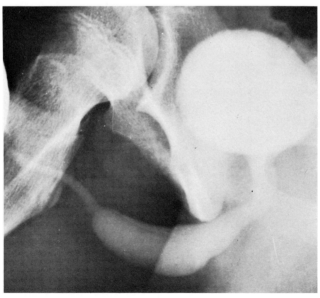

Figure 9–319. Saccular diverticulum of urethra. *Micturition cystourethrogram* showing outline of oval distended diverticulum (From Dorairajan, T.)

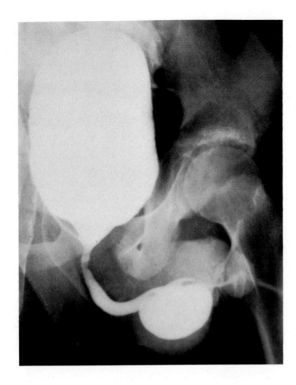

Figure 9–320. *Expression urethrogram.* Saccular diverticulum of anterior urethra in boy aged 14 years.

urethroscopy may be difficult, but voiding or expression urethrograms will often give a clear picture of the condition (Figs. 9–319, 9–320, and 9–321), and a plain roentgenogram will demonstrate calculi, which often form within the diverticulum

(Abeshouse). Simple surgical excision is curative (Fig. 9–322).

Diffuse Form. In the diffuse form, the orifice is so wide that it may be difficult to identify with certainty any true neck to the diverticulum, and the corpus spongiosum

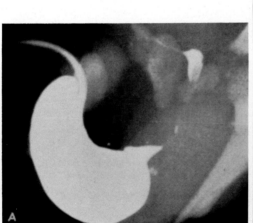
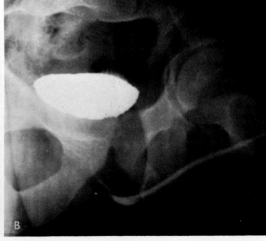

Figure 9–321. Saccular diverticulum of urethra. **A,** *Urethrogram* of 2-day-old boy, after emptying diverticulum with catheter and injecting contrast medium, shows huge diverticulum. (From Demos, N. J., Gillis, D. A., and Barber, K. E.) **B,** *Voiding urethrogram* demonstrates small saccular diverticulum in bulbous portion of urethra of another patient. (Courtesy of Major James Gilbaugh, M.C., U.S.A.F.)

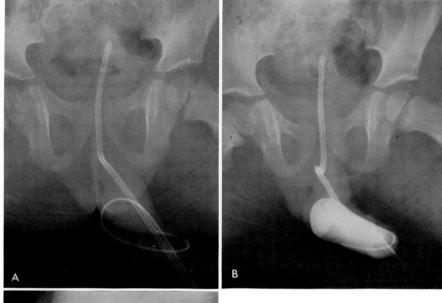

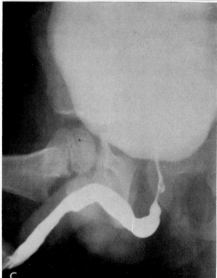

Figure 9–322. Congenital diverticulum of pendulous urethra in boy 3 years of age. **A,** *Plain film.* Urethral catheter in place; tip is in bladder. Opaque ureteral catheter is coiled in urethral diverticulum. **B,** Diverticulum has been outlined with contrast medium injected through ureteral catheter. **C,** *Postoperative retrograde urethrogram* shows good result after diverticulectomy and urethroplasty.

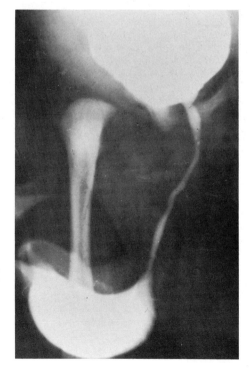

Figure 9–323. *Micturition cystourethrogram.* **Scaphoid megalourethra.** Scaphoid expansion of penile urethra. (From Dorairajan, T.)

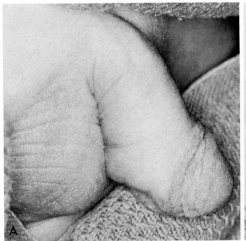
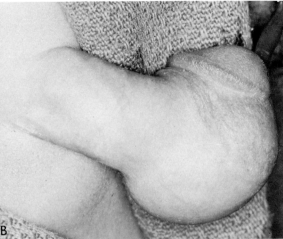
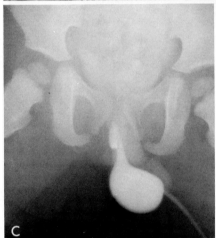

Figure 9–324. Melagourethra. Boy aged 2½. **A** and **B**, Dorsal curvature of penis with deficiency of distal corpus spongiosum. Filling of urethra produces ballooning of distal penis. **C**, *Retrograde urethrogram.* Scaphoid expansion of distal penile urethra. (From Masik, B. K., and Brosman, S. A.)

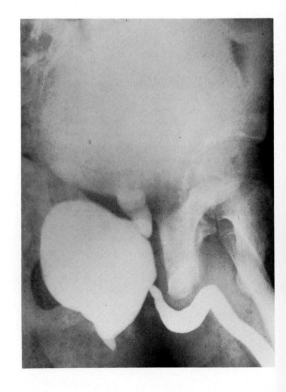

Figure 9–325. *Retrograde cystourethrogram.* Post-traumatic diverticulum of prostatic urethra in male aged 17 (3 months after pelvic injury). Large diverticulum arising from prostatic urethra, extending into adductor compartment of right thigh and distorting posterior urethra. (From Omo-Dare, P.)

may be deficient (Dorairajan) (Figs. 9–323 and 9–324). This type of diverticulum has been described as *megalourethra* and is often associated with anomalies elsewhere in the urinary tract (Dorairajan; Nesbitt; Stephens). A retrograde urethrogram outlines the anomaly well, but surgical correction is difficult.

Diverticula of the Prostatic Urethra. These are extremely rare and are nearly always acquired defects (Knox; Omo-Dare) (Fig. 9–325).

DEEP PELVIC CYSTS

Cysts arising in the male pelvis are extremely rare, and *almost without exception represent remnants of the müllerian duct* (Deming and Berneike; Wesson). In the male, the müllerian duct becomes obliterated after the sixth week of fetal life, and normally the only representations in the adult are the appendix testis and the prostatic utricle (Davies). If the ducts would persist in their entirety, each would follow the vas deferens from the scrotum through the inguinal canal and through the substance of the prostate gland, medial to the ejaculatory ducts, to join its mate to form the utricle. Cystic dilatation may occur at any point along a duct which has failed to undergo normal regression. Although cysts of the müllerian remnant have been found in the inguinal canal, most have arisen deep within the pelvis between the bladder and rectum (Landes and Ransom).

CYSTS OF THE MÜLLERIAN DUCT

Cysts of the müllerian duct usually are encountered in men 20 to 40 years of age, but they also have been found in boys and in elderly men (Begg; Culbertson; Deming and Berneike; Hennessey; Landes and Ransom; Lloyd and Bonnett; Rusche and Butler; Senger and Morgan; Smith and Strasberg; Spence and Chenoweth). Clinical features vary with the size of the cyst and the presence or absence of infection. They include symptoms of urinary obstruction, dysuria, hematuria, suprapubic or rectal pain, and the presence of a lower abdominal mass. Digital rectal examination usually discloses a large midline symmetrical mass arising from the upper margin of the prostate gland but not contiguous with it.

The contents of the cysts have been variously described as serous, mucoid, purulent, and hemorrhagic and as clear, brown, or green. The fluid never contains spermatozoa. Calculi, although rare, may be present within the cyst (Spence and Chenoweth). Cystoscopy reveals encroachment on the vesical neck, trigone, and base of the bladder rather than on the prostate gland. Occasionally cystoscopy is unsuccessful because of severe posterior urethral angulation (Begg; Hennessey; Senger and Morgan). Brownish or bloody fluid may emerge from the verumontanum, especially after digital rectal massage of the cyst (Landes and Ransom). Two approaches to the urographic diagnosis have been used: (1) catheterization of the cyst with a ureteral catheter through the utricle, if possible, and injection of contrast medium (Fig. 9–326) and (2) transrectal or transperineal needle aspiration of the cyst and injection of contrast medium (Fig. 9–327). One successful attempt at suprapubic aspiration and injection of contrast material has been reported (Neustein and Schutte). Retrograde urethrography will not outline the cyst but may be used in conjunction with air cystography to show the posterior vesical position of the cyst (Lloyd and Bonnett; Spence and Chenoweth). Oblique or lateral roentgenographic views will show the mass posterior to the bladder. The cyst rarely becomes so huge that it displaces the ureters (Coppridge; Neustein and Schutte) (Fig. 9–328).

DILATATION OF PROSTATIC UTRICLE

The prostatic utricle is derived from the fused ends of the müllerian ducts and is the homologue of the female uterus and upper part of the vagina (Davies). It varies

Fig. 9–326

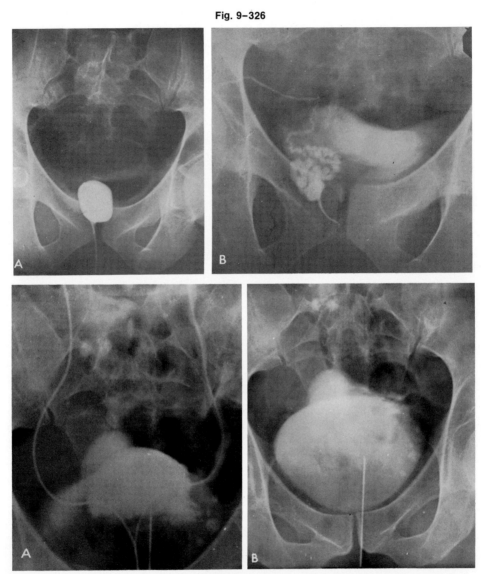

Fig. 9–327

Figure 9–326. Müllerian duct cyst. A, Cyst injected with contrast medium by means of ureteral catheter passed through sinus pocularis of utricle. B, *Right seminal vesiculogram* made by injecting contrast medium through vasotomy incision. Seminal vesicle displaced laterally by cyst. (From Culbertson, L. R.)

Figure 9–327. Müllerian duct cyst. A, Cyst has been injected with contrast medium by means of needle introduced through perineum at time of making *bilateral retrograde pyelograms.* Bladder partially filled with medium. Cyst can be seen lying behind bladder. B, Same plus *retrograde cystogram.* (From Deming, C. L., and Berneike, R. R.)

in size and shape, with its length ranging from 8 to 10 mm, and its width ranging from 1 to 2 mm near the opening and increasing to 4 to 6 mm at the blind end (Edling). The utricle undergoes senile involution similar to that of the prostate gland and, except for an occasional calculus or cystic dilatation, never attains clinical significance (Moore) (Figs. 9–329 and 9–330).

The association of hypospadias and incomplete testicular descent with an enlarged prostatic utricle has been recognized for many years (Arnold; Young and Cash). In fact, the size of the utricle has been used to substantiate the intersex theory of hypospadias as opposed to the theory of a mere fusion defect (Howard; Shopfner). Since routine endoscopy and genitography are rarely performed in cases of hypospadias, it is not suprising to find only occasional references to anomalies of the utricle (Edling; Moore; Shopfner).

There has been a tendency in the literature to include the dilated utricle with the general category of müllerian duct cyst (Landes and Ransom; Slocum; Spence and Chenoweth). Although sharing a common embryologic origin, these two rare entities should be differentiated on the basis of the following clinical and pathologic findings (Myers and associates): (1) cysts of the utricle most often are detected clinically in the first and second decades, whereas most müllerian duct cysts are detected in the third and fourth decades; (2) the enlarged utricle always is associated with hypospadias and incomplete testicular descent, whereas the müllerian duct cysts occur as isolated anomalies in males with normal external genitalia (Arnold; Campbell; Gullmo and Sundberg; McKenna and Kiefer; Middleton; Myers and associates; Young and Cash); (3) cysts of the utricle can be excised with relative ease, a fact of surgical importance, whereas the excision of müllerian duct cysts is difficult, owing to their dense adherence to the prostate gland, seminal vesicle, and posterior wall of the bladder (McKenna and Kiefer; Myers and associates; Slocum).

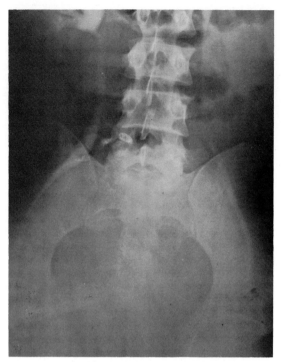

Figure 9–328. *Bilateral pyelogram.* Wide displacement of lower portions of both ureters. Diagnosis of **huge müllerian duct cyst,** proved surgically. (From Coppridge, W. M.)

Routine methods of urethrocystography will seldom outline the utricle in the normal individual (Edling; Gullmo and Sundberg) (Figs. 9–331 and 9–332). Filling of the utricle is of no special diagnostic importance unless it is enlarged or associated with hypospadias (Edling) (Fig. 9–333; see also Fig. 9–353). Utriculography may be accomplished by inserting a ureteral catheter into the dilated orifice or occluding the orifice with a cone-tip ureteral catheter and injecting contrast medium (Fig. 9–334 *B*). In addition to the retrograde or flushing technique used in genitography, one may also use the multiple-channel catheter technique (Edling, Gullmo and Sundberg; Shopfner). Rarely does the utricle become so huge that it displaces the bladder and ureters, but when it does, it may partially be outlined by means of a voiding cystourethrogram (Myers and associates) (Fig. 9–334 *A*, *B*, and *C*).

CYSTS OF THE SEMINAL VESICLES

Cysts of the seminal vesicles rarely attain clinical significance; only about 20 cases have been well documented in the literature. (Deming; Francke; Hart, 1961; 1966; Heetderks and Delambre; Heller and Whitesel; Kimchi and Wiesenfeld; Lawson and MacDougall; Lloyd and Pranke; Lund and Cummings; Stewart and Nicoll; Zinner). The age of the patient, at the time of clinical detection, has ranged from 18 to 59 years, the majority of patients being in the third decade. Irritative symptoms predominate—burning, urgency, and increased frequency of urination. Pain is not in-

Fig. 9–329

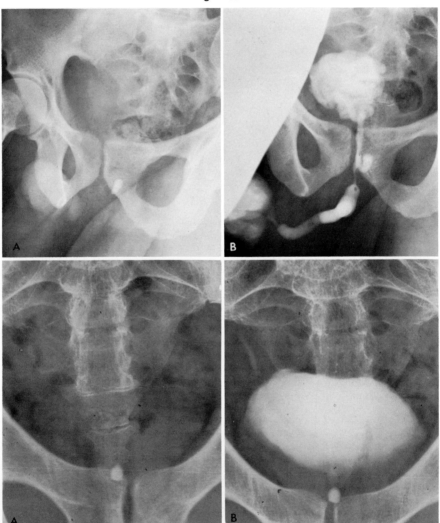

Fig. 9–330

Figure 9–329. Stone in utricle. A, *Plain film.* B, *Retrograde urethrogram,* right semi-oblique position. Communication of utricle with urethra outline. Patient has postoperative contracture of vesical neck with typical toothpaste contour of contrast medium in bladder.

Figure 9–330. Stone in utricle. A, *Plain film.* B, *Excretory cystogram.*

frequent and may be pelvic, urethral, or testicular; it sometimes is associated with ejaculation (Heller and Whitesel; Lund and Cummings; Stewart and Nicoll). Hematospermia does not appear to be a feature of the condition and has been described on only two occasions (Heller and Whitesel; Stewart and Nicoll). Digital rectal examination discloses a monolocular cyst, located to one side of the midline, above the prostate. This lateralization helps differentiate the cyst of the seminal vesicle from the more common müllerian duct cyst.

Seminal vesicle cysts are usually small compared to müllerian duct cysts and, therefore, rarely cause disturbance of ureteral drainage (Deming; Heetderks and Delambre). The excretory urogram is usually normal; however, a presumptive diagnosis of cysts of the seminal vesicle can be made if a solitary kidney is outlined. Several of the reported seminal vesicle cysts have

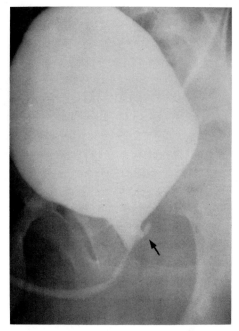

Figure 9–331. *Retrograde cystogram.* **Normal utricle filled with contrast medium.** *(arrow).*

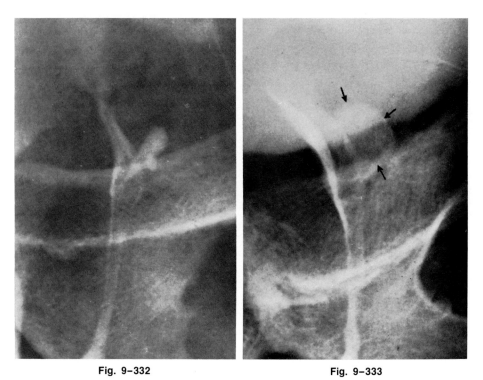

Fig. 9–332   **Fig. 9–333**

Figure 9–332. *Urethrogram* outlining **normal utricle.** Calculus in prostate gland is projected over utricle. (From Edling, N. P. G.)

Figure 9–333. *Urethrogram showing* **enlarged utricle** *(arrows).* (From Edling, N. P. G.)

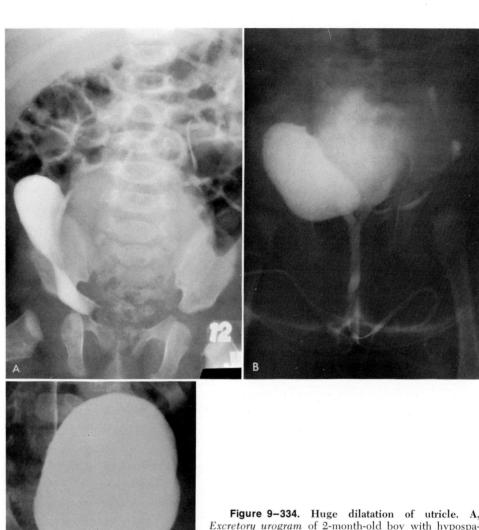

Figure 9–334. Huge dilatation of utricle. **A,** *Excretory urogram* of 2-month-old boy with hypospadias and undescended testes shows large "pelvic mass" displacing bladder and ureters. **B,** *Retrograde cystogram* and *utriculogram* show bladder displaced upward and to right by huge dilated utricle. Note also left ureteral reflux. **C,** *Expression urethrogram* shows only small defect in posterior urethra where utricle had arisen.

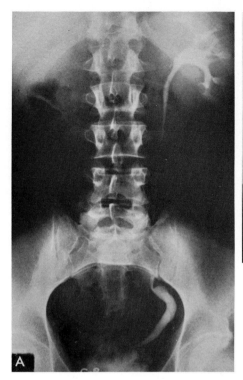

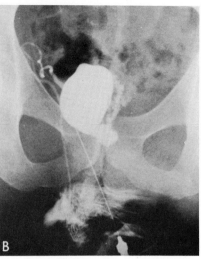

Figure 9–335. Cyst of seminal vesicle. **A,** *Excretory urogram.* Asymptomatic cystic mass above right lobe of prostate gland of 28-year-old man. No visualization of right kidney. **B,** Transperineal aspiration and injection of contrast material into cyst cavity. Contrast material is still present from seminal vesiculogram, which also showed reflux into cyst. (From Hart, J. B., 1966.)

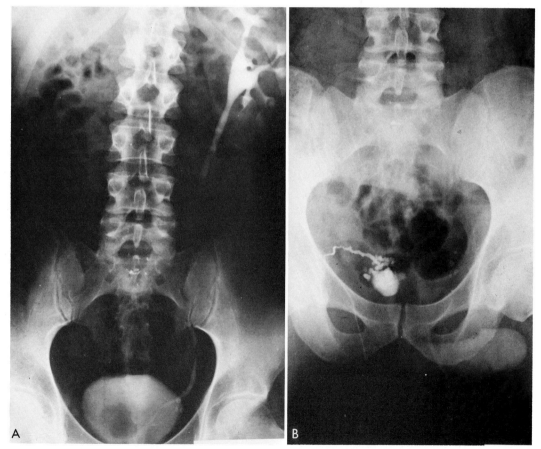

Figure 9–336. Cyst of seminal vesicle with ipsilateral renal agenesis. Man aged 31. Perineal pain with ejaculation. **A,** *Excretory urogram.* Solitary left kidney with hypertrophy. Radiolucent defect right side of bladder. **B,** *Vasovesiculogram.* Cystic dilatation of right seminal vesicle. Further injection of contrast medium resulted in cyst rupture. After cyst rupture, patient no longer had perineal pain. (From Greenbaum, E., and Pearman, R. O.)

been associated with a proved absence of the ipsilateral kidney. In other cases the kidney has been presumed absent, since there was no concentration of media on excretory urography (Hart, 1961; 1966; Heetderks and Delambre; Kimchi and Wiesenfeld; Zinner) (Figs. 9–335 and 9–336). This entity should be distinguished from ectopic ureter opening into the seminal vesicle, a disorder that nearly always is accompanied by cystic dilatation of the involved seminal vesicle. Cystography may disclose a posterior filling defect from the extravesical pressure (Kimchi and Wisenfeld) (Fig. 9–337). Retrograde or antegrade seminal vesiculography is often effective in outlining the cyst (Hart, 1966; Heller and Whitesel; Lund and Cummings; Stewart and Nicoll), but vesiculography by either method may be followed by acute epididymitis (Heller and Whitesel; Stewart and Nicoll). Urethrography, in conjunction with vesiculography, will localize the cyst but is usually not necessary (Heller and Whitesel)

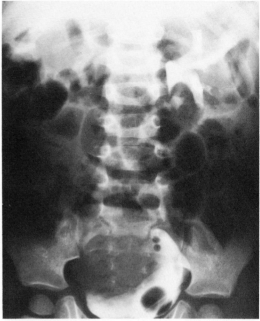

Figure 9–337. **Deep pelvic cyst.** *Excretory urogram.* Nonfunction on the right side with defect in bladder outline produced by cystic mass behind bladder. Vasovesiculography would help indicate origin of cyst. (From Feldman, R. A., and Weiss, R. M.)

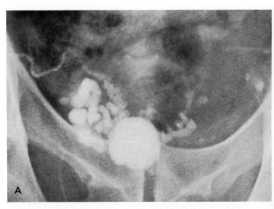

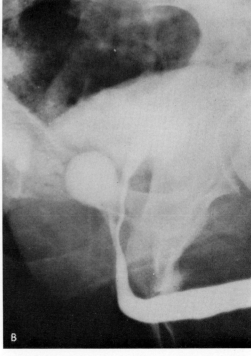

Figure 9–338. Cyst of seminal vesicle. **A,** *Seminal vesiculogram* via right vas deferens shows cyst of seminal vesicle in asymptomatic 55-year-old man. **B,** *Urethrography plus seminal vesiculography* helps localize cyst. (From Heller, E., and Whitesel, J. A.)

(Fig. 9–338). Ultrasonography may also be utilized to outline cysts of the deep pelvis (Fig. 9–339).

Endoscopy is nearly always possible and reveals elevation of the trigone and base of the bladder on the affected side. This elevation may extend into the proximal portion of the prostatic urethra. Catheterization of the ejaculatory duct with a 3-F or 4-F olive-tip catheter permits retrograde vesicu-lography (Fig. 9–340). Aspirating either transvesically during cystography or transperineally will yield the characteristic brownish fluid, which should contain spermatozoa. The presence of spermatozoa helps distinguish this lesion from müllerian duct cyst. Injecting contrast material and taking a roentgenogram after aspiration confirms the presence and cystic character of the lesion.

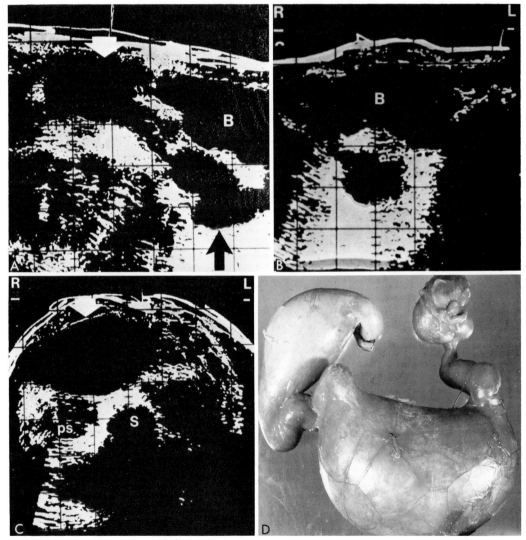

Figure 9–339. Cyst of seminal vesicle. Man aged 34. Asymptomatic palpable abdominal mass. **A** through **C**, *B-scan ultrasonogram.* **A,** *Longitudinal scan* to the right of the midline demonstrates an irregular mass extending from the pelvis *(black arrow)* retroperitoneally into the abdomen *(white arrow).* B = urinary bladder. **B,** *Transverse scan* outlines mass posterior to bladder (B). **C,** *Transverse scan* through the abdominal component of the mass *(white arrow).* S = spine; ps = psoas muscle. **D,** Intact surgical specimen illustrates the pelvic and abdominal components of the mass. (From Walls, W. J., and Lin, F.)

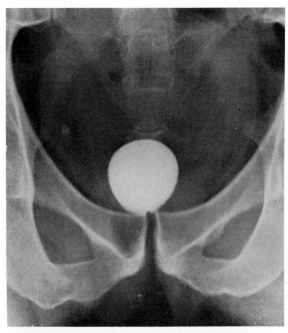

Figure 9–340. Cyst of seminal vesicle. Ejaculatory ducts were catheterized, and catheter entered cyst where contrast medium was injected. (From Stewart, B. L., and Nicoll, G. A.)

CYSTS OF THE PROSTATE GLAND

Cysts of the prostate are usually incidental findings at autopsy, since because of their small size they rarely attain clinical significance (Emmett and Braasch; Wesson). The cysts may be congenital or acquired. Acquired cysts may be classified as follows: (1) retention cysts, which are the result of occlusion of the prostatic ducts; (2) cystic adenoma; and (3) cysts which occur in connection with carcinoma undergoing degeneration (Emmett and Braasch; Kirkland and Bale; Melen). By far the most common prostatic cyst is the simple retention cyst. Obstructive symptoms predominate and occur most often during the fifth and sixth decades of life (Emmett and Braasch). Digital rectal examination reveals a 1-cm to 2-cm cystic mass to one side of the midline and in continuity with the prostate (Melen). Endoscopically the rounded mass may be seen to deform the vesical neck or posterior urethra. The fluid obtained by aspiration does not contain spermatozoa, which helps differentiate prostatic cysts from cysts of the seminal vesicle. Urethrography may demonstrate a curvature or filling defect in the posterior urethra (Rieser and Griffin). Vesiculography will outline the normal seminal vesicle, but there may be alteration in the course of the ejaculatory duct (Figs. 9–341 and 9–342). Other deep pelvic cysts will also displace the ejaculatory duct, so this alone is not a diagnostic sign (see Fig. 9–326).

GARTNER'S DUCT CYST

In the female the remnants of the distal portion of the wolffian duct remaining in the cervical and vaginal walls are known as Gartner's ducts. If the ureter remains connected to Gartner's duct, an ectopic ureteral orifice will open into the vagina or vestibule. Cystic dilatations of Gartner's duct are usually small and of no urologic consequence. Occasionally, however, the cystic dilatation may become large enough to cause urographic abnormalities (Fig. 9–343).

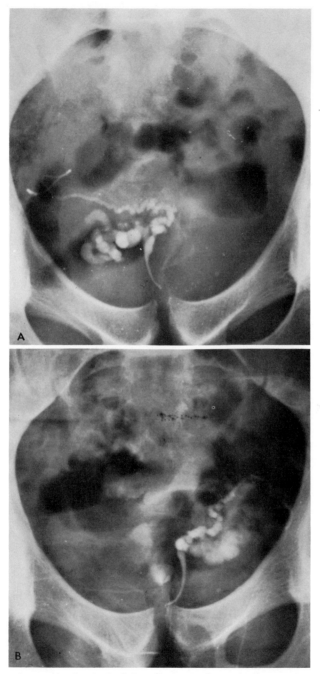

Figure 9–341. Cyst of prostate gland of adult male. **A,** *Right seminal vesiculogram* demonstrates convex course of ejaculatory duct as it passes around cyst. **B,** *Left seminal vesiculogram* with similar convexity. (From Rieser, C., and Griffin, T. L.)

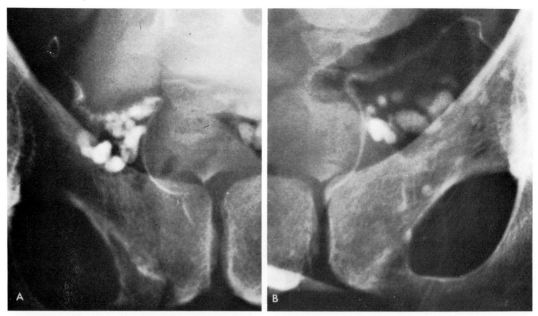

Figure 9–342. Cyst of prostate gland. A, *Right,* and B, *left retrograde seminal vesiculograms* reveal curvilinear lateral deviations of ejaculatory ducts around margins of cyst. (From Rieser, C., and Griffin, T. L.)

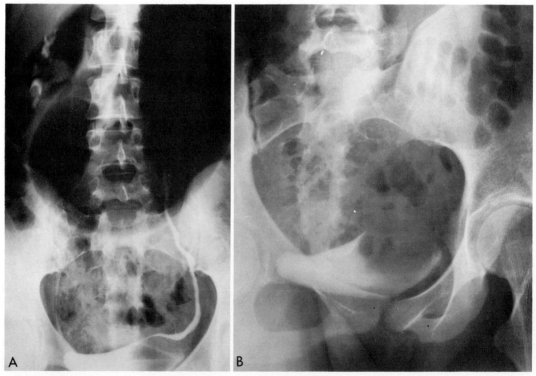

Figure 9–343. Cyst of Gartner's duct. Woman aged 20 with nontender cystic mass palpable in left vaginal fornix. *Excretory urogram.* A, Normal-appearing upper tract with terminal left ureter being pushed upward by rounded mass. B, Radiolucent mass left side of bladder noted on *excretory cystogram.* Exploration revealed cystic mass attached to left side of vagina with intimate relationship to posterior bladder and left lower ureter. (From Rhame, R. C., and Derrick, F. C., Jr.)

CONGENITAL ABSENCE OF THE ABDOMINAL MUSCLES (PRUNE BELLY SYNDROME)

Congenital absence of the abdominal muscles is one part of a triad of abnormalities in which the other two common components are various abnormalities of the urinary tract and undescended testes. Williams and Burkholder found 120 cases in the literature, as of 1967, and added 20 of their own. At about the same time, Bourne and Cerny reported 6 cases, which would bring the total to 146 (140 males and 6 females). The full syndrome is seen only in the male. Approximately 20 per cent of affected persons are stillborn, and 50 per cent die within the first two years of life. Complete or partial absence or deficiency of the transversus abdominis, rectus, internal oblique, and external oblique muscles is usually noted. At times a thin fibrous sheet or even a thin lax muscular layer is found, but often there is nothing but fat between the skin and peritoneum. The skin is wrinkled and lies in redundant folds ("prune belly"). Other associated but less common anomalies are "pigeon breast," malrotation of the gastrointestinal tract, and some form of talipes.

The cause of the absence of abdominal muscles is not clear. It has been suggested (Stumme) that obstruction at, or distal to, the vesical neck exists in utero and results in distention of the bladder with secondary ureteral dilatation and hydronephrosis. As a result of pressure exerted by the distended bladder against the abdominal wall, atrophy of the abdominal muscles occurs. Other workers, on the other hand, have suggested that faulty development of the musculature is the primary defect and that the urinary abnormalities are secondary. Proponents of this theory have expressed the belief that absence of the abdominal muscles, which constitute accessory muscles of urination, permits incomplete emptying of the bladder with resultant dilatation of the bladder, ure-

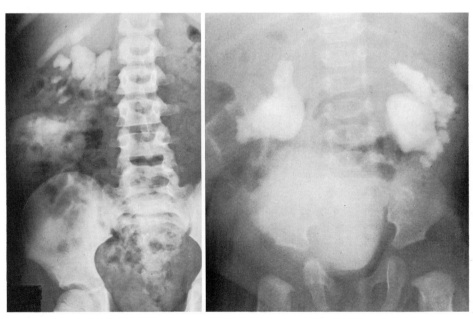

Fig. 9–344   **Fig. 9–345**

Figure 9–344.   Congenital absence of abdominal muscles in boy, 3½ years of age. *Excretory urogram, anteroposterior view.* No function in left kidney. Marked dilatation of right ureter which follows contour of relaxed abdominal wall down to bladder.

Figure 9–345.   Congenital deficiency of abdominal muscles in boy, 4 months of age. *Excretory urogram,* 3-hour film. Bladder is partially filled with medium, and fundus can be seen projecting up toward relaxed abdominal muscles. (Courtesy of Dr. B. I. Levatin.)

ters, and kidneys. More recently, however, Nunn and Stephens advanced an embryologic theory which suggests that the three systems involved in this triad may have been subjected at a certain stage of development to stimuli that have set in motion this series of anomalies: imperfect muscularization of the abdominal wall, imperfect musculariza-

Fig. 9–346

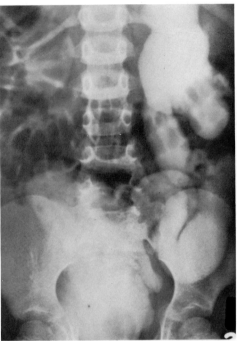

Figure 9–346. Congenital absence of abdominal musculature. *Excretory urogram.* Atrophic hydronephrotic kidney on right and huge pyeloureterectasis with tortuous ureter on left. (Courtesy of Dr. L. R. Devanney.)

Figure 9–347. Congenital absence of abdominal musculature. *Retrograde cystogram.* Large smooth bladder. Vesicoureteral reflux outlines tortuous and widely dilated ureters.

Figure 9–348. Congenital absence of abdominal musculature in young male. *Voiding cystogram.* Large smooth-walled bladder with wide-open funnel-shaped vesical neck.

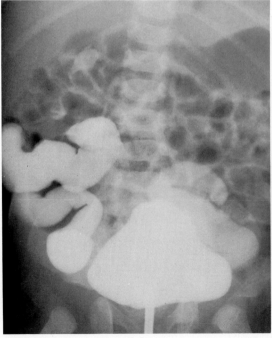

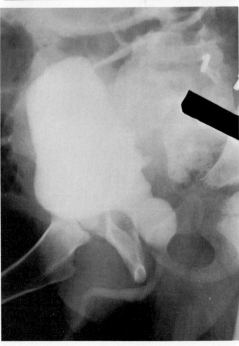

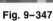

Fig. 9–347   Fig. 9–348

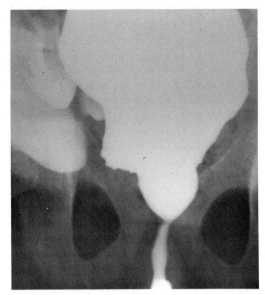

Figure 9–349. Congenital absence of abdominal musculature. *Voiding cystourethrogram* (spot film). Large distended bladder with reflux up huge dilated tortuous right ureter. Dilatation of prostatic urethra suggested possible obstruction from urethral valves, but none was found.

tion and control of growth of the walls of the urinary tract, and imperfect descent of the testes.

Because of the multiple systems involved, and because the syndrome is found almost exclusively in males, Williams and Burkholder think there is reason for a strong suspicion that the condition is due to a sex-linked recessive trait. They assess the urinary problem as primarily one of imperfect development of the entire urinary tract; they think obstruction is rarely a significant factor.

Visualization of the upper part of the urinary tract by excretory urography is usually unsatisfactory in patients with this condition because renal function is impaired. In isolated instances, varying degrees of hydronephrosis or atrophy will be demonstrated, particularly in delayed films taken 2 to 4 hours after the initial injection of contrast medium. The ureters may be visualized and appear dilated, elongated, and tortuous. The ureters frequently are best visualized as a result of vesicoureteral reflux, which occurs during retrograde cys-

tography. The bladder appears large, smooth, and grossly irregular. In some instances a patent urachus may be demonstrated. Gross dilatation of the prostatic urethra, attributable to deficiency of muscle and prostatic tubules, may be demonstrated by voiding cystourethrography (Lattimer) (Figs. 9–344 through 9–349).

INTERSEXUALITY: GENITOGRAPHY IN THE INTERSEXUAL STATE

by Charles E. Shopfner

An infant is reared in the sex assigned at birth on the basis of the genital anatomy. It is important that the sex of rearing be proper because it is the most potent single factor in determination of gender or psychosexual orientation.

The resolution of a clinical intersex problem requires two acts: (1) the prompt assignment of a practical sex before gender role is established, and (2) subsequent treatment if necessary to give the patient sexual adequacy in the assigned sex. The following general principles serve as a guide:

(1) The sex of rearing must be assigned before the gender role is established.

(2) It is easier to make a sexually ambiguous individual into a female than into a male.

(3) The assigned sex must be in accordance with the anatomic capabilities rather than with the chromatin pattern and gonadal biopsy.

(4) Sex of rearing should be assigned on the basis of the anatomy of the entire genital tract rather than on the appearance of the external genitalia alone.

(5) Genitography, done accurately and promptly, provides the necessary information concerning the internal genital passages.

The demonstration of nuclear sex chromatin by Davidson and Smith and Moore and Barr and improved techniques of human chromosomal analysis by Tjio and Puck have resulted in the clinical concept that the sex of rearing is to be in accordance with the chromosomal pattern. Testicular biopsy has also been used as a guide in the assignment of sex for ambiguous individuals. The multiplicity and complexity of the irregularities of sexual differentiation do require that an entire series of clinical studies be done for a precise final diagnosis and treatment. These studies include determination of (1) the sex chromatin pattern, (2) the anatomy of the external genitalia, (3) the anatomy of the internal genitalia, (4) urinary hormonal excretion, and (5) gonadal nature (on the basis of biopsy). Errors in the management of intersex problems have been difficult to avoid in the past, not only because of incomplete understanding of the intersex problem itself but also because of the erroneous impression that the assigned sex must be in accordance with the chromatin pattern and the gonadal nature. An individual functions sexually with his internal and external genitalia and not with chromosomes and gonads. The assignment of the sex of rearing must be a practical one and as close to the anatomic capabilities as possible rather than to the chromatin pattern and gonadal nature.

Knowledge of the anatomy of the genital make-up is essential in the assignment of a practical sex, and only the anatomic make-up of the external genitalia is known from the physical examination. In regard to the internal genital anatomy, knowing the nature of the gonads is not required, but it is necessary to know the anatomic state of the internal genital passages, in particular to establish the presence of a vagina or a urogenital sinus or both. Genitography is the simplest and best procedure for providing this information. Many physicians are not aware that it provides anatomic information frequently not afforded by catheterization, cystoscopy, rectal palpation, or even surgical exploration. For genitography to take its rightful place in the management of the intersex problem, radiologists must assume an active consulting role, must have some knowledge of the basic problem, and must be familiar with

the altered embryology responsible for the genitographic anatomy in the various abnormal conditions.

The Nature of Sex

Hampson, Money, and Hampson listed seven components of sex (Table 9–1).

COMPONENTS OF SEX

Chromosomal Sex

Chromosomal sex is determined by the presence or absence of chromatin bodies beside the nuclei of epithelial or other somatic cells. Only chromosomal females (XX) possess such paranuclear satellites, and Barr (1955) has shown that these bodies are formed by the adherence of two X chromosomes. Chromosomal males (XY) are termed chromatin-negative and chromosomal females chromatin-positive (XX) (Barr, 1955).

The chromosomal sex does not indicate clinical or practical sex, and Plunkett and Barr admonish that

it is premature to equate female-type nuclei with genetic femaleness or male-type nuclei with genetic maleness, as a generalisation in errors of sex development, for our present methods give no direct information concerning the genes that are concerned with sex determination and sex differentiation.

Gonadal Sex

Normally the gonads differentiate in accordance with the chromosomal sex. The undifferentiated gonad has a cortex, which can only become an ovary, and a medulla, which can only become a testis (Grumbach, Blanc, and Engle). Testicular differentiation is recognizable by the beginning of the seventh week in human embryos, but ovarian differentiation occurs somewhat later (Boyd and Hamilton, 1955; Gillman; Grumbach, Van Wyk, and Wilkins). It must be emphasized that gonadal and chromosomal sex do not always agree and that micro-

Table 9–1.   **Seven Components of Sex According to Hampson, Money, and Hampson***

COMPONENT	VARIABLES	COMMENT
Chromosomal sex	Chromatin positive (XX)	
	Chromatin negative (XY)	
Gonadal sex	Testes Neither or both	Morphologic intersex
	Ovaries	
Internal genital anatomy	Müllerian (female)	
	Wolffian (male)	
External genital anatomy		
Hormonal sex	Androgenic	Effect at puberty
	Estrogenic	
Rearing sex	Sex assignment	Governed by genital anatomy
Gender	Sex orientation	Governed by rearing sex

*Modified from Shopfner, C. E., 1964.

scopic study of the gonads does not provide the answer to the question of the practical sex.

Internal Genital Sex

The internal genital ducts are neuter till the eighth week, when sexual differentiation begins (Jones and Scott). If there is testicular differentiation, masculine (wolffian-duct) development occurs. Feminine (müllerian-duct) growth takes place in the absence of testicular differentiation and before the appearance of ovarian differentiation (Boyd and Hamilton, 1948).

External Genital Sex

The external genital structures are derived from the urogenital sinus, genital tubercle, and labioscrotal folds. It is significant that their development begins at 12 weeks, when internal ductal differentiation is being completed (Boyd and Hamilton, 1948). As will be seen later, the development of the external genitalia appears to be directed by a stimulus different from that directing development of the internal genitalia.

Hormonal Sex

Hormonal sex is manifest at puberty and is determined by the hormonal output of the gonads. Healthy testes produce a male (androgenic) puberty, ovaries produce a female (estrogenic) puberty, and gonadal absence or abnormality may result in hormonal failure and absence of pubescence.

Rearing Sex

An infant is reared in the sex assigned at birth in accordance with the genital anatomy. The sex of rearing is the most potent single factor in determining the psychosexual orientation or gender.

Gender

Gender is determined by the sex of rearing and therefore is not determined at birth but becomes gradually evident during early life. Gender is not determined by chromosomes, gonads, hormones, or other somatic factors. Hampson, Money, and Hampson define gender as indicated by the things a person does and says to disclose himself or herself as a man or woman.

From the preceding it is evident that the sex of rearing must be made on the basis of the assignment of a practical sex which, in turn, will ensure the best possible gender role.

NORMAL SEXUAL DIFFERENTIATION

An understanding of genitographic anatomy is enhanced by familiarity with the factors that control normal sexual differentiation. Embryologic development

Table 9–2. **Genetic, Gonadal, and Hormonal Determinants and Inductors of Sex***

INDUCTOR	STRUCTURES DETERMINED BY INDUCTOR	SEXUAL DIFFERENTIATION	
		Normal	*Abnormal*
Primary-genetic, from ovum and sperm	Gonadal primordium	Ovaries Testes	Turner's syndrome Klinefelter's syndrome True hermaphrodite
Secondary, presence of testes (local)	Male internal genitalia	Absence yields normal female Presence yields normal male	Male pseudohermaphrodite (müllerian duct remnants)
Tertiary, hormonal: androgens from testes or extragonadal source	Male external genitalia	Absence yields normal female Presence yields normal male	Female pseudohermaphrodite (adrenocortical, iatrogenic, and idiopathic; also type associated with anal atresia)

*Modified from Shopfner, C. E., 1964.

and sexual differentiation of the genital tract can be considered as being under the control of inductors: primary (genetic), secondary (gonadal), and tertiary (hormonal) (Table 9–2) (Grumbach, Van Wyk, and Wilkins; Hampson, Money, and Hampson; Jones and Scott).

Primary induction is genetic, coming from the ovum and sperm of the mother and father. It determines the gonadal primordium. Normal primary induction produces ovaries in the female and testes in the male. Errors in primary induction result in gonadal dysgenesis, in such conditions as Klinefelter's and Turner's syndromes, and in true hermaphroditism.

Secondary induction determines the male internal genitalia and is in reality the presence of testes. Absence of secondary induction (testes) results in a normal female whereas the presence of secondary induction produces a normal male. Male pseudohermaphroditism in which there are remnants of the müllerian ducts is the result of imperfect secondary induction. Jost has demonstrated that early intrauterine castration of certain animals is invariably followed by feminine genital tract differentiation, whether the gonads have been destined to become ovaries or testes. In other words, wolffian (male) development requires induction by a functioning

testis, but müllerian (female) growth will occur in the absence of such induction regardless of the presence or absence of ovaries. Jost has also shown experimentally that a single testis is capable of directing wolffian growth only on its own side. Thus, there is only a male inductor and its action is local and not hormonal. This local action is best illustrated in human beings by the lateral true hermaphrodite, an intersexual person with a testis on one side and an ovary on the other, in whom wolffian development is restricted to the testicular side.

Jost has also disclosed that removal of one embryonal testis does not alter full bilateral masculinization of the urogenital sinus and external genitalia. This indicates that masculinization of the lower genital tract is the result of pervasive and not locally acting inductors. That these pervasive inductors are androgens is inferred from the fact that the lower genital tract of female embryos is masculinized after exposure to androgens, either iatrogenically or in the condition of adrenal hyperplasia. The testis thus produces an inductor, apparently androgenic, that directs the development of the lower genital tract. This is *tertiary induction.* Absence of it produces a normal female and normal presence of it, a normal male. Imperfect tertiary induction causes female pseudohermaphroditism, which is found idiopathically and in association with adrenal cortical hyperplasia, anal atresia, and administration of steroids to the mother.

EMBRYOLOGY

It is to be understood that the present state of our knowledge of the embryology of the genital system is replete with uncertainties, but detailed and complete information of genital-tract embryology is not necessary for the understanding of intersexual anatomy. It is important to recognize that the genital tract of every human being is in an indifferent state until the embryo reaches the 15- to 20-mm size (Blechschmidt), when differentiation into testis first becomes evident. The prior embryologic anatomy of the male and female embryo is identical. Development from this indifferent stage is determined by the previously

mentioned inductors, and both normal and abnormal anatomy can be traced directly back to this stage (Fig. 9–350). Testicular differentiation from the gonadal primordium begins when the embryo is approximately 6 to 8 weeks old (15- to 20-mm stage), but ovarian differentiation occurs considerably later, perhaps as late as the 40-mm stage.

At the time of the indifferent state the internal genital duct system consists of the wolffian and müllerian ducts and the urogenital sinus (Fig. 9–350). At this time the embryologic male or female internal genitalia will develop, depending on the presence or absence of testes (secondary induction). In the female, wolffian ducts do not become sexual structures. On the contrary, the müllerian ducts persist to differentiate into the uterine tubes, the uterus, and the upper part of the vagina. In the male, the wolffian ducts become the

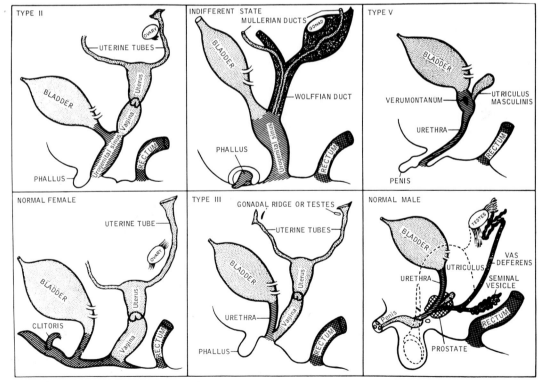

Figure 9–350. Sketches of embryologic anatomy illustrating development of normal and abnormal conditions from indifferent state. Stippling and cross-hatching are used to indicate contribution of müllerian ducts, wolffian ducts, and urogenital sinus in formation of normal as well as abnormal anatomic structures. Types II, III, and V are those referred to in genitographic classification (see Fig. 9–353). (From Shopfner, C. E., 1964.)

vasa deferentia and seminal vesicles, the müllerian ducts retrogress, and the urogenital sinus produces the prostate gland and the posterior part of the urethra.

Like other parts of the genital system, the external genitalia pass first through a period of indifference. At these early stages, the precursors of the external genitalia are the phallus, the urethral groove and folds, and the labioscrotal swellings. In the male, the phallus continues to develop to form a penis; the labioscrotal folds fuse in the midline to cover the urogenital sulcus, resulting in the formation of the scrotum and posterior urethra; and the tissues on the undersurface of the phallus develop and fuse across the midline to form the penile urethra. In the female, the urethral groove remains open and becomes the vulva, the urethral folds form the labia minora, the labioscrotal swellings elongate and become the labia majora, the urethral groove remains open, and the urogenital sinus makes a shallow vestibule containing the orifices of the urethra and vagina.

Technique of Genitography

The objective of genitography is to fill all of the internal genital passages adequately. It makes no difference what method is used as long as the objective is accomplished. In performing genitography, the radiologist should first examine the external genitalia carefully in search of openings. They may occur anywhere on a line from the tip of the phallus to the anus, but usually are located at the base of the phallus or in the perineum. There are many pits, depressions, and dimples that are not true openings, but each should be explored by probing.

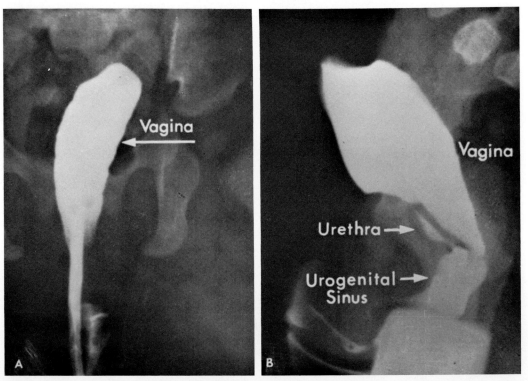

Figure 9–351. Female pseudohermaphrodite. *Genitography.* **A,** Injection was made with single catheter, and only normal vagina was filled. **B,** Injection of same patient was made by flushing method through blunt-nosed syringe. Tip of syringe is in urogenital sinus. Normal vagina and urethra enter sinus near end of syringe. Anatomy of female pseudohermaphrodite was not shown by single-catheter injection in **A.** (If catheter is used, its end should be just within perineal opening and flushing method should be employed to ensure filling of other passages.) (From Shopfner, C. E., 1964.)

Fluoroscopy is the essential feature in obtaining adequate genitography. Blind probing of openings and blind filling of cavities are inappropriate. Fluoroscopy ensures the control and motivation necessary for adequate filling and accurate positioning for spot-film documentation.

Either of two methods may be employed to ensure adequate filling of all genital cavities with opaque material: (1) the flushing technique and (2) the multiple-catheter technique.

FLUSHING TECHNIQUE

A leakage seal between the syringe and the perineum is necessary for the success of the flushing technique, previously described by Tristan and associates and by Shopfner (1964). Obtaining a leakproof seal allows the opaque material to be flushed into all cavities rather than into just one, as when catheter instillation is employed (Fig. 9–351). Flushing can best be accomplished by the use of a blunt-nosed syringe, with the tip of the syringe just inside the skin of the perineal opening and the glass of the barrel held firmly against the perineum to prevent leakage. Injection of opaque material under these conditions usually results in successful filling of all cavities.

MULTIPLE CATHETER TECHNIQUE

The multiple catheter technique is used only when the flushing technique fails. A hazard in this procedure is in placing the catheter in one cavity and missing others. If only one passage is found by probing under fluoroscopic monitoring, the tip of the catheter is withdrawn to a point just inside the skin of the perineum, which is held tightly around it, and the opaque material is injected again. When the catheters enter more than one passage, each is injected simultaneously by means of the flushing technique.

Selection of opaque media is not critical. Both oily and aqueous preparations have been used. Each has its advantages and disadvantages. An aqueous medium is easier to work with and fills the passages more readily. On the other hand, it will leak around the syringe and drain out of the passages more easily. It is suggested that an aqueous medium be tried first and that an oily medium be employed if success is not obtained.

Classification of Anatomy

Numerous classifications for intersex have been given (Jones and Scott; Wilkins; Wilkins and associates), but none can be used for genitographic findings. The simplest classification and also the best one for correlating with genitographic findings is morphologic. The categories are (1) true hermaphroditism, (2) female pseudohermaphroditism, and (3) male pseudohermaphroditism.

MORPHOLOGIC CLASSIFICATION

True Hermaphroditism

In true hermaphroditism, ovarian and testicular tissues are present in the same person. These may be joined together in ovotestes, or an ovary may occur on one side and a testis on the other. The internal and external genitalia are variable and ambiguous.

Female Pseudohermaphroditism

The female pseudohermaphrodite has ovaries, but the lower genital tract and external genitalia are masculinized.

Male Pseudohermaphroditism

The patient with male pseudohermaphroditism has testes and feminized genitalia.

GENITOGRAPHIC CLASSIFICATION

A classification has been proposed for genitography which assists in the interpretation of genitographic findings (Shopfner, 1964) (Fig. 9–352). The classification, originally based on the information obtained from genitographic findings in the case of 25 patients with ambiguous genitalia, remains as valid as when originally proposed. Its chief value is that anatomic information of assistance in assigning a practical sex is provided. Specifically, it affirms the existence of a vagina or urogenital sinus or both and shows the relationship of the urethra to them. It does not include those instances of true hermaphroditism or male pseudohermaphroditism with atretic or hypoplasic structures which do not communicate with the exterior of the body. Even so, the demonstration of only those parts communicating with the exterior is important

because of the principle that it is easier to transform a sexually ambiguous person into a cosmetically and coitally acceptable female than into a satisfactory male (Hamblen; Wilkins and associates).

A general survey of the classification (Fig. 9–352) reveals that a process of progressive masculinization is involved from type I through the intermediate types to type VI and that a process of progressive feminization is involved from type VI through the intermediate types to type I. Before individual examples of each of the types are considered, a few general comments are pertinent. Types I and II are due to imperfect tertiary induction, because development of the müllerian and wolffian ducts is that of the normal female, indicating absence of secondary induction. Types III, IV, and V have abnormal müllerian-duct remnants, indicating imperfect secondary induction. This can be primary or it

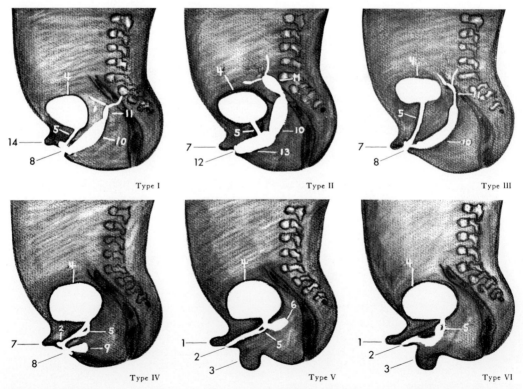

Figure 9–352. This **classification of intersex anatomy** is based strictly on genital passages filled at genitography. Numbers designate structures, as follows: 1, penis; 2, urethral orifice; 3, scrotum; 4, bladder; 5, urethra; 6, utriculus masculinus; 7, phallus; 8, vestibule orifice; 9, hypoplastic vagina; 10, normal-size vagina; 11, uterus; 12, orifice of urogenital sinus; 13, urogenital sinus; 14, hypertrophied clitoris. (From Shopfner, C. E., 1964.)

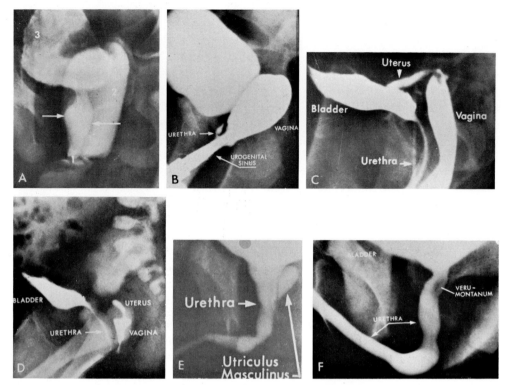

Figure 9–353. *Genitograms* of six different individuals for comparison with classification types in Figure 9–352. **A,** Type I; **B,** type II; **C,** type III, **D,** type V; and **F,** type VI. In **A,** urethra is marked 1, vagina, 2, and bladder, 3. (From Shopfner, C. E., 1967.)

can be associated with defective primary induction in a male embryo. Type VI, simple hypospadias, is imperfect tertiary induction, the same as type I but modified by normal secondary induction.

Progressive masculinization could produce any number of variable intermediate types between I and VI. However, correlation of clinical material has shown that the anatomic types have adhered very closely to the classification types (Fig. 9–353).

Type I Intersexuality

Type I (simple clitoral hypertrophy) is the simplest form of intersex anatomy (Fig. 9–353 *A*). The clitoris exists as an actual phallus. Normal female labioscrotal fusion has occurred, and there is a vestibule into which a urethra and vagina open in the usual location. There has been no secondary induction, and therefore no wolffian duct structures exist and the müllerian

duct structures are fully developed. Genitography shows the relationship of the urethra and vagina to each other and to the vestibule. Sometimes the uterus is opacified or an indentation caused by the uterine cervix is evident. These individuals have ovaries and should be raised as females. If the female gender is properly established, they lead perfectly acceptable sexual lives as females and can bear children. The only possible subsequent treatment required is revision of the phallus for cosmetic reasons. This condition is caused by an androgenizing effect on the genital tubercle.

Type II Intersexuality

Type II (Fig. 9–353 *B*) is the classical anatomy of the female pseudohermaphrodite. It represents an androgenizing effect not only on the genital tubercle as in type I but also on the urogenital sinus. The müllerian-duct structures are well developed and the wolffian ducts have regressed, indicating no secondary induction. There is a phallus, and the urogenital sinus orifice typically is located at its base. The urogenital sinus contains the catheter adaptor in the example and, entering into its upper portion, is the urethra and a fully formed vagina. The slight indentation at the top of the vagina is an indication of the uterine cervix. The presence of the normal-sized vagina is an indication for assignment of the female sex. These individuals have ovaries, result in reality from masculinized female fetuses, lead sexually acceptable lives, and can bear children. If necessary, the phallus can be cosmetically revised at a later date. A search must be made for the cause of the androgenization, because if it is adrenal cortical hyperplasia, the condition is life-threatening in itself.

Type III Intersexuality

Type III (Fig. 9–353 C) represents more masculinization. There is a phallus with the opening usually located in the perineum. Secondary induction has caused the urogenital sinus to grow into the formation of a longer, more male type urethra than in type II. The urethra can open separately or together with the fully formed vagina that has descended downward from the site of the old müllerian duct tubercle to the perineum. The uterus is fully formed. These individuals have had secondary induction, indicating the presence of some type of testicular tissue. They, therefore, are either male pseudohermaphrodites or true hermaphrodites.

The patient illustrated in Figure 9–353 C is a good example of the principle that the presence of a vagina of almost any size is an indication for the assignment of the female sex because of its being easier to transform a sexually ambiguous individual into a cosmetically and coitally acceptable female. The patient was first seen at birth, at which time the chromatin pattern, erroneously, was found to be female and the female sex was assigned on that basis.

When genitography was performed at age 7 months, it became obvious that this patient did have testicular tissue of some type; thus, the patient was a male pseudohermaphrodite. Fortunately, the female sex had been assigned on the basis of the erroneous interpretation of the chromatin pattern; for, despite the actual male chromatin pattern and the presence of testicular tissue, the presence of a fully formed vagina was adequate indication for the assignment of the female sex. If this is assigned early enough, permitting establishment of the female gender, such individuals function as sexually adequate females. However, they will be sterile, will need to have the testicular tissue removed, and possibly will require phallic revision at a later date.

Type IV Intersexuality

In type IV, with its greater degree of masculinization, the müllerian-duct structures are hypoplastic and their descent from the site of the müllerian tubercle is reduced. The patient has a phallus and a single perineal opening. The urogenital sinus has formed a longer, more male-type urethra than is found in type II. The hypoplastic müllerian-duct structures (the vagina and uterus) can open anywhere along the urethra from a point at the site of the old müllerian-duct tubercle to the perineum. Inadequate secondary induction is indicated by the presence of the müllerian-duct structures and indicates the presence of testicular tissue of some type, either male pseudohermaphroditism or true hermaphroditism. The vaginal structure will dilate with use and the assignment of the female sex approaches the anatomic capabilities. Assuming that a female gender has been established properly, these individuals function as sexually adequate females. They will be sterile and will need to have removal of testicular tissue and phallic revision at a later date.

Type V Intersexuality

Additional masculinization in type V has reduced the müllerian-duct development and descent so that a small saccular structure exists at the original site of the old müllerian tubercle. Such a patient has a phallus and commonly presents with hypospadias and testicles in the groin. It is important to demonstrate the müllerian-duct remnant (utriculus masculinus) because it has diagnostic significance. Some true hermaphrodites also present with hypospadias and groin testicles, and the surgeon is amazed to find a hypoplastic uterus and fallopian tubes in the hernial sac at the time of operation; these findings characterize lateralized true hermaphrodites. The demonstration of the utriculus masculinus indicates that a patient cannot be a true lateralized hermaphrodite because the müllerian duct cannot perform a dual function in forming the utriculus masculinus and the hypoplastic structures in the hernial sac. The urethra, longer and more the male type than that of type IV patients, has a perineal or subphallic orifice.

Type VI Intersexuality

Howard states that the association of a utriculus masculinus with hypospadias (type VI) is much more common than generally is believed, but few people regard it as an intersexual problem. However, it does truly represent incomplete masculinization of the external genitalia. The penis is characteristically underdeveloped and the orifice may be located anywhere on a line from the glans penis to the perineum. These patients present with a hypospadic penis and frequently have undescended testicles. The urethra is shortened but is of the male type with a verumontanum. No müllerian-duct remnant is present, and assignment of the male sex is necessary

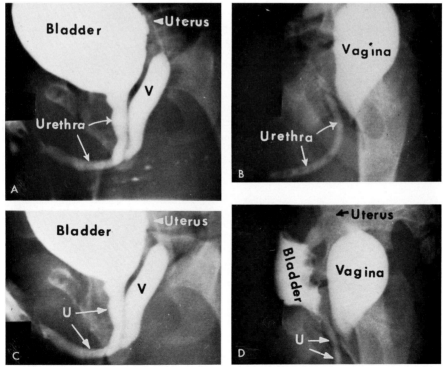

Figure 9–354. *Genitograms* of 18-month-old "male" (**A** and **C**) and 2½-year-old "male" (**B** and **D**), who were admitted to hospital for surgical correction of third-degree hypospadias. Each had **marked hypoplasia of penis** which in reality was nothing more than phallus. Fully formed vagina was present in each case, indicating that sexual function could be performed more adequately as female, if this sex and gender had been established at birth. (From Shopfner, C. E., 1967.)

unless reconstruction of the penis appears too formidable. In this event the female sex can be assigned if this is done early enough and if responsibility is accepted for surgical creation of a vagina at a later date.

That hypospadias must be considered an intersex problem is dramatically illustrated by the patients whose genitograms are shown in Figure 9–354.

Comment

Intersex problems cannot be ignored because of their rarity. They occur once in every 1,000 births (Young) and are even more common when one rightfully in-

cludes hypospadias which alone occurs in 1 out of 650 births (Williams). The importance of the intersex condition is emphasized by the realization that it is more common than such conditions as coarctation of the aorta (1:1,500) (Keith, Rowe, and Vlad), anal atresia (1:5,000) (Young), and esophageal atresia (1:1,600) (Feldman). Intersex is not a problem limited to children's hospitals and pediatric radiologists. These infants are born in general hospitals, and adequate prompt genitography needs to be performed regardless of whether or not there is a children's hospital nearby.

The early assignment of a practical sex as near the anatomic capability as possible cannot be sufficiently emphasized. There is

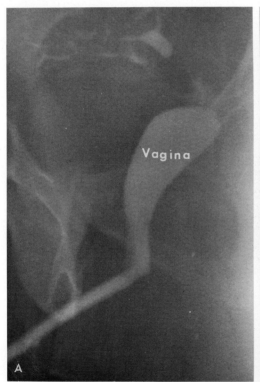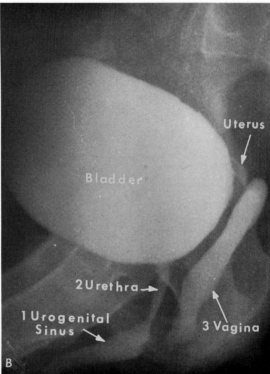

Figure 9–355. Female pseudohermaphrodite. *Genitograms* of 38-year-old "male" admitted to hospital because of hematuria which had been recurrent at monthly intervals since age of 13 years. He had had feeding problem as infant and had had episodes of weakness, nausea, vomiting, and near prostration at ages 8 and 13 years. He professed no interest in female sex. Physical examination revealed phallus, partial labioscrotal fusion, single perineal opening at base of phallus, sparse beard, and minimal breast development. **A,** This shows inadequacy of method of simply inserting catheter and injecting medium which fills only vagina and uterus. **B,** Better filling is obtained with flushing technique, demonstrating urogenital sinus (1) containing openings of urethra (2) and vagina (3). This anatomy is of so-called female pseudohermaphrodite. Patient has mild adrenal hyperplasia which caused masculinization of genital tract. Such persons can lead sexually acceptable lives as females and can bear children. This 38-year-old "male" should have been raised as female, but instead is being forced to live as male because of improper assignment of sex. (From Shopfner, C. E., 1967.)

much uncertainty concerning the age at which gender is established and when the sex of rearing can be successfully changed. These questions arise only when an error in medical management has been committed. There is no uncertainty about the principle that the sex of rearing must be properly assigned in accordance with the anatomic capabilities at birth—when it is *known* that gender is not established—thus avoiding the necessity of a change at a later date.

Genitography should not replace any previously used diagnostic methods. It is a requisite for the demonstration of the internal genital passages, knowledge of which is vital to the early assignment of a practical sex. It should be performed during the first days of life, and certainly no commitment as to sex assignment should be made until it has been done. Proper application of genitographic findings to intersex problems can prevent many tragic errors of sex assignment such as have been made in the past (Fig. 9–355).

UROLOGIC ASPECTS OF ECTOPIC ANUS (IMPERFORATE ANUS; ANAL ATRESIA)

by Charles E. Shopfner

The time-honored inverted films of the abdomen can no longer be accepted as providing adequate roentgenographic examination in an infant with ectopic anus. In 1930, Wangensteen and Rice described the method of taking roentgenograms of the inverted infant. The purpose of this method is to allow the gas to rise to the termination of the rectum and indicate the distance between the skin and the end of the rectum (Fig. 9–356). Ladd and Gross first recommended surgical treatment based on roentgenologic findings. They suggested perineal repair if the rectal air was within 1.5 cm of the anus and intraperineal repair if the distance was greater than this. Scott and Swenson advocated treatment based

on high and low lesions as determined by roentgenologic identification of the relationship of the rectal air to the pubosacral line.

Advancing knowledge and experience have shown that these concepts, based on the inverted film, are no longer tenable. *Imperforate anus* is a broad term applied to various obstructive malformations of the terminal bowel, but most lesions to which it is applied are obviously not imperforate. Imperforate anus is an obvious finding, but it is not the essential feature of this condition. *Urogenital fistula* is the most important associated abnormality to investigate, since its location and extent determine the surgical procedure required to correct the anomaly (Bill and Johnson; Brayton and Norris; Winslow, Litt, and Altman).

Inverted films not only are incapable of demonstrating the ectopic anus (fistula) but also provide inaccurate information 40 per cent of the time (Shopfner, 1965b). Fac-

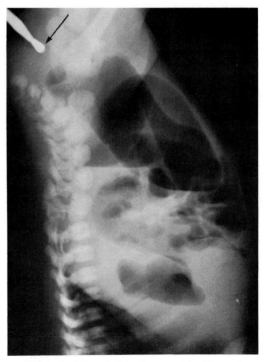

Figure 9–356. Infant born with "imperforate anus." *Plain film* (lateral view) with infant suspended by feet. Gas outlines rectum terminating about 2 cm proximal to anal dimple marked by thermometer (*arrow*). (Courtesy of Dr. C. D. Creevy.)

tors responsible for the diagnostic inaccuracy of the inverted film are: (1) presence of packed meconium in terminal portion of the blind segment, (2) improper placement of the anal marker, (3) mistaken interpretation of gas in the vagina or small bowel as being within the rectum, (4) roentgenologic magnification and distortion, (5) spasm of the levator ani muscle, (6) insufficient time for air to reach the distal blind segment, (7) inaccurate identification of pubosacral line, and (8) ascent and descent of levator sling with crying and straining. There is a sound embryologic basis for expecting that all children lacking an obvious anal opening in the normal location will have an ectopic opening either in a "high" or "low" location. Therefore, the terms *imperforate anus* and *anal atresia* should be discarded and replaced by the anatomic descriptive term of *ectopic anus*.

Embryology

The rectum and the urogenital system have their origin from the cloaca in both sexes (Blechschmidt; Shopfner, 1965b). The cloaca initially contains openings through which enter the allantoic and mesonephric ducts and the hindgut (Fig. 9–357 A). The urorectal septum grows downward to separate the cloaca into the urogenital sinus anteriorly and the rectum posteriorly (Fig. 9–357 B). The descent of the urorectal septum makes the rectal (hindgut) aperture descend steadily lower in the posterior part of the cloaca until finally it is brought to the perineal area, where it is prevented from showing externally by that portion of the cloacal membrane known as the *anal plate* (Fig. 9–357 C and D). The anal plate is formed by the ingrowth of mesodermal tissue between the urogenital

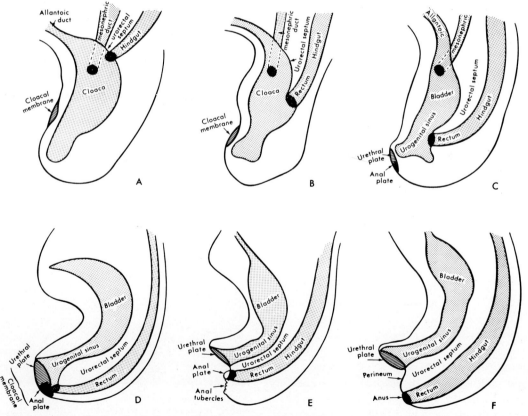

Figure 9–357. Embryologic descent (A through F) of urorectal septum that separates cloaca into anterior urogenital sinus and posterior hindgut (rectum). Early arrest of descent results in high ectopic anus (**C**). Late arrest produces ectopic anus either at posterior fourchette (**D**) or in perineum (**E**). (From Shopfner, C. E., 1965b.)

and rectal epithelial surfaces of the urorectal septum, separating the anal plate from the posterior portion of the cloacal membrane. The remaining portion of the cloacal membrane is the *urethral plate*. The lower end of the rectum at this stage is positioned above the independently developing anus and its musculature. Further descent of the rectum coincides with that of the anal tubercles, placing the rectal aperture at its definitive site in the perineum (Fig. 9–357 E and F). Failure of adequate caudad migration of the rectal aperture down the posterior wall of the cloaca leads to a connection between the pars pelvina of the urogenital sinus and the rectum (Bill and Johnson; Shopfner, 1965b; Winslow, Litt, and Altman).

After the urorectal septum has fully descended, only a small channel, the cloacal duct or duct of Reichel, connects the hindgut with the urogenital sinus. It closes by the time the hindgut aperature reaches its definitive site and joins with the independently developing anal tubercle (de Vries and Friedland).

Since the pars pelvina gives rise to the prostatic and membranous portions of the male urethra, the so-called rectourethral fistula associated with imperforate anus opens into this posterior portion of the urethra. An equivalent failure of caudad migration of the rectal opening in the female results in persistence of the urogenital sinus, and an ectopic anus is created which opens anywhere on a line along the path of caudad descent of the urorectal septum, but is usually located at the superior (Fig. 9–357 C) or inferior (Fig. 9–357 D) extremity of the persistent urogenital sinus. This is the explanation for the so-called high-vaginal and posterior-fourchette fistulas traditionally described as occurring in females with imperforate anus. Strictly speaking, the "fistula" is not a fistula but an ectopic anus, and it does not communicate with the vagina but rather with a persistent urogenital sinus.

Large numbers of infants, in reported series of cases of imperforate anus, are known definitely to have had abnormal communications ("fistulas") between the rectum and the derivatives of the urogenital sinus or perineum (Bradham; Hamm and Harlin; Ladd and Gross; Scott and Swenson). Bill, Johnson, and Foster reported such a connection in 64 of 68 cases. They also think that this connection represents an ectopic rectal opening or anus and that it may occur anywhere along the course of rectal descent, which *in the male* is from the bladder neck to the urethra and perineum and *in the female* is from the high portion of the vagina to the fourchette and perineum.

Doubts as to the "fistulous" nature of the openings also have been raised by Gans and Friedman. They made histopathologic observations indicating that these tracts are lined in part by transitional epithelium identical to that seen in the normal anorectal canal. Therefore, they think the normal anorectal canal is a junctional "cloacal" zone between rectal mucosa and anal epidermis, which contains genitourinary glandular appendages that routinely may be seen as one studies microscopically all the tissue removed at hemorrhoidectomy. Recent studies of de Vries and Friedland confirm the descent of the urorectal septum and its arrest as the embryologic explanation for ectopic anus. They also offer persistence of the cloacal duct or duct of Reichel as the explanation for the rare "H-type" of anorectal fistula without anal atresia. Arrest of urorectal septum growth and descent prior to closure of Reichel's duct leads to the formation of a fistula opening into the dorsal wall of what becomes the membranous urethra in the normal embryo.

Technique of Roentgen Examination

The radiologist should first inspect the perineum in search of openings. There will be a dimple, not a deep pit, where the anus would normally be expected. This dimple will usually pucker on stimulation by pinprick because the independently developing anal musculature is present in a hypoplastic if not a normal state.

A perineal ectopic anus may be located anywhere on a line between the scrotum and anal dimple in the male, and between the fourchette and the anal dimple in the female. This opening will not respond to pinprick. If such an opening is found, it should be injected by the flushing technique, usually best accomplished with a blunt-nosed syringe, its tip being just inside the perineal opening. The barrel of the syringe is pressed firmly against the skin of the perineum to obtain a leakproof seal, and the opaque material is flushed into the tract leading to the rectum. A small catheter or cannula may be employed if the opening is too small to receive the tip of the syringe. It is important that the contrast medium not be instilled into the rectum, because a true picture of the anatomy may not be obtained (Fig. 9–358). In the event that there is no perineal opening, a search

is made for an opening in the vagina of the female and the urethra of the male. *Vaginography* is performed by the flushing technique, using a blunt-nosed syringe with its barrel pressed firmly against the skin to obtain a leakproof seal. *In the male, urethrography* is performed in the same manner with the syringe pressed against the glans penis. Sometimes the opaque material goes into the bladder so easily that an ectopic anus is not filled. A Foley catheter inserted into the bladder with the balloon pulled tightly against the bladder neck may divert the contrast agent into the ectopic opening.

The choice of an opaque material is not critical. An aqueous medium will usually suffice. Occasionally an oily material is injected because its increased viscosity keeps the cavities filled longer and more clearly.

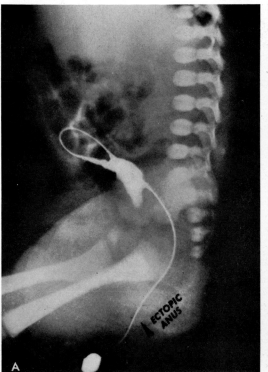 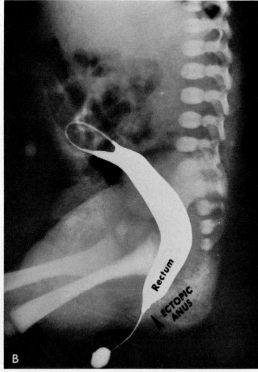

Figure 9–358. Perineal ectopic anus. A, Catheter has been inserted good distance through ectopic anus, and instillation of opaque material caused erroneous impression of high rectal pouch. Rectum distal to opaque material is packed with meconium. **B,** Overlay of **A,** showing rectum as it was demonstrated by flushing technique, with tip of catheter just inside skin of perineal ectopic anus. (From Shopfner, C. E., 1965a).

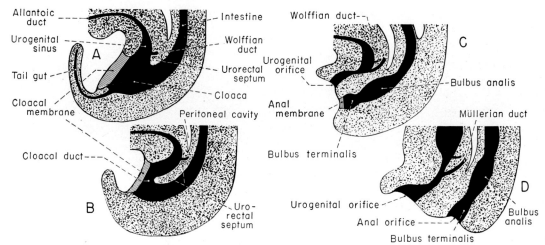

Figure 9–359. A to D, Normal development of rectum and anus. (Adapted from Ladd, W. E., and Gross, R. E.)

Classification of Roentgen Findings

The classification of imperforate anus as given by Ladd and Gross (see Figs. 9–359 through 9–363) is not applicable as a guide for roentgenologic findings, because it does not take into consideration the presence of an ectopic opening. Some physicians simply classify imperforate anus as "high" or "low" on the basis of physical examination (Berdon and associates). Classifications based on the essential feature, the

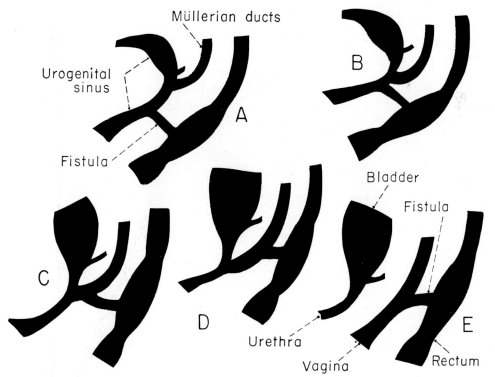

Figure 9–360. Method of production of rectovaginal fistulas. As müllerian ducts descend, they encounter and acquire any existing rectal fistula. A, 22-mm stage (7 weeks). B, C, D, and E, Successive stages in development of müllerian system and its separation from urinary apparatus. (Adapted from Ladd, W. E., and Gross, R. E.)

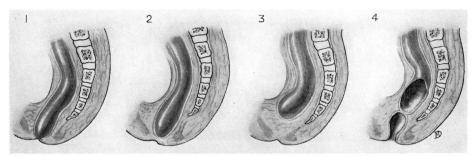

Figure 9–361. Types of anal and rectal abnormalities. **Type 1, Stenosis at anus. Type 2, Imperforate anus.** Obstruction only by persistent membrane. **Type 3, Imperforate anus.** Rectal pouch ending blindly some distance above anus. **Type 4, Anus and anal pouch normal.** Rectal pouch ends blindly in hollow of sacrum. (From Gross, R. E.)

ectopic anus ("fistula"), have been proposed by Scott and Swenson, Gans and Friedman, and Browne. These are unduly complicated and detailed for interpretation of the roentgenographic findings.

A preliminary classification of roentgenographic findings is proposed as an aid to the radiologist (Fig. 9–364). This is based on the findings obtained in 16 cases (Shopfner, 1965a). Subsequent experience has been gained with 13 additional patients, and the classification remains as helpful as when originally proposed. The site of the ectopic opening, the length of the tract leading to the normal-sized rectum, and the presence of a urogenital sinus in the female are the essential features of this classification. Its value lies in the provision of anatomic information of assistance in the surgical management of the infant with imperforate anus.

A tract leading to the rectum was 3 to 4 cm long in two of the males with a rec-

tourethral opening (type IA) (Fig. 9–365 and 9–366) but was 1 cm long in the other two (type IB) (Fig. 9–367). Six of the perineal openings had a tract, approximately 1 cm long, leading to a normal rectum of normal caliber (type IIA). In the other three cases, the tract was about 2 cm long (type IIB). All females with an opening between the urogenital sinus and rectum had a tract 1 cm long (type III). The reason for the difference in length of the tracts or why one is present is not definitely known. There seems to be no relation between the length of the tract and the degree of caudad migration of the opening.

Failure of the urorectal septum to descend below the urogenital sinus causes a persistence of the sinus, with the müllerian duct structures (vagina and uterus) entering it above the site of the ectopic anus (type III (Figs. 9–368 and 9–369). If the urorectal septum descends below the urogenital sinus, the müllerian duct structures sepa-

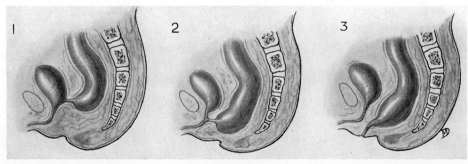

Figure 9–362. Types of fistulas encountered in male patients. **Type 1, Rectovesical fistula. Type 2, Rectourethral communication. Type 3, Rectoperineal fistula** (opening being in front of area where anus should normally open). (From Gross, R. E.)

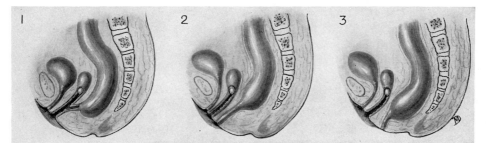

Figure 9–363. Types of fistulas encountered in female patients. **Type 1, Rectovaginal fistula. Type 2, Rectofossa navicularis fistula. Type 3, Rectoperineal fistula.** (From Gross, R. E.)

rate from it and descend to the perineum. The ectopic anal opening is then located anywhere on a line from the posterior fourchette to the independently developing anal tubercles. All females observed to have the ectopic anal opening above the fourchette have had a persistent urogenital sinus and type III anatomy. There have been numerous reports of low rectovaginal openings with a separate urethral orifice, and these are in the category of the fourchette ectopic anus. The high rectovaginal fistulas reported can probably be classified type III on the basis of current experience. Many patients have been described as having a rectovesical fistula, but the existence of such a lesion should be questioned on the basis of current knowledge. Accurate

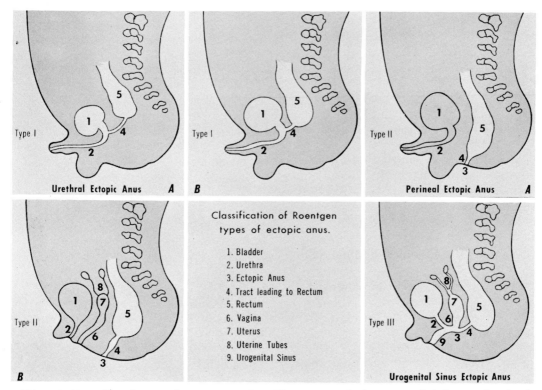

Figure 9–364. Classification of ectopic anus. Type IIB represents both posterior fourchette and perineal ectopic anus in female. They are considered synonymously because, in each, urorectal septum descent has separated ectopic anal opening from urogenital sinus, thus allowing normal development of vestibule, urethra, and vagina. (From Shopfner, C. E., 1965a.)

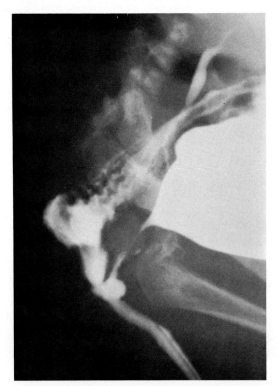

Figure 9–365. Posterior urethral ectopic anus (type IA). *Urethrogram.* Newborn boy with multiple congenital anomalies including myelomeningocele, patent omphalomesenteric duct, posterior urethra, ectopic anus, solitary left kidney with vesicoureteral reflux, and probable crossed fused renal ectopia (Courtesy of Department of Urology and Department of Radiology [Dr. V. C. Payne, Jr., Pediatric Radiologist], Harbor General Hospital, Torrance, California.)

roentgenographic demonstration of the ectopic anus and its relationship to the other anatomic structures will reduce some of the confusion.

Associated Congenital Anomalies

Other anomalies occur in patients with imperforate anus (Table 9–3) (Shopfner, 1965b). Associated anomalies are much more common in patients who have a high ectopic anus, but they do occur in those who have a low one. This is particularly true for vertebral and renal anomalies. It is well to emphasize that sacral and vertebral anomalies are almost invariably associated

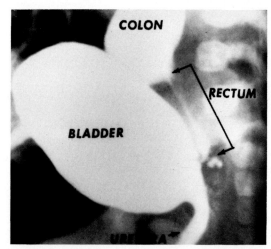

Figure 9–366. Ectopic anus opening at urethrovesical juncture. *Flushing retrograde urethorgram.* The "fistulous" tract from the ectopic anal opening in the posterior urethra to the colon is outlined. (From Shopfner, C. E., 1965b.)

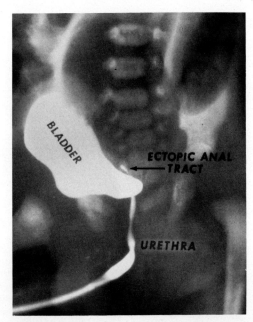

Figure 9–367. Ectopic anus opening in the posterior urethra. Male aged 12 hours. *Flushing retrograde urethrogram.* A, Ectopic anal tract 1 cm long is seen. No contrast material entered the rectum, but this is not essential, because identification of the ectopic anus indicates the need for a colostomy. Definitive demonstration of the tract leading to the rectum can be done later before corrective surgery. (From Shopfner, C. E., 1965a.)

with neurogenic deficiencies of the bladder. It is apparent that such associated anomalies may influence selection of an operative procedure and that they constitute a hazard that will affect the results of treatment.

Suggested Method of Management

On the basis of embryologic, surgical, and associated-anomaly considerations, the roentgenologic evaluation of the infant with imperforate anus has two objectives: (1) demonstration of an ectopic anus and (2) detection of associated anomalies. If either a perineal or a fourchette ectopic anus exists, demonstration of it and the associated "fistulous" tract can be accomplished very easily in the neonatal period.

Table 9–3. **Associated Anomalies in 68 Cases of Imperforate Anus***

ANOMALY	NO.	%
Hypoplasia of sacrum	13	19
Hypoplasia of long bones	3	4.4
Club foot	1	1.5
Congenital heart disease	10	15
Genitourinary abnormality (absent kidney, fusion anomaly, duplication anomaly, or polycystic kidney)	21	31
Gastrointestinal abnormality (esophageal atresia or small bowel atresia)	6	8.8
Abnormality of nervous system (mongolism, cerebral agenesis, or hydrocephalus)	4	5.9

*Modified from Shopfner, C. E., 1965b.

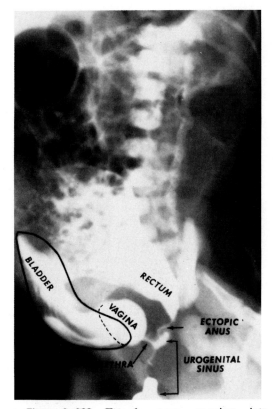

Figure 9–368. Ectopic anus opening into urogenital sinus. Newborn female. *Flushing retrograde urogenital sinogram.* Rectum opens into urogenital sinus, which also receives vagina and urethra. (From Shopfner, C. E., 1965b.)

Roentgenographic demonstration of the urethral or urogenital-sinus ectopic anus and tract is not always so easy. Making certain of a leakproof seal, irrigating the urethra and vagina with sterile water, and using a Foley catheter balloon in the bladder of the male patient to divert the opaque material have been helpful. Actually, the demonstration of the ectopic anus in a high location can be deferred, since most investigators believe that a colostomy is the recommended procedure for this situation. The demonstration of the ectopic anus can be made much easier when the infant is several months old. Some of the lesions have been demonstrated in the neonatal period, but the information is unnecessary if only a colostomy is to be performed. After colostomy, the ectopic anus may be filled either from below or from above via the distal colonic stoma.

For detection of associated anomalies, routine examination of the chest, abdomen, spine, and genitourinary tract is recommended. It is reemphasized that the abdominal film need not be inverted. Of particular importance in this examination is the detection of air in the bladder (Fig. 9–370). Evaluation of the genitourinary tract is very important, and it should be of the entire system, including both a cystogram and an excretory urogram. The method previously described is especially recommended (Shopfner, 1965c).

Comment

The classification of imperforate anus as given by Ladd and Gross is no longer applicable as a guide for roentgenologic findings. Rectal stenosis with a normal anus (type I) may not exist except as Hirschsprung's disease (Bill, Johnson, and Foster) or as congenital stenosis which occurs elsewhere in the colon. Each is on a different embryologic basis than is imperforate anus. Type II, a membrane covering the anus with no ectopic opening, may not exist at all according to Browne, who has never encountered one in a very wide ex-

perience. Type III represents the rectum ending blindly with an ectopic opening and is the type which most patients have had in all reported series. All patients with an absent anal opening must be considered as having this type, which essentially is an ectopic anus.

Patients having atresia of the rectum with a normal anal opening (type IV) should be considered as having atresia of the bowel, such as occurs in other locations of the colon and small bowel. Atresia is a different embryologic entity than is ectopic anus; the latter is not atresia but rather a failure of descent of the rectum.

The flushing injection technique is an innocuous procedure when carefully and properly done. The only complication encountered resulted from the overzealous

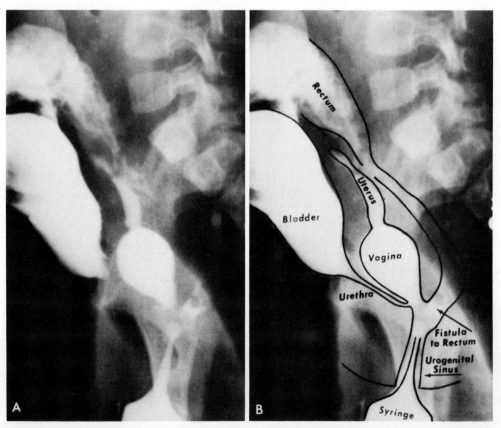

Figure 9–369. Ectopic anus opening into urogenital sinus. Female pseudohermaphrodite. **A** and **B,** *Flushing retrograde urogenital sinogram.* All internal passages including the urogenital sinus, ectopic anus with its "fistulous" tract, vagina, uterus, urethra, and bladder are outlined. **B,** Overlay identifying anatomic structures. (From Shopfner, C. E., 1965a.)

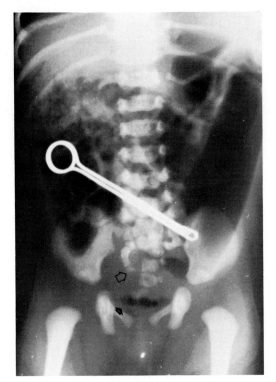

Figure 9–370. Hypoplasia and malformation of sacrum *(upper arrow)*. There is air in bladder *(lower arrow)*. (From Shopfner, C. E., 1965b.)

use of a long metal cannula which penetrated the urogenital sinus of one female patient.

REFERENCES

Abeshouse, B. S.: Diverticula of the Anterior Urethra in the Male: A Report of Four Cases and a Review of the Literature. Urol. & Cutan. Rev. 55:690–707 (Nov.) 1951.

Abeshouse, B. S., and Bhisitkul, I.: Crossed Renal Ectopia With and Without Fusion. Urol. internat. 9:63–91, 1959.

Abrahamson, J.: Double Bladder and Related Anomalies: Clinical and Embryological Aspects and a Case Report. Brit. J. Urol. 33:195–214 (June) 1961.

Abramson, D., Roberts, S. M., and Wilson, P. D.: Relaxation of the Pelvic Joints in Pregnancy. Surg., Gynec. & Obst. 58:595–613 (Mar.) 1934.

Alfert, H. J., and Gillenwater, J. Y.: Ectopic Vas Deferens Communicating With Lower Ureter: Embryological Considerations. J. Urol. 108:172–173 (July) 1972.

Allansmith, R.: Ectopic Ureter Terminating in Seminal Vesicle: Unilateral Polycystic Kidney; Report of a Case and Review of the Literature. J. Urol. 80:425–435 (Dec.) 1958.

Amar, A. D.: Lateral Ureteral Displacement: Sign of Non-Visualized Duplication. J. Urol. 105:638–641 (May) 1971.

Ambrose, S. S., and Nicolson, W. P.: Ureteral Reflux in Duplicated Ureters. J. Urol. 92:439–444 (Nov.) 1964.

Arduino, L. J.: Crossed Renal Ectopia Without Fusion. J. Urol. 93:125–126 (Feb.) 1965.

Arey, L. B.: Developmental Anatomy, Rev. Ed. 7, Philadelphia, W. B. Saunders Company, 1974, pp. 325, 333, and 336.

Arnold, J.: Ein Fall von Uterus masculinus, angeborner Strictur der Harnröhre und hochgradiger Dilatation der Harnblase und Harnleiter. Arch. path. Anat. 47:7–39, 1869.

Arnold, M. W., and Kaylor, W. M.: Double Urethra: Case Report. J. Urol. 70:746–748 (Nov.) 1953.

Ashley, D. J. B., and Mostofi, F. K.: Renal Agenesis and Dysgenesis. J. Urol. 83:211–230 (Mar.) 1960.

Bacon, S. K.: Large Hydronephrosis of a True Supernumerary Kidney. J. Urol. 57:459–466 (Mar.) 1947; Tr. West. Sect., Am. Urol. A. 13:18–25, 1946.

Baggenstoss, A. H.: Congenital Anomalies of the Kidney. M. Clin. North America, July, 1951, pp. 987–1004.

Barr, M. L.: In Bowes, K. (Ed.): Modern Trends in Obstetrics and Gynecology. London, Butterworth and Company, Second Series, 1955, p. 117.

Barr, M. L.: Cytological Tests of Sex. Lancet 1:47 (Jan. 7) 1956.

Barr, M. L.: Sex Chromatin and Phenotype in Man. Science 130:679–685 (Sept. 18) 1959.

Bearman, S., Sanders, R. C., and Oh, K. S.: B-Scan Ultrasound in the Evaluation of Pediatric Abdominal Masses. Radiology 108:111–117 (July) 1973.

Beeby, D. I.: Seminal Vesicle Cyst Associated With Ipsilateral Renal Agenesis: Case Report and Review of Literature. J. Urol. 112:120–122 (July) 1974.

Begg, R. C.: The Urachus and Umbilical Fistulae. Surg., Gynec. & Obst. 45:165–178 (Aug.) 1927.

Begg, R. C.: Colloid Adenocarcinomata of Bladder Vault Arising From Epithelium of Urachal Canal, With Critical Survey of Tumours of Urachus. Brit. J. Surg. 18:422–466 (Jan.) 1931.

Begg, R. C.: Massive Cyst-Adenoma of Müller's Duct Causing Retention of Urine. Brit. J. Urol. 8:105–111, 1936.

Berdon, W. E., Baker, D. H., Santulli, T. V., and Amoury, R.: The Radiologic Evaluation of Imperforate Anus: An Approach Correlated With Current Surgical Concepts. Radiology 90:466–471 (Mar.) 1968.

Berdon, W. E., Hochberg, B., Baker, D. H., Grossman, H., and Santulli, T. V.: The Association of Lumbosacral Spine and Genitourinary Anomalies With Imperforate Anus. Am. J. Roentgenol. 98:181–191 (Sept.) 1966.

Bergqvist, Anna: Ectopic Kidney as a Complication of Pregnancy on Labour. Acta obst. et gynec. scandinav. 44:289–303, 1965–66.

Berman, J. K.: Congenital Anomalies of Rectum and Anus. Surg., Gynec. & Obst. 66:11–22 (Jan.) 1938.

Bill, A. H., Jr., and Johnson, R. J.: Failure of Migration of the Rectal Opening as the Cause for Most Cases of Imperforate Anus. Surg., Gynec. & Obst. 106:643–651 (June) 1958.

Bill, A. H., Jr., Johnson, R. J., and Foster, R. A.: Anteriorly Placed Rectal Opening in the Perineum, "Ectopic Anus": A Report of 30 Cases. Ann. Surg. 147:173–179 (Feb.) 1958.

Blackard, C. E., and Mellinger, G. T.: Cancer in a Horseshoe Kidney: A Report of Two Cases. Arch. Surg. 97:616–627 (Oct.) 1968.

Blechschmidt, E.: The Stages of Human Development Before Birth. Philadelphia, W. B. Saunders Company, 1961, 684 pp.

Boissonnat, P.: Two Cases of Complete Double Functional Urethra With a Single Bladder. Brit. J. Urol. 33:453–462 (Dec.) 1961.

Bonney, W. W., Young, H. H., II, Levin, D., and Goodwin, W. E.: Complete Duplication of the Urethra with Vaginal Stenosis. J. Urol. 113:132–137 (Jan.) 1975.

Bourne, C. W., and Cerny, J. C.: Congenital Absence of Abdominal Muscles: Report of 6 Cases. J. Urol. 98:252–259 (Aug.) 1967.

Boyce, W. H., and Vest, S. A.: A New Concept Concerning Treatment of Exstrophy of the Bladder. J. Urol. 67:503–517 (Apr.) 1952.

Boyd, J. D., and Hamilton, W. J.: British Obstetrics and Gynaecological Practice. London, Heinemann, 1948, pp. 32–38.

Boyd, J. D., and Hamilton, W. J.: In Bowes, K. (Ed.): Modern Trends in Obstetrics and Gynecology. London, Butterworth and Company, Second Series, 1955, p. 60.

Braasch, W. F., and Merricks, J. W.: Clinical and Radiological Data Associated With Congenital and Acquired Single Kidney. Surg., Gynec. & Obst. 67:281–286 (Sept.) 1938.

Bradham, R. R.: Imperforate Anus: Report of 130 Cases. Surgery 44:578–584 (Sept.) 1958.

Brannan, W., and Henry, H. H., III: Ureteral Ectopia: Report of 39 Cases. J. Urol. 109:192–195 (Feb.) 1973.

Brayton, D., and Norris, W. J.: Further Experiences With the Treatment of Imperforate Anus. Surg., Gynec. & Obst. 107:719–726 (Dec.) 1958.

Brooks, R. E., Jr.: Left Retrocaval Ureter Associated With Situs Inversus. J. Urol. 88:484–487 (Oct.) 1962.

Brown, J. J. M.: Lesions of the Anterior Urethra in Infancy and Childhood. Proc. Roy. Soc. Med. 49:891–894, 1956.

Browne, D.: Congenital Deformities of the Anus and the Rectum. A.M.A. Arch. Dis. Childhood 30:42–45 (Feb.) 1955.

Burke, E. C., Shin, M. H., and Kelalis, P. P.: Prune-Belly Syndrome. Amer. J. Dis. Child. 117:668–671 (June) 1969.

Burns, E., Cummins, H., and Hyman, J.: Incomplete Reduplication of the Bladder With Congenital Solitary Kidney: Report of a Case. J. Urol. 57:257–269 (Feb.) 1947.

Butler, D. B., and Rosenberg, H. S.: Sarcoma of the Urachus. A.M.A. Arch. Surg. 79:724–728 (Nov.) 1959.

Campbell, J. E.: Ureteral Peristalsis in Duplex Renal Collecting Systems. Am. J. Roentgenol. 99:577–584 (Mar.) 1967.

Campbell, M. F.: Urology. Philadelphia, W. B. Saunders Company, 1954 vol. 1, p. 483.

Campbell, M. F.: Urology. Ed. 2, Philadelphia, W. B. Saunders Company; 1963, vol. 2, pp. 895–1862.

Campbell, M. F.: Urology. Ed. 2, Philadelphia, W. B. Saunders Company, 1963, vol. 2, pp. 1681–1712.

Carlson, H. E.: Supernumerary Kidney as a Cause of Ureteropelvic Obstruction. J. Urol. 56:179–182 (Aug.) 1946.

Cass, A. S., and Vitko, R. J.: Unusual Variety of Crossed Renal Ectopy With Only One Ureter. J. Urol. 107:1056–1058 (June) 1972.

Charghi, A., Dessureault, P., Drouin, G., Gauthier, G. E., Perras, P., Roy, P., and Charbonneau, J.: Malposition of a Renal Lobe (Lobar Dysmorphism): A Condition Simulating Renal Tumor. J. Urol. 105:326–329 (Mar.) 1971.

Chwalle, R.: Process of Formation of Cystic Dilatations of Vesical End of Ureter and of Diverticula at Ureteral Ostium. Urol. & Cutan. Rev. 31:499–504 (Aug.) 1927.

Collins, D. C.: Congenital Unilateral Renal Agenesia. Ann. Surg. 95:715–726 (May) 1932.

Considine, J.: Retrocaval Ureter: A Review of the Literature With a Report of Two New Cases Followed for Fifteen Years and Two Years Respectively. Brit. J. Urol. 38:412–423, 1966.

Constantian, H. M.: Ureteral Ectopia, Hydrocolpos, and Uterus Didelphys. J.A.M.A. 197:54–57 (July 4) 1966.

Constantian, H. M., and Amaral, E. L.: Urachal Cyst: Case Report. J. Urol. 106:429–431 (Sept.) 1971.

Coolsaet, B., and Cornil, C.: Acute Urinary Retention in Children Caused by Pyoureter. J. Urol. 108:966–968 (Dec.) 1972.

Coppridge, W. M.: Mullerian Duct Cysts: With Report of a Case. South. M. J. 32:248–251 (Mar.) 1939.

Corbus, B. C., Estrem, R. D., and Hunt, W.: Retroiliac Ureter. J. Urol. 84:67–68 (July) 1960.

Counseller, V. S., and Flor, F. S.: Congenital Absence of the Vagina: Further Results of Treatment and a New Technique. S. Clin. North America, August, 1957, pp. 1107–1118.

Cox, C. E., and Hutch, J. A.: Bilateral Single Ectopic Ureter: A Report of 2 Cases and Review of the Literature. J. Urol. 95:493–497 (Apr.) 1966.

Culbertson, L. R.: Müllerian Duct Cyst. J. Urol. 58:134–136 (Aug.) 1947.

Culp, O. S.: Ureteral Diverticulum: Classification of the Literature and Report of an Authentic Case. J. Urol. 58:309–321 (Nov.) 1947.

Culp, O. S.: Heminephro-ureterectomy: Comparison of One-Stage and Two-Stage Operations. J. Urol. 83:369–375 (Apr.) 1960.

Culp, O. S., and Hendricks, E. D.: Potentialities of Partial Nephrectomy. S. Clin. North America 39:887–905 (Aug.) 1959.

Daut, R. V., Emmett, J. L., and Kennedy, R. L. J.: Congenital Absence of Abdominal Muscles With Urologic Complications: Report on a Patient Successfully Treated. Proc. Staff Meet., Mayo Clin. 22:8–13 (Jan. 8) 1947.

Davidson, A. C., and Beard, J. H.: A Seminal Vesicle Cyst: In Association With Ipsilateral Renal Agenesis and Lumbar Scoliosis. South. Med. J. 62:608–610 (May) 1969.

Davidson, W. M., and Smith, D. R.: A Morphological Sex Difference in the Polymorphonuclear Neutrophil Leucocytes. Brit. M. J. 2:6–7 (July 3) 1954.

Davies, J.: Human Developmental Anatomy. New York, The Ronald Press Company, 1963, pp. 177–198.

Davis, L. A., Lich, R., Howerton, L., and Joule, W.: The Lower Urinary Tract in Infants and Children. Radiology 77:445–451 (Sept.) 1961.

Dees, J. E.: Anomalous Relationship Between Ureter and External Iliac Artery. J. Urol. 44:207–215 (Aug.) 1940.

Dees, J. E.: Clinical Importance of Congenital Anomalies of Upper Urinary Tract. J. Urol. 46:659–666 (Oct.) 1941.

Deming, C. L.: Cyst of the Seminal Vesicle. Tr. Am. A. Genito-Urin. Surgeons 28:301–312, 1935.

Deming, C. L., and Berneike, R. R.: Müllerian Duct Cysts. J. Urol. 51:563–568 (June) 1944.

Demos, N. J., Gillis, D. A., and Barber, K. E.: Congenital Diverticula of the Anterior Urethra in Male Infants: Report of Two Cases. J. Urol. 88:252–255 (Aug.) 1962.

de Vries, P. A., and Friedland, G. W.: Congenital "H-Type" Ano-Urethral Fistula. Radiology 113:397–407 (Nov.) 1974.

DeWeerd, J. H., and Litin, R. B.: Ectopia of Ureteral Orifice (Vestibular) Without Incontinence: Report of Case. Proc. Staff Meet., Mayo Clin. 33:81–86 (Feb. 19) 1958.

DeWeerd, J. H.: Urologic Dilemmas Resolved by the Ileal Conduit. J.A.M.A. 178:983–988 (Dec. 9) 1961.

DeWeerd, J. H., and Feeney, D. P.: Bilateral Ureteral Ectopia With Urinary Incontinence in a Mother and Daughter. J. Urol. 98:335–337 (Sept.) 1967.

Dolan, P. A., and Kirkpatrick, W. E.: Multiple Ureteral Diverticula. J. Urol. 83:570–571 (May) 1960.

Dorairajan, T.: Defects of Spongy Tissue and Congenital Diverticula of the Penile Urethra. Australian & New Zealand J. Surg. 32:209–214 (Feb.) 1963.

Duff, P. A.: Retrocaval Ureter: Case Report. J. Urol. 63:496–499 (Mar.) 1950.

Durrani, K. M., Shah, P. I., and Kakalia, G. R.: Interurethral Fenestration for a Case of Double Urethra With Hypospadias. J. Urol. 108:586–590 (Oct.) 1972.

Edling, N. P. G.: The Radiological Aspect of the Utriculus Prostaticus During Urethrocystography. Acta radiol. 32:28–32, 1949.

Ellerker, A. G.: The Extravesical Ectopic Ureter. Brit. J. Surg. 45:344–353 (Jan.) 1958.

Emmett, J. L., and Braasch, W. F.: Cysts of the Prostate Gland. J. Urol. 36:236–249 (Sept.) 1936.

Ericsson, N. O.: Ectopic Ureterocele in Infants and Children: A Clinical Study. Acta chir. scandinav. Suppl. 197, pp. 1–92, 1954.

Fehrenbaker, L. G., Kelalis, P. P., and Strickler, G. B.: Vesicoureteral Reflux and Ureteral Duplication in Children. J. Urol. 107:862–864 (May) 1972.

Felderman, E. S., and Fetter, T. R.: Patent Urachal Cyst. J. Urol. 79:767–770 (Apr.) 1958.

Feldman, M.: Clinical Roentgenology of the Digestive Tract. Ed. 4, Baltimore, The Williams & Wilkins Company, 1957, 776 pp.

Feldman, R. A., and Weiss, R. M.: Urinary Retention Secondary to Müllerian Duct Cyst in a Child. J. Urol. 108:647–648 (Oct.) 1972.

Forgaard, D. M., and Ansell, J. S.: Trifurcation of the Anterior Urethra: A Case Report. J. Urol. 95:785–787 (June) 1966.

Foroughi, E., and Turner, J. A.: Congenital Ureteral Valve. J. Urol. 81:272–274 (Feb.) 1959.

Francke, H.: Ein Fall von multilokulärer Samenbla-senzyste. Centralbl. f. allg. Path. u. path. Anat. 41:145–147 (Dec. 10) 1927.

Friedland, G. W., and Cunningham, J.: The Elusive Ectopic Ureterocele. Am. J. Roentgenol. 116:792–811 (Dec.) 1972.

Friedland, G. W., and DeVries, P.: Renal Ectopia and Fusion: Embryologic Basis. Urology 5:698–706 (May) 1975.

Gans, S. L., and Friedman, N. B.: Some New Concepts in the Embryology, Anatomy, Physiology and Surgical Correction of Imperforate Anus. West. J. Surg. 69:34–37 (Jan.-Feb.) 1961.

Gehring, G. G., Vitenson, J. H., and Woodhead, D. M.: Congenital Urethral Perineal Fistulas. J. Urol. 109:419–421 (Mar.) 1973.

Gettel, R. R., Lee, F., and Ratliff, R. K.: Ureteral Diverticula. J. Urol. 108:392–395 (Sept.) 1972.

Gillman, J.: Development of Gonads in Man, With Consideration of Role of Fetal Endocrines and Histogenesis of Ovarian Tumors. Contrib. Embryol. 32:81–131, 1948.

Gordon, H. I., and Kessler, R.: Ectopic Ureter Entering the Seminal Vesicle Associated with Renal Dysplasia. J. Urol. 108:389–391 (Sept.) 1972.

Goyanna, R., and Greene, L. F.: The Pathologic and Anomalous Conditions Associated With Duplication of the Renal Pelvis and Ureter. J. Urol. 54:1–9 (July) 1945.

Graham, S. D.: Agenesis of Bladder. J. Urol. 107:660–661 (Apr.) 1972.

Gray, S. W., and Skandalakis, J. E.: Embryology for Surgeons. Philadelphia, W. B. Saunders Company, 1972, p. 461.

Greenbaum, E., and Pearman, R. O.: Vasovesiculography: Cyst of the Seminal Vesicle Associated with Agenesis of the Ipsilateral Kidney. Radiology 98:363–364 (Feb.) 1971.

Greene, L. F.: Duplication of the Renal Pelvis and Ureter. S. Clin. North America 24:910–921 (Aug.) 1944.

Greene, L. F., and Kearns, W. M.: Circumcaval Ureter: Report of a Case With a Consideration of the Preoperative Diagnosis and Successful Plastic Repair. J. Urol. 55:52–59 (Jan.) 1946.

Greene, L. F., Emmett, J. L., Culp, O. S., and Kennedy, R. L. J: Urologic Abnormalities Associated With Congenital Absence or Deficiency of Abdominal Musculature. Tr. Am. A. Genito-Urin. Surgeons 43:120–132, 1951.

Gross, R. E., and Moore, T. C.: Duplication of the Urethra: Report of Two Cases and Summary of the Literature. Arch. Surg. 60:749–761 (Apr.) 1950.

Grossman, H., Winchester, Patricia H., and Muecke, E. C.: Solitary Ectopic Ureter. Radiology 89:1069–1072 (Dec.) 1967.

Gruenwald, P., and Surks, S. N.: Pre-ureteric Vena Cava and Its Embryological Explanation. J. Urol. 49:195–201 (Jan.) 1943.

Grumbach, M. M., Van Wyk, J. J., and Wilkins, L.: Chromosomal Sex in Gonadal Dysgenesis (Ovarian Agenesis): Relationship to Male Pseudohermaphrodism and Theories of Human Sex Differentiation. J. Clin. Endocrinol. 15:1161–1193 (Oct.) 1955.

Grumbach, M. M., Blanc, W. A., and Engle, E. T.: Sex Chromatin Pattern in Seminiferous Tubule Dysgenesis and Other Testicular Disorders: Relationship to True Hermaphrodism and to Klinefelter's Syndrome, With a Review of Gonadal Ontogenesis. J. Clin. Endocrinol. 17:703–736 (June) 1957.

Guizzetti, P.: Coexistence of Renal and Genital Anomalies. (abstr.) J.A.M.A. 71:1867, 1918.

Gullmo, A., and Sundberg, J.: A Method for Roentgen Examination of the Posterior Urethra, Prostatic Ducts and Utricle (Utriculography). Acta radiol. 48:241–247, 1957.

Haber, K.: Bifid Ureter with a Blind-Ending Branch Diagnosed by Excretory Urography: Report of a Case. J. Urol. 110:38–39 (July) 1973.

Hamblen, E. C.: The Assignment of Sex to an Individual: Some Enigmas and Some Practical Clinical Criteria. Am. J. Obst. & Gynec. 74:1228–1244 (Dec.) 1957.

Hamm, F. C., and Harlin, H. C.: Imperforate Anus Associated With Urinary Tract Fistula. New York J. Med. 53:561–565 (Mar. 1) 1953.

Hammond, G., Yglesias, L., and Davis, J. E.: The Urachus, Its Anatomy and Associated Fasciae. Anat. Rec. 80:271–282 (July) 1941.

Hampson, Joan G., Money, J., and Hampson, J. L.: Hermaphrodism: Recommendations Concerning Case Management. J. Clin. Endocrinol. 16:547–556 (Apr.) 1956.

Hanley, H. G.: A Horseshoe and a Supernumerary Kidney: A Triple Kidney With a Horseshoe Component. Brit. J. Surg. 30:165–168 (Oct.) 1942.

Harley, L. M., Chen, Y., and Rattner, W. H.: Prune-Belly Syndrome. J. Urol. 108:174–176 (July) 1972.

Harrill, H. C.: Retrocaval Ureter: Report of a Case With Operative Correction of the Defect. J. Urol. 44:450–457 (Oct.) 1940.

Hart, J. B.: A Case of Cyst or Hydrops of the Seminal Vesicle. J. Urol. 86:137–141 (July) 1961.

Hart, J. B.: A Case of Cyst of the Seminal Vesicle. J. Urol. 96:247–249 (Aug.) 1966.

Hartman, G. W., and Hodson, C. J.: The Duplex Kidney and Related Anomalies. Clin. Radiol. 20:387–400 (Oct.) 1969.

Harvard, B. M., and Thompson, G. J.: Congenital Exstrophy of the Urinary Bladder: Late Results of Treatment by the Coffey-Mayo Method of Ureterointestinal Anastomosis. J. Urol. 65:223–234 (Feb.) 1951.

Heetderks, D. R., Jr., and Delambre, L. C.: Cyst of the Seminal Vesicle. J. Urol. 93:725–728 (June) 1965.

Heller, E., and Whitesel, J. A.: Seminal Vesicle Cysts. J. Urol. 90:305–307 (Sept.) 1963.

Hennessey, R. A.: Müllerian Duct Cysts: Report of a Case. J. Urol. 42:1042–1050 (Dec.) 1939.

Herbst, W. P.: Patent Urachus. South. M. J. 30:711–719 (July) 1937.

Heyman, J., and Lundqvist, A.: The Symphysis Pubis in Pregnancy and Parturition. Acta obst. et gynec. scandinav. 12:191–226, 1932.

Higgins, C. C.: Exstrophy of the Bladder: Report of 158 Cases. Am. Surgeon 28:99–102 (Mar.) 1962.

Hinman, F., Jr.: Urologic Aspect of the Alternating Urachal Sinus. Am. J. Surg. 102:339–343 (Aug.) 1961a.

Hinman, F., Jr.: Surgical Disorders of the Bladder and Umbilicus of Urachal Origin. Surg., Gynec. & Obst. 113:605–614 (Nov.) 1961b.

Hock, E., Purkayastha, A. and Jay, B. D.: Retro-iliac

Ureter: A Case Report. J. Urol. 107:37–38 (Jan.) 1972.

Hodson, C. J.: Discussion on Pyelonephritis. Proc. Roy. Soc. Med. 52:669–672 (Jan. 22) 1959.

Hodson, C. J., Drewe, J. A., Karn, M. N., and King, A.: Renal Size in Normal Children: Radiographic Study During Life. Arch. Dis. Child. 37:616–622 (Dec.) 1962.

Hoffenberg, R., and Jackson, W. P. U.: Sex Chromatin and Intersex. (Letter to the Editor.) J. Clin. Endocrinol. 17:454–457 (Mar.) 1957.

Hollinshead, W. H.: Anatomy for Surgeons. New York, Hoeber-Harper, vol. 2, 1956, pp. 556, 564, 567–569, 733, 735, and 753.

Holly, L. E., II, and Sumcad, B.: Diverticular Ureteral Changes: A Report of Four Cases. Am. J. Roentgenol. 78:1053–1060 (Dec.) 1957.

Howard, F. S.: Hypospadias With Enlargement of Prostatic Utricle. Surg., Gynec. & Obst. 86:307–316 (Mar.) 1948.

Hutch, J. A., and Chisholm, E. R.: Surgical Repair of Ureterocele. J. Urol. 96:445–450 (Oct.) 1966.

Idbohrn, H., and Sjöstedt, S.: Ectopic Ureter Not Causing Incontinence Until Adult Life. Acta obst. et gynec. scandinav. 33:457–464, 1954.

Irmisch, G. W., and Cook, E. N.: Double and Accessory Urethra. Minnesota Med. 29:999–1002 (Oct.) 1946.

Johnston, J. H.: Single Ectopic Ureters. Brit. J. Urol. 41:428–433 (Aug.) 1969.

Jones, H. W., Jr., and Scott, W. W.: Hermaphroditism, Genital Anomalies and Related Endocrine Disorders. Baltimore, The Williams & Wilkins Company, 1958, 456 pp.

Jost, A.: Embryonic Sexual Differentiation (Morphology, Physiology, Abnormalities). In Jones, H. W., Jr., and Scott, W. W.: Hermaphroditism, Genital Anomalies and Related Endocrine Disorders. Baltimore, The Williams & Wilkins Company, 1958, pp. 15–45.

Kaplan, N., and Elkin, M.: Bifid Renal Pelves and Ureters: Radiographic and Cinefluorographic Observations. Brit. J. Urol. 40:235–244 (Apr.) 1968.

Keith, A.: Human Embryology and Morphology. Ed. 5, Baltimore, William Wood & Company, 1933, 558 pp.

Keith, J. D., Rowe, R. D., and Vlad, P.: Heart Disease in Infancy and Childhood. New York, The Macmillan Company, 1958, 877 pp.

Kelalis, P. P., Malek, R. S., and Segura, J. W.: Observations on Renal Ectopia and Fusion in Children. J. Urol. 110:588–592 (Nov.) 1973.

Kimchi, D., and Wiesenfeld, A.: Cyst of Seminal Vesicle Associated With Ipsilateral Renal Agenesis: Case Report. J. Urol. 89:906–907 (June) 1963.

Kincaid, O. W.: Renal Angiography. Chicago, Year Book Medical Publishers, Inc., 1966, 275 pp.

King, M. C., Friedenberg, R. M., and Tena, L. B.: Normal Renal Parenchyma Simulating Tumor. Radiology 91:217–222 (Aug.) 1968.

Kirkland, K. L., and Bale, P. M.: A Cystic Adenoma of the Prostate. J. Urol. 97:324–327 (Feb.) 1967.

Kjellberg, S. R., Ericsson, N. O., and Rudhe, U.: The Lower Urinary Tract in Childhood: Some Correlated Clinical and Roentgenologic Observations. Chicago, Year Book Publishers, Inc., 1957, 298 pp.

Klauber, G. T., and Reid, E. C.: Inverted Y Reduplication of the Ureter. J. Urol. *107*:362–364 (Mar.) 1972.

Knox, W. G.: Congenital Diverticulum of the Male Urethra. J. Urol. *58*:344–348 (Nov.) 1947.

Köhler, R.: Solitary Pelvic Kidney Verified by Aortography. Brit. J. Radiol. *36*:448–451 (June) 1963.

Korobkin, M., and Cooperman, L. R.: Vesiculographic Findings in Cysts of the Seminal Vesicle. Radiology *114*:571–574 (March) 1975.

Krasa, F. C., and Paschkis, R.: Das Trigonum vesicae der Säugetiere: Eine vergleichendanatomische Studie. Ztschr. Urol. *6*:1–53, 1921.

Kretschmer, H. L.: Supernumerary Kidney: Report of a Case With Review of the Literature. Tr. Am. A. Genito-Urin. Surgeons *22*:95–118, 1929.

Ladd, W. E., and Gross, R. E.: Congenital Malformations of the Anus and Rectum: Report of 162 Cases. Am. J. Surg. *23*:167–183 (Jan.) 1934.

Landes, R. R., and Ransom, C. L.: Müllerian Duct Cysts. J. Urol. *61*:1089–1093 (June) 1949.

Lattimer, J. K.: Congenital Deficiency of the Abdominal Musculature and Associated Genitourinary Anomalies: A Report of 22 Cases. J. Urol. *79*:343–352 (Feb.) 1958.

Lattimer, J. K., and Smith, M. J. V.: Exstrophy Closure: A Followup on 70 Cases. J. Urol. *95*:356–359 (Mar.) 1966.

Laufer, I., and Griscom, N. T.: Compensatory Renal Hypertrophy: Absence in Vitro and Development in Early Life. Am. J. Roentgenol. *113*:464–467 (Nov.) 1971.

Laughlin, V. C.: Retrocaval (Circumcaval) Ureter Associated With Solitary Kidney. J. Urol. *71*:195–199 (Feb.) 1954.

Lawson, L. J., and MacDougall, J. A.: Multilocular Cyst of the Seminal Vesicle. Brit. J. Urol. *37*:440–442 (Aug.) 1965.

Lenaghan, D.: Bifid Ureters in Children: An Anatomical, Physiological and Clinical Study. J. Urol. *87*:808–817 (June) 1962.

Levisay, G. L., Holder, J., and Weigel, J. W.: Ureteral Ectopia Associated With Seminal Vesicle Cyst and Ipsilateral Renal Agenesis. Radiology *114*:575–576 (Mar.) 1975.

Lloyd, F. A., and Bonnett, D.: Müllerian Duct Cysts. J. Urol. *64*:777–782 (Dec.) 1950.

Lloyd, F. A., and Pranke, D.: Cysts of the Seminal Vesicle. Quart. Bull. Northwestern Univ. M. School *25*:43–46, 1951.

Longo, V. J., and Thompson, G. J.: Congenital Solitary Kidney. J. Urol. *68*:63–68 (July) 1952.

Lowsley, O. S.: Accessory Urethra: Report of Two Cases With a Review of the Literature. New York J. Med. *39*:1022–1031 (May 15) 1939.

Lund, A. J.: Uncrossed Double Ureter With Rare Intravesical Orifice Relationship: Case Report With Review of Literature. J. Urol. *62*:22–29 (July) 1949.

Lund, A. J., and Cummings, M. M.: Cyst of the Accessory Genital Tract: A Case Report With a Review of the Literature. J. Urol. *56*:383–386 (Sept.) 1946.

Luschka, H.: Ueber den Bau des menschlichen Harnstranges. Arch. path. Anat. *23*:1–7, 1862.

Mackie, G. G. and Stephens, F. D.: Duplex Kidneys: A Correlation of Renal Dysplasia With Position of the Ureteral Orifice. J. Urol. *114*:274–280 (Aug.) 1975.

Magri, J.: Solitary Crossed Ectopic Kidney. Brit. J. Urol. *33*:152–156, 1961.

Mahoney, P. J., and Ennis, D.: Congenital Patent Urachus. New England J. Med. *215*:193–195 (July 30) 1936.

Malek, R. S., Kelalis, P. P., and Burke, E. C.: Ectopic Kidney in Children and Frequency of Association with Other Malformations. Mayo Clin. Proc. *46*:461–467 (July) 1971.

Malek, R. S., Kelalis, P. P., Burke, E. C., and Stickler, G. B.: Simple and Ectopic Ureterocele in Infancy and Childhood. Surg., Gynec. & Obst. *134*:611–616 (Apr.) 1972.

Malek, R. S., Kelalis, P. P., Stickler, G. B., and Burke, E. C.: Observations on Ureteral Ectopy in Children. J. Urol. *107*:308–313 (Feb.) 1972.

Maloney, P. K., Jr., Gleason, D. M., and Lattimer, J. K.: Ureteral Physiology and Exstrophy of the Bladder. J. Urol. *93*:588–592 (May) 1965.

Malter, I. J., and Stanley, R. J.: The Intrathoracic Kidney: With A Review of the Literature. J. Urol. *107*:538–541 (April) 1972.

Marshall, V. F., and Keuhnelian, J. G.: Crossed Ureteral Ectopia With Solitary Kidney. J. Urol. *110*:176–177 (Aug.) 1973.

Marshall, V. F., and Muecke, E. C.: Variations in Exstrophy of the Bladder. J. Urol. *88*:766–796 (Dec.) 1962.

Marshall, V. F., and Muecke, E. C.: Congenital Abnormalities of the Bladder. In Encyclopedia of Urology. VII/1. Malformations. Berlin, Springer-Verlag, 1968, pp. 172–176, 176–184; 195–197.

Masik, B. K., and Brosman, S. A.: Megalourethra. J. Urol. *109*:901–903 (May) 1973.

Melen, D. R.: Multilocular Cyst of the Prostate. J. Urol. *27*:343–349 (Mar.) 1932.

Mering, J. H., Steel, J. F., and Gittes, R. F.: Congenital Ureteral Valves. J. Urol. *107*:737–739 (May) 1972.

Mertz, H. O., Hendricks, J. W., and Garrett, R. A.: Cystic Ureterovesical Protrusion: Report of Four Cases in Children and Two in Adults. Tr. Am. A. Genito-Urin. Surgeons *40*:180–190, 1948.

Meyers, M. A., Whalen, J. P., Evans, J. A., and Viamonte, M.: Malposition and Displacement of the Bowel in Renal Agenesis and Ectopia: New Observations. Am. J. Roentgenol. *117*:323–333 (Feb.) 1973.

Middleton, R. P.: A Case of Pyometra in a Male Pseudo-hermaphrodite. New England J. Med. *204*:902–904 (Apr. 30) 1931.

Mills, W. M.: A Case of Supernumerary Kidney. J. Anat. & Physiol. *46*:313–319 (Apr.) 1912.

Mims, M. M.: Multiple Acquired Diverticulosis of the Ureter. J. Urol. *84*:297–299 (Aug.) 1960.

Minniberg, D. T., Montoya, F., Okada, K., Galioto, F., and Presutti, R.: Subcellular Muscle Studies in the Prune-Belly Syndrome. J. Urol. *109*:524–526 (March) 1973.

Mogg, R. A.: Some Observations on the Ectopic Ureter and Ureterocele. J. Urol. *97*:1003–1012 (June) 1967.

Mogg, R. A.: The Single Ectopic Ureter. Brit. J. Urol. *46*:3–10 (Jan.) 1974.

Moore, K. L., and Barr, M. L.: Smears From the Oral Mucosa in the Detection of Chromosomal Sex. Lancet 2:57–58 (July 9) 1955.

Moore, R. A.: Pathology of the Prostatic Utricle. Arch. Path. 23:517–524 (Apr.) 1937.

Moore, T.: Ectopic Openings of the Ureter. Brit. J. Urol. 24:3–18 (Mar.) 1952.

Mostofi, F. K., Thomson, R. V., and Dean, A. L., Jr.: Mucous Adenocarcinoma of the Urinary Bladder. Cancer 8:741–758 (July-Aug.) 1955.

Muecke, E. C.: The Role of the Cloacal Membrane in Exstrophy: The First Successful Experimental Study. J. Urol. 92:659–667 (Dec.) 1964.

Muecke, E. C., and Currarino, G.: Congenital Widening of the Pubic Symphysis: Associated Clinical Disorders and Roentgen Anatomy of Affected Bony Pelves. Am. J. Roentgenol. 103:179–185 (May) 1968.

Mulholland, S. G., Edson, M., and O'Connell, K. J.: Congenital Uretero-Seminal Vesicle Fistula. J. Urol. 106:649–651 (Nov.) 1971.

Myers, G. H., Jr., Lynn, H. B., and Kelalis, P. P.: Giant Cyst of the Utricle. J. Urol. 101:369–373 (Mar.) 1969.

McCauley, R. T., and Lichtenheld, F. R.: Congenital Patent Urachus. South. M. J. 53:1138–1141 (Sept.) 1960.

McDonald, J. H., and McClellan, D. S.: Crossed Renal Ectopia. Am. J. Surg. 93:995–1002 (June) 1957.

McKenna, C. M., and Kampmeier, O. F.: A Consideration of the Development of Polycystic Kidney. J. Urol. 32 37–43 (July) 1934.

McKenna, C. M., and Kiefer, J. H.: Congenital Enlargement of Prostatic Utricle With Inclusion of Ejaculatory Ducts and Seminal Vesicles. Am. A. Genito-Urin. Surgeons 32:305–316, 1939.

Nalle, B. C., Jr., Crowell, J. A., and Lynch, K. M., Jr.: Solitary Pelvic Kidney With Vaginal Aplasia: Report of a Case. J. Urol. 61:862–865 (May) 1949.

Nesbit, R. M., and Bromme, W.: Double Penis and Double Bladder: With Report of a Case. Am. J. Roentgenol. 30:497–502 (Oct.) 1933.

Nesbitt, T. E.: Congenital Megalo-urethra. J. Urol. 73:839–842 (May) 1955.

Neustein, D. H., and Schutte, H.: Müllerian Duct Cysts: With Report of a Case. Brit. J. Urol. 40:72–77 (Feb.) 1968.

Newman, H., Molthan, M. E., and Osborn, W. F.: Urinary Tract Anomalies in Children With Congenital Heart Disease. Am. J. Roentgenol. 106:52–57 (May) 1969.

Newman, L., Simms, K., Kissane, J., and McAlister, W. H.: Unilateral Total Renal Dysplasia in Children. Am. J. Roentgenol. 116:778–783 (Dec.) 1972.

Nix, J. T., Menville, J. G., Albert, M., and Wendt, D. L.: Congenital Patent Urachus. J. Urol. 79:264–273 (Feb.) 1958.

Nordmark, B.: Double Formations of the Pelves of the Kidneys and the Ureters: Embryology, Occurrence and Clinical Significance. Acta radiol. 30:267–278, 1948.

Norman, C. H., Jr., and Dubowy, J.: Multiple Ureteral Diverticula. J. Urol. 96:152–154 (Aug.) 1966.

Nunn, I. N., and Stephens, F. D.: The Triad Syndrome: A Composite Anomaly of the Abdominal Wall, Urinary System and Testes. J. Urol. 86:782–794 (Dec.) 1961.

Omo-Dare, P.: Posterior Urethral Diverticulum in the Male. Brit. J. Urol. 40:445–450 (Aug.) 1968.

Orecklin, J. R., Craven, J. D., and Lecky, J. W.: Compensatory Renal Hypertrophy: A Morphologic Study in Transplant Donors. J Urol. 109:952–954 (June) 1973.

Orquiza, C. S., Bhayani, B. N., Berry, J. L., and Dahlen, C. P.: Ectopic Opening of the Ureter into the Seminal Vesicle: Report of Case. J. Urol. 104:532–535 (Oct.) 1970.

Palmer, J. M., and Russi, M. F.: Persistent Urogenital Sinus With Absence of the Bladder and Urethra. J. Urol. 102:590–594 (Nov.) 1969.

Palmer, J. M., and Tesluk, H.: Ureteral Pathology in the Prune-Belly Syndrome. J. Urol. 111:701–707 (May) 1974.

Passaro, E., Jr., and Smith, J. P.: Congenital Ureteral Valve in Children: A Case Report. J. Urol. 84:290–292 (Aug.) 1960.

Patten, B. M., and Barry, A.: The Genesis of Exstrophy of the Bladder and Epispadias. Am. J. Anat. 90:35–53 (Jan.) 1952.

Peterson, C., Jr., and Silbiger, M. L.: Five Ureters: A Case Report. J. Urol. 100:160–162 (Aug.) 1968.

Petersen, D. S., Fish, L., and Cass, A. S.: Twins With Congenital Deficiency of Abdominal Musculature. J. Urol. 107:670–672 (Apr.) 1972.

Phelan, J. T., Counseller, V. S., and Greene, L. F.: Deformities of the Urinary Tract With Congenital Absence of the Vagina. Surg. Gynec. & Obst. 97:1–3 (July) 1953.

Pick, J. W., and Anson, B. J.: Retrocaval Ureter: Report of a Case, With a Discussion of Its Clinical Significance. J. Urol. 43:672–685 (May) 1940.

Pitt, D. C.: Retrocaval Ureter: Report of a Case Diagnosed Preoperatively by Intravenous and Retrograde Pyelography. Radiology 84:699–702 (Apr.) 1965.

Pitts, W. R., and Muecke, E. C.: Horseshoe Kidneys: A 40 Year Experience. J. Urol. 113:743–746 (June) 1975.

Plunkett, E. R., and Barr, M. L.: Testicular Dysgenesis Affecting the Seminiferous Tubules Principally, With Chromatin-Positive Nuclei. Lancet 2:853–856 (Oct. 27) 1956.

Potter, E. L.: Facial Characteristics of Infants With Bilateral Renal Agenesis. Am. J. Obstet. Gynec. 51:885–888 (June) 1946.

Purpon, I.: Crossed Renal Ectopy With Solitary Kidney: A Review of the Literature. J. Urol. 90:13–15 (July) 1963.

Radasch, H. E.: Congenital Unilateral Absence of the Urogenital System and Its Relation to the Development of the Wolffian and Muellerian Ducts. Am. J. M. Sc. 136:111–118, 1908.

Rank, W. B., Mellinger, G. T., and Spiro, E.: Ureteral Diverticula: Etiologic Considerations. J. Urol. 83:566–569 (May) 1960.

Ravitch, M. M.: Hind Gut Duplication – Doubling of Colon and Genital Urinary Tracts. Ann. Surg. 137:588–601 (May) 1953.

Reddy, Y. N., and Winter, C. C.: Cyst of the Seminal Vesicle: A Case Report and Review of the Literature. J. Urol. 108:134–135 (July) 1972.

Reveno, J. S., and Palubinskas, A. J.: Congenital Renal Abnormalities in Gonadal Dysgenesis. Radiology 86:49–51 (Jan.) 1966.

Rhame, R. C., and Derrick, F. C., Jr.: Gartner's Duct Cyst Involving Urinary Tract. J. Urol. 109:60–61 (Jan.) 1973.

Riba, L. W., Schmidlapp, C. J., and Bosworth, N. L.: Ectopic Ureter Draining Into the Seminal Vesicle. J. Urol. 56:332–338 (Sept.) 1946.

Richardson, E. H.: Diverticulum of the Ureter: A Collective Review With Report of an Unique Example. J. Urol. 47:535–570 (May) 1942.

Rieser, C., and Griffin, T. L.: Cysts of the Prostate. J. Urol. 91:282–286 (Mar.) 1964.

Robson, M. C., and Ruth, E. B.: Bilocular Bladder: An Anatomical Study of a Case; With a Consideration of Urinary Tract Anomalies. Anat. Rec. 142:63–68 (Jan.) 1962.

Rowland, H. S., Jr., Bunts, R. C., and Iwano, J. H.: Operative Correction of Retrocaval Ureter: A Report of Four Cases and Review of the Literature. J. Urol. 83:820–833 (June) 1960.

Rusche, C., and Butler, O. W.: Müllerian Duct Cysts. J. Urol. 59:962–965 (May) 1948.

Saalfeld, J., Walsh, P. C., and Goodwin, W. E.: Ureterovaginoplasty for Vaginal Atresia (Unique Technique in Treatment): A Case Report With Description of Associated Arterial Anomalies and Retroiliac Artery Ureters. J. Urol. 109:1039–1045 (June) 1973.

Samuels, A., Kern, H., and Sachs, L.: Supernumerary Kidney With Ureter Opening into Vagina. Surg. Gynec. & Obst. 35:599–603 (Nov.) 1922.

Sanders, R. C.: The Place of Diagnostic Ultrasound in the Examination of Kidneys Not Seen on Excretory Urography. J. Urol. 114:813–819 (Dec.) 1975.

Sargent, C. R., Amis, E. S., and Carlton, C. E.: Ectopic Ureter, Ipsilateral Vas Deferens and Seminal Vesicle Agenesis and Associated Dermoid Cyst: A Case Report. J. Urol. 103:298–299 (Mar.) 1970.

Satter, E. J., and Mossman, H. W.: A Case Report of a Double Bladder and Double Urethra in the Female Child. J. Urol. 79:274–278 (Feb.) 1958.

Schmidt, J. D.: Congenital Urethral Duplication. J. Urol. 105:397–399 (Mar.) 1971.

Schnitzer, B.: Ectopic Ureteral Opening Into Seminal Vesicle: A Report of Four Cases. J. Urol. 93:576–581 (May) 1965.

Schwartz, S. J., and Shaheen, D. J.: Unusual Configuration of Crossed Fused Renal Ectopia: Case Report. J. Urol. 109:491 (March) 1973.

Scott, J. E. S., and Swenson, O.: Imperforate Anus: Results in 63 Cases and Some Anatomic Considerations. Ann. Surg. 150:477–486 (Sept.) 1959.

Segura, J. W., Kelalis, P. P., and Burke, E. C.: Horseshoe Kidney in Children. J. Urol. 108:333–336 (Aug.) 1972.

Seitzman, D. M., and Patton, J. F.: Ureteral Ectopia: Combined Ureteral and Vas Deferens Anomaly. J. Urol. 84:604–608 (Nov.) 1960.

Selvaggi, F. P., and Goodwin, W. E.: Incomplete Duplication of the Male Urethra. Brit. J. Urol. 44:495–498 (Aug.) 1972.

Senger, F. L., and Morgan, E. K.: Large Congenital Prostatic Diverticulum. J. Urol. 51:162–166 (Feb.) 1944.

Shopfner, C. E.: Genitography in Intersexual States. Radiology 82:664–674 (Apr.) 1964.

Shopfner, C. E.: Roentgenologic Demonstration of the "Ectopic Anus" Associated With Imperforate Anus. Radiology 84:464–469 (Mar.) 1965a.

Shopfner, C. E.: Roentgenologic Evaluation of Imperforate Anus. South M. J. 58:712–719 (June) 1965b.

Shopfner, C. E.: Cystourethrography: An Evaluation of Method. Am. J. Roentgenol. 95:468–474 (Oct.) 1965c.

Shopfner, C. E.: Radiology in Pediatric Gynecology. Radiol. Clin. North America 5:151–167 (Apr.) 1967.

Siddall, A. C.: Cyst of Urachus With Calculus Formation. Chinese M. J. 46:894–898, 1932.

Simon, H. B., Culp, O. S., and Parkhill, E. M.: Congenital Ureteral Valves: Report of Two Cases. J. Urol. 74:336–341 (Sept.) 1955.

Slocum, R. C.: Muellerian Duct Cysts. Tr. Southeast. Sect. Am. Urol. A. 1954, pp. 26–33.

Smith, E., and Strasberg, A.: A Müllerian Duct Cyst in a Male. Canad. M.A.J. 52:160–161 (Feb.) 1945.

Spence, H. M., and Chenoweth, V. C.: Cysts of the Prostatic Utricle (Müllerian Duct Cysts): Report of Two Cases in Children, Each Containing Calculi, Cured by Retropubic Operation. J. Urol. 79:308–314 (Feb.) 1958.

Steck, W. D., and Helwig, E. B.: Umbilical Granulomas, Pilonidal Disease, and the Urachus. Surg., Gynec. & Obst. 120:1043–1057 (May) 1965.

Stephens, F. D.: Double Ureter in the Child. Australian & New Zealand J. Surg. 26:81–94 (Nov.) 1956.

Stephens, F. D.: Anatomical Vagaries of Double Ureters. Aust. & New Zeal. J. Surg. 28:27–33 (Aug.) 1958.

Stephens, F. D.: Congenital Malformations of the Rectum, Anus and Genito-urinary Tracts. Edinburgh, E. & S. Livingstone, Ltd., 1963, pp. 233–240.

Stephens, F. D.: Caecoureterocele and Concepts on Embryology and Aetiology of Ureteroceles. Aust. New Zeal. J. Surg. 40:239–248 (Feb.) 1971.

Stewart, B. L., and Nicoll, G. A.: Cyst of the Seminal Vesicle. J. Urol. 62:189–195 (Aug.) 1949.

Stewart, C. M.: True Right Supernumerary Kidney Diagnosed Preoperatively. Tr. West. Sect., Am. Urol. A. 15:52–57, 1948.

Stuber, J. L., Templeton, A. W., and Bishop, K.: Ultrasonic Evaluation of the Kidneys. Radiology 104:139–143 (July) 1972.

Stumme, E. G.: Ueber die symmetrischen kongenitalen Bauchmuskeldefekte und über die Kombination derselben mit anderen Bildungsanomalien des Rumpfes. Mitt. a. d. Grenzgeb. d. Med. u. Chir. 11:548–590, 1903.

Swenson, O., and Oeconomopoulos, C. T.: Double Lower Genitourinary Systems in a Child. J. Urol. 85:540–542 (Apr.) 1961.

Swenson, O., Moussatos, G. H., and Fisher, J. H.: Results of Repair of Exstrophy of the Bladder. S. Clin. North America 43:151–161, 1963.

Swick, M.: A Quadruple Kidney With a Horseshoe Component Demonstrated With the Aid of Excretion Urography. J. Mt. Sinai Hosp. 4:7–11 (May–June) 1937.

Tabrisky, J., and Bhisitkul, I.: Solitary Crossed Ectopic Kidney With Vaginal Aplasia: A Case Report. J. Urol. 94:33–35 (July) 1965.

Takaha, M., Nakaarai, K., and Ikoma, F.: Complete Reduplication of the Urinary Bladder Associated With Hindgut Duplication: Report of a Case. Acta Urol. Japonica 17:401–414 (June) 1971.

Takahashi, A., and Iwashita, K.: Crossed Renal Ectopia. Jap. J. M. Sc. & Biol. 2:93–111 (Dec.) 1940.

Tanagho, E. A.: Anatomy and Management of Ureteroceles. J. Urol. 107:729–736 (May) 1972.

Tench, E. M.: Development of the Anus in the Human Embryo. Am. J. Anat. 59:333–343 (July) 1936.

Thevathasan, C.: Accessory Urethra in the Male Child: Report of Two Cases. Aust. & New Zeal. J. Surg. 31:134–136 (Nov.) 1961.

Thompson, G. J., and Greene, L. F.: Ureterocele: A

Clinical Study and a Report of Thirty-seven Cases. J. Urol. 47:800–809 (June) 1942.

Thompson, G. J., and Pace, J. M.: Ectopic Kidney: A Review of 97 Cases. Surg., Gynec. & Obst. 64:935–943 (May) 1937.

Thompson, I. M., and Amar, A. D.: Clinical Importance of Ureteral Duplication and Ectopia. J.A.M.A. 168:881–886 (Oct. 18) 1958.

Thompson, W., and Grossman, H.: The Association of Spinal and Genitourinary Abnormalities With Low Anorectal Anomalies (Imperforate Anus) in Female Infants. Radiology 113:693–698 (Dec.) 1974.

Tjio, J. H., and Puck, T. T.: The Somatic Chromosomes of Man. Proc. Nat. Acad. Sc. 44:1229–1236 (Dec. 15) 1958.

Trimingham, H. L., and McDonald, J. R.: Congenital Anomalies in the Region of the Umbilicus. Surg., Gynec. & Obst. 80:152–163 (Feb.) 1945.

Tristan, T. A., Eberlein, W. R., and Hope, J. W.: Roentgenologic Investigation of Patients With Heterosexual Development. Am. J. Roentgenol. 76:562–568 (Sept.) 1956.

Uson, A. C., and Donovan, J. T.: Ectopic Ureteral Orifice: A Report Based on Seventeen Cases. A.M.A. J. Dis. Child. 98:153–161 (Aug.) 1959.

Uson, A. C., Lattimer, J. K., and Melicow, M. M.: Ureteroceles in Infants and Children: A Report Based on 44 Cases. Pediatrics 27:971–983 (June) 1961.

Uson, A. C., and Schulman, C. C.: Ectopic Ureter Emptying into the Rectum: Report of a Case. J. Urol. 108:156–158 (July) 1972.

Vakili, B. F.: Agenesis of the Bladder: A Case Report. J. Urol. 109:510–511 (Mar.) 1973.

Vanhoutte, J. J.: Ureteral Ectopia into a Wolffian Duct Remnant (Gartner's Duct or Cysts) Presenting as a Urethral Diverticulum in Two Girls. Am. J. Roentgenol. 110:540–545 (Nov.) 1970.

Vaughan, G. T.: Patent Urachus: Review of the Cases Reported. Operation on a Case Complicated With Stones in the Kidneys: A Note on Tumors and Cysts of the Urachus. Tr. Am. S. A. 23:273–294, 1905.

Vinstein, A. L., and Franken, E. A.: Unilateral Hematocolpos Associated With Agenesis of the Kidney. Radiology 102:625–627 (Mar.) 1972.

Wall, B., and Wachter, H. E.: Congenital Ureteral Valve: Its Role as a Primary Obstructive Lesion; Classification of the Literature and Report of an Authentic Case. J. Urol. 68:684–690 (Oct.) 1952.

Walls, W. J., and Lin, F.: Ultrasonic Diagnosis of Seminal Vesicle Cyst. Radiology 114:693–694 (March) 1975.

Wangensteen, O. H., and Rice, C. O.: Imperforate Anus: A Method of Determining the Surgical Approach. Ann. Surg. 92:77–81 (July) 1930.

Ward, W. G.: Suppurating Cyst of the Urachus, With Concretion. Ann. Surg. 69:329–330, 1919.

Waterhouse, K.: Anomalies of the Urethra. In Encyclopedia of Urology. VII/1. Malformations. Berlin, Springer-Verlag, 1968, pp. 242–286.

Weiss, J. M., and Dykhuizen, R. F.: An Anomalous Vaginal Insertion Into the Bladder: A Case Report. J. Urol. 98:610–612 (Nov.) 1967.

Welch, K. J., and Kearney, G. P.: Abdominal Musculature Deficiency Syndrome: Prune-Belly. J. Urol. 111:693–700 (May) 1974.

Wesson, M. B.: Cysts of the Prostate and Urethra. J. Urol. 13:605–632 (June) 1925.

Wesson, M. B.: Incontinence of Vesical and Renal Origin (Relaxed Urethra and a Vaginal Ectopic Ureter). J. Urol. 32:141–152 (Aug.) 1934.

Weyrauch, H. M.: Anomalies of Renal Rotation. Surg., Gynec. & Obst. 69:183–199 (Aug.) 1939.

Whittle, C. H., Coryllos, E., and Simpson, J. S., Jr.: Sarcoma of the Urachus. Arch. Surg. 82:443–444 (Mar.) 1961.

Wiggishoff, C. C., and Kiefer, J. H.: Ureteral Ectopia: Diagnostic Difficulties. J. Urol. 96:671–673 (Nov.) 1966.

Wilkins, L.: The Diagnosis and Treatment of Endocrine Disorders in Childhood and Adolescence. Ed. 2, Springfield, Illinois, Charles C Thomas, Publisher, 1957, 526 pp.

Wilkins, L., Grumbach, M. M., Van Wyk, J. J., Shepard, T. H., and Papadatos, C.: Hermaphroditism: Classification, Diagnosis, Selection of Sex and Treatment. Pediatrics 16:287–300 (Sept.) 1955.

Williams, D. I.: Ectopic Ureterocele. Proc. Roy. Soc. Med. 51:783–784, 1958a.

Williams, D. I.: Urology in Childhood: Encyclopedia of Urology. Berlin, Springer-Verlag, 1958b, vol. 15, 353 pp.

Williams, D. I.: Urology in Childhood. Berlin, Springer-Verlag, 1958, p. 105.

Williams, D. I., and Burkholder, G. V.: The Prune Belly Syndrome. J. Urol. 98:244–251 (Aug.) 1967.

Williams, D. I., and Lightwood, R. G.: Bilateral Single Ectopic Ureters. Brit. J. Urol. 44:267–273 (Apr.) 1972.

Williams, D. I., and Woodard, J. R.: Problems in the Management of Ectopic Ureteroceles. J. Urol. 92:635–652 (Dec.) 1964.

Williams, J. L., and Goodwin, W. E.: Congenital Multiple Diverticula of the Ureter. Brit. J. Urol. 37:299–301, 1965.

Willmarth, C. L.: Ectopic Ureteral Orifice Within an Urethral Diverticulum: Report of a Case. J. Urol. 59:47–49 (Jan.) 1948.

Wines, R. D., and O'Flynn, J. D.: Transurethral Treatment of Ureteroceles. Brit. J. Urol. 44:207–216 (Apr.) 1972.

Winslow, O. W., Litt, R., and Altman, D.: Imperforate Anus From a Roentgenologic Viewpoint. Am. J. Roentgenol. 85:718–725 (Apr.) 1961.

Wojewski, A., and Kossowski, W.: Total Diphallia: A Case of Plastic Repair. J. Urol. 91:84–86 (Jan.) 1964.

Wrenn, E. L., Jr., and Michie, A. J.: Complete Duplication of the Male Urethra. Ann. Surg. 145:119–122 (Jan.) 1957.

Wulfekuhler, W. V., and Dube, V. E.: Free Supernumerary Kidney: Report of a Case. J. Urol. 106:802–804 (Dec.) 1971.

Young, H. H.: Genital Abnormalities, Hermaphroditism and Related Adrenal Disease. Baltimore, The Williams & Wilkins Company, 1937, 649 pp.

Young, H. H., and Cash, J. R.: A Case of Pseudohermaphrodismus Masculinus, Showing Hypospadias, Greatly Enlarged Utricle, Abdominal Testis and Absence of Seminal Vesicles. J. Urol. 5:405–430 (May) 1921.

Zellermayer, J., and Carlson, H. E.: Congenital Hourglass Bladder. J. Urol. 51:24–30 (Jan.) 1944.

Zinner, A.: Ein Fall von intravesikaler Samenblasenzyste. Wien med. Wchnschr. 64:605–609, 1914.

Chapter 10

INFECTIOUS DISEASES
OF THE
GENITOURINARY TRACT

ACUTE PYELONEPHRITIS

by

Glen W. Hartman, Joseph W. Segura,
and Robert R. Hattery

Acute bacterial pyelonephritis is a common clinical problem; however, patients with this disorder infrequently have excretory urograms taken during the acute episode. In series of patients with acute pyelonephritis reported by Little and associates and by Silver and associates, 24 per cent and 28 per cent, respectively, had abnormal excretory urograms. These and other authors have recently emphasized the radiographic manifestations of acute pyelonephritis (Bailey and associates; Cameron and Azimi; Davidson and Talner; Evans and associates).

Acute bacterial infection involving the renal parenchyma may produce changes made manifest by a wide variety of clinical and laboratory, urographic and angiographic, and histologic findings. The appearance of the excretory urogram or angiogram depends on the severity of the infection and its duration, the virulence of the organism, the alterations produced by antibiotic treatment, and the presence of underlying renal disease. Discrepancies between roentgenographic and histologic findings may in part be due to these variables.

Heptinstall emphasizes that most of the pathologic information on the acute stage of pyelonephritis is derived at autopsy from severe cases of infection often associated with obstruction.

Gross Pathologic Appearance in Acute Pyelonephritis

The kidney is usually enlarged because of inflammatory edema. Multiple abscesses, varying in size from minute to several millimeters, may be observed, mainly in the cortex. The abscess may be rounded or may assume a wedge shape similar to the appearance of an infarct. Tissue between the areas of infection may appear normal. Yellowish streaks, representing collecting tubules filled with pus, may be seen to extend from the cortex into the medulla and the papillae. Reduction in the thickness of parenchyma, papillary necrosis, calyceal blunting, dilatation of the collecting system, and exudates of the pelvic mucosa may be seen. Associated perinephric abscess is uncommon unless the infection is caused by *Staphylococcus aureus*.

Microscopic Findings in Acute Pyelonephritis

The acute inflammatory process is associated with extensive tissue destruction,

809

particularly in the cortex. All renal elements may be destroyed in the areas of abscess, but the arteries, arterioles, and glomeruli show considerable resistance to infection. In the areas adjacent to an abscess, it is common to find that various numbers of proximal convoluted tubules are lost, but there are no arterial changes and few or no glomerular changes. Uncommonly, however, glomeruli may show invasion of inflammatory tissue. In less severely involved areas, large numbers of polymorphonuclear leukocytes are seen in the interstitial tissues and collecting tubules. Chronic inflammatory cells (lymphocytes, plasma cells, and eosinophils) may also be seen. Experimentally, chronic inflammatory cells have been observed within a few days in the rabbit and rat. Abscesses in the medulla are seen in the outer part, whereas the presence of polymorphonuclear leukocytes in the collecting ducts is characteristic of the inner part. Necrosis of the papillae may also be seen. The patchy distribution of normal areas of renal parenchyma interspersed with areas of acute inflammation is an important feature of acute pyelonephritis.

Bailey, Little, and Rolleston reported a patient on whom a renal biopsy was performed 19 days after the onset of acute pyelonephritis. The biopsy revealed extensive polymorphonuclear infiltration of the interstitial spaces, and the tubules were packed with cellular debris. An excretory urogram taken on the second day revealed that both kidneys were enlarged when compared with their size on a urogram done before the episode of acute pyelonephritis. The left kidney was otherwise normal. The right kidney failed to excrete any contrast medium. At 9 days, however, a urogram revealed diminished and delayed excretion of contrast medium in the right kidney. A urogram performed 10 weeks later was normal except for a 1-cm decrease in size of the right kidney compared with its size before the episode of acute pyelonephritis.

Two of the five patients with acute bacterial nephritis reported by Davidson and Talner had nephrectomies. In one case, the kidney was totally involved with an inflammatory process consisting of polymorphonuclear infiltrate in the interstitial tissues and multiple small abscesses. There was little accumulation of infiltration in the tubules, and the tubules were not dilated. The glomeruli were preserved but depleted of red cells. Lymphocytes, plasma cells, and lipid-containing histiocytes were also found. In the other case, the resected kidney revealed numerous areas, varying in diameter from a few millimeters to 3 centimeters, which extended into the subcapsular region and papillae, exuded pus, and were golden tan in color. Acute and chronic inflammatory cells and lipid-laden histiocytes were present without evidence of tumefaction or granuloma formation.

Roentgen Findings in Acute Pyelonephritis

THE EXCRETORY UROGRAM IN ACUTE PYELONEPHRITIS

The findings on excretory urography consist primarily of alterations in the nephrogram, delayed appearance time of contrast medium in the calyces, decreased density of contrast medium in the collecting system, attenuation and distortion of the calyces and infundibula, pyelocaliectasis and ureterectasis, renal enlargement, and occasionally papillary ulceration (Figs. 10–1, 10–2, and 10–3).

The nephrogram may be of normal density, but the duration of the nephrogram may be longer on the involved side. More frequently, however, the nephrogram is diminished in intensity. This diminished nephrogram may be generalized throughout the entire kidney or may have a segmental distribution. The density of the nephrogram is usually uniform, but it may have a striated appearance.

Delayed appearance time of contrast medium may be observed throughout the calyces, or a segmental delay in appearance time may occur in an area of a segmental abnormality of the nephrogram. Similarly,

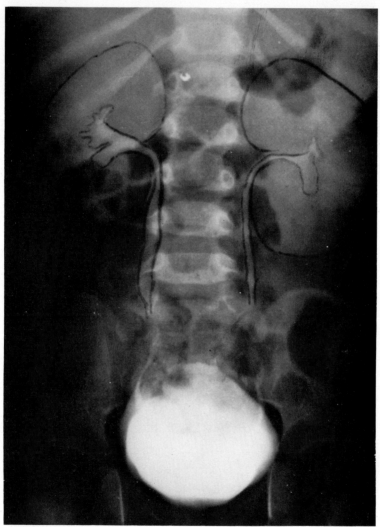

Figure 10–1. *Excretory urogram* of a 2½-year-old girl with **acute pyelonephritis.** Marked bilateral renal enlargement.

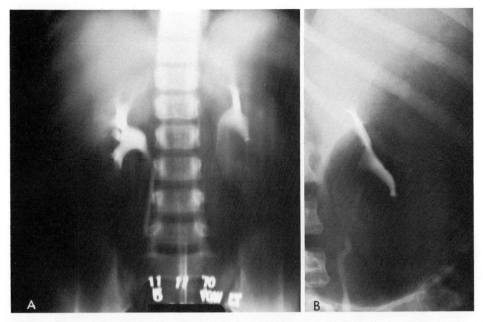

Figure 10–2.   Nine-year-old boy with localized **acute pyelonephritis. A,** *Excretory urogram.* Swelling of lower pole of left kidney with compression of collecting system. **B,** *Nephrotomogram.* Heminephrectomy revealed multiple microscopic abscesses throughout swollen portion of left kidney.

the density of the contrast medium within the calyces may be decreased.

Renal enlargement is usually generalized, but segmental enlargement of the parenchyma may occur in association with the segmental distribution of the nephrogram and density of contrast medium within the calyces. Distortion and attenuation of the calyces and infundibula are associated with enlargement of the kidney secondary to edema of the parenchyma. Renal size on an excretory urogram made during an episode of acute pyelonephritis should be compared with urograms done before the acute episode and on follow-up examinations.

Pyelocaliectasis and ureterectasis may be associated with the changes in the parenchyma, but other, unrelated, causes for dilatation may be present and should not be overlooked. Shopfner (1966) emphasized the association of dilatation of the collecting system with infection and vesicoureteral reflux.

Four of 16 patients reported by Silver and associates had radiographic changes in both kidneys. The most common abnormality on the clinically uninvolved side was renal enlargement. Davidson and Talner and Little and associates also described renal enlargement on the clinically uninvolved side.

THE RENAL ANGIOGRAM IN ACUTE PYELONEPHRITIS

Four patients described by Silver and associates had selective renal arteriograms (Figs. 10–4 and 10–5). In two patients, the arteriograms were normal. The most striking abnormalities observed in the other two patients were a striated nephrogram in the cortex in one patient and mottled parenchymal lucencies in the other. The angiographic findings reported by Davidson and Talner consisted of a decrease in the caliber and number of branches of the interlobar arteries, some stretching of vessels, no neovascularity, abnormal distribution of intrarenal blood flow, and an abnormal nephrogram.

Text continued on page 817

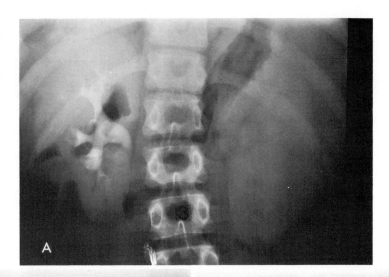

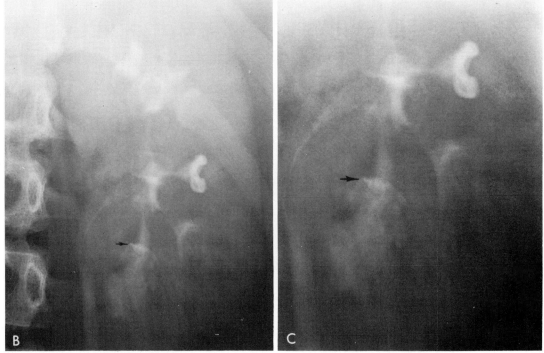

Figure 10–3. Acute pyelonephritis. An 18-year-old male with chronic granulomatous disease of childhood. **A,** *Excretory urogram (3-minute film).* Delay in excretion of contrast medium on left. Enlarged left kidney. **B,** *Excretory urogram (10-minute film).* Contraction of left renal pelvis. Caliectasis in midportion of left kidney. Papillary necrosis of upper-pole calyces. Communicating abscess in lower pole of left kidney medially which faintly opacifies. *Arrow* points to level of lower-pole calyx. **C,** *Excretory urogram (magnification view).* Linear nephrogram involving lower pole. (From Forbes, Hartman, Burke, and Segura.)

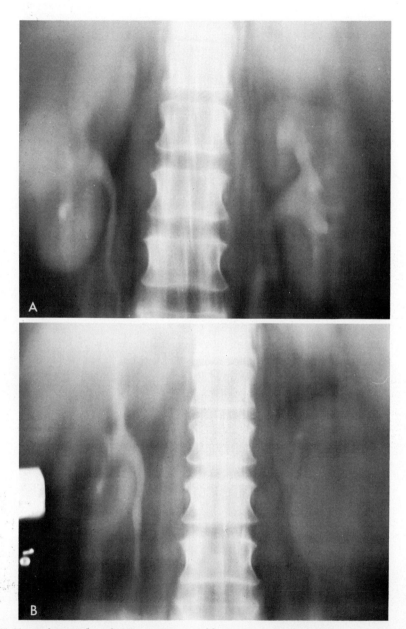

Figure 10–4.   **Acute bacterial nephritis** in a 57-year-old woman. **A,** *Nephrotomogram* obtained 2 years before admission. Scarring of upper pole secondary to pyelonephritis with blunting of underlying calyx. **B,** *Nephrotomogram* reveals diminished opacification of swollen left kidney during an acute episode.

Legend continued on opposite page

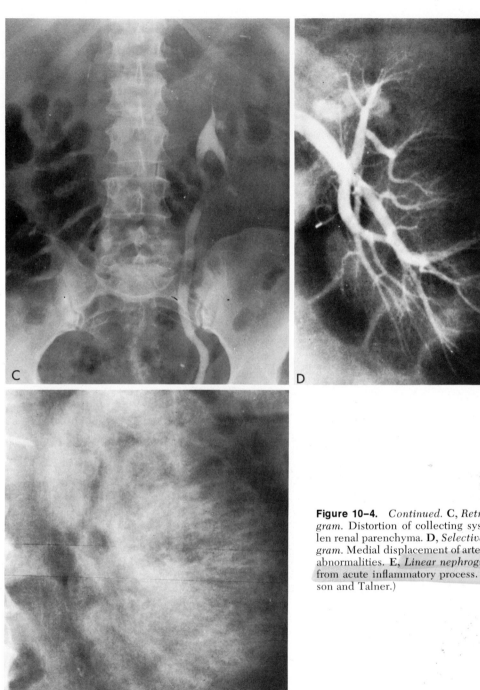

Figure 10–4. *Continued.* **C,** *Retrograde pyelogram.* Distortion of collecting system by swollen renal parenchyma. **D,** *Selective renal arteriogram.* Medial displacement of arteries with focal abnormalities. **E,** *Linear nephrogram,* resulting from acute inflammatory process. (From Davidson and Talner.)

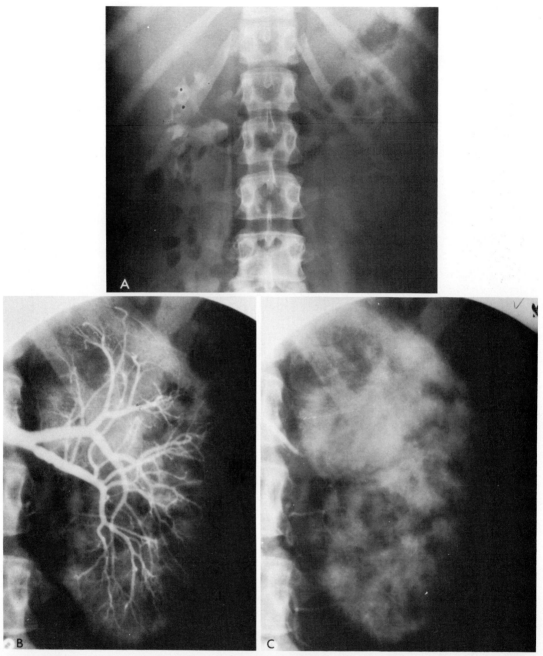

Figure 10–5.   **Acute bacterial nephritis** in a 23-year-old woman. **A,** *Excretory urogram.* Marked enlargement of left kidney with faint opacification of parenchyma and without dilatation of collecting system. **B,** *Selective renal arteriogram, arterial phase.* There is some stretching of upper-pole vessels and slight decrease in branching of intralobar arteries. **C,** *Selective renal arteriogram, nephrographic phase.* A mottled nephrographic pattern is present. **D,** *Excretory urogram* performed 7 days after initial study. Left kidney has decreased in size, and there is prompt opacification. (From Davidson and Talner.)

Illustration continued on opposite page

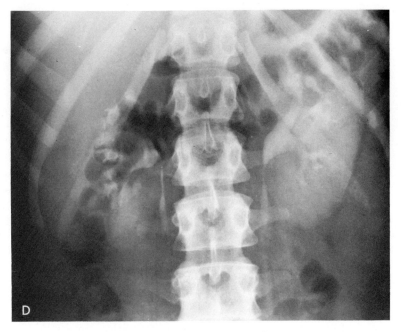

Figure 10–5. *Continued.*

THE FOLLOW-UP EXCRETORY UROGRAM IN ACUTE PYELONEPHRITIS

Three of five patients reported by Davidson and Talner were treated conservatively. In these cases, there was prompt excretion of contrast medium on excretory urograms obtained at 7, 10, and 25 days after the initial examinations. Five patients reported by Silver and associates had follow-up urograms. Three patients with multiple abnormalities during the acute episode of pyelonephritis had the same but less severe changes on follow-up. One patient had a normal follow-up urogram and one had only renal enlargement on the follow-up exam. Bailey and associates reported generalized renal parenchymal wasting without calyceal distortion in a patient examined by urography three months after an episode of acute pyelonephritis.

DIFFERENTIAL DIAGNOSIS

The differential diagnostic possibilities for the excretory urographic findings include acute pyelonephritis, obstructive uropathy, acute arterial or venous vascular occlusive disease, and infiltrative neo-plasm. If the kidney does not excrete sufficient contrast medium to opacify the collecting system, retrograde pyelography may be required to rule out obstruction. In some cases, however, high-dose urography with tomography may allow adequate visualization of the collecting system to exclude an obstructive etiology. Angiography may be required to exclude vascular occlusive disease and infiltrative neoplasm as the cause for the urographic findings.

CHRONIC PYELONEPHRITIS

The term "chronic pyelonephritis" is often loosely applied by pathologists, urologists, and radiologists to various renal conditions regardless of their cause (Braasch; Emmett and associates). Hodson (1967b) has emphasized that it is essential that "chronic pyelonephritis" be defined specifically as "those changes in the kidney which result directly from bacterial infection." Beeson lists the following as the most reliable criteria in establishing the clinical diagnosis: (1) repeated episodes of febrile illness associated with pain and tenderness in the region of the kidney, pyuria,

and bacteriuria; (2) presence of a pathologic condition known to predispose to
urinary tract infection such as vesicoureteral reflux or obstruction; (3) impaired
renal function; and (4) characteristic urographic findings. If one accepts Hodson's
definition, it is also necessary to limit the
radiographic diagnosis of chronic pyelonephritis to renal changes that result only
from bacterial infections of the kidney and
to avoid using the term for various nonspecific renal abnormalities of unknown etiology.

Routes of Infection

Bacteria are thought to reach the kidney by three separate routes, namely, (1)
hematogenous, (2) ascending (via the
ureter), and (3) lymphatic.

The hematogenous route has been
studied by the intravenous injection of bacteria into experimental animals. Renal infection occurs consistently with the intravenous injection of cocci, but bacillary
pyelonephritis does not result experimentally unless special conditions prevail
such as previous scarring of the kidney
produced by infection or fulguration, or
urinary stasis produced by ureteral ligation
(Beeson and associates; de Navasquez,
1950, 1956). Because the great majority of
urinary tract infections in humans are
caused by bacilli, it has appeared unlikely
that the hematogenous route is the primary
one. However, Shopfner (1970) expressed a
different view. He studied 69 infants suffering from sepsis and found that 33 per
cent had radiographic evidence of urinary
tract infection, as evidenced by such findings as obstruction and atony of the calyces, pelves, and ureters, vesicoureteral reflux, and "nonobstructive" hydronephrosis.
He concluded that the hematogenous route
of renal infection is the common one and
that the ureters and bladder are infected
simultaneously.

It is generally accepted that severe
parenchymal infections, such as solitary
abscess (renal carbuncle), multiple cortical

abscesses, diffuse cortical infection, and
perinephritic abscess, are blood-borne.
These are usually coccal infections (frequently *Staphylococcus aureus*) initiated
by foci of infection elsewhere in the body.

The ascending route (via the ureter) is
generally thought to be responsible for the
large majority of renal infections, both
acute and chronic (Hutch and associates,
1962, 1963). Responsible organisms are
usually normal fecal flora such as gram-
negative bacilli or *Streptococcus faecalis*.
In the past, the ascending theory was opposed because it was thought to depend in
part on the "swimming upstream" concept,
but since vesicoureteral reflux has been
demonstrated to occur in 50 to 80 per cent
of children with chronic pyelonephritis, a
method of transport of bacteria from bladder to kidney is apparent (Hinman and
Hutch; Hodson and Edwards).

The lymphatic route is probably rare,
but theoretically it is possible for bacteria
to reach the kidneys via lymphatics draining the bladder, sigmoid, or rectum.

Gross Pathologic Changes in Chronic
Pyelonephritis
(Fig. 10–6)

It is important for the physician to appreciate that the changes seen on the urogram are an excellent reflection of the gross
pathologic changes caused by chronic pyelonephritis (Hodson, 1959; 1967a).

Gross pathologic changes are localized,
and in the chronic stage they consist of a
large area of fibrosis or scarring that involves the entire thickness of the kidney.
The scars are irregular in distribution and
the underlying calyx is blunted, but the
corresponding papillae, although fibrous
and retracted, are not excavated or
sloughed as in papillary necrosis. The involved kidney is small (atrophied), and the
collecting system may be dilated and have
a thickened fibrosed wall. Linear tomography has been extremely helpful as a
method of detecting and evaluating renal
scarring that may be missed on conventional urograms.

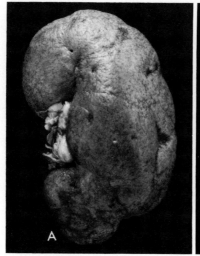 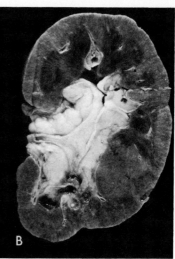

Figure 10-6. *Pathologic specimen* of kidney in **chronic atrophic pyelonephritis. A,** Surface of kidney reveals deep cortical scar involving entire lower pole of kidney. **B,** Cut surface reveals marked thinning of parenchyma of lower pole with associated calyceal blunting typical of chronic atrophic pyelonephritis.

Microscopically, pyelonephritis can be difficult or impossible to differentiate from other renal abnormalities, especially the sequelae of renal vascular disease and interstitial nephritis, as indicated by Kimmelstiel and colleagues. Heptinstall states that it is "doubtful if the renal biopsy can be used for making the diagnosis of chronic pyelonephritis unless use is made of information from the radiologist on the status of the calyceal system and from the clinician on the presence of urinary tract infection."

Characteristic features of bacterial chronic atrophic pyelonephritis are:

1. Onset (usually) during first 5 years of life.

2. Common association with vesicoureteral reflux.

3. Large scars (tissue damage involving several lobes).

4. Polar distribution of scars.

5. Small scars sometimes occurring in otherwise normal areas.

6. Islands of normal tissue sometimes found in large scars.

7. Depressed kidney surface and retracted papillae; involvement of whole thickness of the renal parenchyma.

8. Absence of necrosis and sloughing of papilla.

9. Associated calyceal blunting.

Intrarenal Reflux and the Role of Infection
(Fig. 10-7)

The occurrence of intrarenal reflux has been described by Hodson (1972), Mellins, and Rolleston and associates. Rolleston and associates reported the occurrence of intrarenal reflux associated with vesicoureteral reflux in 16 patients (20 kidneys). Intrarenal reflux was not observed in patients over the age of 4 years, was present in 6.7 per cent of patients examined, and was seen only in conjunction with moderate or severe degrees of vesicoureteral reflux. Renal damage with the radiographic appearance of the scarring seen in atrophic pyelonephritis was shown in 13 of the 20 kidneys showing intrarenal reflux. The renal scarring in 12 of 13 kidneys corresponded precisely to the anatomic area of the kidney into which intrarenal reflux had occurred. Fifty-eight cases of renal damage were found in an analysis of 365 refluxing ureters in children under age 5 years. Intrarenal reflux was present in 24 per cent of these damaged kidneys. Bacteriuria was present initially in all 16 children with intrarenal reflux, but in 5 of these patients there was no episode of illness suggestive of urinary tract infection, nor were bacteria detected on follow-up examinations of the

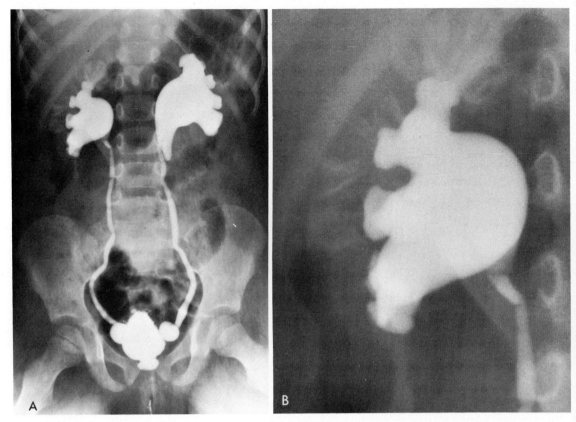

Figure 10–7. **A,** *Voiding cystourethrogram.* Marked contracture of the bladder and large bilateral congenital periureteral diverticula in a 6-year-old child. **B,** Close-up view of right kidney. Intrarenal reflux with contrast medium filling intrarenal tubules.

urine. In three of the patients with moderate vesicoureteral reflux associated with intrarenal reflux, the kidneys continued to grow normally despite proven episodes of bacteriuria in the follow-up period.

An excellent monograph by Hodson and associates (1975) reports that the relationship between vesicoureteral reflux and coarse renal scarring (atrophic pyelonephritis) has been studied in swine and related to the scars observed in atrophic pyelonephritis in man. Intrarenal reflux was produced in the experimental model by a combination of vesicoureteral reflux and raised bladder pressure. In the model, gross intrarenal reflux and the more severe degrees of vesicoureteral reflux occurred at bladder pressures of higher than 45 mm Hg, whereas intrarenal reflux was uncommon when bladder pressures were 35 mm Hg and below. The combination of pro-

longed raised intravesical pressure (50 mm Hg or more) with intrarenal reflux eventually produced features of obstructive nephropathy and focal scarring that are also found in man. These authors stress the importance and interrelationships of intrarenal reflux, vesicoureteral reflux, infection, and the pressure within the urinary tract as factors in scar formation in their experimental model. It was found that infection was not an essential factor, but the presence of infection appeared to intensify the process.

In the experimental model, infected and uninfected chronic scars could only be differentiated histologically. This differentiation was not always possible, however, if the infection had been cleared for more than two weeks before the histologic specimen was obtained. Macroscopically, the infected and uninfected scars were similar in size, nature, and distribution. Bacterial invasion of the kidney was confined to areas in which intrarenal reflux was shown to occur. Except for a single case, intrarenal reflux and infection always resulted in scar formation, and a single episode of bacteriuria in the presence of intrarenal reflux is likely to result in an acute inflammatory lesion, which, if untreated, may later result in a scar. On the other hand, the role of infection in initiating intrarenal reflux remains unclear.

Lesions ranging from focal scarring with normal adjacent papilla and focal scarring with generalized obstructive nephropathy were found in the model and were similar to those observed in human beings. The dominant factors that determine the renal changes are bladder pressure and the duration and severity of vesicoureteral reflux.

Hodson and associates also point out that in the animal model, prolonged moderate or severe sterile intrarenal reflux eventually produces severe fibrosis, extending from the subcapsular surface to the papillary tip, in the segment of the kidney into which the reflux occurred. Contraction of the fibrous segments causes scars that closely resemble the scars of chronic atrophic pyelonephritis that are observed in children (and adults).

In studies of vesicoureteral reflux using barium sulfate, the contrast medium was observed fluoroscopically to enter the renal substance over a period of 20 to 30 seconds. On histologic examination, barium particles were observed in dilated collecting ducts, loops of Henle, and, in some instances, in Bowman's capsule. In animals with changes of obstructive nephropathy and focal fibrosis, barium was found in lymphatics over the lower pole of the kidney, in periureteral tissues, in the renal fascia and thickened capsule, or in paraaortic nodes. Intrarenal reflux represents a form of pyelotubular backflow into the renal parenchyma via the ducts of Bellini and eventually into collecting ducts and nephrons. It is postulated that the resulting fibrosis results from rupture of the tubular system within the cortex and leakage of urine into the interstitial renal tissue.

Intrarenal reflux, which has been documented and defined radiographically, usually accompanies the more severe degree of vesicoureteral reflux occurring during voiding cystourethrography. It is observed mostly in children, usually occurs at the renal poles, and extends from the papilla to the cortex, involving the entire thickness of the renal parenchyma.

Roentgen Diagnosis in Chronic Pyelonephritis

Uroradiographic techniques adequate to demonstrate the renal parenchyma and calyces clearly are essential for the diagnosis of chronic pyelonephritis (Figs. 10–8 through 10–26); retrograde pyelography is rarely indicated, and then only to supplement excretory urography in instances of severely impaired or absent renal function. Even when renal function is considerably impaired, the renal parenchyma and collecting system may be satisfactorily visualized by using a large initial dose of contrast medium, infusion, reinjection, ureteral compression, or tomography.

The anatomic features of the scars observed by Hodson and associates in their animal model and those seen in children are strikingly similar. The major macroscopic and gross anatomic characteristics of the scars are (1) flat depressions with irregular rolled edges at the interface of the scar and normal parenchyma, (2) linear clefts, and (3) deep punctate pits. The large flat scars are commonly located at the renal poles and usually involve the entire renal parenchymal substance. The renal papillae are contracted, apparently by contraction of fibrous tissue, and islands of normal interspersed renal tissue are commonly observed.

The urographic hallmark of chronic pyelonephritis is the coarse focal renal scar with clubbing of the underlying calyx (Filly and associates). These scars can be either unilateral or bilateral, and although

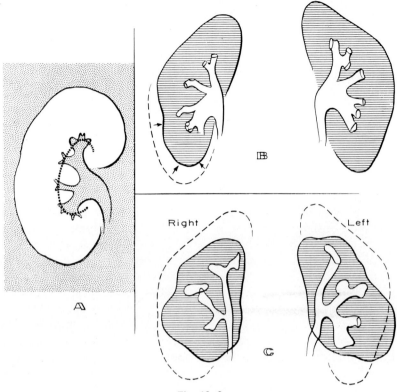

Fig. 10–8

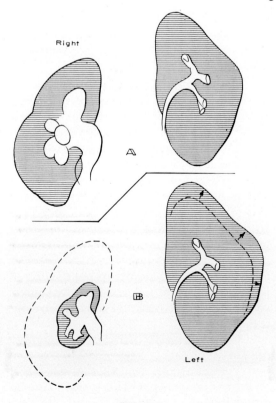

Fig. 10–9

Figure 10–8. A, **Normal kidney** showing interpapillary line used for measurement of thickness of renal substance. B, Tracing of excretory pyelogram of woman, 21 years of age. In two regions of lower half of right kidney there is localized narrowing of renal substance and clubbing of adjacent calyces. **Early focal pyelonephritis.** Left kidney is normal. C, Tracing of excretory pyelogram of woman, 29 years of age. **Advanced bilateral chronic pyelonephritis.** Note small size of kidneys, irregular outlines, and marked variations of thickness of renal substance with calyceal clubbing. Dotted lines indicate normal contour of kidney. (Modified from Hodson, C. J., 1959.)

Figure 10–9. Diagrammatic presentation of **chronic atrophic pyelonephritis of right kidney** following transvesical meatotomy for removal of ureteral stone. A, Preoperative condition. Right pyelocaliectasis caused by obstruction from ureteral stone. B, Same case, 11 years after meatotomy. Atrophy of right kidney and compensatory hyperplasia of left kidney. Dotted lines indicate contour of kidneys in their normal state. (Modified from Hodson, C. J., and Edwards, D., 1960.)

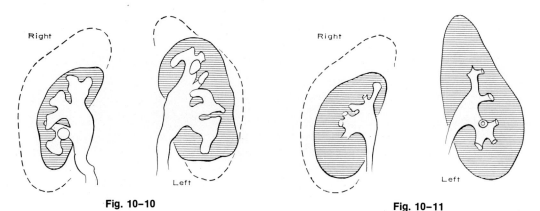

Fig. 10–10   Fig. 10–11

Figure 10–10. Diagrammatic presentation of **bilateral atrophic pyelonephritis** in girl, 7 years of age, with bilateral vesicoureteral reflux. Dotted lines indicate contour of kidneys in their normal state. (Modified from Hodson, C. J., and Edwards, D., 1960.)

Figure 10–11. Diagrammatic presentation of **unilateral (right) atrophic pyelonephritis** in girl, 10 years of age, who had 6-year history of recurring infection. (Modified from Hodson, C. J., and Edwards, D., 1960.)

no constant pattern of distribution can be described, the poles are usually involved (Hodson and Wilson). The scars may be so extensive that the blunted calyx appears to lie directly beneath the renal capsule, and marked atrophy is common in advanced stages of the disease.

Less prominent scarring and blunting may be difficult to detect, but careful comparison of the relationship of the calyces to the renal outline will reveal minor pathologic changes. The "interpapillary line" is an excellent means of dramatizing this relationship of the renal cortical margin to the

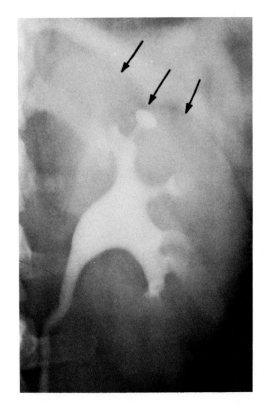

Figure 10–12. *Excretory urogram.* **Minimal chronic pyelonephritis.** Localized parenchymal scar (*arrows*) with underlying calyceal blunting. Far-advanced atrophic pyelonephritis was present in right kidney.

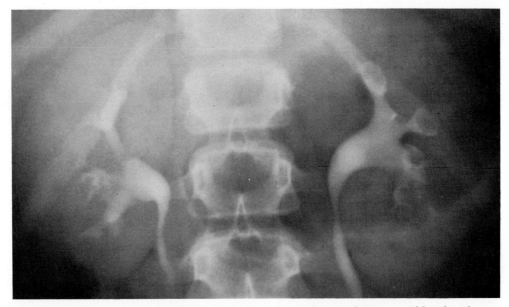

Figure 10–13. *Excretory urogram.* **Minimal chronic pyelonephritis.** Eleven-year-old girl with scarring of lower pole of right kidney and blunting of underlying calyces. Upper pole of right kidney and both poles of left kidney are approximately equally thick.

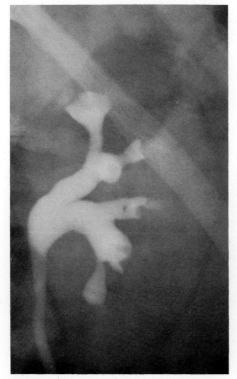

Figure 10–14. *Excretory urogram.* **Unilateral chronic pyelonephritis.** Blunting involving only lower-pole calyx with thinning of parenchyma of medial aspect of lower pole of left kidney.

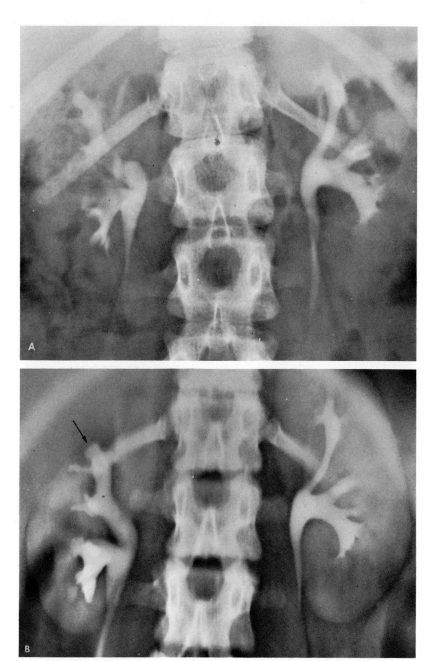

Figure 10–15. Chronic pyelonephritis of right kidney. History of recurring urinary infection since childhood in girl, 15 years of age. **A,** *Excretory urogram.* Suggestion of atrophy of cortex of upper pole of right kidney, but renal outline indistinct. **B,** *Nephrotomogram.* Excellent visualization of both renal outlines. Gross cortical scar of upper pole with blunting of underlying calyces (*arrow*). Less marked changes are present in lower pole. Compensatory hypertrophy, left kidney.

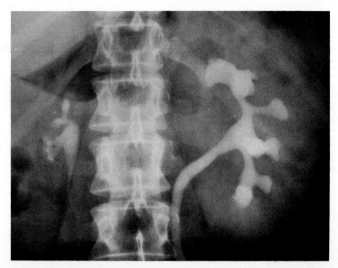

Figure 10–16. *Excretory urogram.* **Chronic pyelonephritis.** Marked atrophy of right kidney and compensatory hypertrophy of left kidney with minimal calyceal blunting.

calyces. The thickness of the parenchyma in relationship to the calyces is greatest at the renal poles. Frequently, the parenchymal thickness of the poles is nearly equal in both kidneys if the collecting systems are bilaterally symmetrical. The parenchyma is often less thick along the upper lateral margin of the left kidney because of "splenic impression." A similar appearance may be seen in the right kidney because of the liver.

Localized areas of normal parenchyma remaining in grossly scarred kidneys may undergo compensatory hypertrophy and result in a pseudotumor (King and associates). It is extremely important to recognize a pseudotumor because it may resemble a solid renal tumor on urography, nephrotomography, or angiography, and misdiagnosis may result in unnecessary nephrectomy. The absence of tumor vessels on vascular studies and awareness of the pos-

Text continued on page 837.

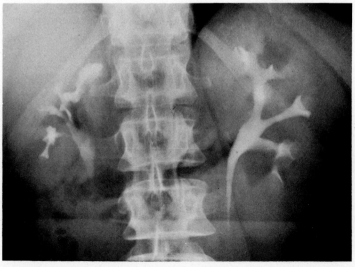

Figure 10–17. *Excretory urogram.* **Advanced chronic pyelonephritis** of right kidney. Compensatory hypertrophy of left kidney.

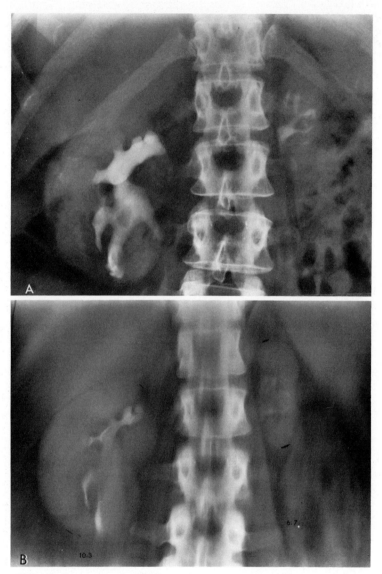

Figure 10-18. Bilateral chronic atrophic pyelonephritis. **A,** *Excretory urogram.* Marked atrophy of left kidney. Typical deep cortical scars involving both poles of right kidney. **B,** *Nephrotomogram.* Degree of parenchymal loss is better demonstrated on tomography.

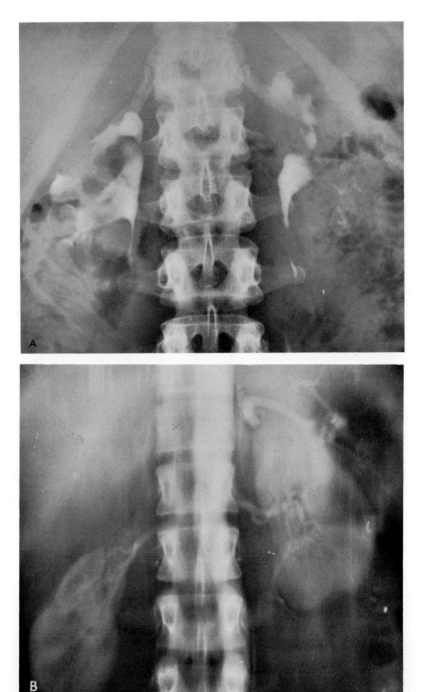

Figure 10–19. *See opposite page for legend.*

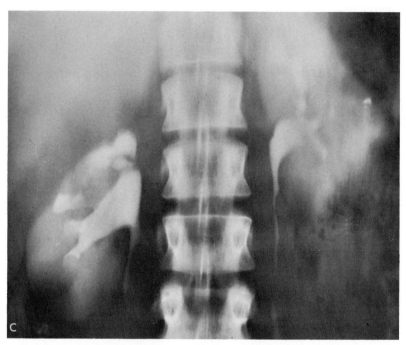

Figure 10–19. Chronic bilateral atrophic pyelonephritis. Thirty-six-year-old woman with long-standing history of urinary tract infection and hypertension for 10 years. **A,** *Excretory urogram.* Calyceal clubbing and deformity, but renal outlines not demonstrated. **B,** *Arterial phase of nephrotomogram.* Scarring of upper pole of right kidney and lower pole of left kidney. **C,** *Nephrographic phase of nephrotomogram.* Entire right kidney in "focus" at this level. Typical findings of calyceal blunting associated with cortical atrophy are well demonstrated.

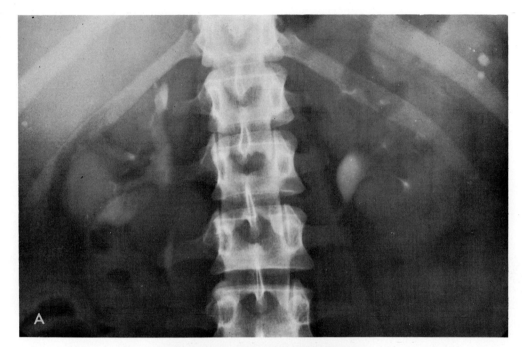

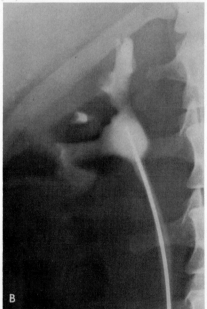

Figure 10–20.   *See opposite page for legend.*

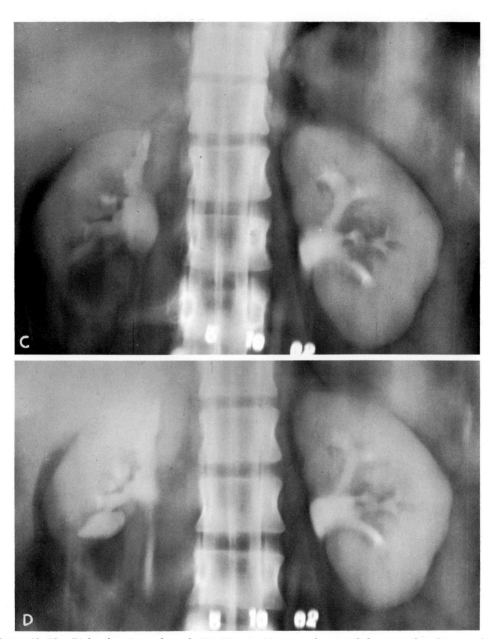

Figure 10–20.   Right chronic pyelonephritis. Woman 39 years of age with long-standing history of urinary tract infection and hypertension. **A,** *Excretory urogram.* Renal outlines only partially demonstrated. Marked deformity of lower-pole calyx of right kidney. **B,** *Right retrograde pyelogram.* **C** and **D,** *Nephrotomograms at 6-cm and 8-cm levels, respectively.* Cortical scarring of upper pole of right kidney is well shown at 6 cm. Lower pole is best seen at 8 cm.

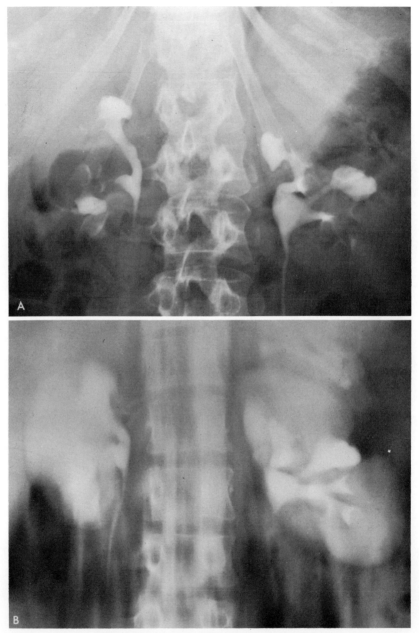

Figure 10–21. *See opposite page for legend.*

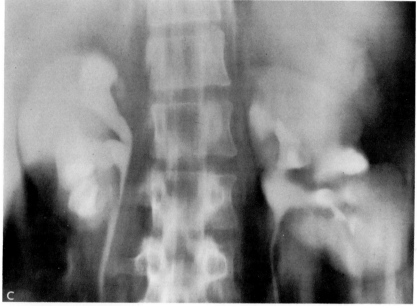

Figure 10–21.   **Bilateral atrophic chronic pyelonephritis.** Forty-nine-year-old woman. **A,** *Excretory urogram.* Marked calyceal blunting, but renal cortex not outlined. **B,** *Nephrotomogram (5-cm "cut").* Left kidney best seen at this level, with marked localized scarring. **C,** *Nephrotomogram (7-cm "cut").* Right kidney shows best in this "cut." Abnormal irregular dilated calyces with complete loss of cortex above upper calyx and marked atrophy of lower pole of kidney.

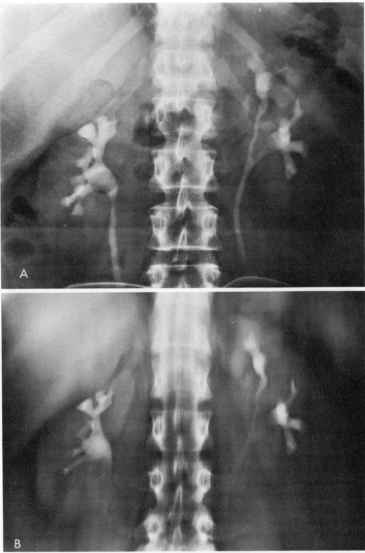

Figure 10–22. Chronic bilateral atrophic pyelonephritis. **A,** *Excretory urogram.* Blunting of upper-pole calyces on right with overlying cortical scarring. **B,** *Nephrotomogram.* Parenchymal scars are better visualized. **C,** *Selective right renal arteriogram, arterial phase.* Deep cortical scar involving upper pole of right kidney with otherwise normal vascularity. **D,** *Selective left renal arteriogram, arterial phase.* Cortical scars in upper pole of left kidney.   *Illustration continued on opposite page.*

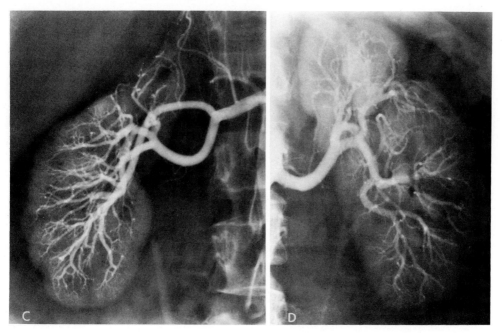

Figure 10–22. *Continued.*

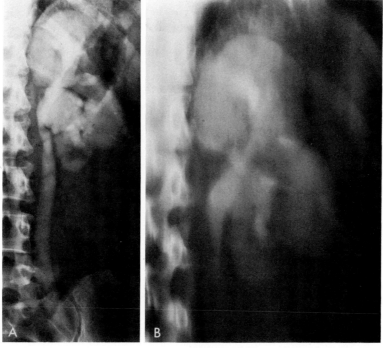

Figure 10–23. **Chronic atrophic pyelonephritis, left kidney. A,** *Excretory urogram.* Cortical scarring with blunting of underlying calyces associated with ureterectasis. Vesical ureteral reflux was present on left. **B,** *Nephrotomogram.* Marked cortical scarring of left kidney with a large pseudotumor in lower portion of left kidney laterally.

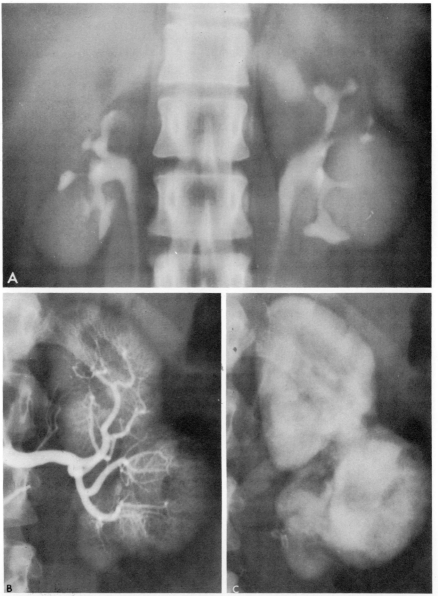

Figure 10–24.   Bilateral atrophic pyelonephritis. "Pseudotumor." **A,** *Excretory urogram.* Marked parenchymal scarring with associated calyceal blunting. Prominent lower poles bilaterally raise question of intrarenal mass lesions. **B,** *Selective left renal arteriogram.* Island of normal parenchyma in left lower pole has undergone compensatory hypertrophy (pseudotumor). **C,** *Arteriogram, nephrographic phase.*

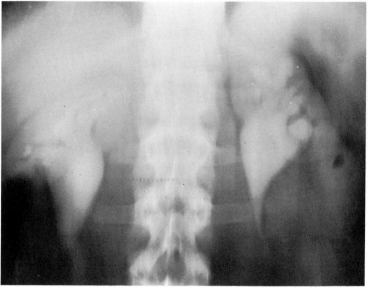

Figure 10-25. *Infusion with tomography.* **Bilateral pyelonephritis and chronic renal failure.** Twenty-two-year-old male with repeated urinary tract infections and gross bilateral reflux. Blood urea, 105 mg/100 ml; serum creatinine, 4.85 mg/100 ml. High-dose excretory urography adequately demonstrates advanced renal disease despite renal failure.

sibility of localized hypertrophy help prevent this error. In certain cases, renal radionuclide scans may be helpful by demonstrating normal uptake in the pseudotumor.

Severe cicatricial changes of the calyces and pelvis are usually due to tuberculosis. These seldom occur in bacterial pyelonephritis, but they may cause bizarre deformities and obliteration of the collecting system.

Vesicoureteral Reflux in Adults

The role of vesicoureteral reflux and its association with pyelonephritis in children and adults has been emphasized in numerous articles in the literature. Recently, Berquist and associates stressed the importance of obtaining fluoroscopically monitored voiding cystourethrograms in adults with a history of recurrent urinary tract infections or with uroradiographic evidence

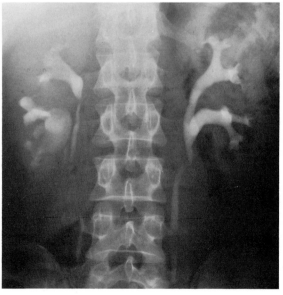

Figure 10-26. *Excretory urogram.* **Complete duplication of right collecting system with pyelonephritis** involving lower segment. (Vesicoureteral reflux was present in lower-pole ureter.)

of renal parenchymal scarring, ureteral dilatation, or mucosal striations. In their series of 200 adults with reflux, renal parenchymal scarring was seen on excretory urograms with tomograms in 62 per cent of the patients. The scarring was localized in 40 per cent of the patients and generalized in 60 per cent. Ureteral dilatation was seen in 20 per cent and mucosal striations were seen in 10 per cent. Clinically, the patients were divided into three groups: (1) those whose excretory urograms were positive but who had negative urine cultures and no history of urinary tract infections, (2) those who had had recurrent urinary tract infections with and without positive urine cultures, and (3) those with reflux related to previous genitourinary or pelvic surgery. The history of urinary tract infection may begin in childhood, although in 87 per cent of the patients reported by Berquist and associates, urinary tract infections did not occur until adulthood.

The association of complete duplication of the collecting system and reflux into the lower-segment ureter is well established. Parenchymal atrophy and scarring of the lower segment of the duplex kidney may be difficult to ascertain on conventional excretory urograms; therefore, tomography is valuable for visualization of the parenchyma.

Chronic Pyelonephritis in Children

Chronic atrophic pyelonephritis is primarily a disease of children, although the persistent scarring that it causes may not be demonstrated until adulthood. This concept is supported by the demonstration of a high incidence of associated vesicoureteral reflux in pediatric patients. The characteristic urographic findings of chronic pyelonephritis are virtually diagnostic during childhood, but in adults the scars resulting from segmental infarction may at times be indistinguishable. Chronic pyelonephritis occurring in childhood may interfere with renal growth, and Hodson (1967b) empha-

sizes that measurement of the kidney is a very sensitive method of detecting or excluding renal damage. He has established a clinical scale that correlates the relationship between normal kidney length and child height; it is very helpful in the clinical follow-up of children who have chronic pyelonephritis. Hodson has also emphasized that in children, the ratio of the thickness of the renal parenchyma at the poles to the overall renal length is higher than in adults. This ratio may also be helpful in evaluating parenchymal changes in children. The association of reflux and urinary tract infection in children makes the voiding cystourethrogram as essential as the excretory urogram in evaluating children who have urinary tract infection.

DIFFERENTIAL DIAGNOSIS IN CHRONIC PYELONEPHRITIS

Segmental renal infarction resulting in a gross renal scar may at times be impossible to differentiate from chronic pyelonephritis. In most instances, however, the papilla underlying an infarct undergoes less scarring and retraction and, therefore, the calyx retains normal cupping. The appearance of a normal calyx is very helpful in diagnosis, since blunting is a constant feature of chronic pyelonephritis. Extensive renal infarction or ischemia causes smooth overall renal atrophy; however, the calyces retain their normal cupped appearance. The calyces may be difficult to visualize because of decreased renal function even with high-dose or infusion urography, and retrograde pyelography may be required for adequate visualization of calyceal anatomy.

Back pressure renal atrophy (hydronephrotic atrophy) is a relatively common manifestation of temporary obstruction of the collecting system and has been described in detail by Hodson and Craven. Diffuse parenchymal atrophy with dilatation of the collecting system and blunted calyces may also be seen in patients with complete vesicoureteral reflux.

Obstruction of the ureteropelvic juncture or the ureter may cause no permanent renal abnormality but may result in diffuse calyceal blunting associated with generalized thinning of the renal cortex if relief of the obstruction is delayed. Obstruction of a single major calyx or infundibulum causes similar changes in the related calyceal tips and localized scarring. In the latter instance the changes closely resemble the scar of chronic pyelonephritis, although localized cicatricial changes of the collecting system are more often due to renal tuberculosis.

Renal atrophy from various causes, including chronic pyelonephritis, may result in fibrolipomatosis. In this condition a substantial amount of fat is accumulated in the renal sinus, replacing atrophied renal parenchyma. Urography reveals attenuation, elongation, compression, and distortion of the infundibula, suggesting peripelvic masses. Slight calyceal blunting may be present. Bolus or infusion nephrotomography reveals an accumulation of renal sinus fat that appears radiolucent when compared with the density of the opacified atrophied renal parenchyma. Computerized tomographic scanning of the kidneys may be very useful in differentiating renal sinus fat from parapelvic cysts or solid tumors. Ultrasound has also been used to differentiate fat in the renal sinus from peripelvic masses.

Irregularity of the parenchyma related to persistent fetal lobulation should not be confused with scarring due to renal infarcts or chronic pyelonephritis. Fetal lobulations produce indentations or clefts *between* normal calyces. These clefts overlie the normal septa of Bertin between renal lobes.

Atrophy of the kidney may result from numerous other noninflammatory conditions, but rarely is calyceal blunting a predominant feature. Nephrosclerosis and chronic glomerulonephritis cause both kidneys to be equally reduced in size, with anatomically normal collecting systems. Radiation nephritis is usually unilateral and at times may closely resemble chronic pyelonephritis. The urographic picture of tuberculosis or papillary necrosis usually has little in common with that of chronic pyelonephritis because cortical scarring is not a prominent feature of these conditions.

Congenital hypoplasia of the kidney is relatively uncommon; the term "hypoplastic" should be reserved for uniformly small (usually less than 60 g) kidneys with smooth cortical margins. The hypoplastic kidney may have a reduced number of calyces, but the calyces are normally cupped.

XANTHOGRANULOMATOUS PYELONEPHRITIS

Xanthogranulomatous pyelonephritis is an unusual form of renal infection characterized by abscess formation. Microscopically, the abscesses are usually multiple with central necrosis, and chronic inflammatory cells (plasma cells, lymphocytes, and multinucleated giant cells) and lipid-laden histiocytes are commonly seen adjacent to them. An intense fibrous tissue reaction is often seen at the periphery of the lesions. Depending on the extent of the infection, the inflammatory process may be confined to the kidney or may involve the perinephric and paranephric spaces (Elliott and associates).

Xanthogranulomatous pyelonephritis is more common in females (Anhalt and associates; Gammill and associates; Noyes and Palubinskas), although Gingell and associates and Malek and associates reported an equal sex distribution. Most patients have a long history of urinary tract infection (months to years), and 7 of the 13 patients with xanthogranulomatous pyelonephritis described by Gammill and associates were diabetics. *Proteus mirabilis* is the most common uropathogen, although *Escherichia coli, Pseudomonas, Aerobacter, Staphylococcus aureus, Klebsiella,* and *Staphylococcus faecalis* have been identified as pathogens. In 7 of 18 patients with xanthogranulomatous pyelonephritis described by Malek and associates, there was an association of reversible hepatic dysfunction similar to the hepatic dysfunction observed in some patients with renal cell carcinoma.

Radiographic Findings in Xanthogranulomatous Pyelonephritis

Xanthogranulomatous pyelonephritis may present either as a diffuse process involving the kidney or as a localized renal abscess (Figs. 10–27, 10–28, and 10–29). Perinephric extension of the inflammatory process may produce an ill-defined renal margin and alterations of the perinephric space. The radiographic manifestations and the rate of incidence reported in the literature vary because of the spectrum of gross anatomic and microscopic changes produced by the inflammatory process.

In the review of xanthogranulomatous pyelonephritis reported by Noyes and Palubinskas, 85 per cent of the cases were associated with a nonfunctioning kidney, whereas 15 per cent of the patients presented with a renal mass. Ureteropelvic juncture obstruction with a nonfunctioning kidney may be associated with an opaque calculus (80 per cent), inflammatory stricture, or tumor, or with a nonopaque calculus (Noyes and Palubinskas). Nine of these patients had localized disease (six unilocular and three multilocular) and four had diffuse disease. Eight of the patients with localized or segmental involvement of the kidney had little or no impairment of function on the excretory urogram. Excretory urograms on the five patients with diffuse involvement demonstrated poor visualization of the collecting system in three and nonvisualization in two.

The excretory urogram may reveal a nonfunctioning or poorly functioning pyonephrotic kidney (Beachley and associates), renal enlargement with diffuse parenchymal involvement, or segmental involvement presenting as a renal mass or abscess (tumefactive form of xanthogranulomatous pyelonephritis). Nephrolithiasis is commonly associated with xanthogranulomatous pyelonephritis (22 to 80 per cent of cases) and may manifest as an obstructing stone or a staghorn calculus, or as calcification within the parenchyma. Eight of 13 patients with xanthogranulomatous pyelonephritis (60 per cent) reported by Gammill

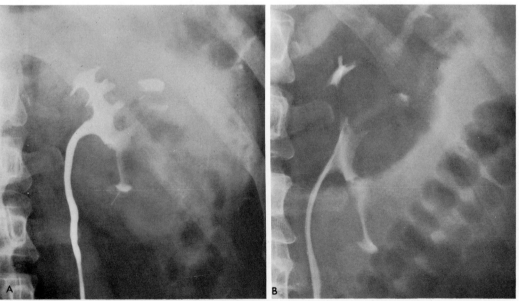

Figure 10–27. Tumefactive xanthogranulomatous pyelonephritis. **A,** *Retrograde pyelogram.* Mass lesion of lower pole of left kidney. **B,** *Three months later.* Enlargement of mass with greater compression and deformity of calyces, and kidney displaced against spinal column. Nephrectomy done at this time.

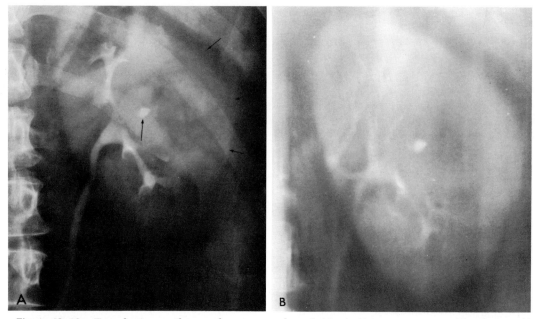

Figure 10–28. Tumefactive xanthogranulomatous pyelonephritis. **A,** *Excretory urogram.* Mass lesion of left kidney with calyceal deformity and renal calculus (*vertical arrow*). **B,** *Nephrotomogram.* This delineates outline of mass better than does **A** and demonstrates that the mass is solid. Preoperative diagnosis: hypernephroma.

Figure 10–29. *Excretory urogram.* **Tumefactive xanthogranulomatous pyelonephritis.** Large mass occupying upper pole of left kidney. Underlying calyces distorted and blunted. Urine culture revealed *Proteus* organisms. Resected specimen: xanthogranulomatous pyelonephritis.

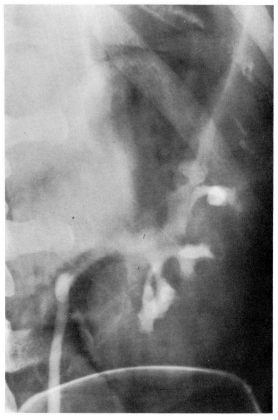

and associates had calculi; six of these had staghorn calculi, one had an obstructing ureteral stone, and one had calculi within the inflammatory lesion.

In the 18 cases of xanthogranulomatous pyelonephritis reported by Malek and associates, urographic studies demonstrated a renal mass in twelve patients, a nonfunctioning kidney in three, and a hydronephrotic kidney in three. Nephrolithiasis was found in four patients, and in three patients the inflammatory mass contained calcification.

The angiographic appearance of xanthogranulomatous pyelonephritis, like the urographic appearance, varies according to the extent that the kidney is involved by the inflammatory process. Gammill and associates suggest that some cases of xanthogranulomatous pyelonephritis can be differentiated angiographically from renal cell carcinoma, but they point out that the vascular pattern produced by squamous cell carcinoma and by a solitary avascular xanthogranulomatous mass cannot be definitely distinguished from renal cell carcinoma. Vinik and associates and Becker have emphasized the difficulty in angiographically differentiating xanthogranulomatous pyelonephritis from renal cell carcinoma.

RENAL AND PERIRENAL ABSCESS

by H. Peter Jander

Renal and perirenal abscesses are considered together because their radiographic and clinical features are so similar that a separate description would be redundant. Presently available evidence suggests, however, that in many instances a significant difference in pathophysiology and etiology exists between these two entities. This is outlined subsequently.

Inflammation of the renal and perirenal space represents an unusually difficult and often frustrating problem for the clinician and radiologist alike. This is particularly disturbing because delayed diagnosis is associated with prolonged morbidity and high mortality (Thorley and associates) and frequently leaves no alternative but to resect an irreversibly damaged, nonfunctioning kidney. Early and accurate diagnosis, on the other hand, allows intensive parenteral antibiotic therapy that results, at times, in complete morphologic and functional recovery of the organ. The diagnostic application of improved understanding of the pathophysiologic events and morphologic changes involved in renal and perirenal abscess formation (Hill and Clark), combined with a clearer demonstration of the pathologic process through improved conventional urographic techniques, angiography, radionuclide studies, sonography, and computerized axial tomography, is an important step toward this end.

Etiology of Renal and Perirenal Abscesses

Prevalent current concepts about the source and mechanism of renal abscess formation are best discussed separately from those concerned with perirenal abscess formation.

Renal abscesses are uncommon disorders accounting for no more than 2 per cent of all renal masses (Pollack and associates). Renal tissue is thought to become infected by one of three mechanisms: (1) hematogenous spread from a distant infected focus, (2) ascending infection from the bladder, and (3) lymphatic spread from nearby organs.

In the preantibiotic era, 80 per cent of renal abscesses were thought to be hematogenous in origin (Campbell). The pathogens entered the blood stream from a preceding and often forgotten superficial or deep infection elsewhere in the body, for example, from a furuncle or carbuncle, or from paronychia, tonsillitis, endocarditis, otitis media, or other source. Staphylococci and streptococci were the usual offending organisms. During the last 25 years, gramnegative organisms have been implicated much more often and are now identified as the causative organism in 80 per cent of adults and 50 per cent of children (Murphy and Koehler; Timmons and Perlmutter).

ASCENDING infection - gm - abscess

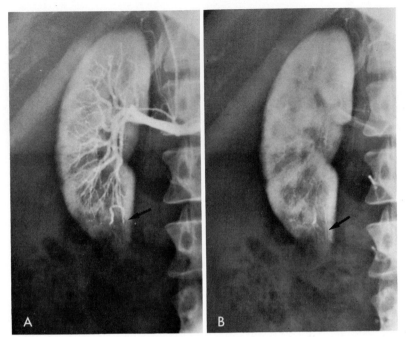

Figure 10–30. *Arteriogram.* **Renal and perirenal abscess** involving lower pole and perirenal space of right kidney (*arrows*). Infection had spread from chronic ulcerative colitis of ascending colon. **A,** *Arterial phase.* **B,** *Parenchymal phase.*

Since clinical evidence of preceding gram-negative septicemia is rare and since it is nearly impossible to produce gram-negative hematogenous pyelonephritis experimentally unless the kidney is traumatized or completely obstructed (Cotran), it seems likely that the route of spread in the majority of today's patients is ascending from the bladder via the ureter to the kidney, where pyelonephritis and cortical abscesses develop. Vesicoureteral reflux is thought to provide a convenient vehicle for the upstream transport of pathogens. Staphylococcal and streptococcal infection are still encountered, especially in patients with diabetes mellitus and, with increasing frequency, in drug addicts who maintain their habit through "mainlining."

The lymphatic spread of infection to the kidney has never been actually demonstrated, but theoretically, lymphatics originating in the bladder and rectum could provide a bacterial pathway to the kidneys.

Perirenal abscesses can form when a renal cortical abscess breaks through the true renal capsule. If the process continues on to break through the renal (Gerota's) fascia, it theoretically represents pararenal extension even though the distinction between peri- and pararenal location is usually not made clinically. In Altemeier and Alexander's series of 160 patients with retroperitoneal abscess, 76 (43 per cent) of the abscesses were perinephric (Altemeier and associates). Seventy per cent of these abscesses were of renal origin, with pyelonephritis the most common preceding renal affliction. Twenty-five per cent had no known etiology. If the abscess is situated in a pararenal location anterior to the renal fascia, direct extension from duodenal, biliary-duct, pancreatic, and colonic lesions becomes a likely cause (Fig. 10–30). Less than 5 per cent of abscesses in this location are thought to have a hematogenous origin (Thorley and associates).

Pathophysiology of Renal and Perirenal Abscesses

Accumulated experimental and clinical data provide a substantial body of basic information concerning the functional and morphologic changes associated with renal and perirenal abscess formation.

Combined angiographic, microangiographic, and histologic studies of experimental pyelonephritis done in chronologic sequence delineate the following events (Hill and Clark).

During the first week of hematogenous gram-negative pyelonephritis, there is progressive vasoconstriction of segmental renal arterial branches, arcuate arteries, interlobular arteries, and afferent arterioles localized in the region of acute inflammation. The postglomerular peritubular capillary plexus in the involved areas is clogged with polymorphonuclear leukocytes and is progressively destroyed by the inflammatory process. It appears that this vasoconstrictive response to inflammation is unique to the vascular bed of the renal cortex and sets it apart from vascular beds in other sites, including the perirenal space, which respond with vasodilatation rather than vasoconstriction (Zweifach and associates) (see Figure 10–63). The cause of this vasospasm remains speculative. In 1966, Hill suggested that locally released renin could be responsible through the renin-angiotensin mechanism. Trueta and associates showed that systemic application of bacterial endotoxins (made up of the phospholipid fraction of the cell walls of gram-negative organisms) will cause this phenomenon, and Palmiero and associates suggested that endotoxins act through catecholamine release.

By the end of the first week the kidney is markedly swollen. Mononuclear cells and fibroblasts begin to join the predominantly polymorphonuclear infiltrate at this point. Papillary necrosis of a variable extent can be seen on microangiographs and histologic sections but cannot be identified by clinical imaging procedures at this stage.

By two weeks the kidney size has returned to normal. The arterial spasm has subsided but has given way to mild tortuosity and kinking of arteries as a result of newly formed fibrous tissue replacing the destroyed parenchyma. In cases with papillary necrosis, the sequestration of the necrotic papilla is largely complete, and ingrowth of fibrous tissue and re-epithelialization of the raw surface have begun.

After one month of untreated infection, the main renal artery and its branches are diminished in caliber, probably as a response to diminished blood demand in a partially destroyed kidney. If the infectious process continues unchecked and leads to complete destruction of the kidney, the corresponding renal artery will be completely lost while the renal vein may still be demonstrated angiographically (Fig. 10–31). At the same time, new vascular growth appears in the region of the renal pelvis and in the periphery of cortical and medullary abscesses. These new vessels may be too small and too few in number to be identified in clinical radiographic studies but may sometimes be demonstrated in microangiograms (Fig. 10–32). Others, particularly those in the periphery of the abscess, give rise to the inflammatory blush seen in angiograms of some patients (Fig. 10–33). Over the ensuing two months, the tortuosity and kinking of arteries and arterioles become much more prominent, and their caliber decreases further in response to further contraction of the fibrous scar tissue that now replaces destroyed parenchyma. Glomeruli are most resistant to the infectious process, but eventually they exhibit all stages of glomerulosclerosis with eventual complete destruction. Few tubular elements survive in involved areas.

Clinical Aspects of Renal and Perirenal Abscess

There is no sex predilection for renal and perirenal abscesses. Predisposing factors such as renal calculi, neurogenic bladder, urinary tract obstruction and intravenous drug abuse are very common. Diabetes was found in 67 per cent of the patients in one series (Cotran). Early manifestations of the disease are nonspecific and nonlocalizing and consist of low-grade fever, general

Text continued on page 848

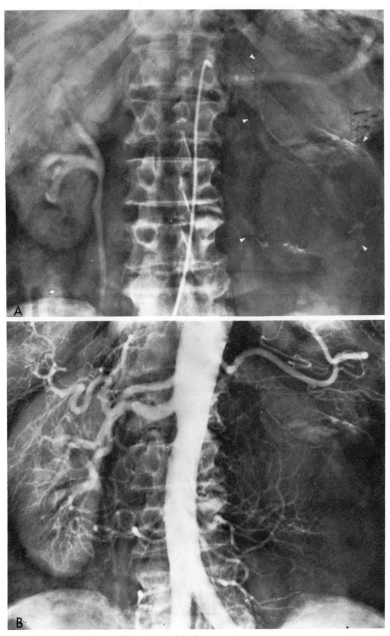

Figure 10–31. **End stage of chronically infected kidney. A,** *Excretory urogram.* Multilocular calcified mass in left upper quadrant *(arrows).* **B,** *Arteriography* reveals absence of left renal artery and "absence" of left kidney.

Illustration continued on following page

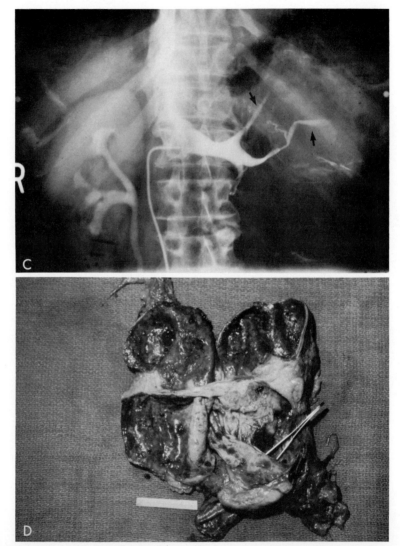

Figure 10–31 *Continued.*   C, *Venography* demonstrates presence of the compressed left renal vein *(arrows)*. D, *Surgical specimen.* At surgery, a huge cystic mass containing dark brownish fluid with tissue debris and blood was found. The cut surface revealed complete replacement of the normal renal parenchyma. Histologic diagnosis: multicystic kidney with chronic pyelonephritis.

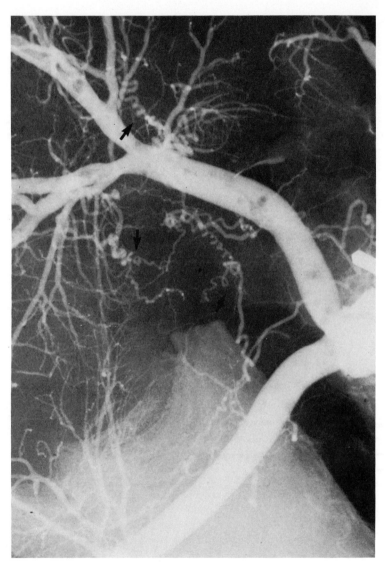

Figure 10–32. *Injected specimen* of a **chronically infected kidney with a staghorn calculus.** Note the "corkscrew" arteries in the region of the inflamed pelvis *(arrow).*

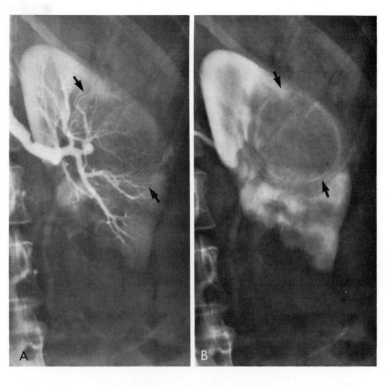

Figure 10–33. Renal cortical abscess with peripheral inflammatory blush. **A,** *Arteriogram, arterial phase.* Note displacement and splaying of arteries around abscess (*arrows*). Arterial caliber is reduced. Accessory artery to lower pole is not opacified. **B,** *Arteriogram, capillary phase.* Peripheral inflammatory blush in late parenchymal phase (*arrows*).

malaise, increased sedimentation rate, high white blood cell counts, and abdominal pain. As the infection progresses, dysuria, chills, and flank pain become the predominant symptoms, and on physical examination flank tenderness, abdominal muscle guarding, abdominal mass, and limitation of hip motion due to irritation of the psoas muscle may be found. It must be emphasized that urine cultures are often negative throughout the entire course of the disease even when pathogenic organisms can be cultured from the surgical specimen.

Roentgen Findings in Renal and Perirenal Abscesses

The earliest phases of renal or perirenal infection leave no radiographic traces. A plain film with its inherent low radiographic sensitivity only allows detection of advanced and virulent forms of infection, usually with substantial perirenal spread. The changes observed result from two principal factors: mass effect and host response to bacterial toxins.

A mass within or adjacent to the kidney such as a renal or perirenal abscess manifests itself by displacement of the kidney or by deviation of adjacent structures such as the hepatic and splenic flexures of the colon and the duodenum (Fig. 10–34). Depending on the location of the abscess, the kidney may be pushed medially against the spinal column, laterally, downward, or upward. It must be remembered, however, that normal kidneys are subject to wide variations of position. The additional finding of a soft-tissue mass (representing an abscess situated in a position to cause displacement) is valuable evidence that the renal displacement is due to a pathologic process.

Bacterial products elicit a radiographically recognizable host reaction in the kidney and adjacent structures in some patients. The earliest recognizable effect on the kidney itself is diffuse enlargement that is probably the result of renal edema (see Figure 10–1). Renal calculi have been reported to be associated with perirenal abscess in 20 to 30 per cent of patients (Altemeier and associates; Trueta and associates; Zweifach and associates). In patients in whom inflammation spreads

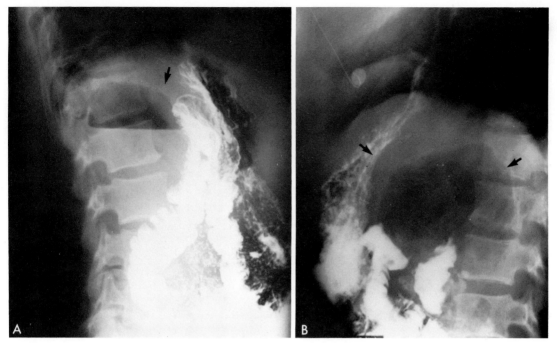

Figure 10–34. Perinephric abscess simulating subdiaphragmatic abscess and displacing adjacent structures. **A,** *Barium enema and lateral view.* Large (peri-) renal abscess represented by air-fluid level displacing splenic flexure of colon anteriorly *(arrow).* **B,** *Upper gastrointestinal series.* Body of the stomach is pushed anteriorly by gas-filled abscess *(arrows).*

beyond the true renal capsule, psoas and renal margins may become hazy and indistinct (Fig. 10–35), and lumbar scoliosis with the concavity to the side of the lesion may ensue (Fig. 10–36). Extension of the process superiorly into the subphrenic area

causes elevation of the ipsilateral hemidiaphragm with subsegmental atelectasis, and pleural effusion may be observed (Figs. 10–37 and 38). Occasionally, a gas-containing abscess may form, simulating subdiaphragmatic abscess of nonrenal ori-

Figure 10–35. *Plain film.* Perinephric abscess involving right kidney. Note haziness of shadow on right, with absence of normal outline of psoas muscle, which is considered characteristic of perinephric abscess.

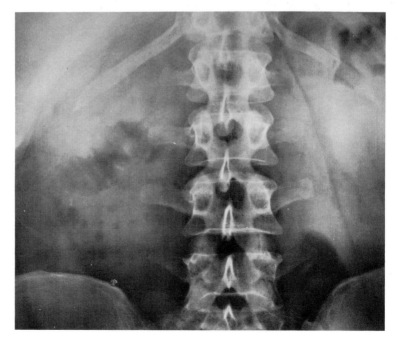

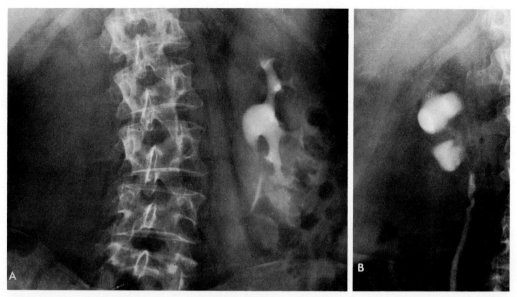

Figure 10–36.   Cortical abscess of right kidney **with perinephric abscess. A,** *Excretory urogram.* Large perinephric abscess of right kidney, which has no function. Scoliosis of lumbar portion of spinal column, with concavity toward right and absence of normal psoas outline. Left kidney normal. **B,** *Right retrograde pyelogram.* Cortical abscess has eroded into pelviocalyceal system.

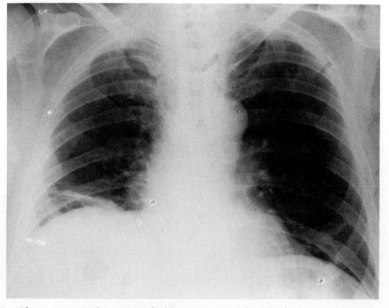

Figure 10–37.   *Chest x-ray.* **Right perirenal abscess** associated with elevation of right hemidiaphragm and subsegmental atelectasis.

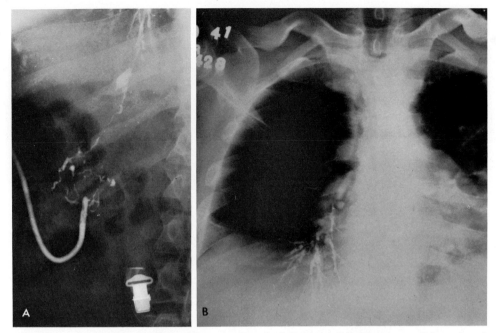

Figure 10–38. Perinephric abscess with nephrobronchial fistula. A, Medium injected through catheter inserted in draining lumbar sinus outlines irregular cavity in right renal region with communication through diaphragm to lower part of bronchial tree. **B,** Film of chest shows contrast medium outlining lower small bronchi. Note: This condition originated from branched calculus in right kidney, complicated by multiple cortical abscesses and perinephric abscess. Subcapsular nephrectomy was done for this condition. Draining sinus continued and incision was explored about 4½ months later. A piece of stone and a fragment of renal pelvis were removed and sinus was curetted. These films were made 1 month after curettage.

gin (Fig. 10–39). Paralysis and dilatation of bowel loops adjacent to the abscess are seen more rarely. In severe necrotizing infections associated with obstruction or diabetes, air in the kidneys and perirenal space may be detected on the plain film (Fig. 10–40). These forms of infection carry a mortality rate of 40 per cent or more but fortunately are rare (Love and associates; Stadalnik and Dublin).

All these findings, including perirenal gas, are nonspecific in that they can be the result of duodenal perforation (Fig. 10–41), emphysematous pancreatitis, or lesser-sac abscess as well as renal and perirenal abscess, but their detection may be a great help in diagnosis when properly correlated with the clinical data at hand.

THE UROGRAM IN RENAL AND PERIRENAL ABSCESSES

With contrast opacification of the renal parenchyma and collecting system, specific abnormalities are made more obvious, and plain film findings such as haziness of the renal outline and renal displacement become more easily recognizable. One of the earliest changes seen is evidence of pressure on one or more calyces, which may be caused by either a perirenal accumulation of pus or a cortical abscess in the vicinity of the calyx (Figs. 10–42 through 10–48). The involved calyx or calyces may fill incompletely during excretory urography, but if pressure on the calyx from the abscess is minimal, they may be filled during retrograde pyelography. If this happens, the calyx may appear almost normal or only slightly dilated on the retrograde pyelogram, and the findings may be dismissed as being of no importance unless the physician is keenly aware of the possibilities. If the process is advanced, however, incomplete calyceal filling or even complete obliteration may be evident from the retrograde pyelogram.

The sign of "fixation" or decrease in

Text continued on page 856

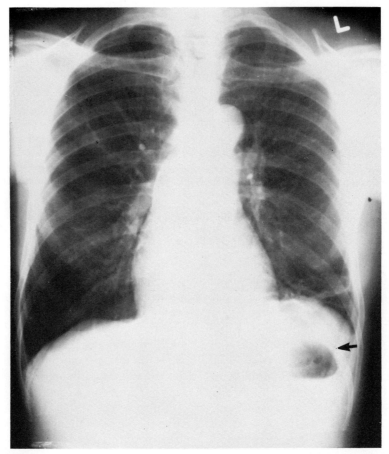

Figure 10–39. *Chest x-ray.* **Left renal abscess** *(arrow)* containing gas and fluid and simulating a left sub-diaphragmatic abscess.

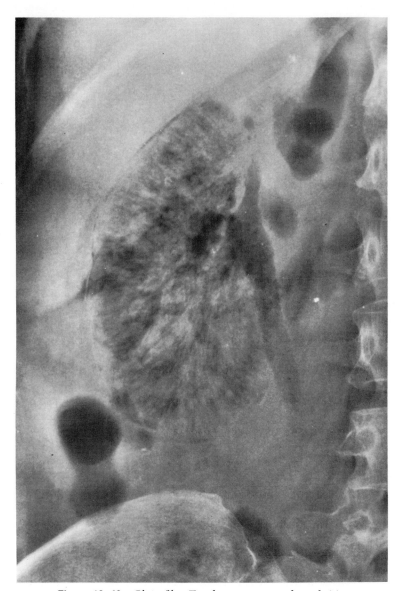

Figure 10–40. *Plain film.* Emphysematous pyelonephritis.

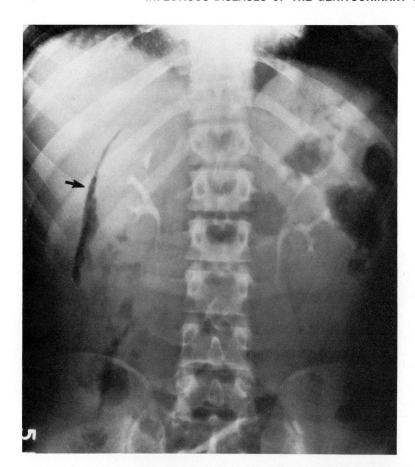

Figure 10–41. *Excretory urogram.* **Ruptured duodenum with perirenal air** *(arrow).*

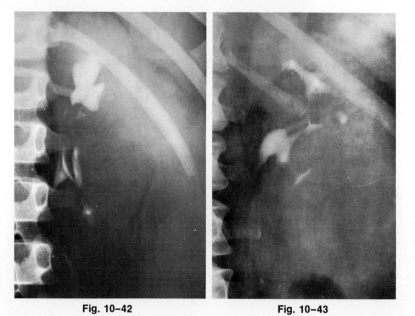

Fig. 10–42   Fig. 10–43

Figure 10–42. *Excretory urogram.* **Cortical abscess,** left kidney. Large, sharply outlined mass causing crescentic deformity of pelvis and lower-pole calyces.

Figure 10–43. *Excretory urogram.* **Large cortical abscess,** lower pole of left kidney. Ureter displaced medially and lower-pole calyces slightly deformed.

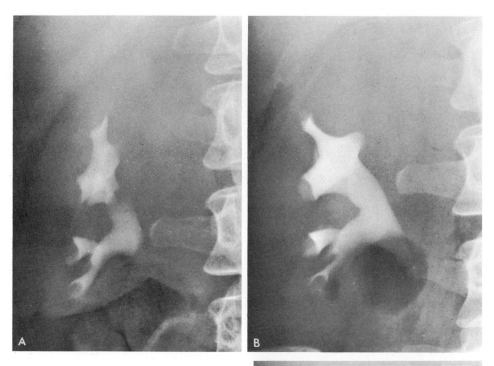

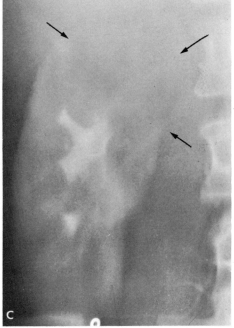

Figure 10–44. Cortical abscess (renal carbuncle) in upper pole of right kidney of woman, 52 years of age. Progress films. Diagnosis proved surgically. **A,** *Excretory urogram.* Little or no deformity of upper calyx, but outline of upper pole of kidney poorly delineated. **B,** *Excretory urogram,* 6 weeks later. Marked change in contour of upper calyx, which is now definitely pathologic and suggests expanding lesion in cortex distorting calyx. **C,** *Nephrotomogram.* Abscess can be seen as translucent round area 6 cm in diameter in upper pole (*arrows*). Simulates solitary cyst.

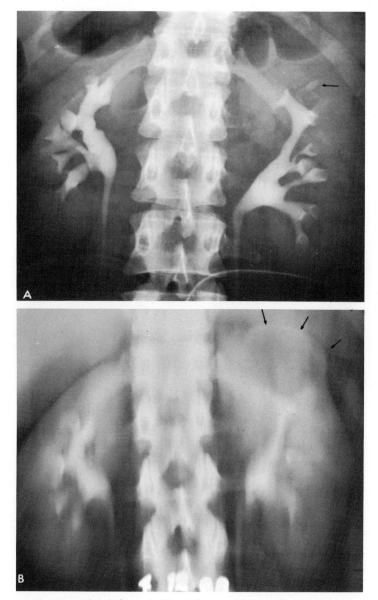

Figure 10–45.   Renal abscess, left kidney. A, *Excretory urogram.* Small parenchymal calculus (*arrow*). Renal outline of upper pole of left kidney is ill defined. **B,** *Nephrotomogram.* Thick-walled mass lesion (*arrows*) in upper pole of left kidney. Preoperative diagnosis: renal abscess versus necrotic hypernephroma.

mobility of a kidney, which has been stressed by Mathé, is a fairly common and important finding. Fixation can be demonstrated by exposing films during both phases of respiration or by obtaining a film with the patient upright (Fig. 10–49). A normal kidney should have an excursion of the width of one lumbar vertebra. If the kidney is fixed in its position, perirenal inflammation should be suspected.

A cortical abscess may erode into and communicate with the collecting system of the kidney so that the resulting urogram will show irregular cavities simulating tuberculosis (Figs. 10–50 through 10–53). A cortical abscess may also "point" toward the periphery and rupture through the renal capsule into the perinephric fat rather than into the pelviocalyceal system. Occasionally this rupture can be suspected on

Text continued on page 860

NORMAL KIDNEY EXCURSION - 1 LUMBAR vert.

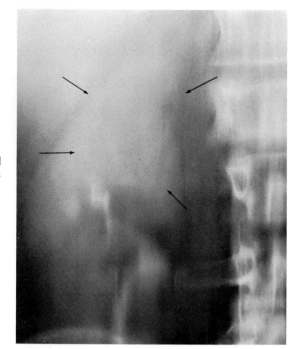

Figure 10–46. *Nephrotomogram.* **Cortical renal abscess.** Mass lesion, upper pole of right kidney. Margins of abscess (*arrows*) indistinct.

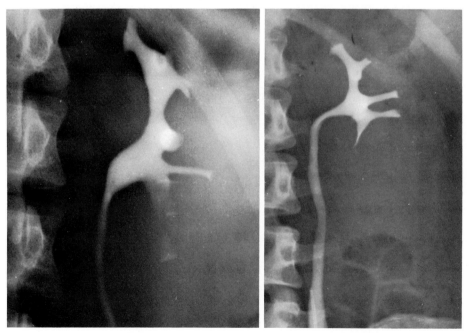

Fig. 10–47   Fig. 10–48

Figure 10–47. *Retrograde pyelogram.* **Cortical abscess,** lower pole of left kidney. Distortion and incomplete filling of the lower-pole calyx result.

Figure 10–48. *Left retrograde pyelogram.* **Cortical abscess** in lower pole of left kidney, causing crescentic deformity of lower calyces of left kidney, simulating tumor or cyst.

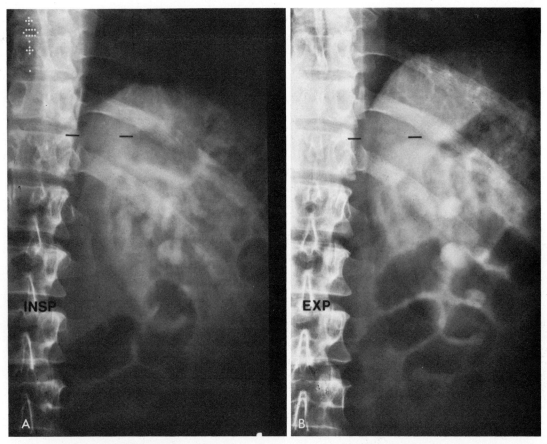

Figure 10–49. *Excretory urogram.* **Perinephric abscess.** Fixation of right kidney in deep inspiration (**A**) and expiration (**B**) due to perinephric inflammation.

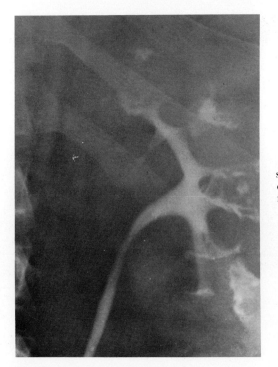

Figure 10–50. *Retrograde pyelogram.* **Cortical abscess, left kidney.** Left retrograde pyelogram demonstrates communication between abscesses and calyces, with marked calyceal deformity.

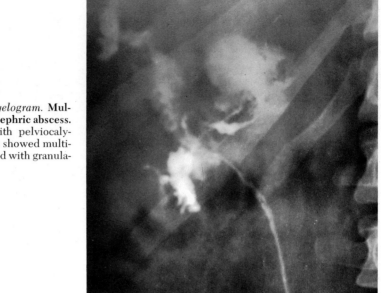

Figure 10–51. *Retrograde pyelogram.* **Multiple abscesses of kidney and perinephric abscess.** Abscess pockets communicate with pelviocalyceal system. Incision and drainage showed multilocular pockets in renal region filled with granulation tissue.

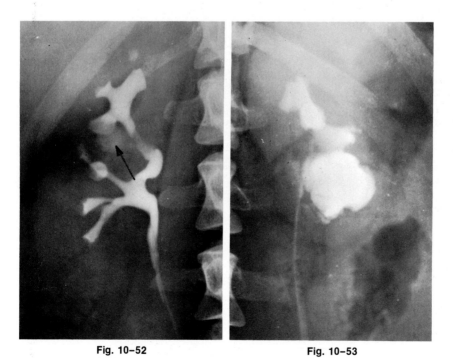

Fig. 10–52   Fig. 10–53

Figure 10–52. *Retrograde pyelogram.* **Cortical abscess** that has eroded through infundibulum of upper calyx and communicates with pelviocalyceal system.

Figure 10–53. *Retrograde pyelogram.* **Cortical abscess** involving lower pole of left kidney and communicating with lower group of calyces, causing marked deformity and cortical necrosis.

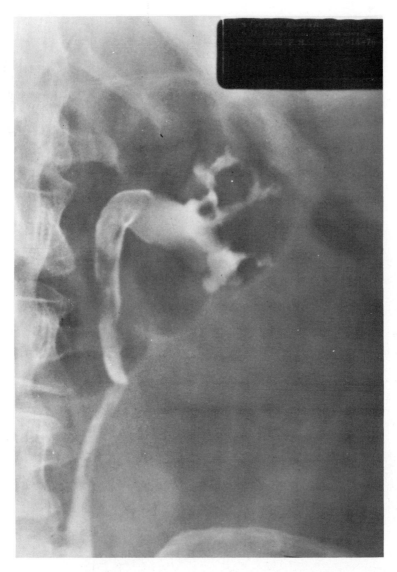

Figure 10–54. *Retrograde pyelogram.* Dispersion of contrast medium throughout pus in collecting system of **pyonephrotic kidney.**

both the plain film and the excretory urogram owing to a loss in clarity of the renal margin and to the extension of a mass opacity beyond the confines of the kidney.

The clinical manifestations of pyonephrosis are similar to those of cortical abscess. It is a separate pathologic entity, however, because the infection is predominantly within the pelvis and calyces. Obstruction is a constant feature, and an inflammatory exudate accumulates within a dilated pelviocalyceal system. All or part of the involved kidney invariably fails to function during excretory urography, and

the renal shadow may appear enlarged. Retrograde pyelography demonstrates either complete obstruction (usually at the ureteropelvic juncture) or a peculiar pyelographic picture resulting from dispersion of the contrast medium throughout exudate and debris that has accumulated in the dilated pelvis and calyces (Fig. 10–54).

The diagnostic endpoint of renal and perirenal abscesses, with rare exceptions, is a "renal mass" or "perirenal mass," and further differentiation can only be achieved by additional imaging procedures (Figs. 10–55 and 10–56).

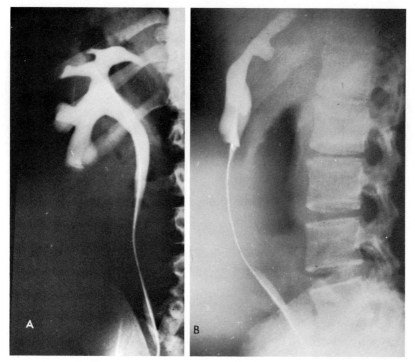

Figure 10-55. Cortical infection of right kidney with perinephric abscess. **A,** *Right retrograde pyelogram, anteroposterior view.* Deformity of upper calyces, with flattening and crescentic outline, suggesting pressure from cortical abscess. **B,** *Lateral view.* Marked anterior displacement of kidney from perinephric abscess. (From Menville, J. G.: The Lateral Pyelogram as a Diagnostic Aid in Perinephric Abscess. J.A.M.A. *111*:231–233 (16 July) 1938.

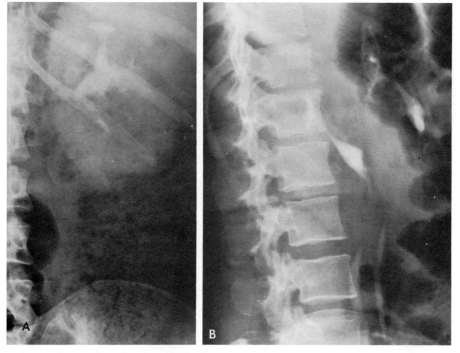

Figure 10-56. Perinephric abscess with displacement of kidney. **A,** *Excretory urogram.* Upward and lateral displacement of left kidney with poor filling. **B,** *Lateral view.* Marked anterior displacement of left kidney caused by perinephric abscess. (Courtesy of Dr. S. J. Arnold and Departments of Urology and Radiology, Jewish Hospital of Brooklyn.)

RADIONUCLIDE IMAGING IN RENAL AND PERIRENAL ABSCESSES

Edwards and Hayes in 1970 were the first to draw attention to the potential of gallium citrate ^{67}Ga as a tumor localizing agent when they reported its preferential uptake in a variety of malignant neoplasms. Subsequent reports confirmed the tumor affinity of gallium citrate but pointed out an "annoying" propensity to localize in inflammatory lesions as well (Higasi and associates; Langhammer and associates; Lavender and associates). Recent attempts to take advantage of this "annoying" quality have met with some success and it appears that under appropriate clinical conditions, the uptake of ^{67}Ga in inflammatory lesions can be helpful in detection and differential diagnosis of renal abscesses (Fratkin and Sharpe; Hopkins and associates; Koehler; Kumar and associates; Littenberg and associates; Love and associates; Obrant; Rabinowitz and associates).

Intravenously administered gallium citrate labels leukocytes and macrophages. This property explains its reported accumulation in processes such as rheumatoid arthritis, fractures, and infections, and in surgical incisions (Bell and associates). Gallium citrate also binds to plasma proteins and is actively excreted in the bile, and by the gastrointestinal tract and the kidneys. Unfortunately, the accumulation of gallium citrate in an area is an indication of a septic process only if tumors (particularly those rich in leukocytes, such as Hodgkin's lymphoma) can be excluded and the process can be separated from the lumina of the gut, the urinary tract, and the biliary tree. Fortunately, the concentration of isotope in normal tissue rapidly decreases, whereas the accumulation in inflammatory areas first increases and then decreases slowly. Because of this, scanning is most successful at 48 to 72 hours after the administration of the isotope and after the bowel and bladder have been evacuated. Figure 10–57 depicts a renal and perirenal abscess demonstrated on gallium scan. Refinement of the procedure, e.g., by selective labeling of leuko-

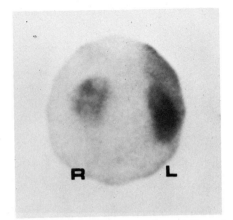

Figure 10–57. *Gallium scan.* **Large left renal and perirenal abscess.** Increased accumulation of gallium citrate ^{67}Ga in left kidney.

cytes, may enhance its specificity and reduce nonspecific accumulation of the isotope in the biliary tree, gut, and urinary tract. A gallium scan is a readily performed, noninvasive procedure, and when closely correlated with the history, the physical examination, and other imaging procedures, it can provide helpful information in this difficult diagnostic area.

THE RENAL ANGIOGRAM IN RENAL AND PERIRENAL ABSCESSES

The imaging procedures described so far, singly or in various combinations, usually allow one to establish unequivocally the presence or absence of a renal or perirenal pathologic process. Correlation of these data with the clinical findings and physical examination will favor a presumptive diagnosis of abscess in many patients. In others, uncertainty may still persist with regard to whether a process is inflammatory or malignant in nature. In our experience, renal angiography, though not infallible, is a very sensitive diagnostic tool for distinguishing these two entities.

Angiographic differentiation is based on those unique morphologic and dynamic vascular changes characteristic of inflammatory lesions that are described in the pathophysiology section of this discussion.

It will be remembered that in early infection, postglomerular, peritubular capillaries in the inflamed area are clogged with neutrophilic leukocytes, and larger proximal arteries are in vasospasm. This vasospastic response to inflammation is a unique characteristic of renal vessels and sets them apart from vessels in other anatomic regions, including the perirenal space, which respond with vasodilatation. The occluded capillaries and constricted arteries cause slow flow of contrast in the inflamed areas that results in persistent arterial filling while the remainder of the normal parenchyma is already in the nephrographic phase. Often these arteries will be stretched and displaced around the abscess (Fig. 10–58). A consequence of the capillary occlusion and destruction is a mottled nephrogram and loss of distinctness of the corticomedullary margin and renal outline (Fig. 10–59).

In later states of the disease process, the slow flow persists as a result of vascular luminal compromise due to fibrous encasement of renal vessels. This process, together with the associated contraction of the fibrous scar tissue, leads to development of tortuous or "corkscrew" arteries (Fig. 10–60).

Inflammatory neovascularity characterized by an increased number of fine, regular, often parallel-running, and normally tapering vessels is often seen in the periphery of the abscess (Fig. 10–61). In our experience, these vessels can be distinguished from tumor vessels, which exhibit an irregular course and caliber with puddling and pooling of contrast material—although the difference can at times be quite subtle.

Trueta and coworkers convincingly demonstrated that the renal blood has two potential pathways of flow. One is cortical, the other medullary. Under normal circumstances, most blood circulates through the cortical route. It appears that certain experimental and clinical conditions, ranging from systemic application of bacterial en-

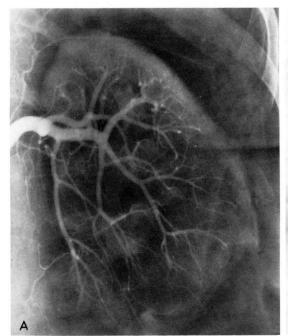 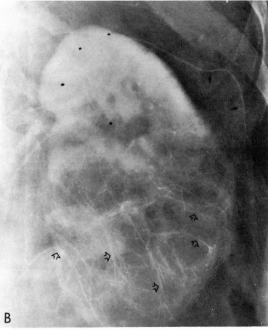

Figure 10–58. *Selective left renal arteriogram.* **Renal abscess. A,** *Arterial phase.* Interlobar branches in inflamed area are stretched and displaced and fine cortical branches fail to opacify. **B,** *Parenchymal phase.* Arteries in infected lower half of kidney (*open arrows*) are still filled with contrast medium, indicating slow flow. Note also displaced capsular artery (*dark arrows*).

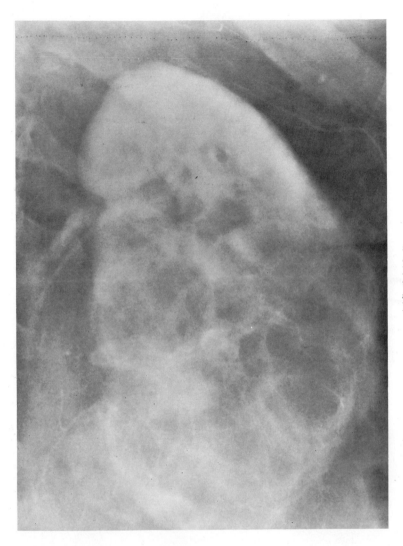

Figure 10–59. Renal abscess. *Late nephrographic phase of selective left renal arteriogram.* Renal outline of infected lower two-thirds of kidney is indistinct, and corticomedullary junction is lost.

dotoxin to the crush syndrome, lead to spasm of interlobular arteries and force the blood through the medullary pathway with a resultant shortened intrarenal circulation time (Trueta phenomenon). Reports of angiographic findings in renal and perirenal abscesses occasionally mention early venous opacification and usually attribute this finding to the Trueta phenomenon (Becker, Kanter, and Perl; Coombs and associates). Our own review of 32 selective renal angiograms of renal and perirenal inflammatory lesions did not reveal early-draining veins. Neither did most other reports in the field (Caplan and associates; Koehler; Rabinowitz and associates). It

seems that this phenomenon is nonspecific and may be limited to advanced cases of renal inflammation (Becker, Kanter, and Perl).

If the abscess extends into the perirenal space, the capsular arteries will be displaced and may show a vasodilatory response to inflammation (Figs. 10–62 and 10–63). Lumbar arteries and veins may contribute to the vascular supply of a perirenal abscess.

In a recent review of 32 cases in which arteriography was done at our institution, the angiographic changes described in the preceding discussion were observed as shown in Table 10–1.

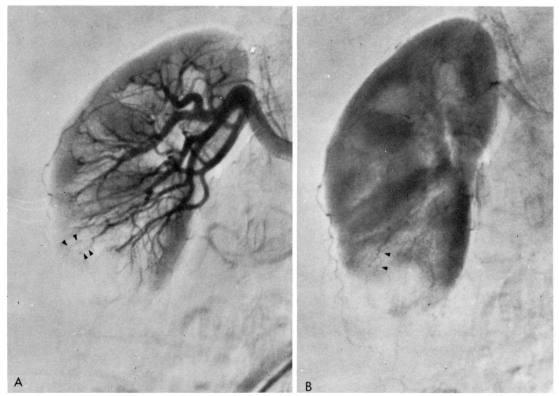

Figure 10–60. Perinephric abscess. *Selective arteriography.* **A,** *Arterial phase.* Lack of filling of smaller branches in lower pole abscess and "corkscrew" arteries in same area (*arrowheads*). Note also prominent capsular artery. **B,** *Parenchymal phase* reveals slow flow through "corkscrew" arteries (*arrowheads*), and displaced and prominent capsular artery indicates perirenal extension. There is loss of cortical and corticomedullary margins.

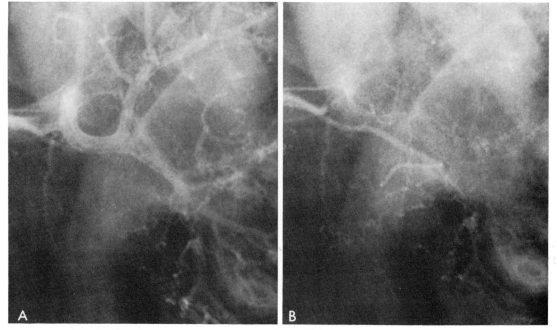

Figure 10–61. Inflammatory neovascularity in a chronically infected kidney. **A,** *Late arterial phase.* **B,** *Parenchymal phase.*

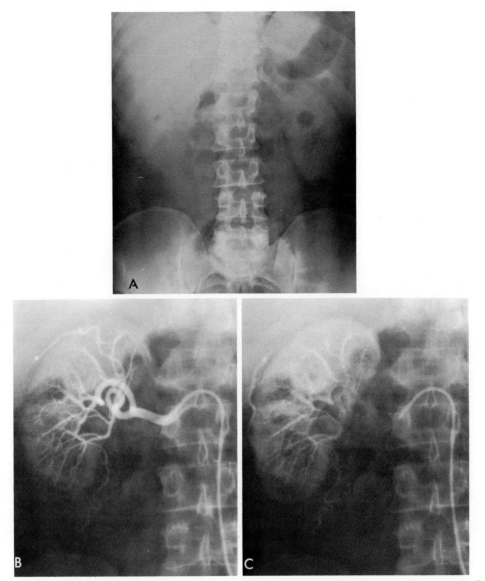

Figure 10–62. Perinephric abscess. Fifty-one-year-old man. **A,** *Plain film.* Absent right psoas shadow. Indistinct outline, right kidney. **B,** *Arteriogram.* Capsular arteries enlarged and tortuous, especially over lower pole. **C,** *Arteriogram, late arterial phase.* Capsular arteries supply tangle of vessels in abscess overlying lower pole.

Epinephrine has been employed infrequently in our patients, but when used, it invariably gave the expected response of vasoconstriction in abscesses and lack of constriction in tumors. Whether reported inconsistencies are related to technical problems such as inadequate mixing of epinephrine with saline or the use of inappropriate dosages, or to true abnormal response of the target vessels remains an open question.

It is our experience that careful evaluation of all dynamic and morphologic changes on high-quality angiograms will allow diagnosis of renal and perirenal inflammatory lesions with a level of confidence that approaches that possible in distinguishing cysts from neoplasms.

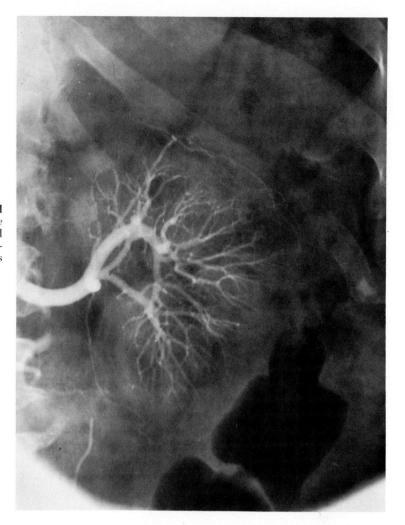

Figure 10-63. Acute renal and perirenal abscess. *Selective arteriogram.* While peripheral renal arteries are in spasm, capsular artery is dilated and reveals prominent flow.

Table 10-1. **Angiographic Changes Found in 32 Cases of Renal and Perirenal Abscess**

ANGIOGRAPHIC FINDINGS	NUMBER OF CASES	PER CENT OF CASES
Slow flow	12	37.5
Reduced or absent peripheral arterial filling	26	81
Stretching of intrarenal vessels	23	72
Capsular artery displacement	16	50
Capsular artery enlargement	7	22
Inflammatory neovascularity	15	47
Tumor neovascularity	0	0
Delayed nephrogram	11	34
Mottled nephrogram	23	72
Loss of cortical definition	30	94
Inflammatory stain	15	47
Early venous filling	0	0

RESPONSES OF THE COLLECTING SYSTEM TO INFECTION

DILATATION

Ureteral infection may be associated with chronic pyelonephritis. Dynamic factors such as atony, abnormal peristalsis, and dilatation have been observed in patients with vesicoureteral reflux and attributed to active ureteral infection Following successful antibiotic therapy, the ureteral dilatation may disappear and normal peristalsis may return (Shopfner, 1970). Improvement is less likely if the infection is chronic and neglected or inadequately treated.

Vesicoureteral reflux accentuates the degree of ureteral dilatation, and therefore ureters that appear normal on excretory urograms may be found to be grossly dilated during voiding cystography. The lower third of the ureter is frequently dilated on the urogram when reflux is present. Ureteral compression is a helpful adjunct during excretory urography because undue distensibility of the upper ureter may be demonstrated by this means.

MUCOSAL STRIATION

Linear mucosal striations of the renal pelvis and ureter may be associated with

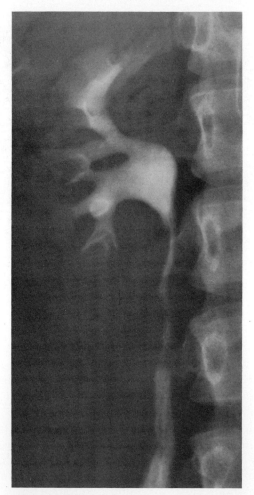

Figure 10–64. *Excretory urogram.* **Inflammatory linear striations,** upper right ureter. Twenty-two-year-old woman with active urinary tract infection. After 6 weeks of antibiotic therapy, striations were no longer evident.

active infection and can result from mucosal edema (Gwinn and Barnes), but they are most frequently demonstrated in dilated or unduly distensible ureters that are incompletely distended during urography (Fig. 10–64). In the latter instance, the findings will usually persist on subsequent urograms, but mucosal edema resulting from active infection will disappear during adequate therapy. The typical fine linear pattern allows easy differentiation from other mucosal abnormalities such as ureteritis cystica and neoplasm.

STRICTURES AND OBSTRUCTION

Severe or chronic ureteral infection (Figs. 10–65 through 10–74) may cause isolated ureteral strictures as areas of alternate constriction or dilatation, but stricture formation is much more likely to occur in tuberculous infection. The diagnosis of

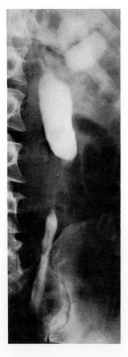

Figure 10–65. *Left retrograde pyelogram.* **Advanced chronic pyelonephritis with ureteral stricture.** Marked inflammatory changes in ureter associated with stricture of middle portion of ureter and dilatation above and below. Advanced caliectasis.

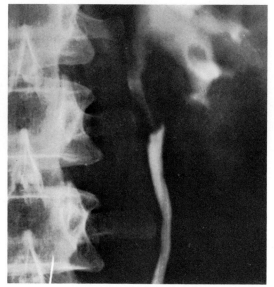

Figure 10–66. *Retrograde pyelogram.* **Chronic pyelonephritis with ureteral stricture.** Marked inflammatory changes in upper third of ureter, with area of narrowing 3 cm below ureteropelvic juncture. Left nephrectomy: definite thickening of ureter below ureteropelvic juncture.

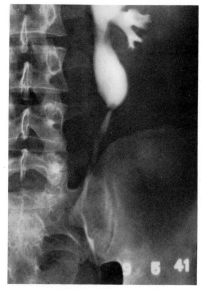

Figure 10–67. *Retrograde pyelogram.* **Ureteral stricture.** Plastic operation done on ureter for stricture.

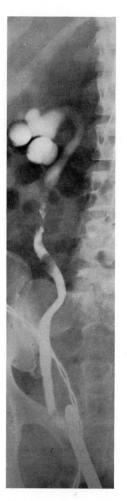

Figure 10–68. *Retrograde pyelogram.* **Ureteral stricture.** Obstruction 2.5 cm below ureteropelvic juncture. Pyelocaliectasis.

ureteral catheter is not sufficient to warrant a diagnosis of stricture, since either finding may result from ureteral peristalsis or spasm.

Ureteral obstruction may result from retroperitoneal abscess formation. The infection is usually secondary to inflammatory bowel disease and perforation. Regional enteritis with perforation of the terminal ileum is the most common (Schofield and associates). In this instance, the site of obstruction is usually the mid-right ureter. Chronic ulcerative colitis and diverticulitis of the colon may also result in perforation, retroperitoneal abscess formation, and ureteral obstruction.

stricture can be established by urography only when the collecting system is definitely dilated above the area in question. Urographic demonstration of a narrowed ureteral segment and inability to pass a

Text continued on page 873

Retroperitoneal aast.

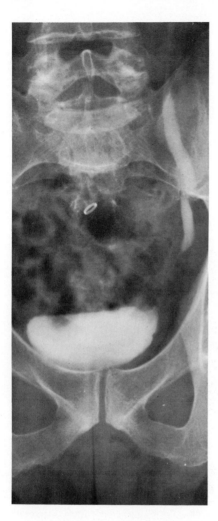

Figure 10–69. *Excretory urogram.* **Inflammatory ureteral stricture,** lower left ureter.

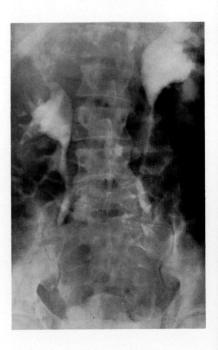

Figure 10–70. *Excretory urogram.* **Regional ileitis** (Crohn's disease) with inflammation in the retroperitoneum resulting in bilateral partial ureteral obstruction. (From Schofield, P. F., Staff, W. G., and Moore, T.)

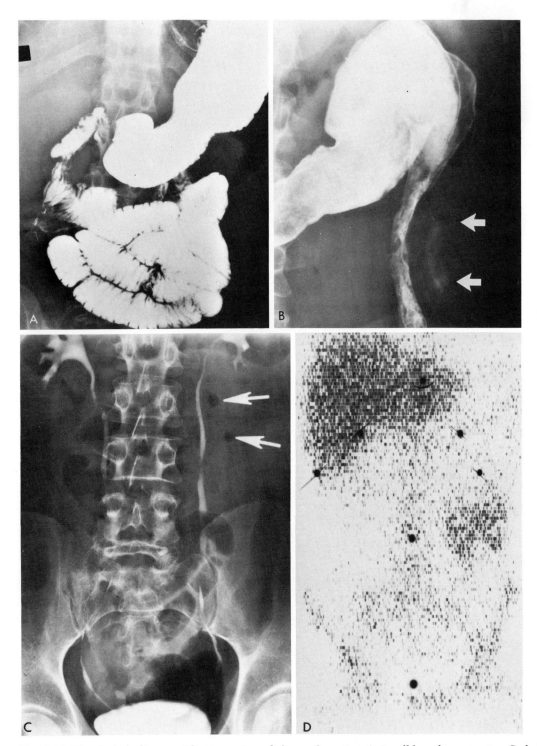

Figure 10–71.   Crohn's disease with retroperitoneal abscess formation. **A,** *Small bowel examination.* Crohn's disease involving second portion of duodenum with multiple associated fistulas (*arrows*). **B,** *Colon examination.* Crohn's disease involving splenic flexure of colon. Barium in fistulous tract (*arrows*). **C,** *Excretory urogram.* Small collections of gas in retroperitoneal abscess (*arrows*). **D,** *Gallium scan.* Increased uptake at site of left retroperitoneal abscess.

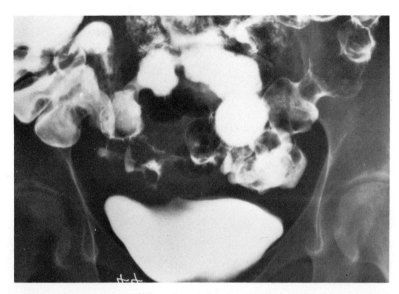

Figure 10–72.   Regional enteritis. *Small bowel examination.* Bladder is filled with barium via fistulous connection between distal ileum and urinary bladder. Note indentation on dome of bladder secondary to extravesical inflammatory response.

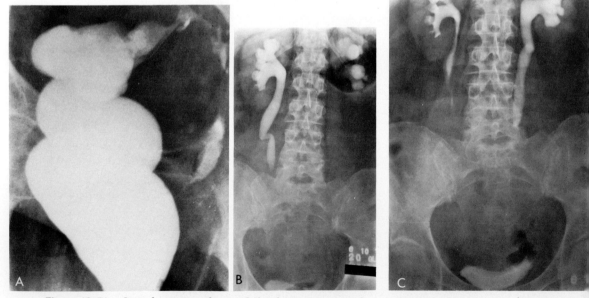

Figure 10–73.   Granulomatous colitis with fistulous tracts. A, *Colon examination.* Extensive Crohn's disease of sigmoid colon with multiple fistulous tracts. **B** and **C,** *Excretory urographic series* demonstrating bilateral pyelocaliectasis and ureterectasis, more marked on left, extending to level of pelvic inlet. Obstructive changes due to retroperitoneal abscess. Deformity of bladder secondary to paravesical inflammatory response.

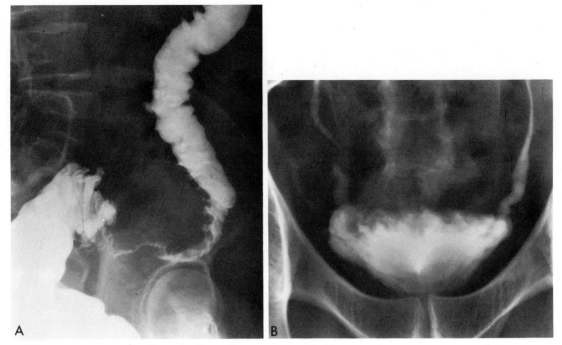

Figure 10–74. Diverticulitis of colon, affecting urinary bladder. **A,** *Colon examination.* Typical findings of diverticulitis involving sigmoid colon. **B,** *Excretory urogram.* Irregularity of dome of bladder secondary to extension of pelvic inflammatory process.

PYELOURETERITIS AND CYSTITIS CYSTICA

Cystitis and pyeloureteritis cystica are benign processes consisting of suburothelial cysts that elevate the urothelial mucosal layer (Figs. 10–75 through 10–78). Grossly, the cysts are smooth and rounded, and they contain colorless or yellowish serous fluid with a consistency of mineral oil. The cysts may range in size from microscopic to as large as 2 cm in diameter. They are usually multiple; however, a solitary cyst may be seen occasionally. The cysts may be clustered but remain discrete, or coalescence of lesions may make it difficult to visualize the complete circumference of individual cysts.

The pathogenesis of cystitis and pyeloureteritis cystica remains unknown. The lesions are submucosal, and it is possible that they represent nests of epithelium resulting from downward proliferation of transitional epithelium (Bothe and Cristol;

von Brunn). Such nests might subsequently separate from the surface of the epithelium and might develop the appearance of cysts after central degeneration had occurred. This concept does not, however, explain the clear association between cystitis cystica and recurrent or chronic urinary tract infection.

Stirling and Ash thought that metaplasia of the glands of the surface epithelium is the cause of cystitis cystica. In this view, cystitis cystica is only one of several possible epithelial reactions, including cystitis glandularis and cystitis follicularis.

Uehling and King thought that the submucosal glandular cysts and lymphoid follicles associated with this disease raise questions of an immunologic role in cystitis cystica. Uehling and Steihm found that levels of secretory IgA are elevated in children with urinary tract infections, and they speculated that cyst formation may be related to an immune response whereby the lymphoid follicles strive to produce antibod-

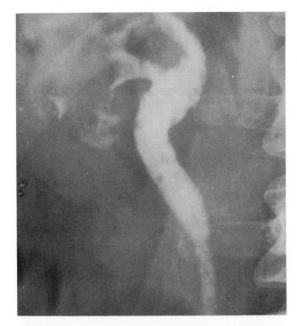

Figure 10–75. Pyelitis and ureteritis cystica. Marked inflammatory changes in calyces from long-standing infection, with pyelitis cystica involving pelvis and ureter. Cysts produce small negative shadows which suggest air bubbles. (Courtesy of Dr. E. D. Busby.)

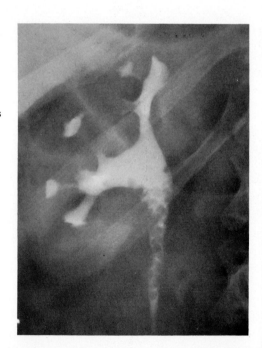

Figure 10–76. *Excretory urogram.* Pyelitis and ureteritis cystica.

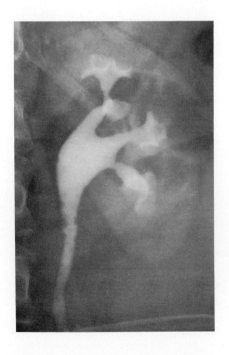

Figure 10–77. *Excretory urogram.* Pyelitis and ureteritis cystica.

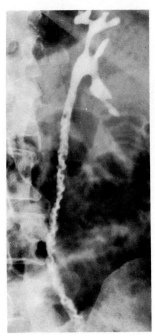

Figure 10–78. Advanced ureteritis cystica and renal cyst. Calyceal blunting of left kidney. Renal cyst distorts lower-pole calyces. (From Loitman, B. S., and Chiat, H.)

ies. As of this writing, however, this concept remains unsubstantiated.

The urographic findings are usually diagnostic. The typical appearance consists of multiple, small, smooth, rounded, discrete lucent defects that produce a characteristic scalloping when viewed in profile. The common causes of radiolucent filling defects usually are easily differentiated from pyeloureteritis cystica. Air bubbles may occasionally cause some confusion; however, they do not have a constant position, tend to coalesce into larger defects with change in position, and do not produce a scalloped appearance of the pelvis or ureter. A single cyst or a few scattered cysts seen in the renal pelvis or ureter, or coalescent cysts in the renal pelvis, may be difficult to distinguish from transitional cell tumor. Since pyeloureteritis cystica may persist and remain unchanged over several years of follow-up, comparison with previous excretory urograms is extremely helpful in differentiating these benign cysts from transitional cell tumor. Pyeloscopy, brush biopsy, and cytologic examination of the urine may also be helpful in excluding neoplasm

The excretory urograms of 30 patients with pyeloureteritis cystica were studied by Fierke and associates. Seventy per cent of the patients had a history of urinary tract infection or an active urinary infection at the time the excretory urogram was performed, and 50 per cent had evidence of urolithiasis. Seventy per cent had unilateral involvement. Thirty per cent of the patients had radiographic changes of chronic pyelonephritis in the parenchyma and calyces. In 95 per cent, the cysts occurred in the renal pelvis or upper ureter. However, the cysts may occur in a calyx or infundibulum, or one segment of a duplicated collecting system may be involved with the other being spared.

Follow-up excretory urograms may show that the cysts increase or decrease in number and size, disappear, or remain unchanged. Two of 30 patients reported by Fierke and associates had persistent evidence of pyeloureteritis cystica during 5 and 7 years of follow-up. One patient had a decrease in the number of cysts over a 5-year period, and the other had no detectable change in the appearance of the cysts over a 7-year period.

Cystitis cystica is a manifestation of chronic cystitis in which cystoscopic examination reveals multiple yellowish-brown cysts, usually 1 to 5 mm in diameter, seen most commonly over the trigone and base of the bladder. Although the lesions may occur throughout all parts of the bladder, they are more sparse when located away from the base. These lesions are found most often in women, probably because urinary tract infection occurs more often in women, and they are occasionally found in children. Kaplan and King reported a rate of incidence of 2.7 per cent in a group of children with urinary tract infection. They found that the presence of cystitis cystica in children usually indicated a poor prognosis for control of chronic urinary tract infection.

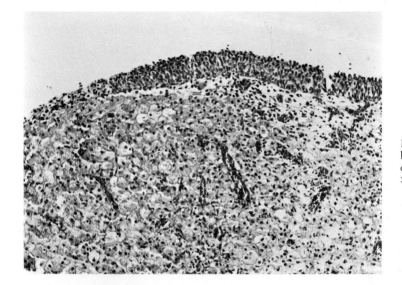

Figure 10–79. Malacoplakia. Histiocytic inflammatory collection beneath intact transitional mucosa. (Hematoxylin and eosin; ×140.)

MALACOPLAKIA

Malacoplakia is a histiocytic inflammatory reaction found most often in the bladder but also occurring elsewhere in the urinary tract (Figs. 10–79 through 10–83). Lesions have also been found in the testis, prostate, retroperitoneum, colon, and stomach (Halpern and associates; Miller and Finck). About 140 cases have been reported. Clinically, most patients present with hematuria and symptoms suggestive of vesical irritation. Most have a history of recurrent or chronic urinary tract infection, and women predominate in a ratio of 4 to 1. The average age at diagnosis is about 51 years (Smith). When the disease is in the bladder, cystoscopy will reveal raised, soft, yellowish lesions up to 3 cm in diameter. These lesions can be discrete or confluent and can involve any part of the bladder. The diagnosis is established by biopsy. Microscopic examination will demonstrate the large histiocytic Hansemann cells, many of which contain the deeply basophilic calculospherules (Michaelis-Gutmann bodies) that are pathognomonic of the disease.

In some 25 per cent of cases of malaco-

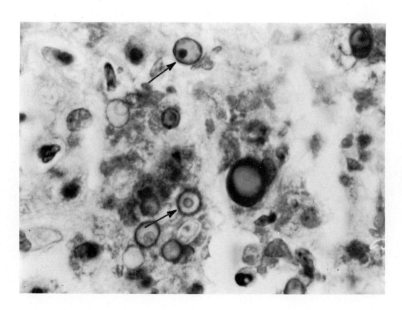

Figure 10–80. Malacoplakia. Michaelis-Gutmann bodies (*arrows*) within cytoplasm of histiocytes. Note characteristic internal structure. (Periodic acid–Schiff stain; ×1070.)

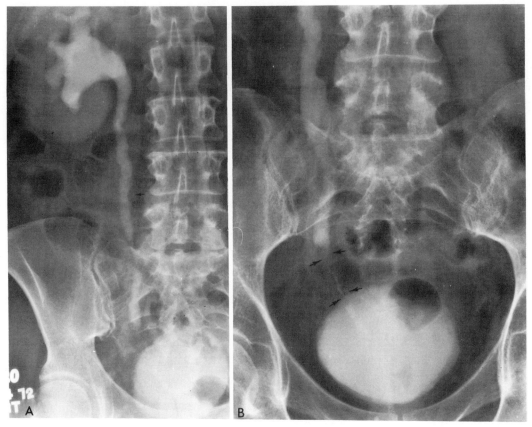

Figure 10–81. Malacoplakia. **A,** *Excretory urogram.* Ureterectasis, with multiple flat filling defects throughout course of ureter. *Arrow* points to typical lesion of malacoplakia. **B,** *Excretory urogram.* Close-up of right lower ureter. *Arrows* point to area of narrowing in lower ureter caused by extensive malacoplakia.

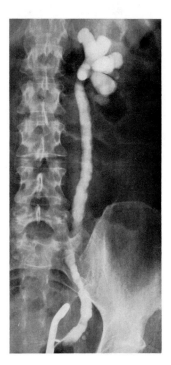

Figure 10–82. *Left retrograde pyelogram* in woman aged 48 with chronic urinary infection. **Malacoplakia of ureter** with filling defects, irregularity of entire left ureter, and associated ureterectasis and pyelocaliectasis. Surgical exploration and resection of lower ureter revealed extensive malacoplakia. (From Kolodny, G. M.)

plakia in the urinary tract, the kidney and renal pelvis are involved. The gross and microscopic picture may strongly suggest renal cell carcinoma (Miller and Finck). Halpern and colleagues reported bilateral ureteropelvic juncture obstruction secondary to malacoplakia of both renal pelves.

The cause of malacoplakia is unknown. An association with sarcoidosis was noted in two cases by Redewill in 1943, and since then four other instances of concurrence of these two diseases in the same patient have been reported (Brownstein and associates). The strongest association is with recurrent urinary tract infections, and support for the causative role of bacteria comes from the study of Terner and Lattes. They have documented that the Michaelis-Gutmann bodies are the products of phagocytized bacteria that have become calcified.

If the upper urinary tract is not involved, the excretory urogram is usually normal. If the lesions involve the ureter, they may cause obstruction with a defect simulating a primary ureteral tumor or stricture (Schneiderman and Simon). A generalized dilatation with multiple filling defects or a scalloping appearance may occur. In patients with extensive involve-

ment of the bladder, the cystogram may show multiple filling defects that cannot be distinguished from cystitis glandularis or carcinoma. In most cases, however, the diagnosis is made by cystoscopic examination and biopsy.

GAS-PRODUCING INFECTIONS OF THE URINARY TRACT

Gas in the renal substance, perirenal areas, bladder wall, or lumen of the collecting system may result from infection, penetrating trauma, fistulous connection with the intestinal tract, penetrating posterior-wall duodenal ulcer, and various diagnostic and surgical procedures (Figs. 10–84 through 10–91). The exact location of the gas is usually obvious because of its distribution.

Gas-producing infections of the urinary tract are usually a rare manifestation of ordinary urinary aerobic pathogens such as *Escherichia coli*. Bacterial generation of gas occurs more commonly in the patient with severe diabetes, and this finding promotes speculation that hyperglycemia may produce a special situation in which excess glucose in the tissue is fermented by the bacteria. The urinary tract and perirenal areas are rarely involved with anaerobic gangrenous infection caused by clostridial organisms unless the infection is part of a generalized process.

Gas within the wall of the bladder or within the renal substance is seen only when infection involves the kidney or bladder, but large amounts of gas may also accumulate within the collecting system. Gas within the collecting system may result from small-intestinal or colonic fistulas, but gas is not then seen within the bladder wall or kidney substance because there is sufficient inflammatory reaction adjacent to the fistula to prevent air from dissecting along soft-tissue planes. Fistulas are usually secondary to carcinoma or diverticulosis of the colon with secondary involvement of the bladder.

Cystitis emphysematosa may be sus-

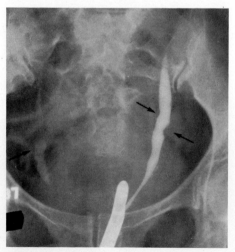

Figure 10–83. *Left retrograde ureterogram.* Malacoplakic stump of left ureter (left kidney and upper ureter had been removed previously elsewhere for malacoplakia of renal pelvis and upper ureter).

Text continued on page 883

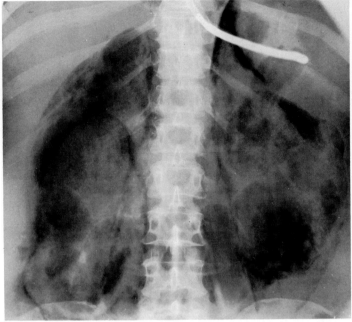

Figure 10–84. *Plain film.* **Extensive renal and perirenal emphysema with urinary infection in diabetic patient.** Kidneys and adrenal glands outlined on both sides. No gas could be seen within renal pelves. (From Gillies, C. L., and Flocks, R.)

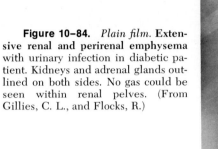

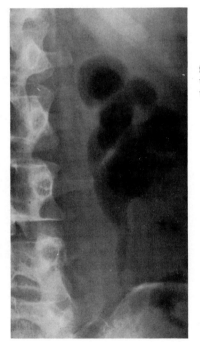

Figure 10–85. *Plain film.* **Gas-filled left ureter, pelvis, and calyces from ureterosigmoidostomy.** Forty-six-year-old female with previous left ureterosigmoidostomy. Left collecting system dilated. Left kidney failed to function on excretory urography.

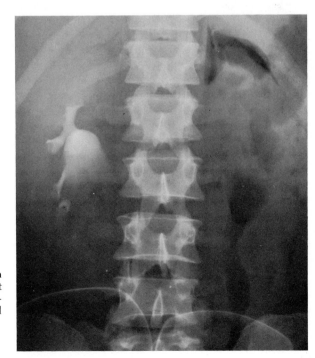

Figure 10–86. *Excretory urogram.* **Air in renal and ureteral bed** 11 days after surgery. Left nephrectomy and ureterectomy for hydronephrosis. Gas outlines ureter and upper portion of renal bed.

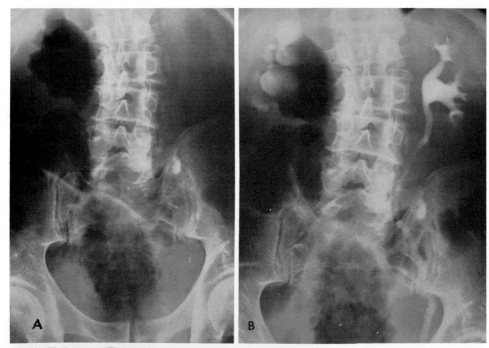

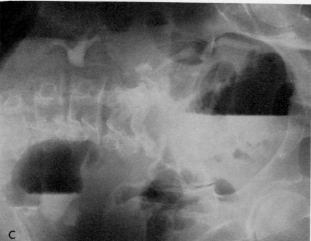

Figure 10–87. Emphysematous cystitis associated with gas filling of right collecting system and bladder. Nondiabetic man aged 70 years. Bilateral vesicoureteral reflux demonstrated on cystogram, and *E. coli* isolated from urine. **A,** *Plain film.* Gas outlines dilated right pelviocalyceal system, ureter, and bladder. Multiple locules of gas within bladder wall. **B,** *Excretory urogram.* Both kidneys excrete medium. **C,** *Lateral decubitus view.* "Air-fluid" levels in right renal pelvis and in bladder.

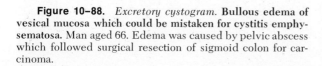

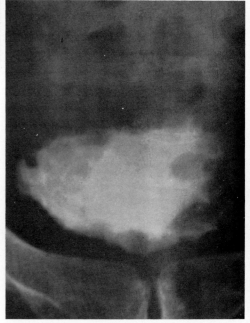

Figure 10–88. *Excretory cystogram.* Bullous edema of vesical mucosa which could be mistaken for cystitis emphysematosa. Man aged 66. Edema was caused by pelvic abscess which followed surgical resection of sigmoid colon for carcinoma.

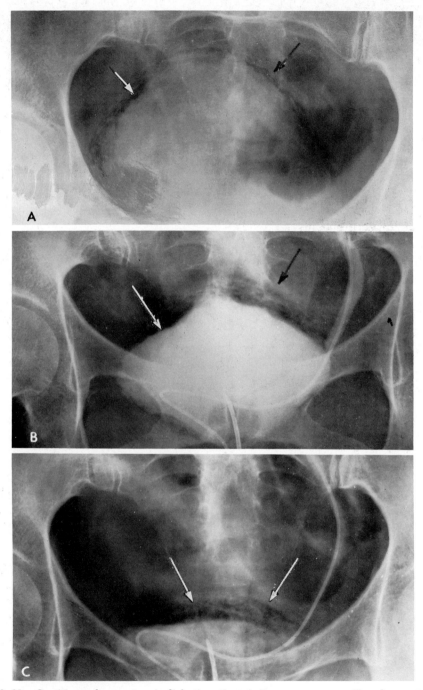

Figure 10-89. Cystitis emphysematosa in diabetic patient. **A,** *Excretory urogram.* Translucent ring of negative air or gas shadows surround bladder (*arrows*). **B,** *Retrograde cystogram.* Same (*arrows*). **C,** Bladder incompletely filled with contrast medium which has run back from making a left pyelogram. Ring of gas shadows seems to maintain same relation to collapsed wall of bladder. (From Teasley, G. H.)

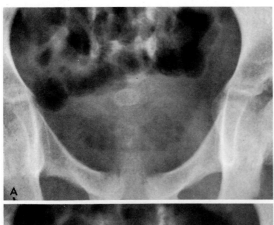
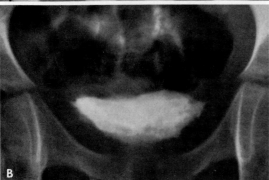

Figure 10–90.   Air in bladder of 4-year-old girl with *E. coli* infection. **A,** *Plain film.* Multiple air bubbles in region of bladder. **B,** *Excretory urogram.* Multiple views demonstrated that bubbles of air were within bladder lumen.

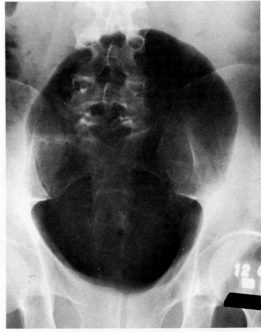

Figure 10–91.   *Plain film.* Distention of bladder from spontaneous generation of gas in severely diabetic male aged 30. Severe urinary tract infection (*E. coli*) resulting in marked production and accumulation of gas.

pected on the basis of the cystoscopic appearance of the bladder. In reported cases, the vesical mucosa has been described by such terms as "marked acute cystitis," "bladder mucosa fiery red, velvety, granular, shaggy, and rough," and "mucosa thrown into folds or rugae, between which are hundreds of transparent silvery globules, vesicles, or cysts, having the appearance of air bubbles." These cysts may be easily ruptured by the heel of the cystoscope. The diagnosis can be suspected on the plain film from the distribution of the gas bubbles in the region of the bladder. Excretory urography establishes the diagnosis by confirming the location of the gas in the bladder wall, especially if films are made with the bladder in various degrees of distention. In rare instances, a severe urinary infection may generate sufficient gas to outline the bladder in a manner similar to that occurring in air cystography.

The most common causes for gas in the urinary collecting system are iatrogenic. Careless technique frequently results in the injection of air during retrograde pyelography or voiding cystourethrography, and gas occasionally accumulates in the renal pelvis and ureter in patients who have had ureterosigmoidostomy (see Figure 10–85). In the latter instance the accumulation is accompanied by reflux of fecal material, and infection ensues.

CYSTITIS

The diagnosis of cystitis is suggested by symptoms of vesical irritability and confirmed by cystoscopic examination. Changes in the vesical mucosa may range from a mild diffuse erythema confined to the mucosa to a more severe generalized hemorrhagic cystitis characterized by widespread areas of bleeding, edema, and redness. The term *areal cystitis* refers to patchy, more or less discrete areas of inflammation.

In general, urography has only a limited role in the diagnosis of cystitis. The ex-

cretory or retrograde cystogram may reveal irregularities of the vesical mucosa owing to bullous edema, and sometimes small, contracted bladders are seen, but these changes are present only in extreme cases. (See "Cystitis Cystica" and "Malacoplakia.")

Bacterial Cystitis

The majority of cases of cystitis occur in adult women, although other peaks of incidence are in older men and in young children, particularly young girls. When cystitis occurs in older men, it is usually related to obstruction from benign prostatic enlargement. In children, urinary tract infection is a danger signal and frequently is associated with a high incidence of abnormalities in the urinary tract, particularly vesicoureteral reflux. Urologic evaluation usually reveals no anatomic abnormalities in adult women with cystitis. Most cases are caused by gram-negative bacilli, usually *Escherichia coli.* Frequency, urgency, and dysuria are the common presenting complaints and are frequently accompanied by gross hematuria. Uncomplicated cystitis responds rapidly to appropriate antibacterial therapy but is recurrent in many individuals. Most patients who have had cystitis, particularly children, should have excretory urography and voiding cystourethrography as part of the evaluation of the urinary tract. These studies are directed toward discovery of underlying anatomic abnormalities, however, and play no part in the diagnosis of cystitis itself.

Interstitial Cystitis

Interstitial cystitis is a rare disease of unknown cause that is almost always found in women and is characterized by symptoms of urinary frequency and suprapubic pain when the bladder is full (Lapides) (Figs. 10–92 and 10–93). The pain is usually relieved by voiding. Bladder capac-

Fig. 10–92

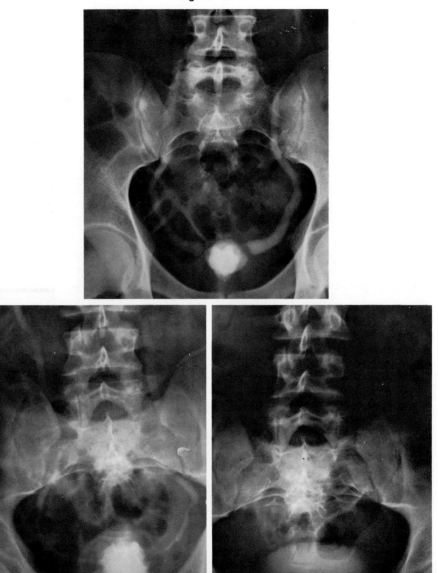

Fig. 10–93

Figure 10–92. *Excretory urogram.* Interstitial cystitis with marked contraction of bladder, causing obstruction of both ureters, with ureterectasis.

Figure 10–93. *Excretory urograms.* Interstitial cystitis with marked contraction of bladder. A and B, Contraction of bladder causes obstruction of both ureters, with moderate ureterectasis.

ity is small, frequently no more than 100 to 150 ml, and the symptoms are usually progressive.

Suggestions that the disease is related to bladder autoantibodies have never been confirmed (Gordon and associates; Silk). Urine is regularly sterile, and microhematuria is usually present. The diagnosis is established by cystoscopic examination. The characteristic lesion appears as a well-circumscribed reddish area with a small central ulcer. A mucosal tag may frequently be present at the center of the lesion. Any number of lesions may be found in the bladder, but frequently only one to four lesions are present. They are exquisitely tender and will bleed readily when the bladder is overdistended. If the lesions are surgically excised, typical lesions will appear elsewhere in the bladder mucosa. In long-standing cases, bladder capacity is severely reduced, occasionally to less than an ounce.

Treatment of interstitial cystitis remains unsatisfactory. Overdistention of the bladder under general anesthesia to the point that the bladder mucosa splits and bleeding occurs, followed by silver nitrate irrigations, will afford temporary symptomatic relief. Recurrence of symptoms within months to a year is the rule, however, and many of these individuals end up as bladder cripples and ultimately require urinary diversion (Wallack and associates). Urography is of limited value in the diagnosis, except late in the disease when the excretory cystogram will reveal a small, contracted bladder.

Cyclophosphamide Cystitis

Bleeding caused by the urinary metabolites of cyclophosphamide can be minimal but may progress to the point of life-threatening hemorrhage. Hemorrhagic cystitis occurs in three to 40 per cent of patients treated with cyclophosphamide and may be expected to remain a clinical problem as long as cyclophosphamide is a mainstay of chemotherapy for lymphoprolifera-

tive and myeloproliferative disorders (Forni and associates; Hutter and associates; Johnson and Meadows; Lawrence and associates). Symptoms may occur at any point in the course of cyclophosphamide therapy and usually appear after several weeks of treatment. Frequency and urgency are followed by hematuria of any degree of severity. The bladder may fill with clots that occasionally require cystotomy for removal. Rarely, cystectomy is indicated as a life-saving procedure. Formalin instillations into the bladder have successfully stopped the bleeding in some instances, but this treatment itself may carry a significant hazard. Cystoscopy may reveal mild telangiectasia, or the entire vesical mucosa may be inflamed. The disease can progress to the point where only a small, fibrotic bladder remains.

Eosinophilic Cystitis

Rarely, cystoscopic examination of the bladder reveals a severe inflammatory reaction with red, raised lesions and sometimes pseudopolyp formation (Fig. 10–94) (Frensilli and associates; Rubin and Pincus). Biopsy specimens show pronounced eosinophilic infiltration of the mucosa, submucosa, and bladder wall.

Patients complain of frequency dysuria, and urgency with some hematuria. Eosinophilic cystitis is found at all ages, and one-third of the cases reported occurred in childhood. The cause is unknown, although the pathologic process and the eosinophilia frequently found in the peripheral blood smear strongly suggest that this disease is an allergic reaction. Treatment is empiric, with steroids, antihistamines, and antibiotics. Urography has shown hydronephrosis, reflux, and small, contracted bladders (Goldstein; Palubinskas; Wenzl and associates).

Cystitis Glandularis

Cystitis glandularis is a rare proliferative condition of the bladder epithelium

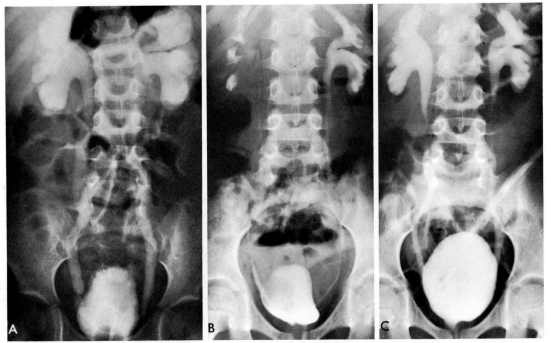

Figure 10–94. **A,** *Retrograde cystogram.* **Eosinophilic cystitis** in girl aged 2 years. Note irregularity and contraction of bladder with extensive bilateral vesicoureteral reflux. **B,** *Excretory urogram* following treatment (which included temporary suprapubic cystostomy). Marked improvement in kidneys and bladder. **C,** *Cystogram.* Bilateral reflux still present. (From Champion, R. H., and Ackles, R. C.)

that is of significance primarily because its cystoscopic appearance resembles that of carcinoma and because it probably is a premalignant lesion, eventually leading to mucinous adenocarcinoma (Figs. 10–95 through 10–97). Most cases have occurred in patients with bladder exstrophy, but occasional examples may be found in otherwise normal bladders.

According to Mostofi, cystitis glandularis is the result of a second line of evolution leading from the subepithelial nests of transitional cells (von Brunn's nests) as described in the section on cystitis cystica. The first line of evolution forms cysts and evolves into cystitis cystica. In the second line, there is true gland formation, and cystitis glandularis develops. Although the initiating factors are unknown, they may simply be metaplastic changes resulting from chronic irritation.

Emmett and McDonald recognized two types of glands: (1) the intestinal type of gland resembling goblet cells of the intestine, and (2) the subtrigonal glands of Albarron, which are lined by multiple layers of cells and which also contain mucus. They thought that these cells might originate in ectopic nests of intestinal epithelium and that adenocarcinoma could originate in either of these types of cells. This theory does not, however, explain the predilection of cystitis glandularis for the exstrophied bladder. Inasmuch as it is known that bladder epithelium is normal in newborn infants with bladder exstrophy, cystitis glandularis must be an acquired disease.

Recently, Yalla and associates reported an intriguing association between cystitis glandularis and pelvic lipomatosis. The majority of the patients with lipomatosis who were examined cystoscopically also had cystitis glandularis. This strong association of two rare entities suggests a common etiology, or at least a cause-and-effect relationship. Yalla and associates suggest that stasis of venous blood or lymphedema from the mass of paravesical fat may be the precipitating factor.

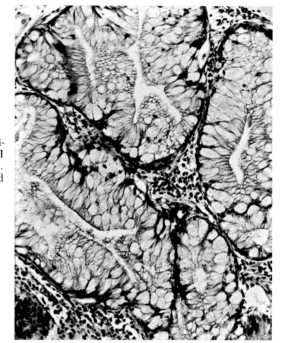

Figure 10–95. *Photomicrograph* from biopsy specimen of bladder in a case of **cystitis glandularis. Intestinal type of glands** with goblet cells (see text for explanation). (Hematoxylin and eosin; ×145.) (From Emmett, J. L., and McDonald, J. R.)

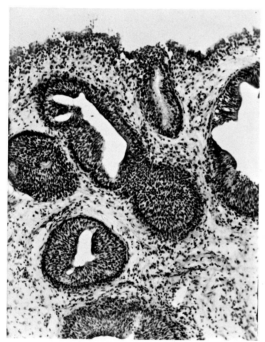

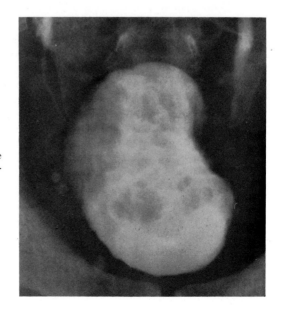

Figure 10–96. *Photomicrograph* from biopsy specimen of bladder in a case of **cystitis glandularis. Subtrigonal type of glands** lined by several layers of cells (see text for explanation). (Hematoxylin and eosin; reduced from ×95.) (From Emmett, J. L., and McDonald, J. R.)

Figure 10–97. *Excretory urogram.* Multiple negative filling defects in cystogram from **extensive cystitis glandularis** in man aged 33.

Diagnosis is made by biopsy of the suspicious lesions. Urography is of little help unless the filling defects from bullous edema are seen or there is a mass lesion effect on cystography (Fig. 10–97). These will usually be confused with tumor. Treatment is by transurethral excision and fulguration, and periodic cystoscopic examination should be done to watch for the possible development of carcinoma.

Tubercular Cystitis

Tuberculosis is discussed in detail elsewhere in this chapter. Genitourinary tuberculosis has become uncommon since the availability of effective antituberculosis chemotherapy, yet occasional cases still occur. Tubercular cystitis is important primarily in that it should be included in the differential diagnosis in all cases of cystitis. Cystoscopic examination reveals evidence of acute, mild cystitis, sometimes indistinguishable from acute bacterial cystitis; however, cultures for general bacteria will be negative. A high degree of alertness usually leads to the correct diagnosis.

PROSTATITIS (ACUTE BACTERIAL PROSTATITIS, CHRONIC BACTERIAL PROSTATITIS, CHRONIC PROSTATITIS ["PROSTATOSIS"]; PROSTATIC DUCT ABSCESS)

Urography is not ordinarily useful in the diagnosis of bacterial disease of the prostate (Figs. 10–98 through 10–103). Occasionally, acute prostatitis will cause such swelling of the prostate as to precipitate obstructive symptoms and even urinary retention. The diagnosis of acute prostatitis is usually clinically obvious, and urography is generally not indicated.

Symptoms of chronic perineal pain, intermittent dysuria, and episodes of frequency, together with the finding of *pathogenic bacteria* in the prostatic secretions, establish the diagnosis of chronic bacterial prostatitis. This condition is probably not common, but it is one of the great "wastebasket" diagnoses of modern medicine. Without evidence of pathogenic bacteria in the prostatic secretions, bacterial prostatitis is not an established diagnosis. Meares referred to this clinical situation as

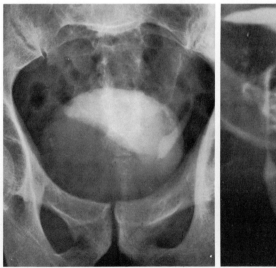

Fig. 10–98

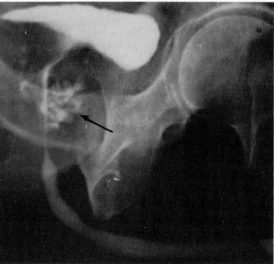

Fig. 10–99

Figure 10–98. *Excretory urogram.* **Acute prostatic abscess causing filling defect in right half of bladder.**
Figure 10–99. *Cystourethrogram.* **Chronic abscesses of prostatic ducts** (*arrow*). **Note width of normal anterior urethra.**

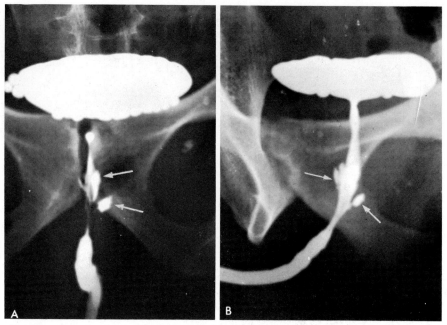

Figure 10–100. Chronic abscesses of prostatic ducts. A, *Cystourethrogram in anteroposterior position.* B, *Oblique view. Lower arrow (arrow on patient's right) points to utricle.*

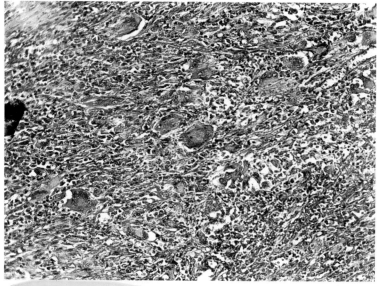

Figure 10–101. Granulomatous prostatitis with giant cells of foreign-body type scattered throughout reaction, which exhibits no particular pattern of distribution. Histiocytes and other inflammatory cells are also present. Note absence of caseation. (Hematoxylin and eosin; ×145.) (From Kelalis, P. P., and Greene, L. F.)

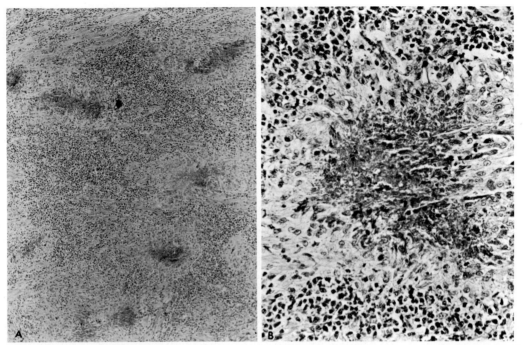

Figure 10–102.   Allergic granuloma of prostate. A, Scattered areas of fibrinoid necrosis with intense infiltration of eosinophils. (Hematoxylin and eosin; ×50.) **B,** Area of fibrinoid necrosis surrounded by palisading histiocytes and abundant eosinophils. (Hematoxylin and eosin; ×200.) (From Kelalis, P. P., Harrison, E. G., Jr., and Utz, D. C.)

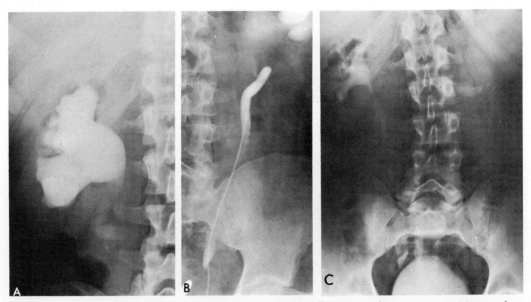

Figure 10–103.   Bilateral ureteral obstruction from extensive allergic granulomatous prostatitis in male aged 28. Successful treatment with prednisone. **A,** *Excretory urogram* demonstrates hydronephrosis and hydroureter on right. No function was seen on left. **B,** *Left retrograde pyeloureterogram* reveals obstruction in distal pelvic ureter. **C,** *Excretory urogram* after 3 months of treatment with prednisone. Right kidney has returned almost to normal. Still no function on left. (From Kelalis, P. P., Harrison, E. G., Jr., and Utz, D. C.)

"prostatosis." This names, but does not explain, a frustrating and common clinical problem.

An acute prostatic abscess occasionally may enlarge to such proportions as to elevate the base of the bladder. Retrograde urethrograms may demonstrate chronic abscess of the prostatic ducts.

Granulomatous Prostatitis

A clinical picture of fever, symptoms of lower urinary tract infection, and a prostate that feels malignant on rectal examination in a middle-aged or elderly man should suggest the possibility of granulomatous prostatitis (Kelalis and Greene). Prostate biopsy, which is mandatory, reveals tissue with marked histiocytic granulomatous reaction. There is no evidence of caseation, and there are no malignant cells. The cause is unknown; however, it seems likely that the disease is a granulomatous reaction to extravasated prostatic secretions made available by destruction of glandular epithelium from severe prostatic infection (Brown). The disorder is treated conservatively with antibiotics and supportive measures. The process will resolve spontaneously, and surgery is not necessary despite transitory obstructive symptoms. Urography is of no value in the diagnosis. The prostatic calculi found in 10 to 15 per cent of cases are nonspecific.

BRUCELLOSIS OF THE URINARY TRACT

In 1886, Sir David Bruce, working on the island of Malta, was the first to isolate and describe the organism responsible for the disease we now know as "brucellosis." He named the organism *Micrococcus melitensis*. In 1918, Alice Evans showed this organism to be similar to *Bacillus abortus* of Bang. She suggested that the name "brucellosis" (in honor of Sir David Bruce) be used instead of the terms "Malta fever" or "undulant fever." The *Brucella* group of organisms now includes the *abortus*, *suis*, and *melitensis* species.

Infection with *Brucella* species has been shown to occur in almost every organ in the human body. It has been stated that in about 50 per cent of cases the *Brucella* organisms may be found in the urine during some stage of the disease. There is a paucity of literature on the subject of brucellosis of the urinary tract. Most of the articles concern probable *Brucella* infections of the testes, epididymides, and prostate. Proved cases of brucellosis of the kidneys and bladder are rare.

Seven cases of brucellosis of the urinary tract have been reported from the Mayo Clinic (Greene and Albers; Greene and associates; Kelalis, Greene, and Weed). In these reports the similarity to tuberculosis was stressed. An amicrobic urinary infection associated with acute cystitis that is refractory to the ordinary types of treatment in a patient who has a past history of brucellosis, or who has worked as a butcher or in a meat-packing plant, should make one suspect the presence of the disease. The urine contains much pus, but no organisms are found with Gram's stain on routine cultures. It usually is necessary to employ special methods of culture identification. Among those more commonly used is incubation at 37° C on hormone blood-agar plates in 10% carbon dioxide. Cystoscopically, the severe, acute ulcerative cystitis suggests tuberculosis, but inoculating urine into guinea pigs produces no evidence of tuberculosis. Occasionally, lesions develop in the spleen, and these lesions on culture will show *Brucella* organisms. A positive agglutination reaction in a high titer (1:400 or more) is suggestive.

Roentgen Findings in Brucellosis
(Figs. 10–104 through 10–107)

Little has been known or written about urographic changes that may occur in kidneys attacked by brucellosis. In the seven Mayo Clinic cases mentioned, the urograms showed varying degrees of cica-

Text continued on page 895

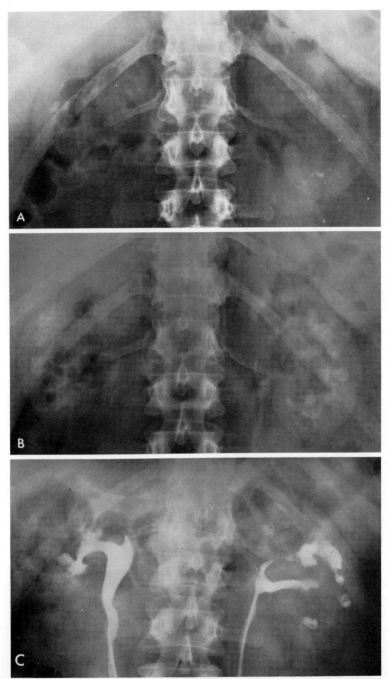

Figure 10–104. Brucellosis. **A,** *Plain film.* Multiple small irregular areas of calcification widely distributed over both renal areas. **B,** *Excretory urogram.* Marked caliectasis, with much cortical destruction. Difficult to localize calcification. Much of it is obscured by dilated calyces that appear irregular and moth-eaten and are suggestive of tuberculosis. **C,** *Bilateral retrograde pyelogram.* Note inability to fill upper group of calyces of either kidney, apparently due to cicatricial narrowing of infundibulum serving upper calyces. Note also extreme deformity of middle and lower calyces characterized by alternate areas of cicatrization and dilatation. (Courtesy of Dr. L. F. Greene.)

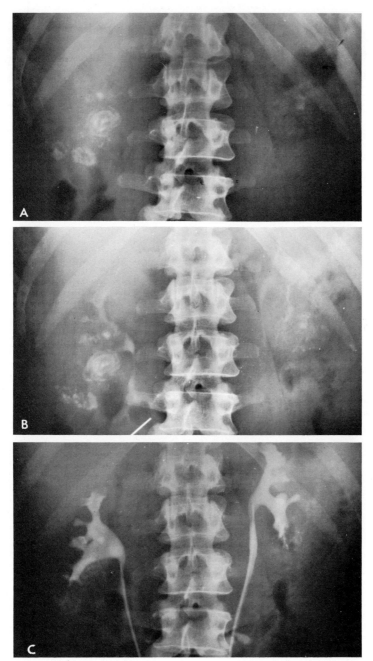

Figure 10–105.   Brucellosis. **A,** *Plain film.* Calcific shadows of irregular size and shape "splashed" over both renal areas, most marked on right. **B,** *Excretory urogram.* Calcific shadows do not outline any definite calyces. Some overlie calyces, whereas others are well removed, suggesting cortical rather than calyceal or pyramidal involvement. **C,** *Bilateral retrograde pyelogram.* Very few, if any, changes in pelvis and calyces.

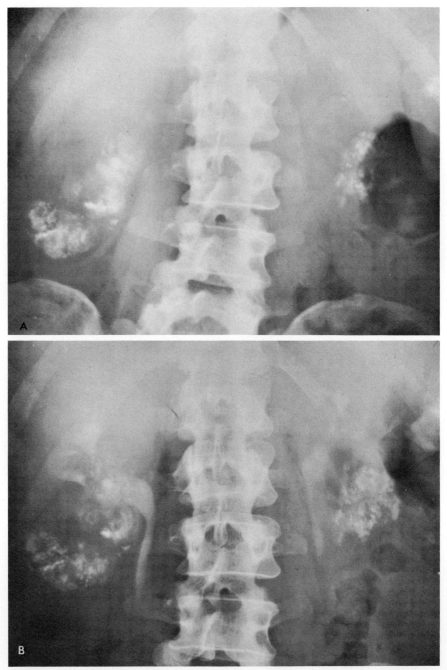

Figure 10–106.   Brucellosis. Same case as Figure 10–105, 10 years later. Marked increase in degree of renal calcification. There is also calcific area in spleen. **A,** *Plain film.* **B,** *Excretory urogram.*

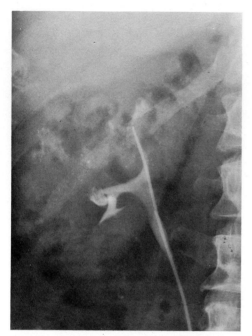

Figure 10–107. Brucelloma simulating hypernephroma. *Retrograde pyelogram* shows space-occupying lesion in lateral aspect of right kidney containing calcium. Hypernephroma suspected. Nephrectomy. Granuloma typical of tuberculosis revealed by both gross and microscopic examination. Tissue culture was positive for *Brucella suis*. (From Kelalis, P. P., Greene, L. F., and Weed, L. A.)

tricial deformity and dilatation of the pelvis and calyces simulating advanced tuberculosis. In one case, cicatricial narrowing of the calyces was sufficient to isolate portions of a calyx so that, although it could be visualized on the excretory urogram, no medium entered it as seen on the retrograde urogram. One of the most interesting findings was calcification of the renal cortex. In one case the calcification was extensive and seemed to be "splashed" over all areas of the kidney without regard to the position of the pelvis and calyces or cortex and medulla. This is in contradistinction to the calcification seen in renal tuberculosis, which usually involves and outlines definite calyces or groups of calyces. The condition must also be differentiated from nephrocalcinosis, in which the calcification usually is limited to the pyramids. It is of interest that in two of the seven cases a granulomatous lesion of the kidney (proved

by tissue culture to be a brucelloma) was incorrectly diagnosed as hypernephroma because the disorder presented as a space-occupying lesion (Fig. 107).

FUNGAL INFECTION OF THE KIDNEY

Renal Candidiasis and Actinomycoses
(Figs. 10–108 through 10–111)

Renal candidiasis is the most common fungal infection of the urinary tract. The incidence of urinary tract involvement with *Candida* has increased in recent years because of prolonged antibiotic therapy, adrenal corticosteroid administration, chemotherapy, and the use of immunosuppressive agents (Holt and Newman). Fungal infections of the urinary tract are also more common in patients with underlying disorders such as diabetes mellitus, neoplasms, blood dyscrasias, or other types of chronic disease. Renal involvement with candidiasis is usually secondary to systemic infection. Rarely, the kidney is the only organ affected, and then the mode of infection is considered to be ascending from the bladder and the ureter instead of hematogenous (Schönebeck and Winblad).

Clark and associates have reported that renal candidiasis may assume three forms that may represent different stages of the same disease process: (1) acute pyelonephritis; (2) disseminated candidiasis that involves several organs including the kidneys; and (3) chronic pyelonephritis and hydronephrosis. The diagnosis of urinary tract candidiasis is established by a history compatible with pyelonephritis, urographic abnormalities, and positive urine cultures.

In the acute stages the kidneys are swollen, as in patients with acute pyelonephritis of bacterial etiology, and they contain multiple parenchymal abscesses and interstitial edema. Renal failure may accompany the acute phase, and excretory urography may demonstrate a significant decrease in or absence of renal excretion.

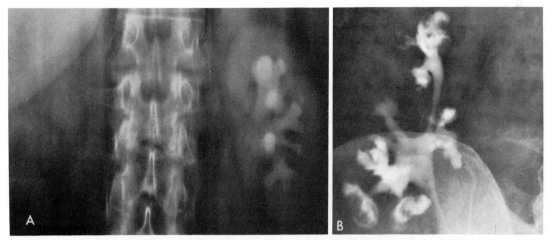

Figure 10–108.   Moniliasis and renal papillary necrosis. A, *Nephrotomogram.* Extensive papillary necrosis involving left kidney in a 39-year-old woman with history of analgesic abuse. Right kidney failed to excrete contrast medium. **B,** *Retrograde pyelogram, right kidney.* Marked irregularity of collecting system with multiple defects in collecting system as a result of monilial infection and papillary necrosis.

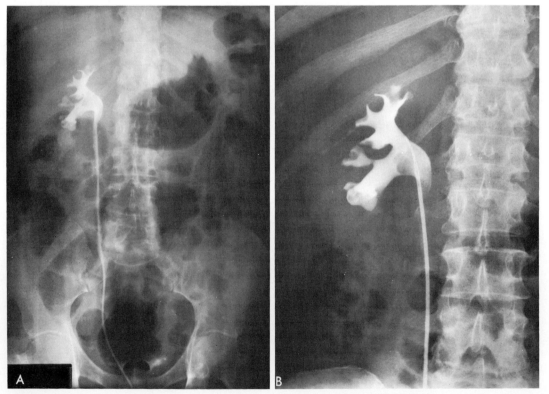

Figure 10–109.   Candidal fungus ball in a 62-year-old woman with solitary right kidney who presented with fever and anuria. *Retrograde pyelogram.* Large filling defect at right ureteropelvic juncture due to candidal fungus ball that caused complete obstruction. (From Turner, Grisby, Enright, Chance, Frazier, Womach, and Long.)

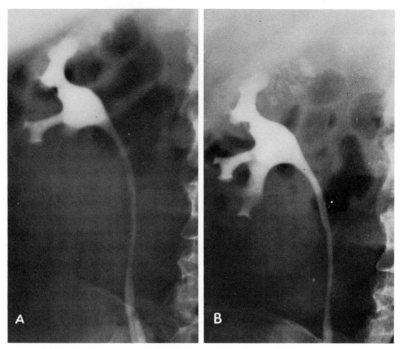

Figure 10–110. Renal actinomycosis. **A,** *Right retrograde pyelogram.* **B,** Second attempt at right retrograde pyelogram. Note difficulty in filling lower calyx because of pressure from lesion in lower pole. Similar to finding of ordinary renal carbuncle.

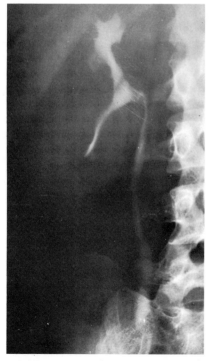

Figure 10–111. Renal actinomycosis. *Right retrograde pyelogram.* Obliteration of middle calyx and elongation of upper and lower calyces with abnormal terminations, suggesting renal tumor. (From Hunt, V. C., and Mayo, C. W.)

Hydronephrosis is a common late finding (Béland and Piette; Harbach and associates; Levin and associates; Turner and associates).

Papillary necrosis may be associated with the more protracted course of renal candidiasis. The findings may be similar to the classic picture of papillary necrosis (Knepshield and associates), but in renal candidiasis there is also a tendency to develop much more irregular cavities with extensive destructive changes. In these instances, multiple filling defects may be seen in the collecting systems due either to sloughed papillae or to *Candida* mycelia (fungus balls).

Renal actinomycosis occurs rarely and usually as a secondary lesion (Baron and Arduino; Davies and Keddie; Hunt and Mayo; Piper and associates; Weese and Smith). The kidney in most such cases becomes involved from the gastrointestinal tract or through the diaphragm from pulmonary disease. Urographically, the resulting lesion is impossible to distinguish from ordinary renal carbuncle, cortical abscess, perinephritic abscess (Boijsen and Reuter), and renal tumor unless the diagnosis can be made by demonstrating the actinomyces organisms or "sulfa bodies" in the urine or in pus draining from a wound or the renal sinuses.

TUBERCULOSIS OF THE GENITOURINARY TRACT

Pathogenesis of Genitourinary Tuberculosis

Tuberculosis of the genitourinary tract is generally considered to be secondary to the hematogenous dissemination of tubercle bacilli from a primary pulmonary lesion and is initially a bilateral disease. As a consequence of its hematogenous origin, numerous tiny miliary tubercles can be found on serial sections in both kidneys. Most of these small lesions tend to heal spontaneously or as the result of chemotherapy instituted for the pulmonary disease.

At first, tuberculous bacillary emboli are located in the glomerular and cortical arterioles, where they cause small tubercles to develop. Healing depends on the number and virulence of the bacteria, on the local and general resistance of the host, and on the sensitivity of the strain of bacteria to chemotherapy. If healing does not occur, a necrotizing lesion develops; bacteria pass down the tubules and may be detected in the urine, with or without pyuria. New tubercles form at the narrow portion of the loop of Henle in the medulla, necrotize, coalesce, and involve the calyceal wall at the tip of the papilla (Lieberthal). This small, irregular, ulcerating cavitation represents the first lesion that can be detected urographically. The ulcerocavernous papillitis may be a solitary lesion in one kidney or may be multiple in one or both kidneys. With progression of the infection, the lesion may enlarge to cause a cavernous process involving the entire pyramid.

The disease spreads by secondary infection of the mucous membrane of the other calyces and the renal pelvis, ureter,

and bladder. Multiple granulomatous lesions of the system may develop and cause edema, round cell infiltration, cavitation, and fibrosis. At the areas of physiologic narrowing in the urinary tract, such as the calyceal infundibula, the ureteropelvic juncture, the ureter overlying the sacroiliac joint, and the vesicoureteral juncture, such lesions cause hydrocalyx, hydronephrosis, or hydroureter, with consequent further destruction of the renal parenchyma.

The healing of extensive tuberculous lesions in the urinary tract is characterized by calcification as well as fibrosis and stricture formation, which may be enhanced by rapid healing on adequate chemotherapy. Calcium deposits may be found in caseating granulomas and in the linings of tuberculous cavities, owing partially to the healing process and partially to sedimentation of urinary calcium salts on necrotic surfaces.

Clinical and Laboratory Findings in Genitourinary Tuberculosis

The most common symptoms related to urinary tract tuberculosis are those commonly related to any type of urinary tract infection (see Table 10–2). Dysuria, frequency, and nocturia occur most often,

Table 10–2. **Clinical Findings in 95 Tubercular Patients With Genitourinary Symptoms**[*]

FINDINGS	NUMBER OF PATIENTS[a]	PER CENT OF PATIENTS
Urinary tract symptoms		
Dysuria	53	56
Frequency	41	43
Nocturia	36	38
Gross hematuria	25	26
Cloudy urine (pyuria, tissue fragments)	25	26
Urgency	20	21
Suprapubic pain	5	5
Total incontinence	2	2
Epididymitis	12	13
Draining scrotal fistula	1	1

[*]From Kollins and associates.
[a]Most had multiple symptoms.

ulcerocavernous papillitis

and most patients have a number of symptoms (Wechsler and associates). The clinical history frequently dates back over several months or years, and frequently the patient has received several unsuccessful courses of antibiotic treatment for suspected nontuberculous infection. Many patients have given a history of chronic, recurrent urinary tract infection associated with pyuria, and repeatedly negative cultures for the common urinary pathogens. Nonspecific systemic symptoms such as fever, anorexia, fatigue, or weakness are often associated.

Urinary tract tuberculosis is usually a disease of adults, and frequently there is a history of prior tuberculosis affecting other organ systems. In a recent Mayo Clinic series, 27 of 98 patients had a known earlier history of clinically apparent tuberculosis involving another part of the body (Kollins and associates). Seventeen of these 27 patients had known skeletal tuberculosis, and 13 had prior symptoms related to pulmonary tuberculosis. Only 52 of the 98 patients had positive chest roentgenograms, including minor changes such as minimal fibrosis or calcified granulomata. Since the primary focus of tuberculosis in these patients was almost certainly pulmonary, it is obvious that pulmonary tuberculosis frequently heals and leaves little or no radiologic evidence of its prior existence. It is also evident that the absence of pulmonary pathology in a patient suspected of having genitourinary tuberculosis should not discourage further work-up for tuberculosis.

Available diagnostic methods are used to (1) establish the tuberculous nature of the disease, (2) estimate the extent of the lesion in each kidney, (3) estimate the remaining amount of functioning renal tissue, (4) follow the progress of healing, and (5) detect complications of the healing process. Tuberculosis of the genitourinary tract can be diagnosed only by demonstrating the presence of *Mycobacterium tuberculosis* in urine or tissue specimens, and only a positive culture or a positive guinea pig inoculation test should be considered as conclu-

sive evidence of tuberculosis. Positive urine cultures are not always obtained initially on patients with active genitourinary tuberculosis. If urographic and clinical findings are highly suggestive of tuberculosis, repeated cultures may be required for verification. In our experience, as many as eight attempts have been necessary before a positive culture has been obtained.

Roentgen Findings in Genitourinary Tuberculosis

THE PLAIN FILM IN GENITOURINARY TUBERCULOSIS

Urographic diagnosis in genitourinary tuberculosis begins with careful examination of the plain film. Deposition of calcium in an attempt to heal tuberculous lesions often provides a major diagnostic clue (Ross), and the detection of tuberculous lesions in the bony structure may be suggestive of genitourinary tuberculosis (Scheinin and Kontturi).

Calcification of the Urinary Tract

Parenchymal calcifications produced by renal tuberculosis tend to be indefinite and irregular in outline and not as dense or well defined as renal calculi (Figs. 10–112 through 10–134) (Crenshaw; Gow, 1965). These indistinct calcifications may involve a relatively large portion of the kidney. The most poorly defined parenchymal opacifications seen in cases of renal tuberculosis are produced by caseation and a limited amount of calcification. Such faint shadows may be recognized only after exceedingly careful examination of the plain film, as they may be only slightly more dense than renal tissue. Tomography is an essential adjunct in the demonstration of these faintly calcified areas of parenchyma. The size of the area involved with calcification may vary from a few minute areas to a cast of the entire kidney. Frequently, the parenchyma is diffusely calcified, and the involved kidney fails to excrete contrast medium (autonephrectomy). The pattern and density of calcifica-

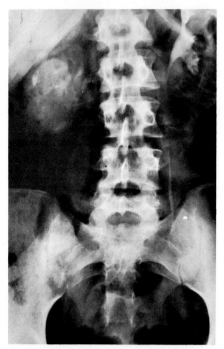

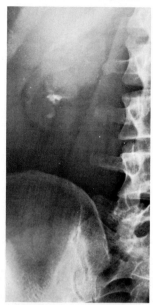

Figure 10–113. *Plain film.* **Diffuse tuberculous calcification** of right kidney in case of **autonephrectomy,** with no function remaining, as demonstrated by excretory urogram (not shown here).

Figure 10–112. Right renal tuberculosis. Patient admitted to hospital with tuberculosis of right sacroiliac joint. On plain film (not shown) a grossly calcified asymptomatic right kidney was seen coincidentally (autonephrectomy). *Excretory urogram.* Left kidney normal. Note irregular areas of decalcification of right sacroiliac joint. Right nephroureterectomy. Ureter was normal and no pathologic relationship was noted between ureter and sacroiliac joint.

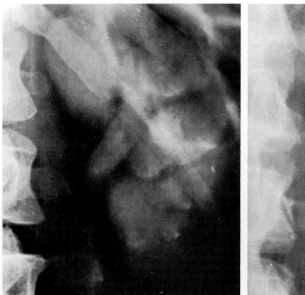

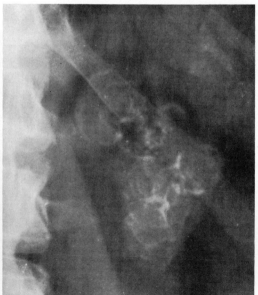

Fig. 10–114   **Fig. 10–115**

Figure 10–114. *Plain film.* **Extensive caseation and necrosis caused by tuberculous left kidney.** Minimal degree of calcification but sufficient to outline pelvis and upper portion of ureter.

Figure 10–115. *Plain film.* **Extensive calcification of nonfunctioning left kidney (autonephrectomy).**

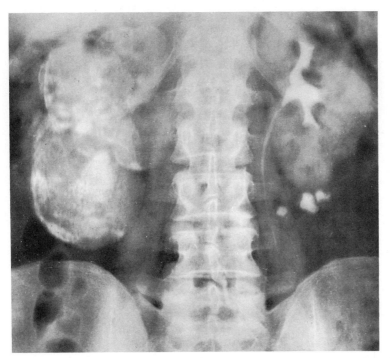

Figure 10–116. *Excretory urogram.* **Autonephrectomy of tuberculous right kidney** with marked calcification of calyceal walls and calcium deposits in contents of collecting system. Marked stricture of ureteropelvic juncture.

tion are highly variable. The kidney may be atrophic, normal in size, or enlarged. Whenever diffuse calcification of the renal parenchyma is encountered in a nonfunctioning kidney, tuberculosis is almost certainly the cause.

Tuberculous calcification of the ureter is not as common as renal calcification, and calcification of the bladder is relatively rare. Calcification of the ureter usually is not difficult to recognize, because of its position and contour, but at times it is difficult to distinguish calcification of the ureteral wall from ureteral calculi. According to Friedenberg, Ney and Stachenfeld, tuberculous calcification of the ureteral wall should be differentiated from calcification due to schistosomiasis (bilharziasis); in the latter case the ureter is dilated and the calcification is limited to the lower ureteral segment. Calcification of the wall of the bladder, although uncommon in tuberculosis, is easily recognized.

Tuberculous calcification of the prostate gland may be impossible to distinguish from nontuberculous calculous prostatitis without additional clinical data. In differential diagnosis, it should be remembered that prostatic calculi occur much more commonly than does tuberculous calcification of the prostate. Demonstration of tubercle bacteria in the urine would, of course, lend weight to the diagnosis of tuberculous calcification, although renal tuberculosis and prostatic calculi of nonspecific origin may occur together. Calcification of the seminal vesicles may occur in tuberculosis but it is not common. Calcification of the vasa deferentia is more commonly encountered. Diabetes, however, is usually the causative factor in calcification of the vasa. King and Rosenbaum have reported that calcification secondary to diabetes occurs primarily in the wall of the vasa, resulting in smooth, sharply defined parallel lines, whereas tuberculous calcification is largely intraluminal and results in an irregular pattern of calcification.

Calcification of splenic granulomata,

Text continued on page 907

Fig. 10–117   Fig. 10–118

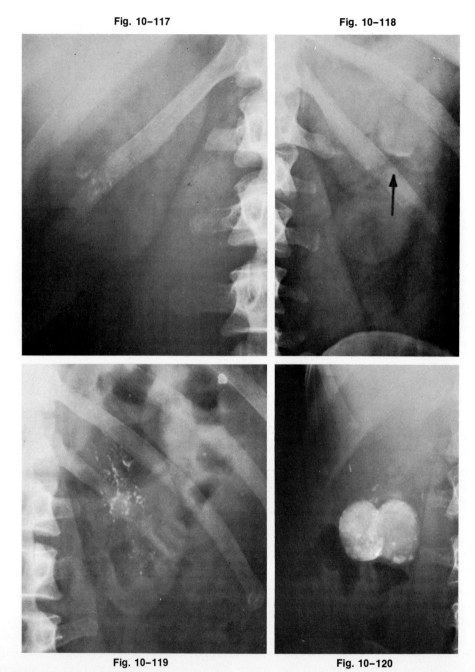

Fig. 10–119   Fig. 10–120

Figure 10–117. *Plain film.* **Tuberculous calcification of right kidney.** Shadows are indefinite and irregular in outline. Distribution of shadows would suggest tuberculous calcification.

Figure 10–118. *Plain film.* **Tuberculous calcification of left kidney.** Irregularity of calcific area and its position near lateral margin of kidney suggest tuberculosis rather than stone.

Figure 10–119. *Plain film.* **Tuberculous calcification of left kidney.** Calcific areas are indefinite and irregular in outline and seem to overlie pelvis and calyces. Differs from nephrocalcinosis in that renal pyramids do not seem to be outlined.

Figure 10–120. *Plain film.* **Tuberculous calcification of right kidney,** of unusual density, which might be confused with renal stone.

Fig. 10–121   Fig. 10–122

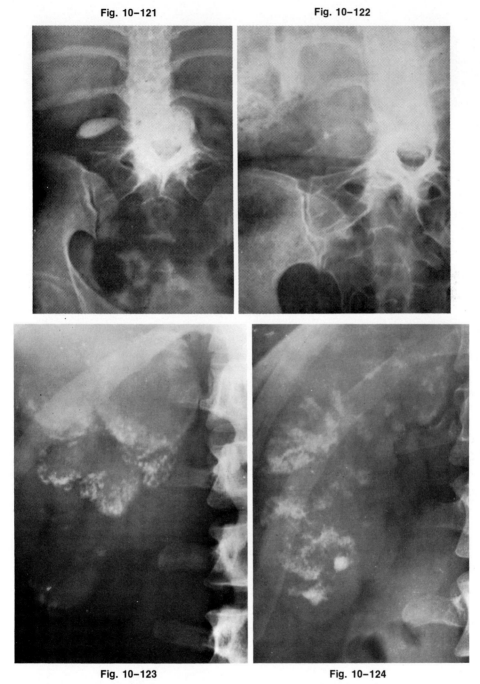

Fig. 10–123   Fig. 10–124

Figure 10–121.   *Plain film.* Calcification of psoas abscess secondary to tuberculosis of lumbosacral vertebrae (Pott's disease). Right kidney was also involved by tuberculosis and showed no function in excretory urogram.

Figure 10–122.   *Excretory urogram.* Same case as in Figure 10–121 but 17 years later. Most of calcium has been absorbed.

Figure 10–123.   *Plain film.* Diffuse tuberculous calcification of right kidney in case of autonephrectomy, with no function remaining.

Figure 10–124.   *Plain film.* Extensive tuberculous calcification of nonfunctioning right kidney (autonephrectomy), which might be confused with advanced stage of nephrocalcinosis.

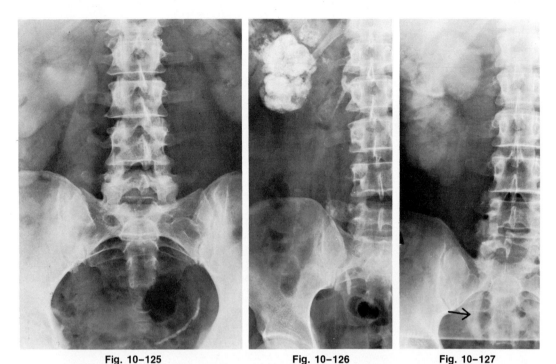

Fig. 10–125   Fig. 10–126   Fig. 10–127

Figure 10–125. *Excretory urogram.* **Bilateral renal tuberculosis** in woman, 57 years of age, with 30-year history of tuberculosis. **Nonfunctioning left kidney with calcification (autonephrectomy) and calcification of lower part of left ureter.** Stricture of terminal part of right ureter produced hydronephrosis. Cutaneous ureterostomy performed on right.

Figure 10–126. *Excretory urogram.* **Long-standing right renal tuberculosis** in man, 38 years of age, **with draining psoas abscess. Nonfunctioning calcified right kidney (autonephrectomy) with calcified psoas abscess and calcification of ureter.** Left kidney was normal.

Figure 10–127. *Plain film.* **Autonephrectomy** of right kidney, from **tuberculosis. Diffuse caseation with calcification of right kidney and calcification of ureter** (*arrow*).

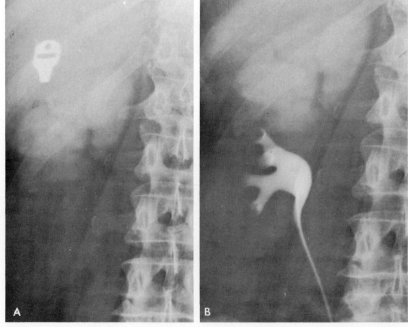

Figure 10–128. Duplicated kidney with **autonephrectomy** of upper segment from old **tuberculosis.** Caseation of upper segment casts dense shadow. **A,** *Plain film.* **B,** *Retrograde pyelogram.* (Courtesy of Dr. R. B. Carson.)

904

Fig. 10–129   Fig. 10–130

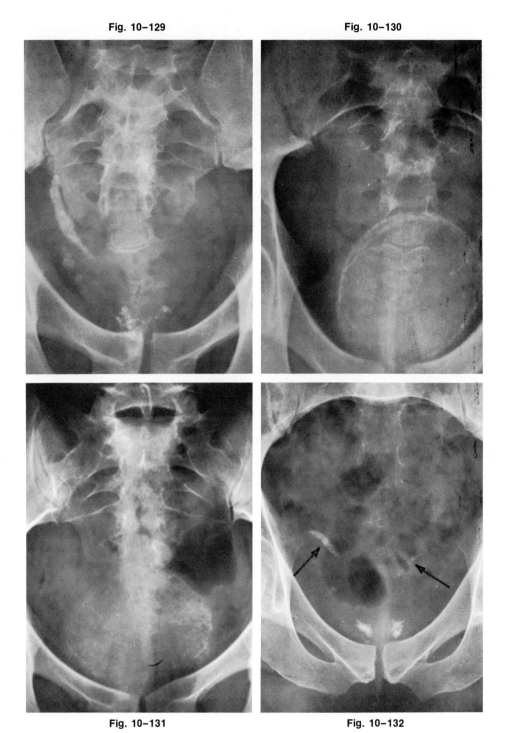

Fig. 10–131   Fig. 10–132

Figure 10–129. *Plain film.* **Tuberculous calcification** of lower part of right ureter and also of prostate gland.
Figures 10–130 and 10–131. *Plain film.* **Tuberculous calcification** of wall of urinary bladder.
Figure 10–132. *Plain film.* **Tuberculous calcification** of vasa (*arrows*) and prostate gland.

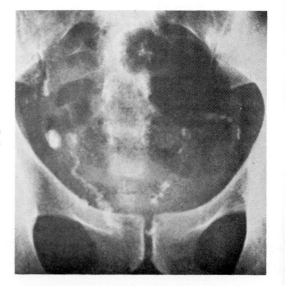

Figure 10–133. *Plain film.* **Tuberculous calcification of vasa and seminal vesicle.** (Courtesy of Dr. T. Leon Howard.)

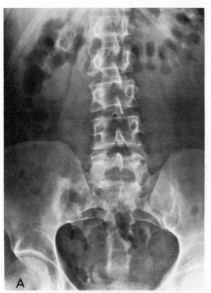

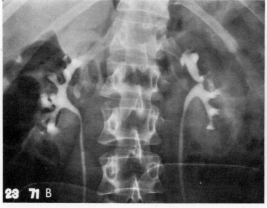

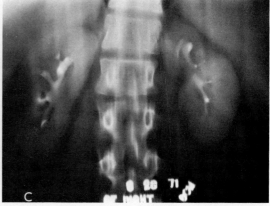

Figure 10–134. *Excretory urogram.* **Tuberculosis with renal and skeletal involvement. A,** Obliteration of right sacroiliac joint secondary to tuberculous arthritis. **B,** *Excretory urogram.* Blunting of upper-pole calyx with dilatation secondary to stricture of infundibulum. **C,** *Nephrotomogram.* Associated parenchymal scarring involving upper pole of left kidney with vague calcification of parenchyma at base of scar.

mesenteric nodes, and psoas abscesses may be helpful contributing evidence if genitourinary tuberculosis is being considered. Calcified mesenteric nodes and splenic granulomata commonly result from other causes, especially histoplasmosis. Calcified psoas abscesses are frequently associated with radiographic evidence of tuberculous spinal involvement (Pott's disease) and are quite specific for tuberculosis.

THE UROGRAM IN TUBERCULOSIS OF THE URINARY TRACT

Urographic Changes in the Kidney
(Figs. 10–135 through 10–150)

Tuberculosis of the kidney is initially a disease of the renal parenchyma (Riddle). It can be diagnosed urographically only if the lesion has ulcerated into a calyx and resulted in a papillary cavity or, eventually, in characteristic changes within the collecting system.

Minimal erosion of a tip of one calyx

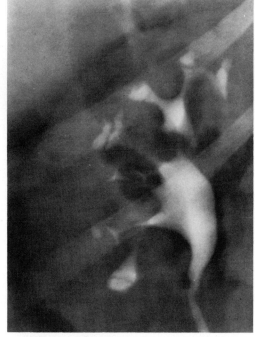

Figure 10–136. *Excretory urogram.* **Renal tuberculosis with papillary cavities.** Active renal tuberculosis with multiple papillary cavities typical of those seen in other causes of renal papillary necrosis.

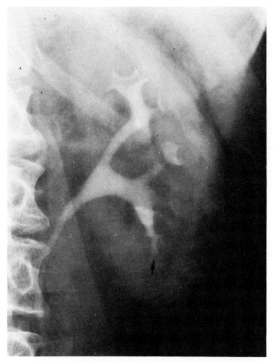

Figure 10–135. Renal tuberculosis. *Excretory urogram.* Small papillary cavity involving lower pole of left kidney (*arrow*).

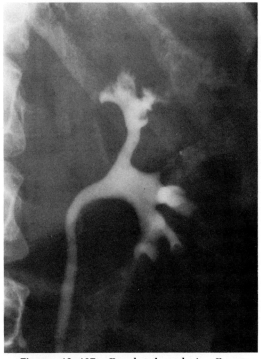

Figure 10–137. Renal tuberculosis. *Excretory urogram.* Extensive destructive changes of papillae involving upper pole of left kidney secondary to necrosis and erosion.

Fig. 10–138

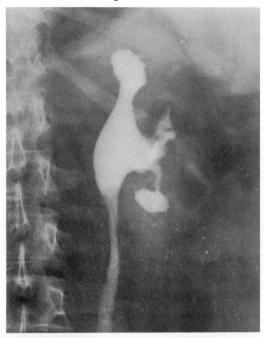

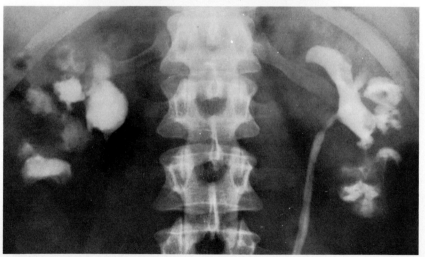

Fig. 10–139

Figure 10–138. *Left retrograde pyelogram.* **Advanced renal tuberculosis.** Destruction of middle calyces. "Pinched-off" lower calyx, which is irregularly dilated, indicating papillary necrosis. Minimal dilatation of upper calyx, pelvis, and ureter.

Figure 10–139. *Bilateral retrograde pyelogram.* **Advanced bilateral renal tuberculosis** with extensive papillary necrosis.

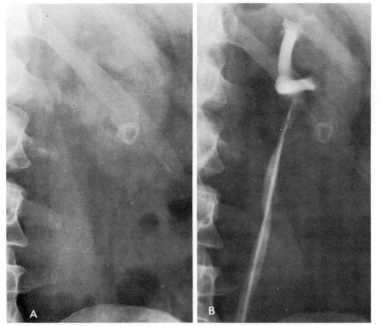

Figure 10–140. Left renal tuberculosis with calcification. **A,** *Plain film.* Calcific shadow over lower pole of left kidney. **B,** Left retrograde pyelogram. Marked cicatrization, erosion, and deformity of pelviocalyceal system. Lower calyx almost obliterated. Calcification of lower papilla. **Tuberculous ureteritis.**

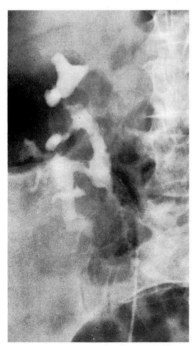

Figure 10–141. *Retrograde pyelogram.* **Far-advanced right renal tuberculosis; nonfunctioning right kidney.** Marked papillary necrosis. Note bizarre outline of collecting system and irregularity of renal pelvis and ureter.

(indicating involvement of the tip of a pyramid) may be the earliest urographic finding. Such minimal calyceal irregularity may be difficult to distinguish from pyelosinous backflow or a variation of the normal. In many such cases, the final decision must rest on clinical and laboratory data rather than on urographic interpretation. As the infection proceeds, greater changes in the calyces occur. Increased caliectasis associated with irregularity in contour indicates erosion of the pyramids and cortical necrosis. These changes have been described by such terms as "fuzzy," "feathery," and "moth-eaten." Depending on the amount of necrosis and on whether the cavity contains caseous or liquid material, deposits of contrast medium in varying densities may be seen outside the calyx. Sometimes such collections are connected with the calyx by a tiny fistulous tract (Kollins and associates).

Cicatrization of calyces and infundibula are common and significant findings in renal tuberculosis (Kollins and asso-

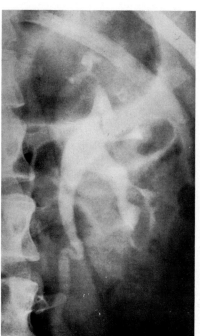
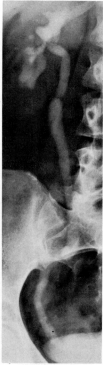
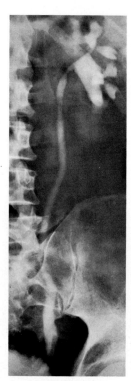

Fig. 10–142

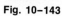
Fig. 10–143

Fig. 10–144

Figure 10–142.   Tuberculosis of upper pole of left kidney. Cicatricial change of upper-pole calyces. Six years previously, right nonfunctioning tuberculous kidney was removed.

Figure 10–143.   *Excretory urogram.* Right renal tuberculosis, with tethering due to moderate strictures of calyceal infundibula at their junction with renal pelvis. Note ureteral strictures opposite third lumbar vertebra and at ureterovesical juncture.

Figure 10–44.   *Excretory urogram.* Left renal tuberculosis. Butterfly type of calyceal pattern in upper pole; ureteral stricture of intramural portion. (Right kidney was normal.)

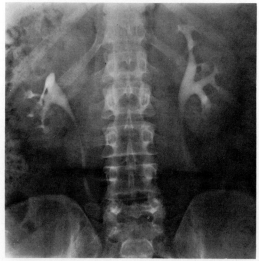

Figure 10–145. *Excretory urogram.* **Renal tuber-culosis.** Infundibular stricture involving upper right renal collecting system with typical tethering at point of stricture. Small focus of parenchymal calcification situated just superior to left renal pelvis.

ciates). The formation of strictures in the collecting system is a common complication of tuberculosis but is relatively uncommon in other bacterial infections. Stricture of the infundibula may incompletely isolate parts of the collecting system, or parts of a calyx may be isolated so that it appears on the urogram as a pinched-off cyst-like structure (Bruce and associates). Indeed, it is sometimes impossible to decide whether such a cavity partially filled with contrast medium represents a diseased and dilated calyx or whether it is a primary cavity ruptured into the collecting system. It is evident that with a severe infectious process almost any bizarre pattern or cicatricial deformity of the calyces might occur. When the process becomes more advanced, a whole group of calyces may become entirely obliterated or destroyed, owing to

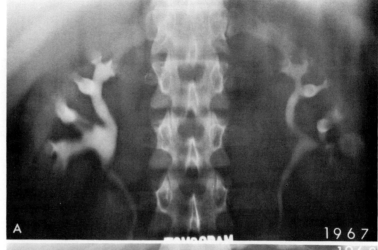

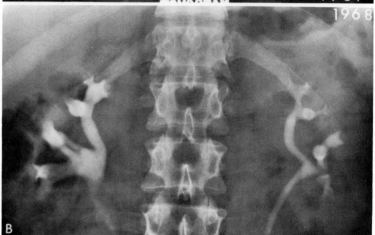

Figure 10–146.   Renal tuberculosis. *Excretory urogram.* **A,** Cicatricial changes of collecting system with retraction of pelvis toward point of stricture. Contrast-filled cavity distal to point of stricture due to localized caliectasis. **B,** *Excretory urogram* about 1 year later. Stricture formation has progressed so that markedly dilated calyx has now been completely obliterated.

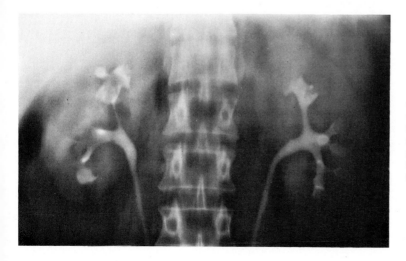

Figure 10–147.   Renal tuberculosis. *Nephrotomogram.* Relatively radiolucent mass occupying midportion of right kidney laterally is due to a large tuberculous granuloma. Inflammatory changes in upper and lower-pole calyces of right kidney.

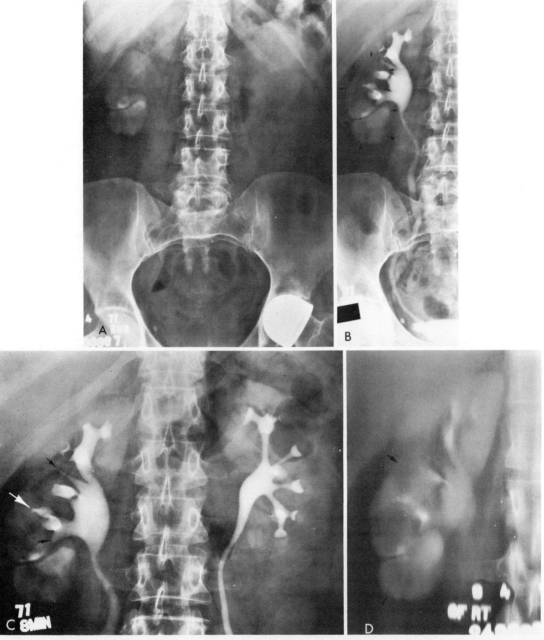

Figure 10–148.   Renal tuberculosis with several classic findings. **A,** *Plain film.* Diffuse calcification throughout lower right kidney. **B,** *Excretory urogram. Arrows* outline extent of calcification in parenchyma. **C,** *Excretory urogram* (localized view). Papillary cavity (*large arrow*). Infundibular strictures (*small arrows*). **D,** *Nephrotomogram.* Multiple radiolucent filling defects throughout parenchyma (*arrows*) due to granulomatous masses.

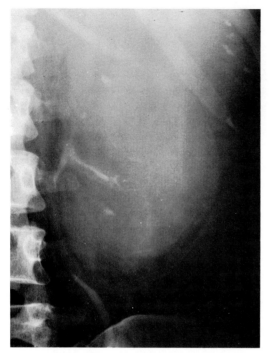

Figure 10–149. *Excretory urogram.* **Left renal tuberculosis simulating tumor.** At operation, extensive caseous tuberculosis with cavitation was found. Right kidney normal.

cicatrization or destruction and caseation of large portions of the kidney (Figs. 10–142, 10–143, and 10–144).

Parenchymal masses are commonly associated with renal tuberculosis. In the Mayo Clinic series, 24 of 98 patients had urographically detectable mass lesions (Kollins and associates). Most, but not all, such lesions will be granulomatous in nature, and they may range up to 5 cm or more in size. Calcification of the mass is a common finding and may be punctate or diffuse, making differentiation from a calcified renal cell carcinoma difficult. Simple cysts occur in tuberculous kidneys at least as frequently as in normal renal units, and occasionally a renal cell carcinoma is found to coexist with renal tuberculosis (Figs. 10–149 and 10–150).

If the ureter is completely obstructed and the bladder is normal, urine cultures may be negative for tuberculosis even though a tuberculous, autonephrectomized kidney is present. In cases of unilateral autonephrectomy and a normal remaining

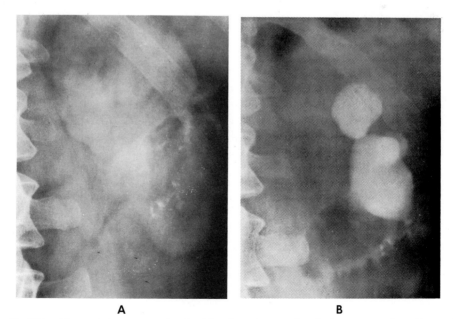

A   B

Figure 10–150. **Adenocarcinoma associated with tuberculosis with calcification. A,** *Plain film.* Enlargement of upper pole of left kidney. Irregular areas of calcification over lower pole. **B,** *Excretory urogram.* Obliteration of lower calyces from tuberculosis with calcification. Irregular dilatation of upper calyces found to be due to adenocarcinoma (hypernephroma) of upper pole. (Courtesy of Dr. T. D. Moore.)

contralateral kidney, calcification of the parenchyma may be the only lead to the correct diagnosis. The tuberculous process in autonephrectomized kidneys may be completely extinguished, but this may be impossible if the contents are still infectious.

Urographic Changes in the Ureter
(Figs. 10–151 through 10–156)

Tuberculous changes in the ureter are always secondary to renal tuberculosis (Rees and Hollands). Early urographic changes are ureteral dilatation and a

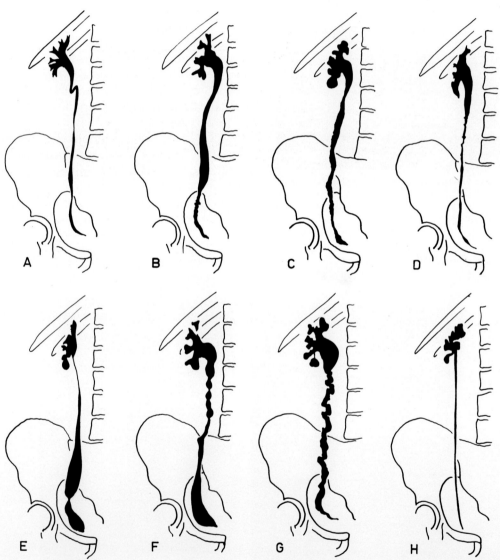

Figure 10–151. Tuberculous urographic changes of ureter. *Schematic drawing.* **A,** Normal ureter; kink in ureter overlying psoas line and different caliber of ureteral outline are due to normal peristalsis; they are not exactly reproducible in all films of same series of urograms. **B,** Irregular outline of pelvic ureter due to tuberculous ulcerations. **C,** Moderately dilated ureter with multiple marginal irregularities representing tuberculous ulcerations. **D,** Long ureteral stricture. **E,** Multiple (two) ureteral strictures in pelvic ureter. **F,** "Beaded" ureter representing alternating strictures and dilatations (see text). **G,** "Corkscrew" ureter (see text). **H,** "Pipestem" ureter (see text).

Fig. 10–152

Fig. 10–153

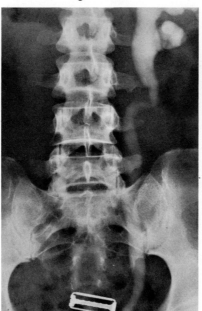
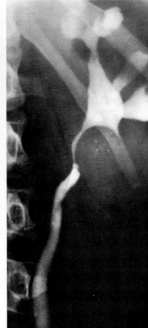

Figure 10–152. *Excretory urogram.* **Solitary left tuberculous kidney.** (Right kidney removed previously for tuberculosis.) Pyeloureterectasis resulting from obstruction from **contracted tuberculous bladder. Tuberculous stricture of intramural portion of ureter** and tuberculous infection of kidney and ureter.

Figure 10–153. *Left retrograde pyelogram.* **Left renal tuberculosis.** Destruction and obliteration of lower calyx. **Stricture of ureter** adjacent to pelvis, with irregular dilatation below.

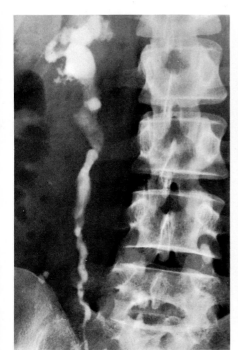
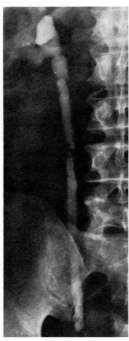

Figure 10–154. *Retrograde pyelogram.* **Advanced tuberculosis. "Pipestem" ureter.** Marked parenchymal destruction of kidney.

Figure 10–155. *Retrograde pyelogram.* **Urinary tuberculosis. "Pipestem" ureter** and marked destruction of kidney. Wall of ureter is thickened and fixed and contains alternate areas of dilatation and narrowing.

Fig. 10–154   Fig. 10–155

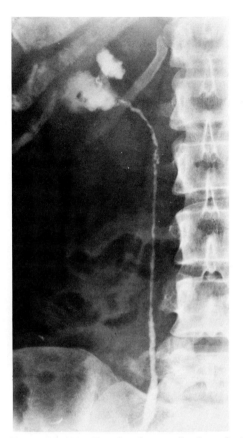

Figure 10–156. Renal and ureteral tuberculosis. *Retrograde pyelogram.* Right kidney failed to excrete contrast medium during excretory urography. Retrograde pyelography revealed marked dilatation of intrarenal collecting system and extensive tuberculous involvement of entire right ureter.

Sometimes areas of stricture and dilatation alternate, giving the characteristic image of a string of pearls ("beaded" ureter) and finally resulting in a tortuous course because of confluent strictures and ulcerations. Such an extremely irregular outline of the ureter ("corkscrew" ureter) strongly suggests tuberculosis. In advanced cases, another variety of ureteral involvement is represented by the thick-walled shortened ureter with a narrow lumen This "pipestem" ureter runs a course almost as straight as a pencil toward the bladder It has no peristalsis and is not dilated. In Figure 10–151 a schematic presentation is given of these ureteral changes. In particular, multiple strictures and the "beaded," the "corkscrew," and the "pipestem" ureter are to be considered almost characteristic of tuberculous ureteritis (Figs. 10–151 through 10–156).

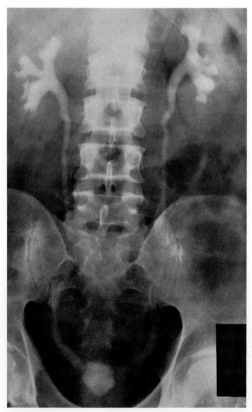

Figure 10–157. *Excretory urogram.* **Bilateral renal tuberculosis.** Moderate caliectasis and ureterectasis. Marked contracture of bladder from active tuberculous cystitis.

slightly irregular outline that often extends from the renal pelvis to the bladder. The dilatation is caused by inflammatory changes with edema and infiltration in the narrow intramural portion, whereas the slight irregularities are due to multiple small ulcerations. As ureteral involvement increases, the wall of the ureter may become thickened so that the ureter loses its normal elasticity and peristaltic capacity Areas of fibrosis, cicatrization, and constriction may alternate with areas of dilatation. Stricture formation may occur in any portion of the ureter but appears most often at the ureteropelvic and ureterovesical junctures (Barrie and associates; Claridge; Friedenberg). Strictures are highly variable in length and may be single or multiple.

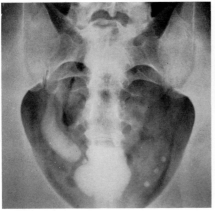 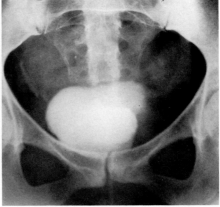

Fig. 10–158   Fig. 10–159

Figure 10–158. *Excretory cystogram.* Marked deformity of vesical outline from **tuberculous cystitis.** Calcareous lesion in region of right ureteral orifice which causes filling defect of bladder and apparent abrupt termination of dilated right ureter.

Figure 10–159. *Excretory urogram.* **Left renal tuberculosis with tuberculous involvement of left half of bladder,** causing marked deformity.

Urographic Changes in the Bladder
(Figs. 10–157 through 10–160)

The most common urographic finding is a contracted, spastic bladder of small capacity (Moonen). At times, however, one encounters cystograms of unusual contour that usually represent a tuberculous lesion that has been confined to one portion of the bladder and has caused localized deformity from spasticity, cicatrization, and fibrosis. Filling defects simulating tumor, stone, or diverticulum may be caused by marked cicatrization with deformity of one portion of the bladder or by a hyperplastic, granular-appearing inflammatory lesion that has the gross appearance of tumor (Figs. 10–157 through 10–160).

ADDITIONAL RADIOGRAPHIC METHODS

Retrograde Pyelography

In many cases of far-advanced renal tuberculosis, the excretory urogram is not adequate for complete evaluation (Emmett and Braasch). This usually results from complete loss of or insufficient function of the diseased kidney Retrograde pyelography is often carried out in such cases to delineate pathologic changes of the collecting system. If retrograde pyelography is performed in patients with proved or suspected renal tuberculosis, prophylactic antibiotic therapy should be given, and if bilateral studies are necessary, one side should be examined at a time, the second side being examined after an interval of 4 to 6 days. In particular, the risk of in-

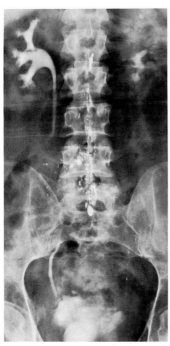

Figure 10–160. *Excretory urogram.* **Left renal tuberculosis and marked tuberculous changes of bladder.** Normal right kidney.

trarenal reflux caused by back pressure with spread of bacteria into the renal tissues, the lymphatic system, or the bloodstream should be considered. Such studies should be made under fluoroscopic control with accurate positioning of the catheter tip and with low-pressure piston injection of a carefully measured amount of contrast material, in order to avoid backflow. Backflow may occasionally even lead to incorrect interpretation or diagnosis with regard to the amount of destroyed renal tissue.

Renal Angiography

Renal angiography has only limited value in the diagnosis of tuberculosis. No significant changes on the arteriogram are seen in early tuberculosis with small calyceal deformities. Although it has been suggested that changes in the small ramifications of the arterial pattern (De Nunno) and obliteration of small vessels (Frimann-Dahl, 1966; Olsson, 1967) are sometimes seen as early changes, most authorities in this field agree that such changes are insignificant and that early renal tuberculosis can be better diagnosed by excretory urography than by renal angiography. In advanced cases, renal arteriography may help particularly in study of vascularization of renal segments that do not show up on excretory urography or retrograde pyelography (Frimann-Dahl, 1955, 1958). Angiography will then permit one to recognize avascular areas where, in the arterial phase, the renal vessels stretch around dilated calyces or granulomatous abscesses (Fritjofsson and Edsman). In the nephrographic phase the areas are seen as filling defects, and the amount of well-vascularized or reasonably well-vascularized renal parenchyma may be judged. Becker, Weiss, and Lattimer stated that, in their experience, renal arteriography only confirmed the findings of nephrotomography in advanced cases but did not yield any additional information. At the present time, it seems correct to say that renal arteriography is usually not appropriate as a method of examination in suspected renal tuberculosis, because it is of no help in detecting early lesions, and it only confirms the findings of nephrotomograms in advanced cases.

Genital Tuberculosis
(Figs. 10–161 through 10–164)

In the male. the prostate gland, seminal vesicles, and epididymis may be affected by tuberculosis. A primary focus in the testis is rare, but the testis may be affected by direct spread from the epididymis. A scrotal fistula from tuberculous epididymitis is not an unusual first sign of urogenital tuberculosis (Ross). It is often located posteriorly or on the lateral border of the scrotum, in contrast to a syphilitic fistula of the testis, which presents anteriorly. The latter lesion has become extremely rare.

Calcifications of the spermatic tract and prostate are visible on a plain film but occur relatively rarely in tuberculosis and are not characteristic. Prostatic calculi are often seen and are usually due to nonspecific chronic low-grade inflammation. They may occur coincidentally in the presence of renal tuberculosis without tuberculous prostatitis. Calcification of the vasa and am-

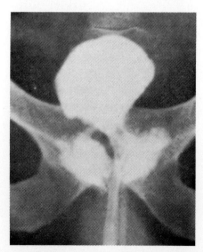

Figure 10–161. *Cystourethrogram.* **Tuberculous abscesses of prostate** which have sloughed and evacuated, leaving large irregular cavities. (Courtesy of Dr. J. K. Lattimer.)

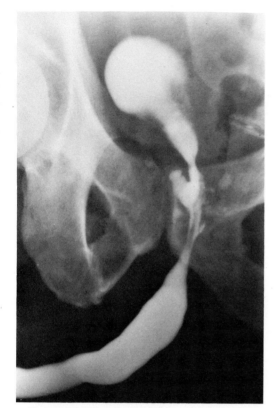

Figure 10–162. *Retrograde urethrogram.* **Tuberculous prostatitis.** Multiple prostatic abscesses that have sloughed and filled with contrast medium.

pullae is associated more often with diabetes than with tuberculosis.

Tuberculous seminal vesiculitis is almost always associated with tuberculous prostatitis. In suspected cases, seminal vesiculography may be carried out by injecting contrast medium into the ductus deferens through a small scrotal incision

Tuberculous prostatitis is an important disease and occurs more often than one would think from studying the literature. It is more resistant to treatment than is renal tuberculosis, it may cause considerable destruction, and it is sometimes difficult to detect because it lacks characteristic symptoms. Retrograde urethrography and micturition cystourethrography are important methods for accurate diagnosis. May and coworkers reported on the roentgenographic diagnosis and the course of the disease in 91 cases. They found definite evidence of prostatic involvement during

urethrography in 22 patients in whom the disorder was not suspected during rectal digital palpation In 38 patients, urethrography confirmed the rectal findings, and in 31 patients with positive rectal palpatory changes, no communication of prostatic cavities with the urethra could be demonstrated by urethrography. They stressed that in the presence of urethrographically demonstrable prostatourethral fistulas, healing may be hastened by performing transurethral prostatic resection in combination with chemotherapy. They advocated routine urethrography in patients with suspected or proven renal tuberculosis.

Genital tuberculosis should be considered in female patients if urinary tuberculosis is present, but only rarely does roentgenographic examination yield results in these instances (Sutherland). Genital tuberculosis may produce pelvic inflammatory masses large enough to displace and distort the lower third of the ureters and the bladder (Sutherland). Fistulous com-

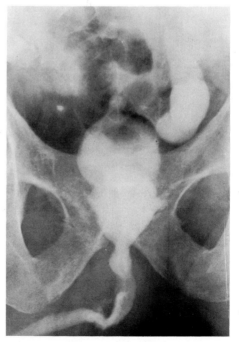

Figure 10–163. *Retrograde cystourethrogram.* Almost complete **sloughing of prostate from extensive tuberculous abscesses.** Vesicoureteral reflux, which increased in severity during chemotherapy.

munications involving the lower parts of the ureters, bladder, and intestine have been reported (see Fistulas and Sinuses, Chapter 15). Menstrual blood samples should be cultured for tuberculosis if possible in all cases of urinary tuberculosis in women. Overbeck and Keller reported that the use of this method disclosed that 9.7 per cent of 187 female patients with renal tuberculosis had positive cultures for otherwise unsuspected genital tuberculosis.

In all patients treated for tuberculosis of the genitourinary tract, careful follow-up roentgen examinations at regular intervals

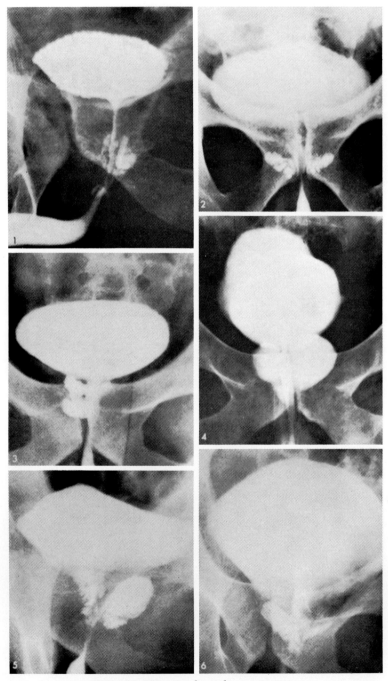

Figure 10–164. *See legend on opposite page.*

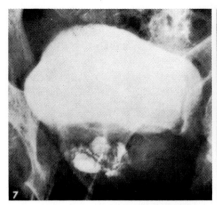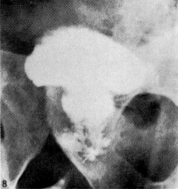

Fig. 10–164. *Continued*

Figure 10–164. **Tuberculous prostatitis.** *Retrograde urethrograms.* **1,** Bilateral periurethral cavities and beginning tuberculous contracture of bladder. **2,** Symmetrical extravasation of contrast medium in prostatic urethra. **3,** Large prostatic cavity on right; small cavities on left. **4,** Complete destruction of prostatic parenchyma. Formation of so-called anterior bladder. **5,** Extensive cavernous prostatitis bilaterally. **6,** Same patient as in **5** after transurethral prostatic resection. **7,** Extensive cavernous prostatitis bilaterally. **8,** Same patient as in **7** after 2 years. Complete liquefaction of prostatic parenchyma, marked "anterior bladder." (From May, P., Hohenfellner, R., König, E., and König, K.)

are mandatory both for evaluation of therapeutic results and for early detection of complications during the healing process (Carr; Roylance and associates). From the outset, it should be explained to all patients that such studies are an essential part of the therapeutic program and that conservative or reconstructive surgical treatment is occasionally necessary as adjunctive treatment.

The particular need for follow-up studies stems from the tendency of tissues affected by tuberculosis to contract from fibrosis in healing. Healing of superficial ulcerations affecting only the mucous membrane produces a small scar that does not cause stricture. Deeper destruction produces considerable fibrosis on healing. Areas of predilection for stricture formation with important consequences are the ureter and more particularly its terminal and intramural portions, the ureteropelvic juncture, and the calyceal infundibulum.

GENITOURINARY BILHARZIASIS (SCHISTOSOMIASIS)

by Abdel Aziz Zaky Hanna

Bilharziasis is probably one of the oldest diseases known to mankind. In 1910,

Ruffer discovered bilharzial ova in the kidneys of mummies dating back to the 20th dynasty (1200 to 1090 B.C.), and historians of medieval Egypt, mostly Arabs, told the story of a disease among the men of Egypt "which made them menstruate like women" (Makar). In 1851, Theodore Bilharz was the first to discover the worms and their relationship to hematuria (Makar). In the past two decades, the disease has spread extensively and has become endemic in different parts of the world, including most of Africa, the southern tips of Europe, Western Asia, the islands on the east coast of Africa, Japan, and even India and Pakistan (Faust and Russell). It is estimated that between 200,000,000 and 300,000,000 people are affected with this disease. Because so many American soldiers have been in these endemic areas and because of the great increase in foreign travel (due to easy access by air transportation), more cases of urinary bilharziasis are being seen in the offices of American urologists. For this reason it is important that the profession become acquainted with this disease.

The disease is related to infestation of the pelvic veins of humans by the parasite *Schistosoma haematobium*. Males, being more often exposed than females, are more often infected, in the ratio of nine males to one female. The urinary bladder is involved in 85 per cent of cases, and the ureters are involved in 44 per cent. In endemic areas, urinary schistosomiasis is commonly seen in older children and adults between the ages of 10 and 30 years. However, most patients, especially those living in the villages, do not seek medical advice until complications set in. Consequently, the actual infestation usually occurs five to ten years before the onset of urinary tract complications, the most important of which are secondary infection, urinary lithiasis, contracted bladder, cancer of the bladder, ureteric stricture, vesicoureteral reflux, and lesions of the bladder neck.

Pathogenesis of Genitourinary Bilharziasis

Bilharziasis is a parasitic disease caused by a blood fluke. Three forms of flukes are responsible: (1) *Schistosoma japonicum*, (2) *S. mansoni* and (3) *S. haematobium.** *S. mansoni* involves chiefly the rectum and liver, whereas *S. japonicum* involves mainly the lungs and liver. *S. haematobium* involves primarily the urinary tract. Vermooten has given an excellent brief account of the life cycle of this parasite, from which the following description is taken: The egg is discharged with the urine (from human beings). When it comes in contact with water it swells, ruptures, and liberates a miracidium. This then penetrates a specific species of snail *(Physopsis africana)* and becomes a sporocyst. Each sporocyst gives rise to a second generation of sporocysts, from which tens of thousands of cercariae are produced. In five to seven weeks they leave the snail and swim free in water for one to seven days, when they die unless they can reach and penetrate the skin or mucous mem-

brane of a human being. Here they enter the venous and lymphatic systems and are carried to the heart and then to the capillaries of the lung. From there they travel via the arterial circulation and eventually reach the portal vein, where they grow into adult worms.

Approximately three weeks after entry through the skin the maturing worms migrate out of the portal vein, traveling against the bloodstream via the inferior and superior mesenteric veins and the hemorrhoidal, spermatic, and retrocecal veins into the vesical, pelvic, and ureteral plexuses, being especially abundant in the veins of the submucosa of the bladder (Makar).

Venous anastomoses between the portal system and the systemic circulation have also been demonstrated around the distal lower third of the pelvic ureter, the vesicoprostatic venous plexus, and the middle rectal veins, probably accounting for the presence of the worm in this region. In the vesical plexus the female worm leaves the male, and because of her smaller size she is able to pass into smaller vessels (where the male cannot go) and to deposit her ova or eggs in the venules beneath the mucous membrane of the bladder. The eggs are laid in a chain of approximately 20, positioned so that their spines engage the vessel wall; this helps their extrusion into the perivenous spaces. Aided by contractions of the muscular wall of the ureter or bladder or both and possibly by the action of lytic enzymes excreted by the ova, the ova reach the lumen of the viscus and are voided with the urine.

Pathology of Genitourinary Bilharziasis

Considerable reaction is initiated in the tissues surrounding the ova. Grossly and cystoscopically the early lesions appear as small areas of hyperemia associated with slight edema. When the ova break through the vesical mucosa, red, granular bleeding areas result which account for the typical "endemic hematuria of Egypt,"

---

*The term "bilharziasis" should refer only to the disease produced by *S. haematobium;* however, in the literature it has been used loosely to include all three varieties.

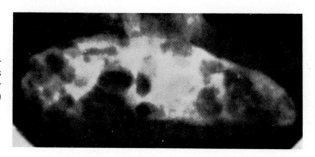

Figure 10–165. Bilharziasis. *Excretory urogram* showing "honeycomb-type" filling defects produced by diffuse involvement of bladder by granulomatous polypi. (From El-Badawi, A. A.)

which is so common in the early stage of the disease.

As the lesions progress, they appear as small, pale, yellowish granules with slightly raised shiny surfaces surrounded by a zone of hyperemia. The lesions simulate tubercles in appearance and are the result of proliferative changes in the tissues, associated with hyperplasia. As the process becomes chronic, lesions enlarge and become nodular. Groups of nodules may coalesce to form bilharzial nodes (bilharziomata); these nodes may undergo necrosis and ulceration or become calcified (Fig. 10–165).

Histologically, the initial lesion is a granuloma *(bilharzioma)* in which an intense cellular reaction containing macrophages, foreign body giant cells, lymphocytes, and plasma cella is seen. Sometimes eosinophils are present in the periphery as well. As the disease progresses, secondary lesions of two main pathologic types develop:

1. *Hyperplastic lesions.* The presence of bilharziomata near the epithelium and in the underlying connective tissue of the vesical or ureteric wall produces prominent nodules and papilloma-like bodies. Sometimes epithelial hyperplasia extends into the submucosa, forming pseudoglandular structures as well. Obstruction at the neck of these "glands" transforms them into a kind of retention cyst producing what are known as *bilharzial cystitis* and *ureteritis cystica.* Squamous metaplasia with leukoplakia formation is common. These hyperplastic mucosal changes are thought to predispose to carcinoma, which is frequently found in bilharzial bladders (Khafagy and associates).

2. *Hypoplastic lesions.* The cellular reaction associated with bilharzial infestation induces fibrosis of a varying degree of severity that involves the full thickness of the infected part of the ureter or bladder. The developing fibrous tissue kills the incarcerated organisms, and stops the process of hyperplasia while at the same time fibrosis proceeds and calcification of the dead ova sets in. The mucous membrane of the involved areas undergoes marked atrophic changes and finally becomes replaced by a thin fibrous layer of tissue. Fibrosis contracts the bladder, interferes with its distensibility, and diminishes its capacity. Severe fibrosis may turn the ureter into an inelastic fibrous tube with areas of stricture and attendant back pressure effects, such as pyelocaliectasis, on the upper tract. The ova that are not removed by the phagocytic action of macrophages remain embedded in the fibrous tissue and undergo calcification. These are often found in immense numbers as calcified sheets in the submucosa and to a lesser extent in the muscularis and adventitia. Fresh lesions continue to develop as long as the parent flukes live. The extent of the damage to the involved tissues is proportional to the number of ova trapped within them.

THE BLADDER

In some cases, because of nonvascularity of the involved bladder regions or the host's defense mechanism atrophy of the mucous membrane occurs. In such a situation old calcified bilharzial ova buried in the submucosal layer present the cystoscopic picture of a typical *sandy patch* (sand under water). If bilharzial ova are trapped in the vesical musculature, they may lead to muscular hyperplasia, but more often they cause fibrosis and atrophy of the muscle bundles with subsequent contraction and deformity of the bladder wall (Makar). In the trigonal area, the bilharzial ova lie in the muscular rather than the submucosal layer; hence they gradually lead to fibrosis of the bladder neck, atrophy of the trigonal muscle, and *clinical* obstruction of the vesical neck. Pericystitis may also occur owing to extension of the disease into the adjacent loose cellular tissues of the pelvis. This leads to a dense, tough perivesical fibrosis that contributes to progressive contraction and deformation of the bladder (Rifaat).

THE URETER

In the ureter, as in the bladder, the ova lying in the subepithelial layer produce hyperplasia of the epithelium with formation of papillomas or nodules that protrude into the lumen of the ureter (Fig. 10–166). It should be noted, however, that papilloma formation is much less common in the ureter than in the bladder. At times, as was pointed out above, epithelial hyperplasia may invaginate into the submucosa to form retention cysts. This condition, termed "ureteritis cystica," may lead to "ureteritis calcinosa" as a result of calcification of the walls of the cysts or calcification of blood within their lumina. The hyperplastic process is followed by atrophy of the subepithelial and epithelial layers and by ulceration of the mucosa with deposition of urate, phosphate, and oxalate crystals on the ulcers. The end result of ureteral bilharziasis is the formation of a granulomatous sclerosing reaction with dense fibrosis involving the entire thickness of the wall of the ureter. In some patients, chronic periureteritis leads to fibrosis of the periureteral tissues, which tends to be more severe around the pelvic segments than in their mid and upper portions (Kamel). The final effect of this combination of mucosal, muscular, and periureteral

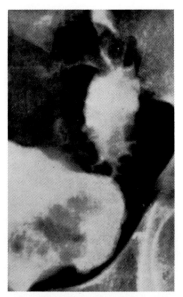

Figure 10–166. Bilharziasis. *Excretory urogram.* Multiple filling defects in bladder and honeycomb-like defects of distal part of pelvic ureter produced by granulomatous polyposis. (From El-Badawi, A. A.)

lesions is scarring, stricture formation, loss of peristaltic activity and elasticity of the involved ureter, calcification of the dead ova in the ureteral wall, and secondary ureteral calculi. The lesions are usually bilateral and may occur in any part of the ureter. Most commonly they are found in the intramural ureter (usually secondary to vesical bilharziasis), next in the distal part of the ureter, and least commonly in the lumbar portion of the ureter, especially at the level of the third lumbar vertebra.

Ureteral stricture is an important complication of ureteral bilharziasis. Strictures are classified into three types: (1) annular, (2) spindle-shaped, and (3) the "third-lumbar ureteral stricture," or Makar s stricture (named after N. Makar of Egypt, who first described it). There are usually advanced degrees of dilatation and tortuosity of the ureter proximal to the stricture; secondary ureteral and renal lithiasis, hydronephrosis, and atrophy of the kidney may ensue. Dilatation and tortuosity of the pelvic ureter associated with a normal lumbar ureter and normal upper urinary tracts were considered by Vermooten to be pathognomonic of bilharziasis.

Vesicoureteral reflux is a complication of bilharziasis found in 11 to 44 per cent of patients (Al-Ghorab and associates, 1966). Historically, Ibrahim was one of the first to recognize this abnormality in 1926, when he demonstrated reflux in bilharzial ureters during cystoscopy. Vermooten, in an experimental study reported in 1937, proved that an incompetent ureterovesical valvular mechanism resulting from bilharziasis allows regurgitation of urine into the ureter. Subsequently, in 1948, Gelfard observed that reflux was an important factor in producing ureteric dilatation without obstruction in patients with bilharzia.

The etiology of bilharzial vesicoureteral reflux is not well understood, but a number of pathologic and physiologic findings associated with the disease have been described that aid in understanding the process. Guindy divided his patients with bilharzia and vesicoureteral reflux into two groups: (1) those with obstruction of the bladder at its outlet and (2) those with disease of the ureterovesical juncture. He pointed out that obstruction at the bladder outlet may be due to bladder neck fibrosis from bilharzial infestation or to obstruction from stone or tumor encroaching on the outlet of the bladder, and he attributed vesicoureteral reflux in these patients to a mechanism similar to that which may cause reflux in patients with nonbilharzial bladder neck obstruction: In the presence of outlet obstruction, a sustained tonus develops in the bladder as it actively resists distention. This causes back pressure and reflux. Both back pressure and reflux may be followed by development of secondary changes in the bladder wall at the uretero-vesical juncture, such as saccules or diverticula. These changes weaken or destroy the detrusor muscle lying under the intramural ureter, thereby causing further aggravation of reflux and rendering it irreversible by destroying the normal antireflux valvular mechanism.

In patients with bilharzial lesions of the ureterovesical juncture itself, Guindy observed a number of abnormalities that interfere with the valvular mechanism that normally prevents reflux, including the following.

1. Bilharzial fibrosis and calcification produce rigidity of the terminal part of the ureter that prevents compression of the terminal ureter by the muscles of the bladder, thus allowing reflux to occur.

2. Stricture of the lower end of the ureter with marked dilatation and tortuosity may pull the intramural part of the ureter into an extravesical location, destroying the normal valvular mechanism at the ureterovesical juncture.

3. Bilharzial fibrosis and calcification in the muscular wall of the bladder around the intramural part of the ureter cause the muscle to lose its function as an actively contracting, firm support against which the intramural ureter can be compressed by the intravesical pressure generated during voiding.

4. A large stone may develop in the intramural part of the ureter and may enlarge the ureteral cavity with destruction of Waldeyer's sheath, weakening of the muscles, and consequent interference with the normal valve-like action that prevents reflux.

Guindy also noted that a combination of two or more of these factors is usually responsible for reflux in bilharziasis. Thus, it is common to find the ureter with its lower end calcified and dilated, a stricture at the ureterovesical juncture, a calcified bladder, and possibly a stone in the lower end of the ureter. These lesions at the ureterovesical juncture may be combined with bilharzial bladder neck obstruction and secondary diverticula or saccules. If cancer complicates bilharzial bladder, it too may produce reflux either by obstructing the bladder at its outlet or by encroaching on the ureterovesical juncture.

Al-Ghorab and associates stated that anatomic factors may be blamed for the occurrence of reflux. Chief among these are fibrosis of the intramural part of the ureter with consequent rigidity, shortening, degeneration and/or fibrosis of trigonal muscle, and gaping of the ureteric orifice caused by surrounding bladder fibrosis. They also mentioned that stenosis of the intramural part of the ureter may be accompanied by reflux.

Other observations pertaining to reflux and its effects include those of Badr and associates and of Safwat. Badr and associates drew attention to patients with spindle-shaped, dilated ureters who did not have ureteral strictures. They suggested that these were caused by regurgitation (reflux) of urine upward through a partially fibrosed and rigid segment of the intramural portion of the ureter that cannot be compressed readily between the contracting bladder muscles. Safwat speculated that destruction of the nerve plexus at the lower end of the ureter and the ureterovesical juncture by bilharziasis may also be a factor contributing to both reflux and dilatation of the bilharzial ureter.

BILHARZIAL BLADDER NECK OBSTRUCTION

Zaher and associates introduced the concept of bilharzial bladder neck obstruction as an explanation for the finding of a dilated spindle ureter when no ureteral obstruction is present.

Study of the bladder neck in this group of patients has shown that bilharziasis in the bladder, though generalized, is more severe in the trigonal plate (Badr and Torky). The trigonal plate is defined as the vascular fibro-areolar layer lying between the trigonal muscles and the fibers of the detrusor vesicae. When bilharzia first infests this area, the trigonal mucosa as well as the supra-montanal part of the posterior urethra becomes congested, edematous, and granular. Later on, when fibrosis becomes established, the trigone becomes shortened in all its dimensions, with concomitant shortening of the supramontanal part of the posterior urethra. This occurs as a result of progressive fibrosis and atrophy of the trigonal musculature caused by interference with its blood supply. The blood vessels that are included in the bilharzial infiltrations are prone to thrombophlebitis and thromboangiitis ending in partial or complete closure of their lumina (Hanna and Saleh).

Badr and Torky described three stages of bilharzial bladder neck obstruction. These are (1) stage of forming stricture (congestive cellular stage), (2) stage of actual or formed stricture (fibrotic stage), and (3) stage of trigonal atrophy (terminal stage). Because the fibrosis is more extensive in the distal half of the trigonal plate, posterior shelving of the vesical outlet results. The vesical outlet itself is narrowed, corrugated, rigid, and nondilatable owing to the fibrotic process.

Bilharzial bladder neck obstruction that leads to obstruction, distension of the bladder, and ureteric reflux was reported by Hassim and associates.

Attia described bilharziasis of the prostate and pointed out that ova are scattered in the prostate and that a cellular reaction may or may not be present around them. In some cases, the main deposition of ova is around the urethra, with the resulting fibrosis causing bladder neck obstruction.

Prostatism that includes the triad of frequency, difficulty in voiding, and abnormal stream of urine is the presenting symptom of bladder neck obstruction, regardless of its etiology. Urinary infection, recurrent colic, recurrent calculosis, renal failure, or delayed closure of postoperative urinary wounds with fistulization may also be seen. Other less common causes of bladder neck obstruction include ball valve action by vesical papilloma at the vesical outlet, fibrosis of the entire prostatic urethra related to submucosal deposition of ova, and obstruction of the vesical neck secondary to bilharzial prostatitis or seminal vesiculitis.

Carcinoma is recognized as a common complication of bilharziasis of the bladder. The disease occurs most often in men (80 per cent or more of the cases) and tends to appear at an earlier age than carcinoma of the bladder in patients who do not have bilharzia, often appearing in patients from 20 to 40 years old. In contrast with the overwhelming preponderance of transitional cell carcinoma in patients with carcinoma of the bladder who do not have bilharziasis, the large majority of these patients have squamous cell carcinoma. Khafagy, El-Bolkainy, and Mansour, for example, reported that in their series of 86 patients with bilharziasis and carcinoma, 66 of the carcinomas were squamous, 18 were transitional, and 2 were adenocarcinomas, while in 90 such patients reported by Dimmette and associates, 50 of the carcinomas were squamous, 33 were transitional, 6 were adenocarcinoma, and 1 was mixed type. The lesions tend to be large and bulky when diagnosed and are usually found on the lateral surfaces, posterior walls, and vault of the bladder. Origin on the trigone is rare. Bladder carcinoma is commonly associated with metaplastic epithelial changes, as was pointed out previously. These include squamous metaplasia (65 per cent), columnar metaplasia (52 per cent), and carcinoma in situ (41 per cent). The ureters, trigone, and urethra are rarely affected by the metaplastic process (Khafagy and associates).

Genital Involvement in Bilharziasis

The genital organs may also be involved with the bilharziasis. Granulomatous sclerosis and fibrosis principally involve the urethra, prostate, and seminal vesicles and more rarely affect the epididymus, spermatic cords, and testicles.

Urethral bilharziasis may take the form of polypi in the fossa navicularis, periurethral abscess, and perineal or scrotal fistulae. Urethral strictures are not common; however, they may occur in association with long-standing bilharzial fistulae. Urethritis cystica occurs very rarely.

Prostatic involvement by bilharziasis leads to enlargement of the gland in the early stages. This may be followed by shrinkage and fibrosis. Occlusion of some of the prostatic ducts and sinuses due to fibrosis may result in the formation of retention cysts. Infection of one of these cysts may then lead to abscess formation. The seminal vesicles may also be involved, resulting in enlarged hard vesicles that may be calcified. The ducts become dilated and may show granulomatous masses. Bilharzial granulation tissue may involve the ampullovesicular angle, causing it to become widened and less acute — in contrast to the reduction or obliteration of the angle that occurs with nonspecific infection. The vesicles themselves become enlarged and hard to palpation. Some may become calcified.

The ejaculatory ducts are rarely involved in the bilharzial process (Mokhless).

Roentgen Diagnosis in Genitourinary Bilharziasis

THE PLAIN FILM

The bladder is involved in 85 per cent and the ureter in 44 per cent of all cases of urinary bilharziasis. As was pointed out above, the end stage of the bilharzial lesion is fibrosis often associated with calcification of the dead ova; these calcific lesions can be seen in the plain film, where they probably represent the most important single diagnostic finding in this disease. Certain findings in the plain film strongly suggest the presence of *Bilharzia*. One of the earlier findings is a curvilinear line of calcification located in the suprapubic region. As the disease progresses, this calcified line extends until it may completely outline the periphery of the bladder (Fig. 10–167). Further deposition of calcium in the wall and epithelial lining of the bladder produces thick calcified bands within the bladder wall (Ragheb) (Figs. 10–168 and 10–169); the bladder may become so heavily calcified and contracted that it may give the appearance of a large vesical calculus (Fig. 10–170). (True calculi are seen in 39 per cent of patients with vesical bilharziasis [Afifi] [Fig. 10–171].) When the vesical wall becomes diffusely calcified, the plain film may look like a cystogram made with contrast medium. In the case of extensive bilharzial tumors of the bladder,

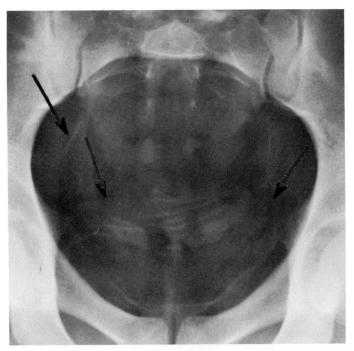

Figure 10–167. Urinary bilharziasis. *Plain film.* Typical bilharzial calcification of bladder and lower part of ureters. Early manifestation. Note smooth, thin, curvilinear calcific line in suprapubic area outlining periphery of bladder. (Courtesy of Dr. F. Shehadeh.)

a pathognomonic finding is obliteration of one side of the bladder as though half of the bladder had been excised or "amputated"—leaving only an irregular serrated margin.

Ureteral bilharziasis is commonly associated with the bladder disease. Changes most frequently seen are linear calcifications involving the distal ureter (Fig. 10–167). As the disease progresses, the whole ureter may become heavily calcified; if the ureter is greatly dilated from an associated stricture, it may look like a calcified loop of intestine (Fig. 10–172). Calcification rarely involves the proximal ureter and the ureteropelvic juncture. Calcified papillomas are commonly seen in the lower third of the ureter and may be difficult to differentiate from ureteral calculi (Fig. 10–171). Ureteritis calcinosa involving the lower third of the ureter appears as spotty, irregular calcifications, which are considered pathognomonic (Fig. 10–173). *Ureteral calculi*

are common in urinary bilharziasis, and evidence of them in the plain film should always lead one to suspect the possibility of distal ureteral stricture.

The kidney is less commonly involved because the venous anastomoses between the renal cortex and the portal system are too small to permit passage of bilharzial ova to the kidney and upper urinary tract. A few cases of bilharzial calcification of the renal capsule have been reported (Atala and Zaher). Renal involvement, however, is usually secondary to vesicoureteral bilharziasis and usually results in the formation of renal calculi, nephrocalcinosis, and obstructive hydro- or pyonephrosis (Fig. 10–174).

In **genital bilharziasis** the most common site of calcification are the seminal vesicles, which provide the typical appearance of a mulberry-shaped calcification seen in the plain film (Fig 10–175). The vas deferens rarely calcifies.

Text continued on page 932

Fig. 10–168

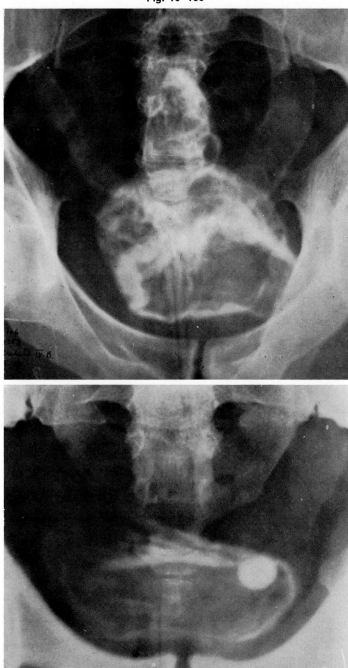

Fig. 10–169

Figure 10–168.   **Bilharziasis.** *Plain film.* Extensive calcification of bladder and both dilated ureters from bilharziasis. (Courtesy of Prof. J. Bitschai.)

Figure 10–169.   **Bilharziasis.** *Plain film.* Calcification of wall of bladder caused by bilharziasis. Also stone in left ureter above ureteral stricture. (Courtesy of Prof. J. Bitschai.)

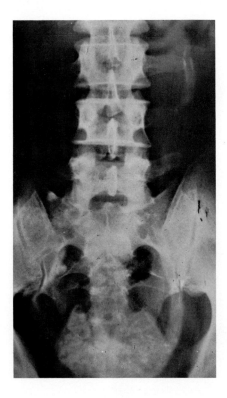

Figure 10–170. Bilharziasis. *Plain film.* Extensive calcification of bladder, entire left ureter, and lower third of right ureter, resulting from bilharziasis. Film is unusual in that calcification of upper part of ureter in this disease is fairly rare. (Courtesy of Prof. J. Bitschai.)

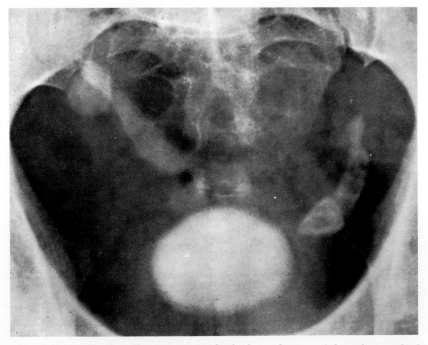

Figure 10–171. Bilharziasis. *Plain film.* Large vesical calculus and primary bilateral ureteral calculi, resulting from bilharziasis. (Courtesy of Prof. J. Bitschai.)

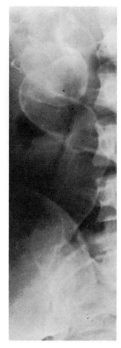

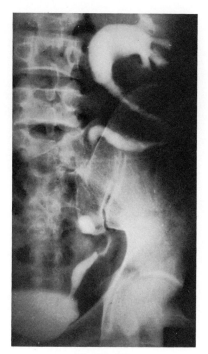

Fig. 10-172   Fig. 10-173

Figure 10-172.   Urinary bilharziasis. *Plain film.* Marked dilatation and tortuosity of entirely calcified right ureter in advanced untreated bilharziasis.

Figure 10-173.   Urinary bilharziasis. *Excretory urogram.* Ureteritis calcinosa involving upper third of left ureter associated with tortuosity and multiple spindle-shaped dilatation of ureter secondary to ureteral strictures.

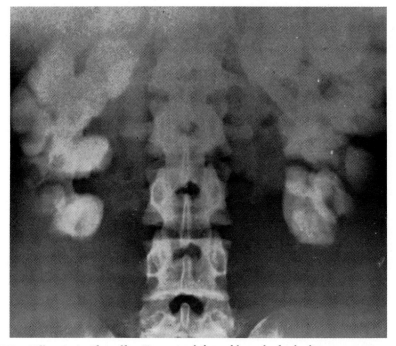

Figure 10-174.   Bilharziasis. *Plain film.* Extensive bilateral branched calculi in young Egyptian man suffering from long-standing bilharziasis. (Courtesy of Prof. J. Bitschai.)

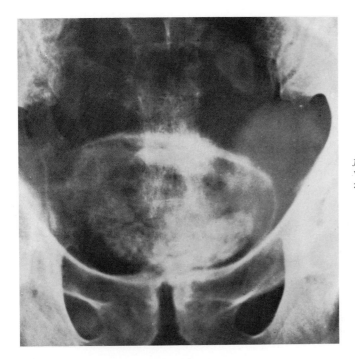

Figure 10–175. Bilharziasis. *Plain film.* Calcification of bladder wall, seminal vesicles, and prostate gland from bilharziasis. (Courtesy of Prof. J. Bitschai.)

THE UROGRAM

The Bladder

The most common finding revealed by the excretory cystogram is a contracted, irregular bladder wall; in some cases large, irregular filling defects produced by multiple bladder tumors are present; this may be considered as the end stage of this disease (Figs. 10–165, 10–166, and 10–176). Elevation of the base of the bladder from bilharzial infection of the prostate is frequently encountered; it is even occasionally seen in children. Vesical calculi are common and may mimic vesical neoplasms. Young and associates reported postvoiding retention of urine in 116 of 128

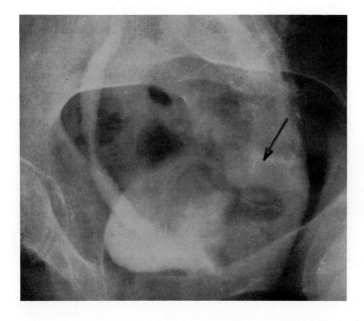

Figure 10–176. Urinary bilharziasis. *Retrograde cystogram.* Right vesicoureteral reflux secondary to urinary bilharziasis. Note filling defect in bladder (*arrow*) suggestive of carcinoma.

patients who had postvoiding films made at excretory urography.

The radiologic assessment of the presence of vesicoureteral reflux in cases of bilharziasis is of great importance to the surgeon from the point of view of management of the cases, as reflux rather than obstruction may be the cause of ureteral dilatation seen on the excretory urogram. The presence of reflux can be confirmed radiologically in many ways, the most important of which are retrograde (ascending) cystography and micturating cystourethrography (see discussion of techniques of cystography and cystourethrography in Chapter 1). Retrograde (ascending) cystography is often not recommended for fear of introducing infection In these patients, the presence of vesicoureteral reflux may be confirmed by the following technique:

An excretory (descending) cystogram is obtained by giving a large intravenous dose of contrast medium. The kidneys and lower ureters are then cleared of contrast medium by induction of diuresis. With the bladder filled and opacified and the ureters emptied by this technique, micturition may then force contrast medium into the ureters, confirming the presence of vesicoureteral reflux.

The Ureter and the Kidney

A "snake head" or spindle-shaped appearance of the terminal (pelvic) ureter is considered pathognomonic (Fig. 10–177); it results from stricture of the intramural ureter. Multiple strictures, usually located in the lower third of the ureter, with multiple spindle-shaped configurations can mimic ureteral tuberculosis (Fig. 10–173). Above the site of the stricture the ureters are often greatly dilated, tortuous, and kinked; vesicoureteral reflux is present in approximately one third of cases (Fig. 10–176). These changes are usually bilateral and involve principally the lower portion of the ureters, but as the disease progresses the pathologic process may extend proximally to involve the upper third of the ureter, the renal pelvis, and the renal calyces; hydronephrosis may result. *Renal*

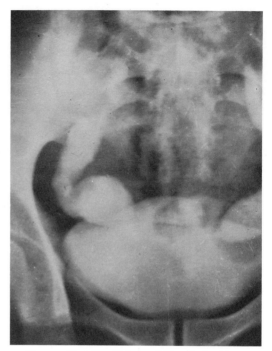

Figure 10–177. Urinary bilharziasis. *Excretory urogram.* Typical "snake head" spindle-shaped appearance of distal lower third of ureters secondary to stricture in intramural ureter.

calculi are not uncommon; they may attain considerable size and form branched (staghorn) calculi (Figs. 10–174 and 10–178). Noncalcified papillomas in the ureter usually appear as smooth filling defects (Figs. 10–166 and 10–179), which may be differentiated from the defects of bilharzial ureteritis cystica by their greater size and smaller number (Fig. 10–180). The calcified honeycomb appearance of ureteritis calcinosa is considered pathognomonic of bilharziasis but must be differentiated from ureteral tumors, which occur only rarely in ureteral bilharziasis (Fig. 10–173). The third-lumbar stricture (Makar's stricture) with its associated ureteral dilatation above and renal secondary hydronephrosis may mimic the urographic appearance of idiopathic retroperitoneal fibrosis (Figs. 10–181 and 10–182). The annular ureteral stricture is the commonest type encountered in this disease (Fig. 10–183), followed in incidence by the spindle-shaped type (Fig. 10–177) and then the third-lumbar stricture (or Makar's stricture). Secondary ureteral cal-

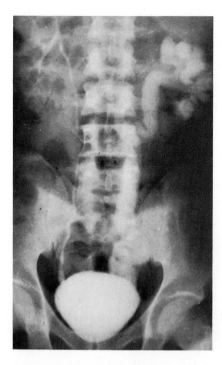

Figure 10–178.   Urinary bilharziasis. *Excretory urogram.* Marked dilatation and tortuosity of whole left ureter secondary to stricture in intramural ureter and resulting in left hydronephrosis and nephrolithiasis.

culi are common findings in urinary bilharziasis (Fig. 10–184).

Obstruction at the ureteropelvic juncture is a rare finding in bilharziasis; it results from fibrous compression and must be differentiated from hydronephrosis caused by vesicoureteral reflux. Scarring and thinning of the renal parenchyma with resultant deformed calyces may be the end result in chronic untreated disease.

Bilharzial changes in the ureter may simulate changes encountered in tuberculous ureteritis in the sense that both lesions are characterized by ureteric stric-

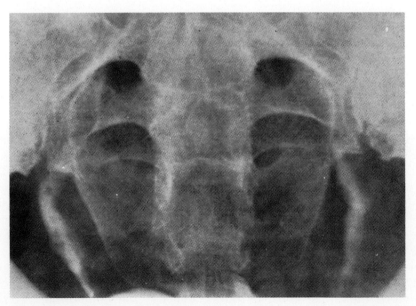

Figure 10–179.   Bilharziasis. *Excretory urogram.* Negative shadows caused by bilharzial papillomatosis of both ureters. (Courtesy of Prof. J. Bitschai.)

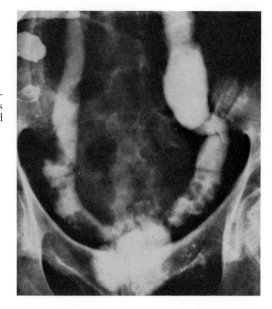

Figure 10–180. Urinary bilharziasis. *Excretory urogram.* Multiple filling defects in lower third of both ureters resulting from bilharzial ureteritis cystica with marked dilatation and tortuosity of proximal parts of ureters.

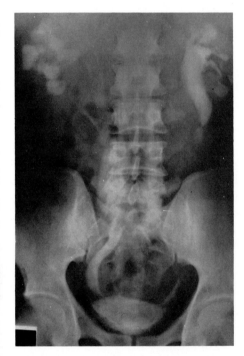

Figure 10–181. Urinary bilharziasis. *Excretory urogram.* General features of urinary bilharziasis in addition to calculi and calcification of bladder wall seen in plain film. Right ureterovesical stricture. **Left ureteral stricture at level of L-3 (Makar's stricture).** (Courtesy of Dr. F. Shehadeh.)

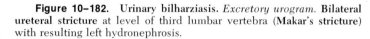

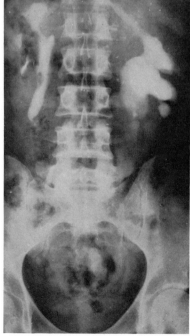

Figure 10–182. Urinary bilharziasis. *Excretory urogram.* Bilateral **ureteral stricture** at level of third lumbar vertebra (Makar's stricture) with resulting left hydronephrosis.

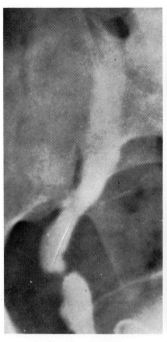 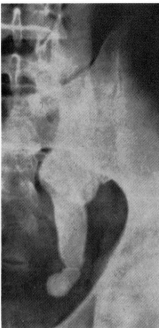

Figure 10–183. Bilharziasis. *Right retrograde pyelogram.* Typical annular type stricture in lower third of ureter with dilatation above and below. (Courtesy of Prof. J. Bitschai.)

Figure 10–184. Bilharziasis. *Plain film.* Giant "primary" ureteral calculus formed in situ in left ureter, which is markedly dilated because of bilharziasis. Stricture in terminal portion of ureter. (Courtesy of Prof. J. Bitschai.)

Fig. 10–183   **Fig. 10–184**

tures. Several important findings seen at urography help distinguish the two:

1. Calcification is uncommon in tuberculosis of the ureter. When seen, it presents a mottled, irregularly scattered pattern in various parts of the ureter, whereas in bilharziasis of the ureter calcification is seen in the majority of cases and is characterized by more or less continuous calcification of the involved area. It is most prominent in the pelvic part of the ureter and is usually associated with calcification of the bladder.

2. Deposits of calcium are common in the kidney with tuberculosis but are seen rarely if ever in bilharziasis.

3. Tuberculous infection causes fibrosis, thickening, and rigidity with straightening or shortening of the ureter, whereas bilharzial infestation causes much more dilatation and lengthening and tends to produce a markedly tortuous ureter without the rigidity seen in tuberculosis.

The Bladder Neck

Micturition and retrograde cystourethrography are important aids in the diag-

nosis of bilharzial obstruction of the bladder neck (Hanna, 1969; Hanna and Saleh). The retrograde cystourethrogram will reveal a shortened and sometimes sacculated prostatic urethra with elevation of its base and shelving of the posterior lip of the vesical neck, which appears stenosed and displaced forward. The remainder of the prostatic urethra is usually normal except for possibly some hypertrophy of the verumontanum or an occasional extravasation of contrast medium into dilated prostatic ducts. The micturition cystourethrogram may be helpful for making the diagnosis of bilharzial obstruction of the vesical neck (Fig. 10–185). It helps visualize the degree of relaxation of the vesical neck during micturition as well as the degree of filling and dilatation of the prostatic urethra. Fluoroscopy with spot films and multiple anteroposterior, oblique, and lateral views may be required.

The Urethra

Retrograde and micturition cystourethrography can reveal fistulous tracts

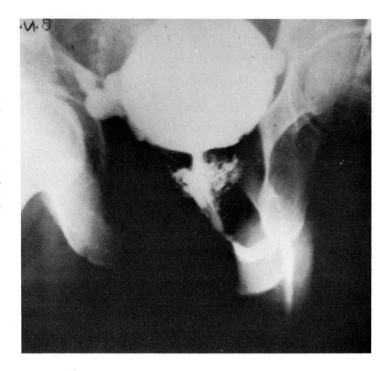

Figure 10–185. Urinary bilharziasis. *Voiding cystogram.* Constriction of vesical neck with dilatation and sacculation of prostatic urethra and extravasation of contrast medium in prostatic ducts. Note cellules and diverticula in bladder.

passing to the perineum. Multiple tracts arising from the bulbous urethra constitute the most common picture seen (Fig. 10–186). The bulbous urethra is often irregular and narrowed owing to external pressure by a fistula-containing inflammatory mass, yet actual stricture is not present (Fig. 10–187). Stricture of the penile urethra, on the other hand, affects a long segment that is usually firm and tortuous, with dilatation and infection of the proximal segment of the urethra. Secondary calculus formation is an ever-present possibility (Rifaat).

Filling defects in the contrast-filled

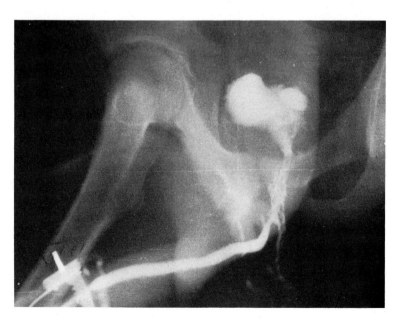

Figure 10–186. *Retrograde urethrocystogram.* **Bilharzial perineal fistula.** (From Hanna, A. A. Z., and Saleh, R.)

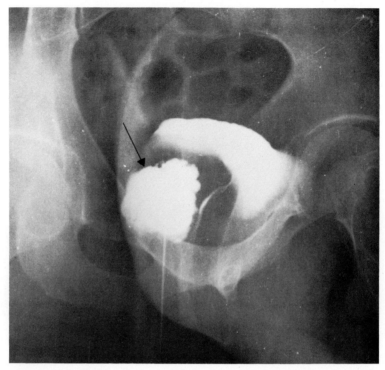

Figure 10–187. Bilharzial prostatic abscess (*arrow*) demonstrated by *transperineal prostatography.* (From Hanna, A. A. Z., and Saleh, R.)

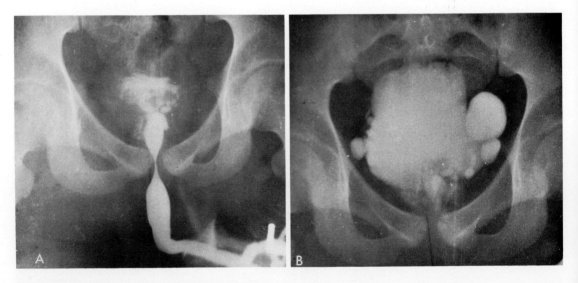

Figure 10–188. Bilharziasis with paracervical papillomata. **A** and **B**, *Retrograde urethrograms.* (From Hanna, A. A. Z., and Saleh, R.)

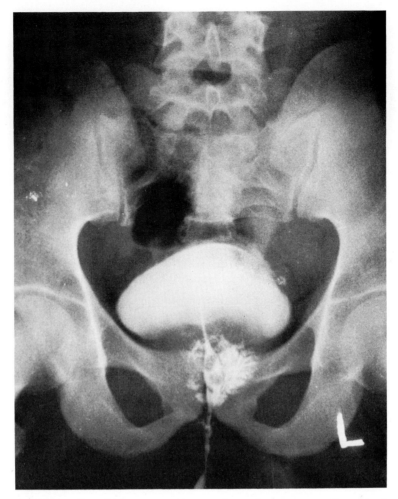

Figure 10–189. **Bilharzial urethritis cystica.** *Retrograde urethrocystogram.* Prostatic ducts are opacified. (From Hanna, A. A. Z., and Saleh, R.)

urethra may be produced by both urethritis cystica and small radiolucent calculi (Figs. 10–188 and 10–189). The lesions of urethritis cystica, lying as they do beneath the mucosa, are never seen completely surrounded by contrast medium and present as filling defects based on the urethral wall. In contrast, small radiolucent calculi lie free in the urethra and are surrounded by contrast medium.

The Prostate

Radiologic evidence of prostatic enlargement and of bladder neck fibrosis may be seen in bilharziasis.

Prostatography (direct injection of contrast medium into the prostatic tissue) may reveal the presence of a prostatic abscess.

The Seminal Vesicle

Seminal vesiculography in bilharziasis reveals dilated seminal vesicles with ill-defined borders, and it may show filling defects due to granulomatous masses. The ejaculatory ducts are patent, and of normal appearance (Fig 10–190). This helps to differentiate enlargement of the prostate due to bilharziasis from malignant enlargement, in which the ejaculatory ducts are stretched, narrowed, or obstructed.

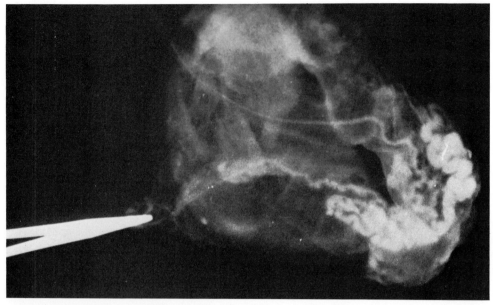

Figure 10–190. Bilharziasis of the seminal vesicles. *Cadaver specimen.* Seminal vesicles outlined by contrast medium. (From Hanna, A. A. Z., and Saleh, R.)

ECHINOCOCCUS CYSTS (RENAL HYDATIDOSIS)

Hydatid disease results from human infestation by two species of the genus *Echinococcus: E. granulosus* and *E. multilocularis.* The disease is highly endemic in sheep- and cattle-raising countries. In the past, most of the cases of hydatidosis in the United States were discovered in immigrants; recent reports, however, indicate an increasing incidence among native-born residents. It is especially common among the Eskimo of Alaska, where the disease is endemic in several areas (Faust and Russell).

Epidemiology of Renal Hydatidosis

The adult tapeworm of *E. granulosus,* the most common species in human hydatidosis, is only 3 to 6 mm long; it inhabits the intestines of dogs and other canines, which constitute the primary hosts in its life cycle. The eggs excreted in the dog's feces are ingested by the intermediate hosts such as human beings, sheep, cattle, and pigs. Dogs are infested by ingesting infected meat, usually mutton or beef, to complete the cycle.

When swallowed by a suitable intermediate host such as a human being, the egg hatches in the duodenum, and the oncosphere migrates through the intestinal wall via the portal system to be lodged in any of several organs, mainly the liver and the lungs. The embryo then begins developing a cystic cavity which may reach a diameter of 1 cm by the fifth month. The covering of the cyst comprises three layers: (1) an outer nonnucleated laminated membrane (ectocyst), (2) an inner layer of germinal membrane (endocyst) that is responsible for the growth of the cyst and from which the brood capsules develop by budding, and (3) an adventitia or pericyst which is contributed by the host (Fig. 10–191). Daughter cysts, which form from the germinal layer of the mother cyst, may remain attached to the endocyst and are encountered outside the cystic cavity only if the cyst ruptures.

Most hydatid cysts in humans are acquired during childhood, possibly because

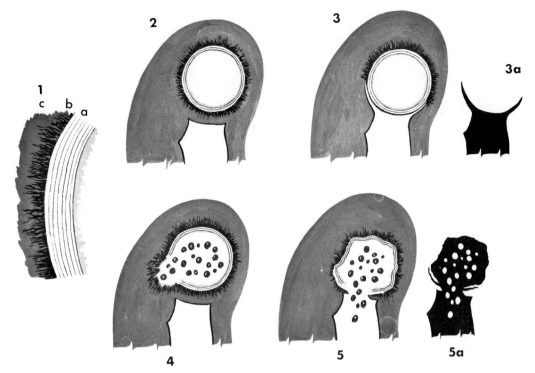

Figure 10–191. Three layers of renal hydatid cyst and its relationship to collecting system. 1, **Endocyst** (a), **ectocyst** (b), and **pericyst** (c) forming three layers. 2, "**Closed**" **cyst** with three membranes intact, overlying major calyx. 3, "**Exposed**" **cyst** with absence of adventitial layer or pericyst; cyst is in close contact with urine. 4 and 5, "**Open cysts**" resulting from rupture and discharge of daughter cysts. (From Kirkland, K.)

of the close contact of children with infected dogs.

Pathogenesis of Genitourinary Infestation in Renal Hydatidosis

The genitourinary system may be involved *primarily* or *secondarily.* Renal hydatidosis comprises 2 per cent to 3 per cent of human cases; it usually is produced during *primary infestation* with the hydatid worms, which reach the kidney via the arterial system.

As illustrated by Kirkland (Fig. 10–191), *secondary infestation* of any part of the genitourinary tract may result from spread of a hydatid cyst located in an adjacent organ or tissue. For instance, the kidney or ureter may be involved by a direct spread from a hepatic, splenic, or retroperitoneal cyst. Rupture of an echinococcus cyst located in the abdomen may result in discharge and

seeding of daughter cysts and scolices in the pelvis with involvement of the retrovesical tissue and organs, such as the prostate gland, vas deferens, and seminal vesicles; these provide new sites for the growth of mature cysts. Vesical irritability, probably the most common symptom of secondary infestation of the genitourinary tract, may be caused by compression of the bladder by a large pelvic cyst. In the kidney, the cyst always originates in the cortex and is invariably subcapsular.

A cyst is considered *closed* if all three layers are intact; when it is no longer protected by the third layer (adventitia or pericyst) or by the lining of the collecting system, it is considered to be an *exposed* cyst. If all three of the layers of the cyst have ruptured, resulting in free communication with the calyces and pelvis, it is described as an *open* or *communicating* cyst (Kirkland).

The renal cyst may grow rapidly, compressing and destroying the kidney, or slowly and insidiously over a period of many years, causing minimal clinical symptoms but eventually resulting in marked distortion of the kidney and loss of renal function. Leakage of the contents of a cyst through incompetent cystic membranes (or layers) or gross rupture of the cyst may produce serious anaphylactic reactions. Some cysts, however, never produce brood capsules, and sometimes the *Echinococcus* is killed by bacterial infection and fibrosis, which may result in calcification of the cyst.

Diagnosis of Renal Hydatidosis

The diagnosis of hydatid disease may be suspected from a history of previous infestation. The passage of grape-like debris in the urine, intermittent dull flank pain, a renal mass with a hydatid thrill, and renal or ureteral colic produced by daughter cysts obstructing the ureter or ureteropelvic juncture are suggestive. Eosinophilia and positive intradermal (Cassoni),

precipitin, complement-fixation, and hemagglutination tests are confirmatory.

ROENTGEN DIAGNOSIS

The Plain Film

The plain film may be of diagnostic help by revealing soft-tissue masses, either calcified or noncalcified, that could represent possible cysts. If calcification is present, daughter cysts may be evident because of a mottled appearance of the calcific distribution or by definite outlining of the various cysts (Figs. 10–192, 10–193, and 10–194).

The Urogram

It is important to remember that echinococcus cysts may be located almost anywhere in the region of the abdomen. They commonly involve organs such as the kidneys, spleen, and liver, but they may occur in other intra-abdominal or retroperitoneal locations, including the pelvis, where they may involve the bladder and genitalia sec-

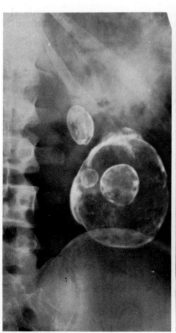 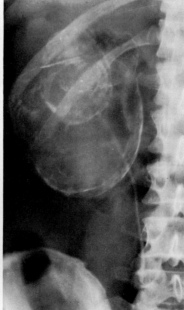

Figure 10–192. *Plain film.* Calcified **echinococcus cyst of left kidney,** showing daughter cysts.
Figure 10–193. *Plain film* with lead catheter in right ureter. **Echinococcus cyst of right kidney** with calcification in walls. Multiple daughter cysts.

Fig. 10–192   **Fig. 10–193**

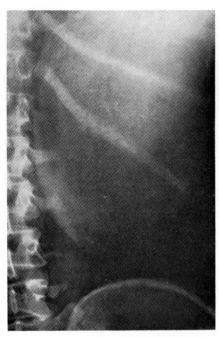

Figure 10–194. Echinococcus cyst of left kidney. *Plain film.* Soft-tissue outline of large cyst with calcific deposits in wall. Some residual barium in transverse colon.

ondarily (Figs. 10–195 and 10–196). In such cases, they may be difficult to distinguish from deep pelvic cysts.

Renal Cysts. The urographic picture of renal hydatidosis may mimic a wide variety of other renal masses or mass-like lesions; and, if possible, they should be differentiated preoperatively because of the hazard of opening the cyst during operation. *Nephrotomography* and *selective renal arteriography* may be of value in making the correct differential diagnosis by demonstrating (1) a thick cyst wall, (2) non-homogeneous radiolucency, as is seen in necrotic tumors, and (3) identification of cysts of extraurinary organs and structures which appear to involve the genitourinary system (Fig 10–197). Baltaxe and Fleming discussed the arteriographic findings in patients with echinococcus cysts and pointed out that in the single patient with a renal lesion studied, the lesion was avascular with a partially calcified rim, and angiography was not sufficient to differentiate it

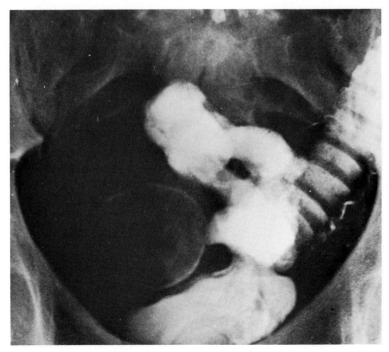

Figure 10–195. *Plain film.* **Genitourinary hydatidosis.** Second infestation of hydatid cyst in bony pelvis, involving vas deferens and lying in close relationship to rectum. (From Kirkland, K.)

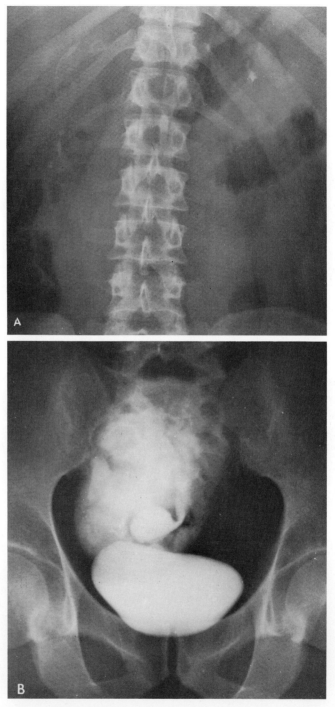

Figure 10–196. *See legend on opposite page.*

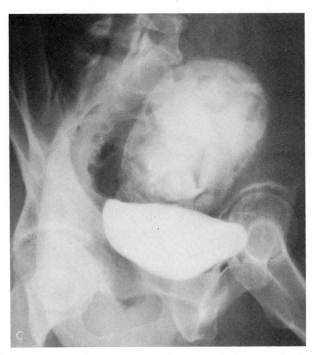

Figure 10–196. Echinococcus cyst of omentum, simulating urachal cyst, and **echinococcus cyst of liver** in man aged 36. Patient complained of large tender mass in lower midportion of abdomen. No residual urine. **A,** *Excretory urogram* demonstrated vaguely outlined ovoid mass extending from symphysis pubis to level of lumbosacral joint (not included in this illustration) and calcified ring in region of liver, which was diagnosed as possible echinococcus cyst. (Needle-puncture aspiration yielded 300 ml clear colorless watery fluid. Microscopy showed only epithelial cells.) **B** and **C,** *Renografin injection, anteroposterior* and *lateral views.* Multiple daughter cysts are outlined. (At operation, freely movable ovoid cyst [12 by 8 cm] was found within omentum; it was attached to dome of bladder by adhesions. Cyst was removed. Pathology: typical cyst with multiple daughter cysts. Microscopy showed typical scolices with hooklets.) (From Constantian, H. M., and Bolduc, R. A.)

from calcified neoplasm They assert, however that angiography helps to determine the extent of the lesion, particularly when more than one cyst is present. If a partially calcified vascular rim is found during the capillary-venous phase, the likelihood that one is dealing with an echinococcus as opposed to carcinoma is increased. They also assert that infected renal abscesses rarely calcify and usually have a thicker and more irregular wall than echinococcus cysts.

Diagnosis is more easily made if the cyst is "open" because its communication with the collecting system then permits direct filling of the cyst with contrast medium (Fig. 10–198). When this is possible, the outlines of daughter cysts (which give the appearance of a cluster of grapes) are pathognomonic. A fluid level, indicating the presence of air, also may be seen oc-

casionally. Surraco has emphasized the "goblet" and "crescent" signs that appear in "closed" or "exposed" cysts (Fig. 10–199); they result from the smooth curvilinear compression of the renal pelvis and spreading and flattening of the calyces. In "exposed" cysts, however, the renal pelvis communicates with the pericystic space (not the cyst itself); thus, contrast medium escapes into the pericystic space, causing an irregular shadow around the cyst (Hanna and Sabry). Compression of a calyx by the cyst produces a crescentic shape that has been described as the sign of the claw (Figs. 10–200 and 10–201).

Diagnostic Needle Puncture

Diagnostic needle puncture of the cyst with direct injection of contrast medium

Text continued on page 949

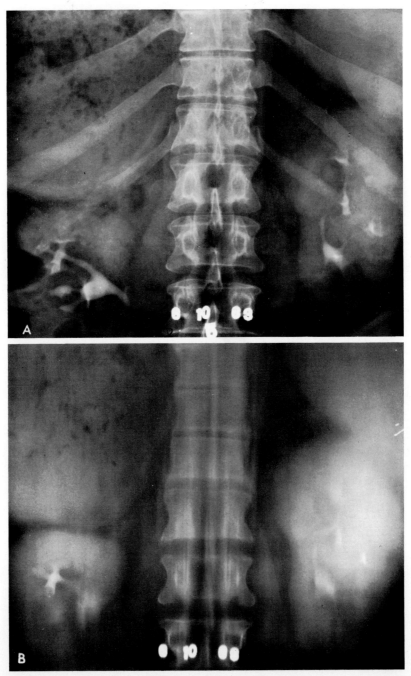

Figure 10–197. Hydatid cyst of liver simulating cyst of kidney. **A,** *Excretory urogram.* Large mass containing a myriad of lucent defects projects over and compresses upper pole of right kidney. This mass was thought to represent renal hydatid cyst. **B,** *Nephrotomogram.* Cyst is shown to be extrarenal, arising from liver. Note increased density and relatively thick wall of hydatid cyst in contrast to simple serous cyst.

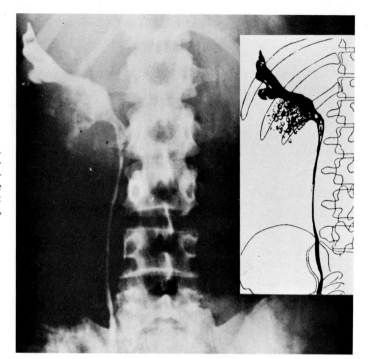

Figure 10–198. *Excretory urogram.* "Open" type renal hydatid cyst in 22-year-old woman. Silent rupture of hydatid cyst in right kidney with discharge of daughter cysts, causing obstruction at ureteropelvic juncture. (From Kirkland, K.)

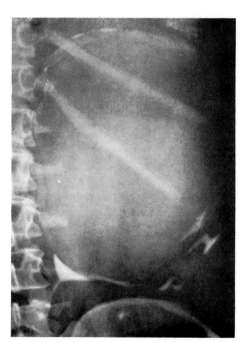

Figure 10–199. Echinococcus cyst of left kidney. *Excretory urogram.* Pelvis and calyces outlined; they are pushed downward and laterally by large "exposed" cyst producing "goblet" or "crescent" sign of Surraco.

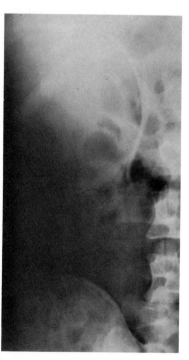

Figure 10–200. *Excretory urogram.* "Exposed" type renal hydatid cyst. Huge uncalcified echinococcus cyst in right kidney, compressing pelvis and calyces. (Arteriography showed mass to be avascular. Nephrectomy performed.) (Courtesy of Dr. F. Shehadeh.)

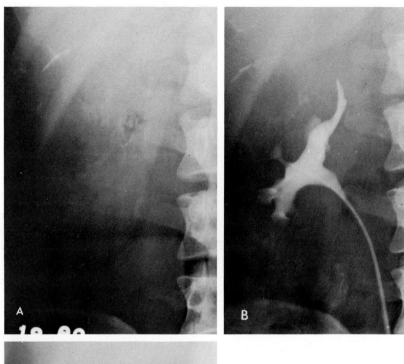

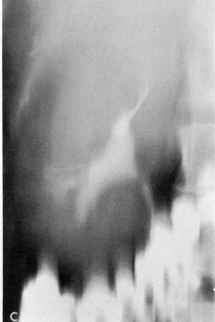

Figure 10-201. "Exposed" type renal hydatid cyst. **A**, *Plain roentgenogram.* Large partially calcified right renal mass. **B**, *Retrograde pyelogram.* Note impression on renal collecting system from cyst. **C**, *Nephrotomogram* confirms cystic characteristics of mass. (Hydatid cyst wall was incised, revealing numerous daughter cysts of various sizes, some of which were collapsed.) (From Henry, J. D., Utz, D. C., Hahn, R. G., Thompson, J. H., Jr., and Stilwell, G. G.)

may provide extremely accurate diagnosis by graphically demonstrating the presence of daughter cysts (see Fig. 10–196). Such a procedure, however, carries a definite risk and must be avoided, because (as mentioned previously under the heading of pathogenesis) the contents of the cyst apparently may be very toxic (Kirkland). If leakage occurs from either spontaneous or surgical rupture of the cyst wall, serious anaphylactic reactions may occur.

REFERENCES

Afifi, M. A.: Roentgenographic Manifestations of Urinary Bilharziasis and Calculus Formations in Egypt, and Intravenous Pyelography. Am. J. Roentgenol. *31*:208–223 (Feb.) 1934.

Al-Ghorab, M. M., El-Badawi, A. A., and Effat, H.: Vesico-ureteral Reflux in Urinary Bilharziasis. A Clinico-radiological Study. Clin. Radiol. *14*:41–47 (Jan.) 1966.

Altemeier, W. A., and Alexander, J. W.: Retroperitoneal Abscess, Arch. Surg. *83*:512–524, 1961.

Altemeier, W. A., Culbertson, W. R., and Fullen, W. D.: Intra-abdominal Sepsis. Adv. Surg. 5:281–333, 1971.

Anhalt, M. A., Cawood, C. D., and Scott, R., Jr.: Xanthogranulomatous Pyelonephritis: A Comprehensive Review With Report of 4 Additional Cases. J. Urol. *105*:10–17 (Jan.) 1971.

Atala, A., and Zaher, M. F.: Bilharzial Calcification of the Renal Capsule: A Case. Report. J. Urol. *101*:125–126 (Feb.) 1969.

Attia, O. W.: Lectures in Pathology. The Scientific Book Centre, Cairo, 1969.

Badr, M. M.: Presentation at the Annual Meeting of the Egyptian Society of Urologists, Cairo, 1972.

Badr, M. M., and Torky, H.: Bilharzial Bladder Neck Obstruction. "A Review." The Medical Journal of Cairo University, Vol. 34, No. 2., 1966.

Badr, M., Safwat, M., Fawzi, R. M., and Zaher, M. F.: Bilharzial Non-obstructive Spindle Shaped Ureter. J. Egypt. Med. Assoc. *39*:213, 1956.

Bailey, R. R., Little, P. J., Rolleston, G. L.: Renal Damage After Acute Pyelonephritis. Br. Med. J. *1*:550–551 (Mar.) 1969.

Baltaxe, H. A., and Fleming, R. J.: The Angiographic Appearance of Hydatid Disease. Radiology *97*:599–604 (Dec.) 1970.

Baron, E., and Arduino, L. T.: Primary Renal Actinomycosis. J. Urol. *62*:410–416 (Oct.) 1949.

Barrie, H. J., Kerr, W. K., and Gale, G. L.: The Incidence and Pathogenesis of Tuberculous Strictures of the Renal Pyelus. J. Urol. *98*:584–589 (Nov.) 1967.

Beachley, M. C., Ranniger, K., and Roth, F. J.: Xanthogranulomatous Pyelonephritis. Am. J. Roentgenol. *121*:500–507 (July) 1974.

Becker, J. A.: Xanthogranulomatous Pyelonephritis: A

Case Report With Angiographic Findings. Acta. Radiol. [Diagn.] *4*:139–144, 1966.

Becker, J. A., Kanter, I. E., and Perl, S.: Rapid Intrarenal Circulation. Am. J. Roentgenol. *109*:167–171 (May) 1970.

Becker, J. A., Weiss, R. M., and Lattimer, J. K.: Renal Tuberculosis: The Role of Nephrotomography and Angiography. J. Urol. *100*:415–419 (Oct.) 1968.

Beeson, P. B.: Urinary Tract Infection and Pyelonephritis. In Black, D. A. K.: Renal Disease. Ed. 2, Philadelphia, F. A. Davis Company, 1967, pp. 382–403.

Beeson, P. B., Rocha, H., and Guze, L. B.: Experimental Pyelonephritis: Influence of Localized Injury in Different Parts of the Kidneys on Susceptibility to Hematogenous Infection. Trans. Assoc. Physicians *70*:120–126, 1957.

Béland, G., and Piette, Y.: Urinary Tract Candidiasis: Report of a Case With Bilateral Ureteral Obstruction. Can. Med. Assoc. J. *108*:472–476 (17 Feb.) 1973.

Bell, E. G., O'Mara, R. E., Henry, C. A., Subramanian, G., McAfee, J. G., and Brown, L. C.: Nonneoplastic Localization of ⁶⁷Ga-Citrate. J. Nucl. Med. *12*:338–339 (June) 1971.

Berquist, T. H., Hattery, R. R., Hartman, G. W., Kelalis, P. P., and DeWeerd, J. H.: Vesicoureteral Reflux in Adults. Am. J. Roentgenol. *125*:314–321 (Oct.) 1975.

Blair, D. C., Carroll, M., Silva, J., and Fekely, F. R.: Localization of Infectious Processes With Gallium Citrate Ga 67. J.A.M.A. *230*:82–85 (Oct.) 1974.

Boijsen, E., Reuter, S. R.: Mesenteric Angiography in Evaluation of Inflammatory and Neoplastic Disease of the Intestine. Radiology *87*:1028–1036 (Dec.) 1966.

Bothe, A. E., and Cristol, D. S.: Cystic Disease of the Upper Urinary Tract: Pyelitis Cystica and Ureteritis Cystica. Am. J. Roentgenol. *48*:787–793 (Dec.) 1942.

Braasch, W. F.: Clinical Data Concerning Chronic Pyelonephritis. J. Urol. *39*:1–25 (Jan.) 1938.

Brown, H. E.: Granulomatous Prostatitis: Its Clinical Significance. J. Urol. *105*:549–551 (Apr.) 1971.

Brownstein, P. K., Mannes, H., and Bogaev, J. H.: Sarcoidosis and Malakoplakia. Urology 6:249–251, (Aug.) 1975.

Bruce, A. W., Awad, S. A., and Challis, T. W.: The Recognition and Treatment of Tuberculous Pyocalyx of the Kidney. J. Urol. *101*:127–131 (Feb.) 1969.

Cameron, D. D., and Azimi, F.: The Value of Excretory Urography in the Diagnosis of Acute Pyelonephritis. J. Urol. *112*:546–549 (Nov.) 1974.

Campbell, M. F.: Perinephric Abscess. Surg. Gynecol. Obstet. *51*:674–682 (Nov.) 1930.

Caplan, L. H., Siegelman, S. S., and Bosniak, M. A.: Angiography in Space-Occupying Lesions of the Kidney. Radiology *88*:14–23 (Jan.) 1967.

Carr, D. T.: The Treatment of Renal Tuberculosis. Med. Clin. North Am. *50*:1137–1139 (July) 1966.

Champion, R. H., and Ackles, R. C.: Eosinophilic Cystitis. J. Urol. *96*:729–732 (Nov.) 1966.

Claridge, M.: Ureteric Obstruction in Tuberculosis. Br. J. Urol. *42*:688–692, 1970.

Clark, R. E., Minagi, H., and Palubinskas, A. J.: Renal Candidiasis. Radiology *101*:567–572 (Dec.) 1971.

Constantian, H. M., and Bolduc, R. A.: Echinococcus

Cyst Simulating Urachal Cyst. J. Urol. 99:755–758 (June) 1968.

Coombs, J. A., Crummy, A. B., and Cossman, F. P.: Angiography in Renal and Pararenal Inflammatory Lesions. Radiology 98:401–403 (Feb.) 1971.

Cotran, R. S.: Experimental Pyelonephritis. In The Kidney. New York, Academic Press., Vol. 2, C. Rouiller and A. F. Muller, Eds., 1969, pp. 269–361.

Crenshaw, J. L.: Renal Tuberculosis With Calcification. J. Urol. 23:515–533 (May) 1930.

Davidson, A. J., and Talner, L. B.: Urographic and Angiographic Abnormalities in Adult-Onset Acute Bacterial Nephritis. Radiology 106:249–256 (Feb.) 1973.

Davies, M., and Keddie, N. C.: Abdominal Actinomycosis. Br. J. Surg. 60:18–22 (Jan.) 1973.

de Navasquez, S.: Experimental Pyelonephritis in the Rabbit Produced by Staphylococcal Infection. J. Pathol. 62:429–436 (July) 1950.

de Navasquez, S.: Further Studies in Experimental Pyelonephritis Produced by Various Bacteria, With Special Reference to Renal Scarring as a Factor in Pathogenesis. J. Pathol. 71:27–32 (Jan.) 1956.

de Nunno, R.: Selective Instrumental Arteriographic Study in the Diagnosis of Renal Tuberculosis. J. Internat. Coll. Surgeons 32:523–529 (Nov.) 1959.

Dimmette, R. M., Sproat, H. F., and Sayegh, E. S.: The Classification of Carcinoma of the Urinary Bladder Associated With Schistosomiasis and Metaplasia. J. Urol. 75:680–686 (Apr.) 1956.

Edwards, C. L., and Hayes, R. L.: Scanning Malignant Neoplasms With Gallium-67. J.A.M.A. 212:1182–1190 (May) 1970.

El-Badawi, A. A.: Bilharzial Polypi of the Urinary Bladder. Br. J. Urol. 38:24–35 (Feb.) 1966.

Elliott, C. B., Johnson, H. W., and Balfour, J. A.: Xanthogranulomatous Pyelonephritis and Perirenal Xanthogranuloma. Br. J. Urol. 40:548–555, 1968.

Emmett, J. L., and Braasch, W. F.: Has Excretory Urography Replaced Retrograde Pyelography in the Diagnosis of Renal Tuberculosis? J. Urol. 40:15–23 (July) 1938.

Emmett, J. L., and McDonald, J. R.: Proliferation of Glands of the Urinary Bladder Simulating Malignant Neoplasm. J. Urol. 48:257–265 (Sept.) 1942.

Emmett, J. L., Alvarez-Jerena. J. J., and McDonald, J. R.: Atrophic Pyelonephritis Versus Congenital Renal Hypoplasia. J.A.M.A. 148:1470–1477 (Apr.) 1952.

Evans, J. A., Meyers, M. A., and Bosniak, M. A.: Acute Renal and Perirenal Infections. Semin. Roentgenol. 6:274–291 (July) 1971.

Faust, E. C., and Russell, P. F.: Craig and Faust's Clinical Parasitology. Ed. 7, Philadelphia, Lea & Febiger, 1964, pp. 553–564.

Faust, E. G., and Russell, P. F.: Echinococcus granulosus. In: Craig and Faust's Clinical Parasitology. Ed. 7, Philadelphia, Lea & Febiger, 1964, pp. 678–688.

Fierke, J., Hartman, G. W., and Hattery, R. R.: Pyeloureteritis Cystica. Presented at the American Roentgen Ray Society Meeting, September, 1975.

Filly, R., Friedland, G. W., Govan, D. E., and Fair, W. R.: Development and Progression of Clubbing and Scarring in Children With Recurrent Urinary Tract Infections. Radiology 113:145–153 (Oct.) 1974.

Forni, A. M., Koss, L. G., and Geller W.: Cytological Study of the Effect of Cyclophosphamide on the Epithelium of the Urinary Bladder in Man. Cancer 17:1348–1355 (Oct.) 1964.

Fratkin, M. J., and Sharpe, A. R.: Nontuberculous Psoas Abscess: Localization Using 67Ga. J. Nucl. Med. 14:499–501 (July) 1973.

Frensilli, F. J., Sacher, E. C., and Keegan, G. T.: Eosinophilic Cystitis: Observations on Etiology. J. Urol. 107:595–596 (Apr.) 1972.

Friedenberg, R. M.: Tuberculosis of the Genitourinary System. Semin. Roentgenol. 6:310–322 (July) 1971.

Friedenberg, R. M., Ney, C., and Stachenfeld, R. A.: Roentgenographic Manifestations of Tuberculosis of Ureter. J. Urol. 99:25–29 (Jan.) 1968.

Frimann-Dahl, J.: Radiological Investigation of Urogenital Tuberculosis. Urol. Internat. 1:396–426, 1955.

Frimann-Dahl, J.: Selective Angiography in Renal Tuberculosis. Acta Radiol. 49:31–41, 1958.

Frimann-Dahl, J.: Angiography in Renal Inflammatory Disease. In Kincaid, O. W.: Renal Angiography. Chicago, Year Book Medical Publishers, Inc., 1966, pp. 230–252.

Fritjofsson, A., and Edsman, G.: Angiography in Renal Tuberculosis. Acta Chir. Scand. 118:60–71, 1959.

Gammill, S., Rabinowitz, J. G., Peace, R., Sorgen, S., Hurwitz, L., and Himmelfarb, E.: New Thoughts Concerning Xanthogranulomatous Pyelonephritis (X-P). Am. J. Roentgenol. 125:154–163 (Sept.) 1975.

Gelfard, M.: Bilharzial Affection of the Ureter. A Study of 110 Consecutive Necropsies Showing Vesical Bilharziasis. Br. Med. J. 1:1228–1230 (26 June) 1948.

Gillies, C. L., and Flocks, R.: Spontaneous Renal and Perirenal Emphysema: Report of a Case in a Diabetic From Escherichia coli Infection. Am. J. Roentgenol. 45:173–174 (Aug.) 1941.

Gingell, J. C., Roylance, J., Davies, E. R., and Penry, J. B.: Xanthogranulomatous Pyelonephritis. Br. J. Radiol. 46:99–109 (Feb.) 1973.

Goldstein, M.: Eosinophilic Cystitis. J. Urol. 106:854–857 (Dec.) 1971.

Gordon, H. L., Rossen, R. D., Hersh, E. M., and Yium, J. J.: Immunologic Aspects of Interstitial Cystitis. J. Urol. 109:228–233 (Feb.) 1973.

Gow, J. G.: Genito-urinary Tuberculosis: A Study of 700 Cases. Lancet 2:261–265 (10 Aug.) 1963.

Gow, J. G.: Renal Calcification in Genito-urinary Tuberculosis. Br. J. Surg. 52:283–288 (Apr.) 1965.

Greene, L. F., and Albers, D. D.: Brucellosis of the Urinary Tract. Mayo Clin. Proc. 25:638–640 (8 Nov.) 1950.

Greene, L. F., Weed, L. A., and Albers, D. D.: Brucellosis of the Urinary Tract. J. Urol. 67:765–772 (May) 1952.

Guindy, A.: Vesico-ureteral Reflux in Bilharzial Affection of the Bladder and Ureter. First International Symposium on Bilharziasis, Ministry of Science and Research, U.A.R., 541, 1962.

Gwinn, J. L., and Barnes, G. R., Jr.: Striated Ureters and Renal Pelvis. Am. J. Roentgenol. 91:666–668 (Mar.) 1964.

Halpern, G. N., Kalies, D. W., Factor, S., and Wein,

A. J.: Malakoplakia Causing Bilateral Ureteropelvic Junction Obstruction. Urology 3:628–631 (May) 1974.

Hanna, A. A. Z.: Urethrographic Aspects in Differential Diagnosis of Bilharzial Bladder Neck Obstruction. Twelfth International Congress of Radiology, Tokyo, Japan, Oct. 6–11, 1969.

Hanna, A. A. Z., and Sabry, Y.: Personal communication to the author.

Hanna, A. A. Z., and Saleh, R.: Radiological Evaluation of Intra-vesical Obstruction. M. D. Thesis, Cairo University.

Harbach, L. B., Burkholder, G. V., and Goodwin, W. E.: Renal Candidiasis: A Cause of Anuria. Br. J. Urol. 42:258–264, 1970.

Hassim, A. M., Carruthers, R. H., and Lucas, C.: Bilharzial Contracted Bladder Treated with Cystoplasty. Br. J. Surg. 55:703–705 (Sept.) 1968.

Henry, J. D., Utz, D. C., Hahn, R. G., Thompson, J. H., Jr., and Stilwell, G. G.: Echinococcal Disease of the Kidney: Report of Case. J. Urol. 96:431–435 (Oct.) 1966.

Heptinstall, R. H.: Limitations of Diagnosis in Chronic Pyelonephritis. In Black, D. A. K.: Renal Disease. Ed. 2. Philadelphia, F. A. Davis Company, 1967, pp. 350–381.

Higasi, T., Nakayama, Y., Murata, A., Nakamura, K., Sugiyama, M., Kawaguchi, T., and Suzuki, S.: Clinical Evaluation of 67 Ga-Citrate Scanning. J. Nucl. Med. 13:196–201 (Mar.) 1972.

Hill, G. S.: Experimental Pyelonephritis: A Microangiographic and Histologic Study of Cervical Vascular Changes. Bull. Johns Hopkins Hosp. 119:79–99, (Aug.) 1966.

Hill, G. S., and Clark, R. L.: A Comparative Angiographic, Microangiographic and Histologic Study of Experimental Pyelonephritis. Invest. Radiol. 7:33–47 (Jan.–Feb.) 1972.

Hinman, F., Jr., and Hutch, J. A.: Atrophic Pyelonephritis From Ureteral Reflux Without Obstructive Signs ("Reflux Pyelonephritis"). J. Urol. 87:230–242 (Mar.) 1962.

Hodson, C. J.: The Radiological Diagnosis of Pyelonephritis: Acute Pyelonephritis. Proc. Roy. Soc. Med. 52:669–672 (Aug.) 1959.

Hodson, C. J.: Radiology of the Kidney. In Black, D. A. K.: Renal Disease. Ed. 2, Philadelphia, F. A. Davis Company, 1967a, pp. 136–169.

Hodson, C. J.: The Radiological Contribution Toward the Diagnosis of Chronic Pyelonephritis. Radiology 88:857–871 (May) 1967b.

Hodson, C. J., and Craven, J. D.: The Radiology of Obstructive Atrophy of the Kidney. Clin. Radiol. 17:305–320 (Oct.) 1966.

Hodson, C. J., and Edwards, D.: Chronic Pyelonephritis and Vesico-ureteric Reflux. Clin. Radiol. 11:219–231 (Oct.) 1960.

Hodson, C. J., Maling, T. M. J., McManamon, P. J., and Lewis, M. G.: The Pathogenesis of Reflux Nephropathy (Chronic Atrophic Pyelonephritis). Br. J. Radiol. Supp. 13: 1–26, 1975.

Hodson, C. J., and Wilson, S.: Natural History of Chronic Pyelonephritis Scarring. Br. Med. J. 2:191–194 (July) 1965.

Hodson, J.: Radiology in Pyelonephritis. Curr. Prob. Radiol. Vol. 2, No. 4 (July–Aug.) 1972.

Holt, R. J., and Newman, R. L.: Urinary Candidiasis After Renal Transplantation. (Letter to the Editor.) Br. Med. J. 2:714–715 (17 June) 1972.

Hopkins, G. B., Hall, R. L., and Mende, C. W.: Gallium–67 Scintigraphy for the Diagnosis and Localization of Perinephric Abscesses. J. Urol. 115: 126–128 (Feb.) 1976.

Hunt, V. C., and Mayo, C. W.: Actinomycosis of the Kidney. Ann. Surg. 93:501–505 (Feb.) 1932.

Hutch, J. A., Hinman, F., Jr., and Miller, E. R.: Reflux as a Cause of Hydronephrosis and Chronic Pyelonephritis. J. Urol. 88:169–175 (Aug.) 1962.

Hutch, J. A., Miller, E. R., and Hinman, F., Jr.: Perpetuation of Infection in Unobstructed Urinary Tracts by Vesicoureteral Reflux. J. Urol. 90:88–91 (July) 1963.

Hutter, A. M., Bauman, A. W., and Frank, I. N.: Cyclophosphamide and Severe Hemorrhagic Cystitis. N.Y. State J. Med. 69:305–309 (15 Jan.) 1969.

Johnson, W. W., and Meadows, D. C.: Urinary-Bladder Fibrosis and Telangiectasia Associated With Long-Term Cyclophosphamide Therapy. N. Engl. J. Med. 284:290–294 (11 Feb.) 1971.

Kamel, M.: Textbook of Urology. First Edition, El-Nasr Modern Bookshop, Cairo, 1962.

Kaplan, G. W., and King, L. R.: Cystitis Cystica in Childhood. J. Urol. 103:657–659 (May) 1970.

Kelalis, P. P., and Greene, L. F.: Carcinoma of the Prostate — or Granulomatous Prostatis? GP 32:86–89, 1965.

Kelalis, P. P., Greene, L. F., and Weed, L. A.: Brucellosis of the Urogenital Tract: A Mimic of Tuberculosis. J. Urol. 88:347–353 (Sept.) 1962.

Kelalis, P. P., Harrison, F. G., Jr., and Utz, D. C.: Allergic Granulomas of the Prostate: Treatment With Steroids. J. Urol. 96:573–577 (Oct.) 1966.

Khafagy, M. M., El-Bolkainy, M. N., and Mansour, M. A.: Carcinoma of the Bilharzial Urinary Bladder. A Study of the Associated Mucosal Lesions in 86 Cases. Cancer 30:150–159 (July) 1972.

Kimmelstiel, P., Kim, O. J., Beres, J. A., and Wellman, K.: Chronic Pyelonephritis. Am. J. Med. 30:589–607 (Apr.) 1961.

King, J. C., Jr., and Rosenbaum, H. D.: Calcification of the Vasa Deferentia in Nondiabetics. Radiology 100:603–606 (Sept.) 1971.

King, M. C., Friedenberg, R. M., and Tena, L. B.: Normal Renal Parenchyma Simulating Tumor Radiology 91:217–222 (Aug.) 1968.

Kirkland, K.: Urological Aspects of Hydatid Disease. Br. J. Urol. 38:241–254, 1966.

Knepshield, J. H., Feller, H. A., and Leb, D. E.: Papillary Necrosis Due to Candida albicans in a Renal Allograft. Arch. Int. Med. 122:441–444 (Nov.) 1968.

Koehler, P. R.: The Roentgen Diagnosis of Renal Inflammatory Masses — Special Emphasis on Angiographic Changes. Radiology 112:257–266 (Aug.) 1974.

Kollins, S. A., Hartman, G. W., Carr, D. T., Segura, J. W., and Hattery, R. R.: Roentgenographic Findings in Urinary Tract Tuberculosis: A 10 Year Review. Am. J. Roentgenol. Radium Ther. Nuc. Med. 121:487–499 (July) 1974.

Kolodny, G. M.: Ureteral Dilatation with Pyuria. J.A.M.A. 197:577–578 (15 Aug.) 1966.

Kumar, B., Coleman, R. E., and Anderson, P. O.: Gallium Citrate Ga 67 Imaging in Patients With Suspected Inflammatory Processes. Arch. Surg. 110:1237–1242 (Oct.) 1975.

Langhammer, H., Gaubitt, G., Grebe, S. F., Hampe, J. F., Haubold, U., Hor, G., Kaul, A., Koeppe, P.,

Koppenhagen, J., Roedler, H. D., and van der Schoot, J. B.: 67 Ga for Tumor Scanning. J. Nucl. Med. *13*:25–30 (Jan.) 1972.

Lapides, J.: Observations on Interstitial Cystitis. Urology 5:610–611 (May) 1975.

Lavender, J. P., Lowe, J., Barker, J. R., Burn, J. I., and Chaudhri, M. A.: Gallium 67 Citrate Scanning in Neoplastic and Inflammatory Lesions. Br. J. Radiol. *44*:361–366 (May) 1971.

Lawrence, H. J., Simone, J., and Aur, R. J. A.: Cyclophosphamide-Induced Hemorrhagic Cystitis in Children With Leukemia. Cancer 36:1572–1576 (Nov.) 1975.

Levin, D. L., Zimmerman, A. L., Ferder, L. F., Shapiro, W. B., Wax, S. H., and Porush, J. G.: Acute Renal Failure Secondary to Ureteral Fungus Ball Obstruction in a Patient With Reversible Deficient Cell-Mediated Immunity. Clin. Nephrol. 9:202–210 (Nov.) 1975.

Lieberthal, F.: Renal Tuberculosis: The Development of the Renal Lesion. Surg. Gynecol. Obstet. 67:26–37 (July) 1938.

Littenberg, R. L., Taketa, R. M., Alazraki, P., Halpern, S. E., and Ashburn, W. L.: Gallium-67 for Localization of Septic Lesions. Ann. Int. Med. 79:403–406 (Sept.) 1973.

Little, P. J., McPherson, D. R., Jr., and de Wardener, H. E.: The Appearance of the Intravenous Pyelogram During and After Acute Pyelonephritis. Lancet *1*:1186–1188 (5 June) 1965.

Loitman, B. S., and Chiat, H.: Ureteritis Cystica and Pyelitis Cystica: A Review of Cases and Roentgenologic Criteria. Radiology 68:345–351 (Mar.) 1957.

Love, L., Baker, D., and Ramsey, R.: Gas Producing Perinephric Abscess. Am. J. Roentgenol. *119*:783–792 (Dec.) 1973.

Makar, N.: Urological Aspects of Bilharziasis in Egypt. Cairo, Société Oriéntale de Publicite, 1955.

Malek, R. S., Greene, L. F., DeWeerd, J. H., and Farrow, G. M.: Xanthogranulomatous Pyelonephritis. Br. J. Urol. *44*:296–308, 1972.

Mathé, C. P. Diagnosis and Treatment of Perinephric Abscess: Renal Fixation: New Roentgenographic Diagnostic Sign. Am. J. Surg. 38:35–49, 1937.

May, P., Hohenfellner, R., König, E., and König, K.: Diagnostik und Therapie der Prostatatuberkulose. Urol. Internat. *21*:329–337, 1966.

Meares, E. M., Jr.: Bacterial Prostatitis Vs. "Prostatosis": A Clinical and Bacteriological Study. J.A.M.A. *224*:1372–1375 (4 June) 1973.

Mellins, H. Z.: Chronic Pyelonephritis and Renal Medullary Necrosis. Semin. Roentgenol. 6:292–309, (July) 1971.

Miller, O. S., and Finck, F. M.: Malakoplakia of the Kidney: The Great Impersonator. J. Urol. 93:407, 1965.

Mokhless, A. S.: Bilharzial Seminal Vesiculitis: A Radiological, Anatomical and Pathological Study. Alexandria Medical Journal 3:285–300 (May) 1962.

Moonen, W. A.: Stricture of the Ureter and Contracture of the Bladder and Bladder Neck Due to Tuberculosis: Their Diagnosis and Treatment. J. Urol. 80:218–228 (Oct.) 1958.

Mostofi, F. K.: Potentialities of Bladder Epithelium. J. Urol. 71:705–714 (June) 1954.

Murphy, J. J., and Koehler, F. P.: Reevaluation of Modern Antibacterial Agents Used for Perirenal Abscess. J.A.M.A. *171*:1287–1291 (Nov.) 1959.

Noyes, W. E., and Palubinskas, A. J.: Xanthogranulomatous Pyelonephritis. J. Urol. *101*:132–136 (Feb.) 1969.

Obrant, O.: Perirenal Abscess. Acta. Chir. Scand. 97:338–353, 1949.

Olsson, O.: Die Kontrastmittel im klinischen Gebrauch. *In* Encylclopedia of Medical Radiology. III. Roentgen Diagnostic Procedures. Berlin, Springer-Verlag, 1967, pp. 583–599.

Olsson, T.: Angiography in Actinomycosis of the Abdomen: Report of 2 Cases. Am. J. Roentgenol. *122*:278–280 (Oct.) 1974.

Overbeck, L., and Keller, L.: Uber den Wert der Menstrualblutuntersuchung bei Frauen mit Nierentuberkulose. Zentralbl. Gynak. 88:1105–1116, 1966.

Palmiero, C., Ming, S. C., Frank, E., and Fine, J.: The Role of the Sympathetic Nervous System in the Generalized Shwartzman Reaction. J. Exp. Med. *115*:609–612, 1962.

Palubinskas, A. J.: Eosinophilic Cystitis: Case Report of Eosinophilic Infiltration of the Urinary Bladder. Radiology 75:589–591(Oct.) 1960.

Piper, J. V., Stoner, B. A., Mitra, S. K., and Talerman, A.: Ileo-vesical Fistula Associated With Pelvic Actinomycosis. Br. J. Clin. Pract. 23:341–343 (Aug.) 1969.

Pollack, H. M., Goldberg, B. B., Morales, J. O., and Bogash, M.: A Systematized Approach to the Differential Diagnosis of Renal Masses. Radiology *113*:653–659 (Dec.) 1974.

Rabinowitz, J. G., Kinkhabwala, M. N., Robinson, T., Spyropoulos, E., and Becker, J. A.: Acute Renal Carbuncle. Am. J. Roentgenol. *116*:740–748 (Dec.) 1972.

Ragheb, M.: The Radiological Manifestation in Bilharziasis. Br. J. Radiol. *12*:21–27 (Jan.) 1939.

Redewill, F. H.: Malakoplakia of the Urinary Bladder and Generalized Sarcoidosis: Striking Similarity of Their Pathology, Etiology, Gross Appearance and Methods of Treatment. J. Urol. 49:401–407 (Mar.) 1943.

Rees, R. W. M., and Hollands, F. G.: The Ureter in Renal Tuberculosis. Br. J. Urol. 42:693–696, 1970.

Riddle, P. R.: Urinary Tuberculosis. Postgrad. Med. J. 47:718–722 (Nov.) 1971.

Rifaat, A. A.: Principles and Practice of Surgery, Vol. 11. Anglo-Egyptian Bookshop, Cairo, 1961.

Rolleston, G. L., Maling, T. M. J., and Hodson, C. J.: Intrarenal Reflux and the Scarred Kidney. Arch. Dis. Child. 49:531–539, 1974.

Ross, J. C.: Calcification in Genito-urinary Tuberculosis. Br. J. Urol. 42:656–660, 1970.

Ross, J. C., Gow, J. G., and St. Hill, C. A.: Tuberculous Epididymitis: A Review of 170 Patients. Br. J. Surg. 48:663–666 (May) 1961.

Roylance, J., Penry, B., Davies, E. R., and Roberts, M.: Radiology in the Management of Urinary Tract Tuberculosis. Br. J. Urol., 42:679–687, 1970.

Rubin, L., and Pincus, M. B.: Eosinophilic Cystitis: The Relationship of Allergy in the Urinary Tract to Eosinophilic Cystitis and the Patho-physiology of Eosinophilia. J. Urol. *112*:457–460 (Oct.) 1974.

Safwat, M.: The Lower Part of Bilharzial Ureter, A Transvesical Approach for Its Management. J. Egypt. Med. Assoc. 44:217, 1961.

Salvatierra, O., Buckley, W. B., and Morrow, J. W.: Perinephric Abscess: A Report of 71 Cases. J. Urol. 98:296–302 (Sept.) 1967.

Scheinin, T. M., and Kontturi, M.: Incidence and Fact of Renal Tuberculosis in Patients with Bone and Joint Tuberculosis. Ann. chir. et gynaec. Finnae 55:36–39, 1966.

Schneiderman, C., and Simon, M. A.: Malacoplakia of the Urinary Tract. J. Urol. 100:694–698 (Nov.), 1968.

Schofield, P. F., Staff, W. G., and Moore, T.: Ureteral Involvement in Regional Ileitis (Crohn's Disease). J. Urol. 99:412–416 (Apr.) 1968.

Schönebeck, J., and Winblad, B.: Primary Renal *Candida* Infection. Scand. J. Urol. Nephrol. 5:281–284, 1971.

Shopfner, C. E.: Nonobstructive Hydronephrosis and Hydrometer. Am. J. Roentgenol. 98:172–180 (Sept.) 1966.

Shopfner, C. E.: Urinary Tract Pathology With Sepsis. Am. J. Roentgenol. 108:632–640 (Mar.) 1970.

Silk, M. R.: Bladder Antibodies in Interstitial Cystitis. J. Urol. 103:307–309 (Mar.) 1970.

Silver, T. M., Kass, E. J., Thornbury, J. R., Konnak, J. W., and Wolfman, M. G.: The Radiological Spectrum of Acute Pyelonephritis in Adults and Adolescents. Radiology 118:65–71 (Jan.) 1976.

Smith, B. H.: Malacoplakia of the Urinary Tract: A Study of Twenty-four Cases. Am. J. Clin. Pathol. 43:409–417 (May) 1965.

Stadalnik, R. C., and Dublin, A. B.: Emphysematous Pyelonephritis. South. Med. J. 67:1425–1426 (Dec.) 1974.

Steyn, J. H., and Logie, N. J.: Coincident Tuberculous Perinephric Abscess and Carcinoma of the Kidney. Br. J. Urol. 38:7–8 (Feb.) 1966.

Stirling, C., and Ash, J. E.: Chronic Proliferative Lesions of the Urinary Tract. J. Urol. 45:342–360 (Mar.) 1941.

Surraco, L. A.: Renal Hydatidosis. Am. J. Surg. 44:581–586 (June) 1939.

Sutherland, A. M: Genital Tuberculosis in Women. Am. J. Obstet. Gynecol. 79:486–497 (Mar.) 1960.

Teasley, G. H.: Cystitis Emphysematosa: Case Report With a Review of Literature. J. Urol. 62:48–51 (July) 1949.

Terner, J. Y., and Lattes, R.: Malakoplakia of Colon and Retroperitoneum: Report of a Case With a Histochemical Study of the Michaelis-Gutmann Inclusion Bodies. Am. J. Clin. Pathol. 44:20–31 (July) 1965.

Thorley, J. D., Jones, S. R., and Sanford, J. P.: Perinephric Abscess. Medicine 53:441–451 (Nov.) 1974.

Timmons, J. W., and Perlmutter, A. D.: Renal Abscess: A Changing Concept. J. Urol. 115(3):299–301 (Mar.) 1976.

Trueta, J., Barclay, A. F., Daniel, P. M., Franklin, K. J., and Prichard, M. M. L.: Studies of the Renal Circulation. Springfield, Ill., Charles C Thomas, 1947, pp. 103–110.

Turner, R. W., Grigsby, T. H., Enright, J. R., Chance, H. L., Frazier, T. C., Womack, C. T., and Lange, E. K.: Anuria Secondary to Mechanical Obstruction Caused by a *Candida* Fungus Ball. J. Urol. 109:938–940 (June) 1973.

Uehling, D. T., and King, L. R.: Secretory Immuno-globulin — An Excretion in Cystitis Cystica. Urology 1:305–306 (Apr.) 1973.

Uehling, D. T., and Steihm, E. R.: Elevated Urinary Secretory IgA in Children With Urinary Tract Infection. Pediatrics 47:40–46 (Jan.) 1971.

Vermooten, V.: Bilharziasis of the Ureter and its Pathognomonic Roentgenographic Appearance. J. Urol. 38:430–441 (Nov.) 1937.

Vinik, M., Freed, T. A., Smellie, W. A. B., and Weidner, W.: Xanthogranulomatous Pyelonephritis: Angiographic Considerations. Radiology 92:537–540 (Mar.) 1969.

von Brunn, A.: Ueber drüsenähnliche Bildungen in der Schleimhaut des Nierenbeckens des Ureters und der Harnblase beim Menschen. Arch. f. mikr. Anat. 41:294–302, 1893.

Wallack, H. I., Lome, L. G., and Presman, D.: Management of Interstitial Cystitis With Ileocecocystoplasty. Urology 5:51–55 (Jan.) 1975.

Wechsler, H., Westfall, M., and Lattimer, J. K.: The Earliest Signs and Symptoms in 127 Male Patients With Genitourinary Tuberculosis. J. Urol. 83:801–803 (June) 1960.

Weese, W. C., and Smith, I. M.: A Study of 57 Cases of Actinomycosis Over a 36 Year Period. Arch. Intern. Med. 135:1562–1568 (Dec.) 1975.

Wenzl, J. E., Greene, L. F., and Harris, L. E.: Eosinophilic Cystitis. J. Pediat. 64:746–749 (May) 1964.

Yalla, S. V., Ivker, M., Burros, H. M., and Dorey, F.: Cystitis Glandularis With Perivesical Lipomatosis. Urology 5:383–386 (Mar.) 1975.

Young, S. W., Khalid, K. H., Farid, Z., and Mahmoud, A. H.: Urinary-Tract Lesions of *Schistosoma haematobium* With Detailed Radiographic Consideration of the Ureter. Radiology 111:81–84 (Apr.) 1974.

Zaher, M. F., Badr., M. M., and Fawzy, R. M.: Bilharzial Urinary Fistula With Report on 50 Cases. J. Egypt. Med. Assoc. 41:412, 1959.

Zweifach, B. W., Lowenstein, B. E., and Chambers, R.: Responses of Blood Capillaries to Acute Hemorrhage in the Rat. Am. J. Physiol. 142:80–93 (Aug.) 1944.

Additional Reading

Al-Ghorab, M. M.: Radiological Manifestation of Genitourinary Bilharziasis. Clin. Radiol. 19:100–111 (Jan.) 1968.

Al-Ghorab, M. M.: Presentation at the Annual Meeting of the Egyptian Society of Urologists, Cairo, 1973.

Hanna, A. A. Z.: A Radiological Study of the Posterior Urethra. Kasr-El Aini Journal of Surgery 10:81–102 (July) 1961.

Hanna, A. A. Z.: The Radiology of the Male Genital Schistosomiasis. Radiology, Vol. 1. (Proceedings of the XIII International Radiology Congress, Madrid, 1 73).

Knutsson, M.: Presentation at the Annual Meeting of the Egyptian Society of Urologists, Cairo, 1972.

Koraitim, M.: A Triple Mechanism for the Production of Bilharzial Bladder Neck Obstruction. J. Urol. 109:393–396 (Mar.) 1973.

Phillips, J. F., Cockrill, H., Jorge, E., and Steiner R.: Radiographic Evaluation for Patients With Schistosomiasis. Radiology 114:31–37 (Jan.) 1975.

Ragab, M. and Hanna, A. A. Z.: A Textbook of Prac-

tical Radiology. Published by the Renaissance
Bookshop, Cairo, 1961.

Safwat, M., El-Sheikh, A., and Hanna, A. A. Z.: Renal
Tuberculosis in Egypt. The Egyptian Journal of
Radiology and Nuclear Medicine *11*:65–78 (Dec.)
1971.

Safwat, M., and Hanna, A. A. Z.: The Child With Difficult Micturition. Kasr-El-Aini Journal of Surgery
10:81–102 (July) 1969.

Saleh, R. W., and Hanna, A. A. Z.: Radiological Evaluation of Infra-vesical Obstruction. M.D. Thesis,
Cairo University, 1975.

Torky, H., Badr, M. M., and Safwat, M.: Place and
Results of Internal Urethrotomy in Treatment of
Anterior Urethral Strictures in the Male. Medical
Journal of Cairo University, Vol. 4, No. 3, p. 39–
46.

URINARY STASIS: THE OBSTRUCTIVE UROPATHIES, ATONY, VESICOURETERAL REFLUX, AND NEUROMUSCULAR DYSFUNCTION OF THE URINARY TRACT

TERMINOLOGY

The nomenclature of upper urinary tract dilatation is confusing. The terms hydronephrosis and hydroureter have customarily been used to describe enlargement of the renal collecting system and the ureter, but they are inaccurate. *Caliectasis*, *pyelectasis*, and *ureterectasis* are more precise words and can be used in combinations such as *pyelocaliectasis* and *ureteropyelectasis* when the dilatation involves associated anatomic structures.

CLASSIFICATION OF STASIS

Obstructive and Nonobstructive Varieties of Stasis

There are two varieties of urinary stasis: *obstructive* and *nonobstructive*. The former is more common, and the obstructive lesion is usually apparent on urographic investigation. Causes of nonobstructive urinary stasis are not as obvious and may be inflammatory, neurogenic, or congenital.

PYELECTASIS (HYDRONEPHROSIS)

Pathophysiologic Changes in the Kidney

The primary effect of the increased pressure of urine in hydronephrosis is parenchymal atrophy. This results from (1) ischemia secondary to compression of the interlobar and arcuate arteries (Figs. 11–1 and 11–2) (Hinman; Widén) and (2) direct parenchymal damage from pressure. Some relief from the increased intrarenal pressure occurs with pyelovenous and pyelolym-

955

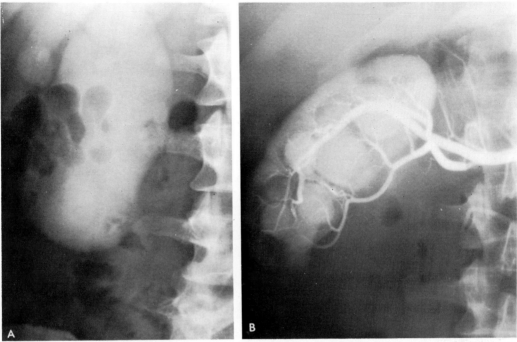

Figure 11–1. Obstruction at ureteropelvic juncture and marked pyelectasis. **A,** *Excretory urogram.* Large distended renal pelvis. Some circular dilated calyces may be seen overlying lateral margin of pelvis near upper pole. **B,** *Selective renal arteriogram.* Marked displacement of branches of renal arteries around dilated calyces. Thinning of renal cortex. (Courtesy of Dr. T. R. Montgomery and Dr. J. H. Gilbaugh.)

phatic backflow of urine. The significance of the phenomenon is measured in terms of the extent of parenchymal damage rather than the degree of pyelocaliectasis. Whereas emphasis has previously been on the degree of pyelocaliectasis, it has now shifted to the degree of atrophy of the renal cortex (Hodson and Craven).

Roentgen Findings in Pyelectasis

As has been mentioned previously (see Chapter 8, "The Normal Urogram"), it is difficult or impossible to distinguish a congenitally large renal pelvis from early pyelectasis. Comparison with the opposite (normal) kidney may supply a reasonable answer because of the tendency to symmetry of the two kidneys (Figs. 11–3, 11–4, and 11–5). In the absence of a normal contralateral kidney, comparison with an earlier urogram will be helpful.

Changes in the Calyces, Renal Papillae, and Renal Pyramids

The first observable radiologic signs of obstructive back pressure occur in the calyces. To appraise early changes accurately, it is important that the variations in appearance of normal calyces be understood (see Chapter 8). The shape of a calyx depends on the contour of the renal papilla. A narrow, pointed papilla presents a narrow, deep, conical calyx; a large, broad, fleshy papilla presents a widely cupped calyx; other papillae may present a sessile, almost flat, contour. In general, the configuration of the normal calyx is that of a "Y." Progressive papillary atrophy and flattening allow more contrast medium to collect at the base of the papilla, finally resulting in a definite clubbing of the calyx. As the process continues, the papilla no longer projects into the calyx but becomes flat and, later, concave; also, the walls of the calyx separate and become widened (Figs.

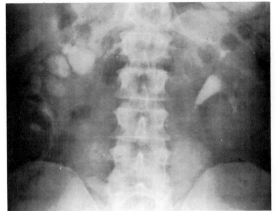

A

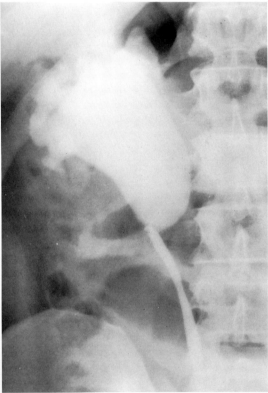

B

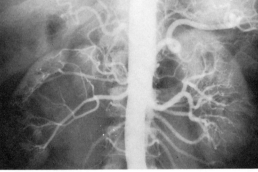

C

Figure 11–2.   Arteriographic demonstration of **displacement and compression of interlobar vessels in hydro-nephrosis** (ureteropelvic juncture obstruction). **A**, *Excretory urogram. Right*—dilatation of calyces; pelvis is not visualized. *Left*—normal. **B**, *Right retrograde pyelogram.* **Marked dilatation of pelvis and calyces.** (At operation, marked narrowing of short segment of ureter adjacent to ureteropelvic juncture found to be cause of obstruction.) **C**, *Midstream arteriogram.* **Two arteries serve right kidney.** Note displacement and reduction in number of arterial branches stretched around dilated calyces and the nephrographic demonstration of thinning of the renal parenchyma. Compare with appearance of normal left kidney. (Courtesy of Dr. T. R. Montgomery and Dr. J. H. Gilbaugh.)

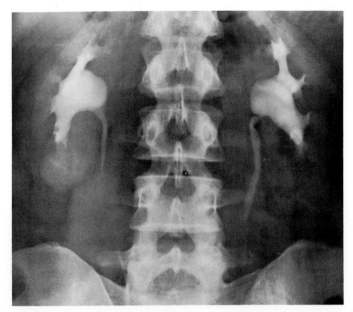

Figure 11–3. *Excretory urogram.* **Minimal bilateral pyelectasis.** Calyces are normal. Difficult to be sure if ureteropelvic junctures are pathologic or variations of normal, but left is not funnel-shaped as is right. Both give impression that retrograde pyelograms might demonstrate greater degree of pyelectasis.

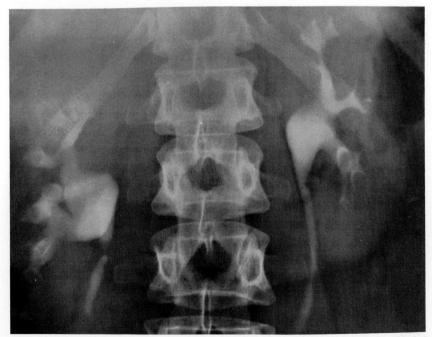

Figure 11–4. *Excretory urogram.* **Mild dilatation of right renal pelvis,** typical of so-called flabby type of pelvis. Ureter not inserted in most dependent position. Compare with left kidney, which is normal.

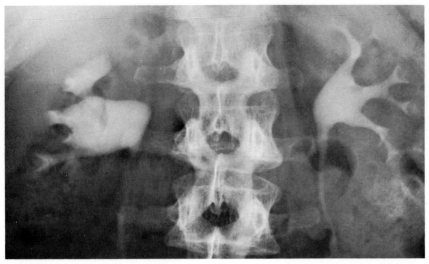

Figure 11–5. *Excretory urogram.* **Minimal pyelectasis on right.** Comparison with left kidney suggests pathologic rather than large normal pelvis.

11–6, 11–7, and 11–8). In the majority of cases, this latter state represents essentially complete atrophy of the renal papilla. Urographically, this lesion simulates renal papillary necrosis after the papilla has separated and been passed. The differential point is that in the case of obstruction all calyces are more or less evenly involved, whereas in papillary necrosis the changes are spotty and uneven with some calyces being involved and others not.

Renal Papillae

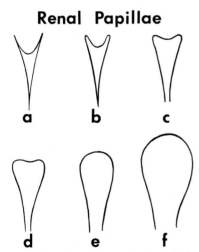

Figure 11–6. Papillary and calyceal changes in obstructive atrophy from normal (*a*) to clubbed (*f*). See text for explanation. (From Hodson, C. J., and Craven, J. D.)

Occasional diagnostic errors are possible if one assumes that a papilla is atrophied just because the calyx is clubbed and dilated. This situation may arise in the case of a rather markedly dilated calyx filled with dense contrast medium that has completely obscured the papilla. Careful radiologic technique with meticulous search for evidence of a papilla in the early film before the contrast medium has become too dense may keep such errors to a minimum (Fig. 11–9).

The process of atrophy is not limited to the renal papillae; rather, it proceeds throughout the entire renal substance. Although the obstructed kidney may appear enlarged, unchanged, or reduced in size, the end result is nearly always some reduction in size and dimensions of the renal cortex (hydronephrotic atrophy) (Fig. 11–10). It should be emphasized that similar parenchymal atrophy also may occur as a result of short intervals of obstruction such as are produced by obstruction from a ureteral stone. In some of these cases, for some unexplained reason, the papilla apparently returns to normal contour despite some degree of definite generalized parenchymal atrophy with decrease in renal size. It seems logical that, in some cases, unexplained renal atrophy that in the past has

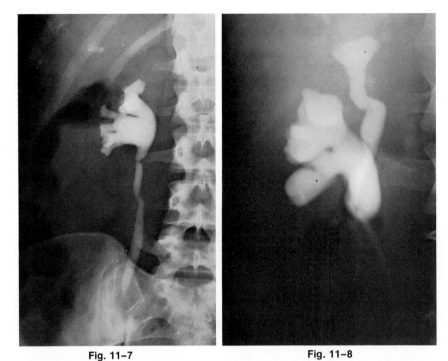

Fig. 11–7   Fig. 11–8

Figure 11–7.   *Right retrograde pyelogram.* **Clubbing of all calyces with associated mild pyelectasis** graded 1. Difficult to say whether pathologic or only result of overdistention.

Figure 11–8.   *Right retrograde pyelogram.* **More advanced clubbing of minor calyces, with broadening of major calyces, in bifid type of pelvis.** Dilatation of pelvis graded 1.

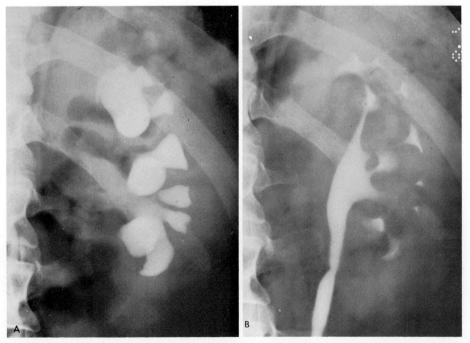

Figure 11–9.   **Obstructive pelviocalyceal dilatation mimicking atrophy.** (Left ureter obstructed from retroperitoneal fibrosis.) **A,** *Preoperative excretory urogram.* Calyceal dilatation and apparent papillary atrophy. **B,** *Excretory urogram* after surgical relief of obstruction. Papillae appear nearly normal once calyceal dilatation has subsided. (From Hodson, C. J., and Craven, J. D.)

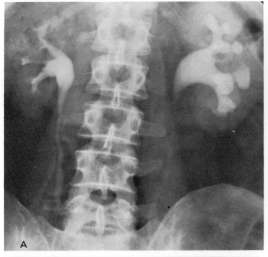
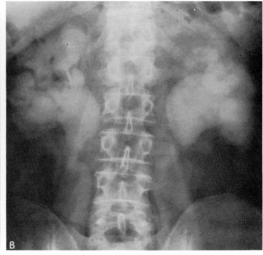
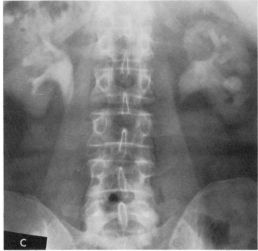

Figure 11-10. Hydronephrotic atrophy of kidney secondary to long-standing urethral stricture with recurring periods of obstruction and vesical distention. **A**, *Excretory urogram*, 1957. **Moderate left pyelocaliectasis**, but left kidney is as large as or larger than right. **B**, *Excretory urogram*, August 1966. Bladder had been distended (6,200 ml residual) for several months because stricture had been neglected. **Advanced bilateral hydronephrosis and hydroureter.** (Stricture dilated and retention relieved.) **C**, *Excretory urogram*, 3 months later. **Minimal left pyelocaliectasis** persists, but there has been reduction in size of kidney—**parenchymal atrophy.**

been attributed to congenital hypoplasia may be the end result of asymptomatic previous episodes of temporary obstruction. It is usually possible to distinguish obstructive parenchymal atrophy from the inflammatory variety (pyelonephritis), because the former tends to be even and symmetrical whereas the latter tends to be focal and spotty. In estimating the degree of renal atrophy, the basis of comparison is usually the "normal" contralateral kidney. This may provide a possible source of error, however; if renal damage is of long standing and the kidney has relatively poor function, compensatory hypertrophy of the normal contralateral kidney may have increased its size.

Changes in the Renal Pelvis

The problem of distinguishing between a large normal renal pelvis and an early pyelectasis has already been discussed (see Figures 11-3, 11-4, and 11-5). Usually, dilatation of the pelvis and calyces proceeds at a fairly uniform rate. In some cases, however, this progression is unequal, and it is not uncommon to see substantial degrees of pyelectasis with entirely normal calyces (Figs. 11-11, 11-12, and 11-13) or significant caliectasis with little or no pyelectasis (Figs. 11-14, 11-15, and 11-16). It has been pointed out that obstruction near the renal pelvis predisposes to dilatation of the pelvis, whereas more

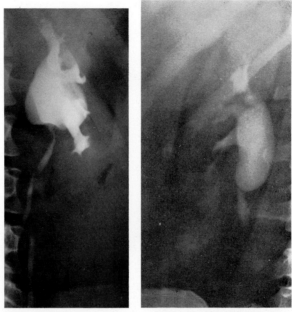

Fig. 11-11   **Fig. 11-12**

Figure 11-11.   *Left retrograde pyelogram.* **Pyelectasis with almost no dilatation of calyces.** Abnormal uretero-pelvic juncture. Ureter is not inserted in most dependent position. (Anomalous vessels found at operation, one in upper and one in lower pole, and angulation of ureter at ureteropelvic juncture.)

Figure 11-12.   *Excretory urogram.* **Extrarenal, elongated type of pelvis, with pyelectasis.** Abnormal uretero-pelvic juncture.

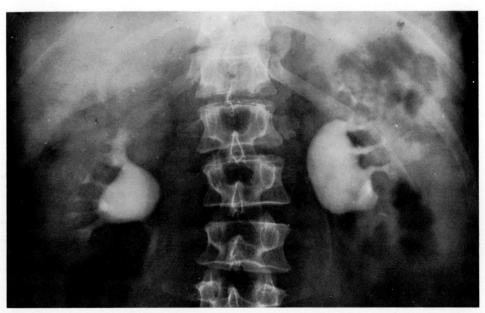

Figure 11-13.   *Excretory urogram.* **Bilateral extrarenal pelves with dilatation, grade 2; no caliectasis.** No surgical exploration.

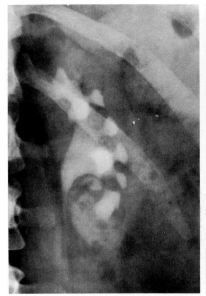

Fig. 11–14

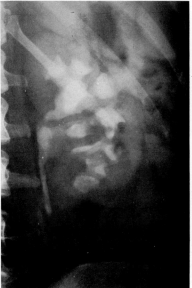

Fig. 11–15

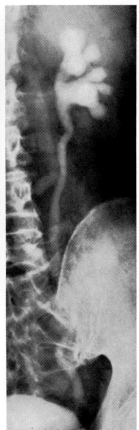

Fig. 11–16

Figure 11–14. *Excretory urogram.* Calyces dilated, grade 1; no pyelectasis.

Figure 11–15. *Excretory urogram.* **Moderate caliectasis with minimal pyelectasis.** Note marked **cortical damage** with **irregular scarring and thinning** of renal parenchyma, resulting from infection or obstruction or both.

Figure 11–16. *Excretory urogram.* **Stricture of terminal portion of left ureter, producing caliectasis and ureterectasis, but minimal pyelectasis.**

distal obstruction produces more dilatation of the calyces than of the pelves. The consistency of this observation, however, is questionable (Figs. 11–17 and 11–18). It is also apparent that an extrarenal type of pelvis dilates more easily than does the intrarenal variety, which is supported and contained within a more rigid and confined space (see Figures 11–11, 11–12, and 11–13). Pyelectasis in the presence of normal calyces may be secondary to a neuromuscular conduction defect rather than to an obstructive lesion. Although this situation may exist on a chronic basis without progressive deterioration, the hazard of infection associated with urinary stasis is a constant concern.

ADVANCED DEGREES OF PYELOCALIECTASIS

In advanced cases of pyelocaliectasis, dramatic urograms may be obtained. Huge, round, dilated calyces may be all that are visualized in an excretory urogram, because there may not be sufficient function to enable one to visualize the large hydronephrotic pelvis (Fig. 11–19). In such a case the pelvis may be visualized only if a 2- to 6-hour delayed film is taken.

The pelvis may become so large that by its own weight the kidney descends and rotates on the anteroposterior axis, thereby accentuating the angle at the ureteropelvic juncture and increasing the degree of obstruction. In far-advanced cases, a huge dilated sac may be all that remains of the kidney and pelvis. Occasionally, the wall of a hydronephrotic sac is calcified, or the interior surface of the sac is covered with an exudate that contains sufficient calcium to cast a shadow (Figs. 11–20 and 11–21). Crescentic collections of contrast material in the renal parenchyma overlying nonopacified dilated calyces are occasionally ob-

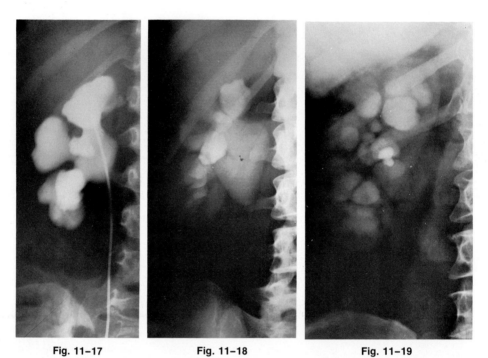

Fig. 11–17   **Fig. 11–18**   **Fig. 11–19**

Figure 11–17. *Right retrograde pyelogram.* Caliectasis, grade 3, and little if any pyelectasis. At operation, ureter was found to be in a nondependent position. A Foley Y-V ureteropelvioplasty was done.

Figure 11–18. *Excretory urogram.* Caliectasis, grade 2, with minimal pyelectasis. At operation **congenital stricture of upper third of ureter** was found.

Figure 11–19. *Excretory urogram.* **Right hydronephrosis with advanced dilatation of calyces.** Not enough medium was excreted to outline pelvis adequately. At operation, anomalous vessels obstructing ureteropelvic juncture were found.

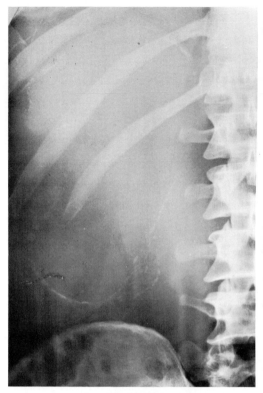 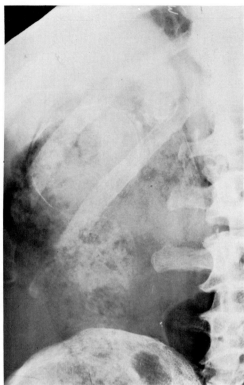

Fig. 11–20   Fig. 11–21

Figure 11–20. *Excretory urogram.* **Advanced pyelectasis on right with no renal function.** Hydronephrotic sac outlined with thin curvilinear shadow of calcium. (Pathologic assessment of nephrectomy specimen showed the pelvis extensively involved with **leukoplakia, containing many focal areas of calcification.**)

Figure 11–21. *Excretory urogram.* **Huge nonfunctioning hydronephrotic right kidney.** Hydronephrotic sac lined with inflammatory exudate, with calcification.

served in cases of severe hydronephrosis (Fig. 11–22). This abnormality, which is termed the crescent sign of hydronephrosis, is detectable during the early phases of excretory urography and then gradually disappears as the calyces and pelvis are opacified. It is attributed to the accumulation of contrast material in collecting tubules that have been flattened and displaced by the hydronephrotic calyces so that they lie parallel to the renal convexity and close to its surface (LeVine and associates).

In advanced hydronephrosis, in which little or no function remains, diagnosis by excretory urography may be impossible even with the use of infusion type excretory urography and delayed films. Angula-

tion of the ureteropelvic juncture from the voluminous pelvis may prevent passage of a ureteral catheter and so preclude retrograde pyelography. In such cases the lesion may easily be confused with tumor (Figs. 11–23 through 11–28).

Blood Clots and Fluid Level

Unusual and bizarre urograms occasionally are encountered in cases of hydronephrosis. Evidence of a fluid level in a large hydronephrotic kidney indicates that air or gas is present (Fig. 11–29). Bleeding is not uncommon in hydronephrosis, and resultant blood clots may present as perplexing filling defects suggesting epithelial cancer (Fig. 11–30).

Text continued on page 969

crescent sign

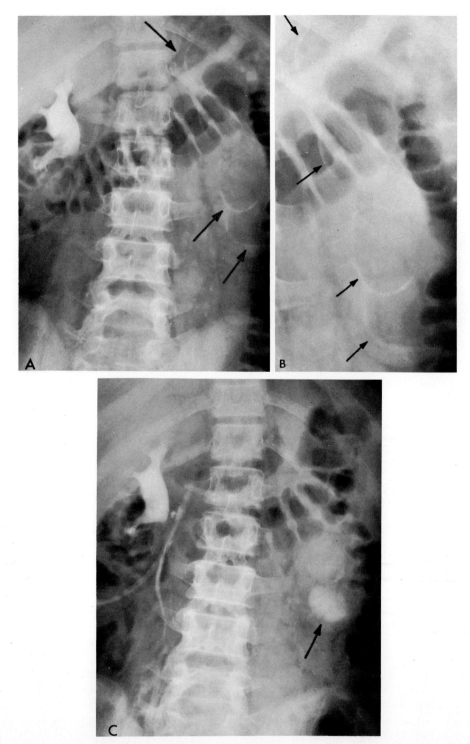

Figure 11-22.   Appearance and disappearance of crescent sign of hydronephrosis. **A,** *Excretory urogram, 5-minute film.* There is good opacification of right renal pelvis and calyces. Pelvis and calyces of left kidney are not opacified, but crescentic collections of medium (crescent sign) are seen in renal parenchyma overlying dilated calyces (*arrows*). **B,** Enlargement of part of film shown in **A.** Crescent sign of hydronephrosis is exaggerated (*arrows*). **C,** *Excretory urogram, 60-minute delayed film.* Some medium has collected in dilated calyces (*arrow*). Crescent sign has almost completely disappeared.

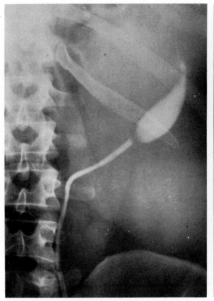
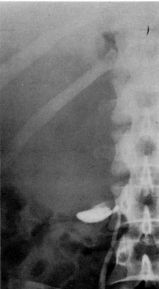

Figure 11–23. *Left retrograde pyelogram.* **Huge hydronephrosis** producing so much pressure at ureteropelvic juncture that only periphery of pelvis and adjacent portion of ureter can be filled. (At operation, **anomalous vessels** were found crossing kidney at ureteropelvic juncture.)

Figure 11–24. *Right retrograde pyelogram.* **Huge hydronephrosis** (pelvis not visualized, as contrast medium will not enter pelvis). Point of obstruction at angulation of ureter in region of ureteropelvic juncture. (At operation, massive hydronephrosis found, secondary to ureteropelvic juncture obstruction.)

Fig. 11–23   Fig. 11–24

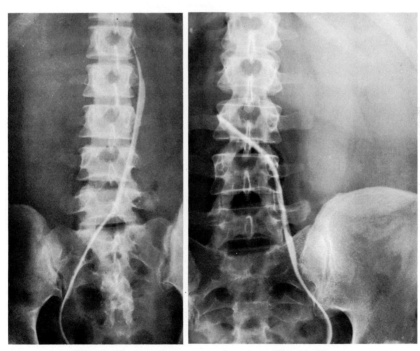

Fig. 11–25   Fig. 11–26

Figure 11–25. *Attempted right retrograde pyelogram.* **Massive hydronephrosis** (pelvis not visualized), **completely displacing right ureter across midline.** Unable to introduce contrast medium into pelvis because of obstruction. Condition could be easily confused with renal tumor. (At operation, huge hydronephrotic kidney was found, filling right side of abdomen.)

Figure 11–26. *Left retrograde pyelogram.* **Massive hydronephrosis, which displaces ureter to right of midline,** obstructing ureter so that contrast medium does not enter pelvis. Could be confused with renal tumor or crossed renal ectopia. (At operation elsewhere, huge hydronephrotic left kidney was found, pelvis extending across vertebral column.)

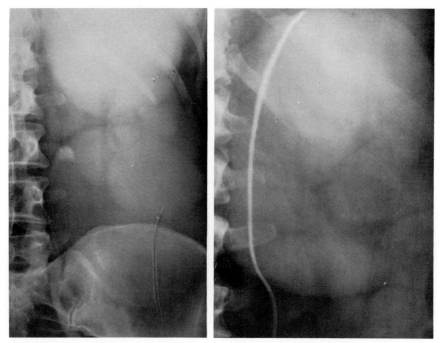

Fig. 11–27   Fig. 11–28

Figure 11–27.   *Excretory urogram.* **Massive hydronephrosis** which on exploration was found to be size of football. **Marked angulation and obstruction at ureteropelvic juncture.**

Figure 11–28.   *Left retrograde pyelogram.* **Massive hydronephrosis** which was not visible on excretory urogram. Contrast medium injected by means of ureteral catheter shows faint outline of huge hydronephrotic sac, the result of congenital ureteropelvic juncture obstruction. Obstruction of undetermined origin at ureteropelvic juncture. In this type of case all other means of diagnosis should be exhausted before retrograde pyelography is attempted. Even then, it should be done with caution.

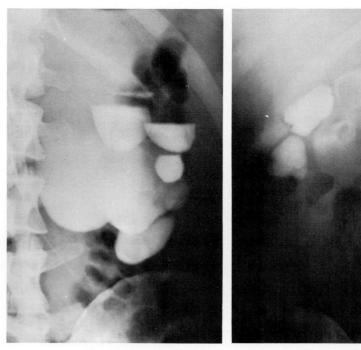

Fig. 11–29   Fig. 11–30

See opposite page for legends

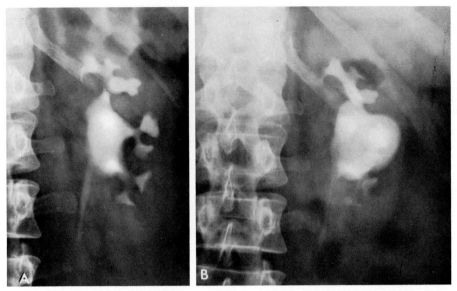

Figure 11–31. *Excretory urograms.* **A,** *Twenty-minute film.* **Apparently mild pyelectasis** of left kidney. **B,** *Sixty-minute film,* with more complete filling. **Pyelectasis of much greater degree** than one would suspect from 20-minute film.

INTERPRETATION OF UROGRAMS: VALUE OF SPECIAL TECHNIQUES

Inconsistencies Between Excretory and Retrograde Urograms

Differences in the size of the renal collecting system as it appears in an excretory urogram and in a retrograde pyelogram can be accounted for by technical factors. In some patients, even a moderate amount of abdominal compression during excretory urography may produce an impressive degree of dilatation of the pelves and ureters. For this reason, this technique should not be used for all exposures. Likewise, if the normal intrarenal pressure is overcome by the introduction of excessive contrast medium during the course of a retrograde study, an acute dilatation of the collecting system will occur. If, however, more than a moderate pyelocaliectasis results, one must consider that a previous insult from obstruction or infection has taken place (Figs. 11–31, 11–32, and 33–33).

Value of Delayed Retrograde Pyelogram

One procedure that may be helpful in distinguishing a large normal pelvis from pathologic dilatation is the delayed retrograde pyelogram, which is made as follows: After the contrast medium has been injected through the catheter and the initial pyelogram has been made, the catheter is withdrawn and the patient is ambulated. Subsequent pyelograms are then made at intervals of 10, 20, and 30 minutes. The degree of obstruction may be assessed from the elapsed time and the amount of medium that is retained in the pelvis. Al-

Figure 11–29. *Left retrograde pyelogram.* **Advanced hydronephrosis with fluid level,** indicating that air is present. (At operation several **anomalous vessels** and **intrinsic obstruction** were found at the ureteropelvic juncture.)

Figure 11–30. *Right retrograde pyelogram.* **Hydronephrosis with dilated calyces.** Two of calyces show **filling defects due to blood clots.** (At operation, congenital obstruction was found at ureteropelvic juncture. Right nephrectomy was done.)

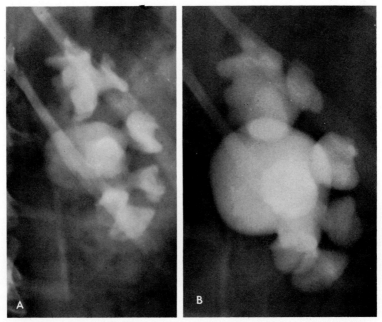

Figure 11–32. A, *Excretory urogram.* Pyelocaliectasis apparently of mild degree. B, *Retrograde pyelogram.* More complete filling shows that degree of pyelocaliectasis is much greater than suspected from excretory urogram.

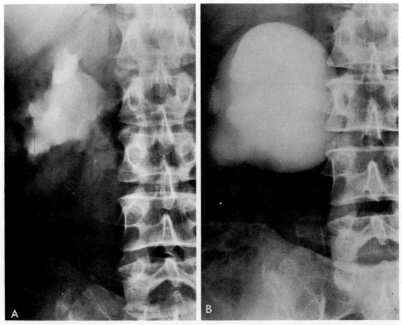

Figure 11–33. Possible diagnostic errors from incomplete filling of pelvis with contrast medium. A, *Excretory urogram, 20-minute film.* Moderately severe hydronephrosis on right. B, *Right retrograde pyelogram.* Complete filling shows pyelectasis to be of much greater degree.

though helpful, this diagnostic procedure is not infallible. The passage of a ureteral catheter may create spasm or edema of the ureter or the ureteropelvic or ureterovesical juncture, and artifactual delayed emptying may then be recorded (Figs. 11–34, 11–35, and 11–36).

Value of Reinjection and Infusion Types of Excretory Urography

In advanced cases of hydronephrosis, function may be so reduced that in the routine series of excretory urograms the usual 20-minute and 45-minute films show nothing. In such cases, the use of reinjection or infusion type excretory urography plus delayed films of several hours may result in visualization sufficient for diagnosis (Figs.

11–37 and 11–38; see also Figure 12–177). As a matter of fact, in occasional cases, urograms made 24 hours after injection of contrast medium may finally visualize sufficient structures for diagnosis (Fig. 11–39).

Renal Radioisotopic Studies in Pyelectasis

In instances of severe renal decompensation from obstructive uropathy, the use of renal imaging, particularly with adjunctive quantitation utilizing radionuclides, will provide more information about the status of the renal cortex than is obtainable by excretory urography. Schlegel and Bakule have not only emphasized the diagnostic

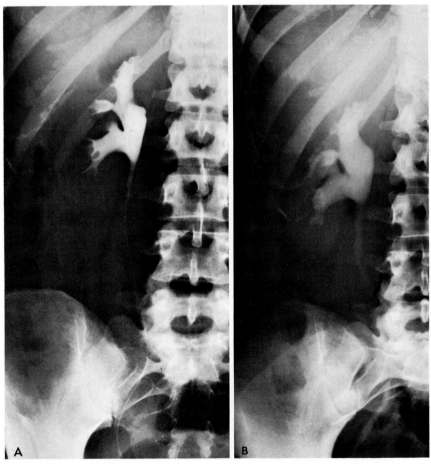

Figure 11–34. *Right retrograde pyelogram and delayed film.* **A,** *Pyelogram.* **Normal. B,** *Twenty-minute delayed pyelogram.* **Pelvis and ureter dilated, grade 1.** Ureter is entirely filled with medium down to bladder because of irritation of ureter during catheterization.

Fig. 11-35

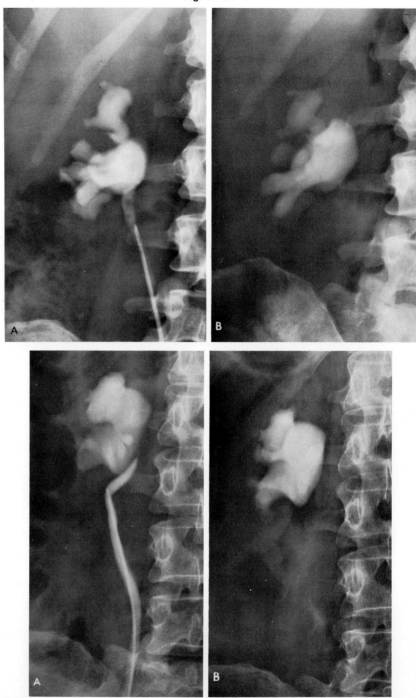

Fig. 11-36

Figure 11-35. *Right retrograde pyelogram with delayed film.* **A,** *Pyelogram.* **Pyelectasis from obstruction of ureteropelvic juncture.** Pelvis is of globular type; it and calyces are dilated, grade 1. **B,** *Twenty-minute delayed pyelogram.* Medium retained in pelvis, none in ureter, indicating obstruction at ureteropelvic juncture.

Figure 11-36. *Right retrograde pyelogram with delayed film.* **A,** *Pyelogram.* **Pyelocaliectasis with high-lying ureteropelvic juncture.** Ureter is not inserted at most dependent portion of pelvis. **B,** *Twenty-minute delayed pyelogram.* Medium is retained in pelvis and calyces; very slight amount in right ureter, indicating obstruction at ureteropelvic juncture.

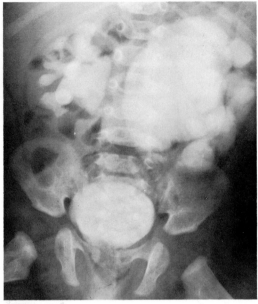

Figure 11-37. *Excretory urogram* of boy, aged 4 months. **Bilateral obstruction at ureteropelvic juncture with pyelectasis,** grade 4 on left and grade 2 on right. This film, made 2½ hours after injection of contrast medium, indicates value of late films.

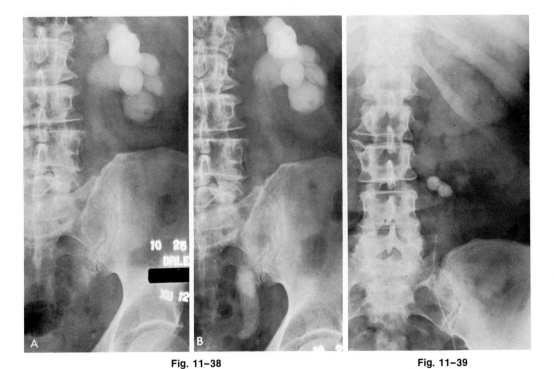

Fig. 11-38   Fig. 11-39

Figure 11-38. Value of delayed or late excretory urogram. (There had been **recently attempted manipulation of left ureteral stone,** and *20-minute excretory urogram* showed suggestion of dilated calyces, but pelvis and ureter were not outlined.) **A,** *Excretory urogram, 2-hour film.* **Pyelocaliectasis with dilatation of upper part of ureter.** Lower part of ureter not outlined. **B,** *Three-hour film.* Entire ureter filled. Obstruction at intramural portion of ureter.

Figure 11-39. Value of delayed or late excretory urogram. *Plain film* with lead catheter in left ureter. (Excretory urogram made 24 hours previously had shown no function.) There is now contrast medium present in kidney. **Hydronephrosis secondary to obstruction at ureteropelvic juncture and calculous obstruction.** (No medium was injected through catheter.)

value of scintigraphic studies in the differentiation of an obstructive process from chronic renal failure but have also pointed out their importance in preoperative evaluation of differential renal function.

LOCALIZED DILATATION OF CALYX (HYDROCALYX, CALYCEAL DIVERTICULUM, AND PYELOGENIC CYST); HYDROCALYCOSIS

Localized dilatation of an entire calyx or a portion of a calyx, a fairly common condition, has caused a good deal of confusion in the literature, especially from the standpoint of terminology and etiology. Bona fide obstruction of a calyx may result from an inflammatory stricture of the infundibulum (Figs. 11–40 and 11–41), stone, tumor, parapelvic cyst (Fig. 11–42), or an intrarenal blood vessel.

When obstruction is not apparent and the etiology is obscure, the condition has been described by such terms as *pyelogenic cyst* (Holm), *calyceal diverticulum* (Prather), and *hydrocalyx* (Figs. 11–43 through 11–56). It has also been suggested that these lesions may represent simple parenchymal cysts or cortical abscesses that have ruptured and drained into a calyx. Holm thinks pyelogenic cysts arise from the wolffian ducts in contradistinction to simple renal cysts, which arise from metanephrogenic tissue. A pyelogenic cyst, in his opinion, must have transitional epithelium. This would distinguish it from a simple cyst or cortical abscess that had ruptured into a calyx. Vermooten suggested that collecting tubule ectasia as seen in sponge kidney is a possible etiologic factor. In all cases, a communication between the cavity and the pelviocalyceal system can be demonstrated either urographically or at operation.

The term *hydrocalyx* should be used to indicate that the entire calyx is involved

Text continued on page 983

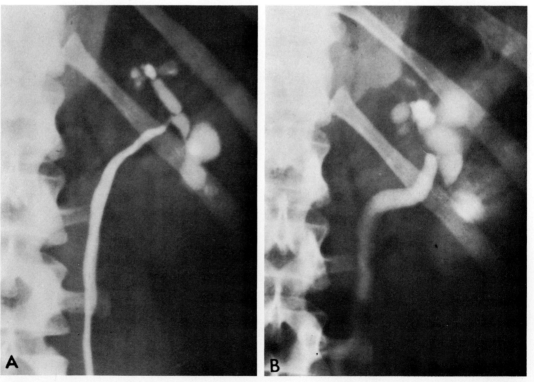

Figure 11–40.   Congenital solitary kidney with stricture at juncture of ureter and calyces. (At surgical exploration there seemed to be no true pelvis.) **A,** *Retrograde pyelogram,* in 1955. **B,** *Retrograde pyelogram,* 1958. **Progression of pyelectasis.** (At operation, cause of stricture was not apparent. Ureterolysis was done.) (Courtesy of Dr. C. D. Creevy.)

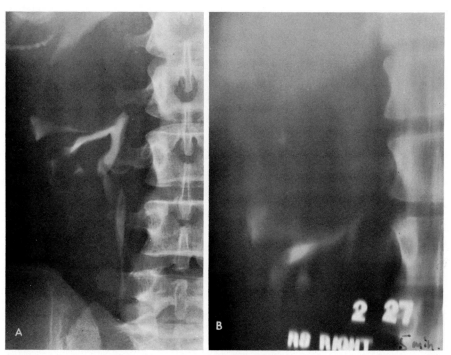

Figure 11–41.   Stricture of infundibulum of upper calyx of right kidney, **producing huge hydrocalyx suggest-ing tumor. A,** *Excretory urogram.* Middle calyx displaced downward by "mass" in upper pole. **B,** *Nephrotomogram.* "Mass" is large negative shadow from dilated calyx. (Nephrectomy done.)

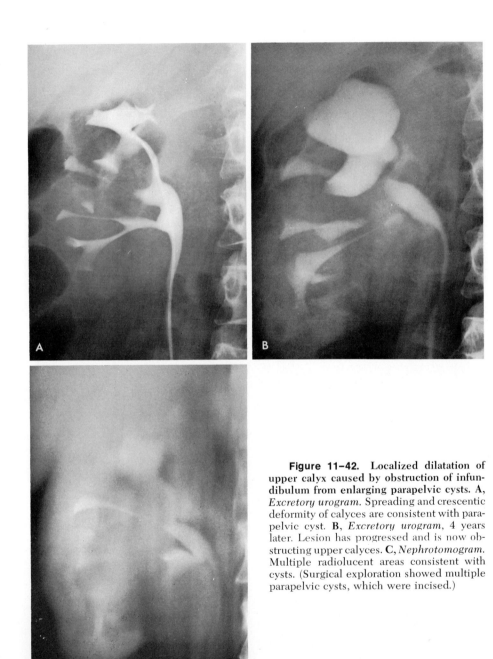

Figure 11–42. Localized dilatation of upper calyx caused by obstruction of infundibulum from enlarging parapelvic cysts. **A,** *Excretory urogram.* Spreading and crescentic deformity of calyces are consistent with parapelvic cyst. **B,** *Excretory urogram,* 4 years later. Lesion has progressed and is now obstructing upper calyces. **C,** *Nephrotomogram.* Multiple radiolucent areas consistent with cysts. (Surgical exploration showed multiple parapelvic cysts, which were incised.)

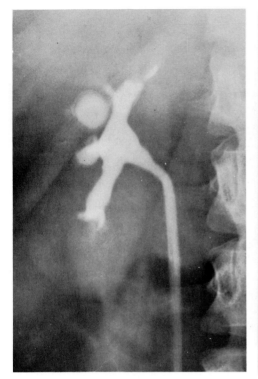

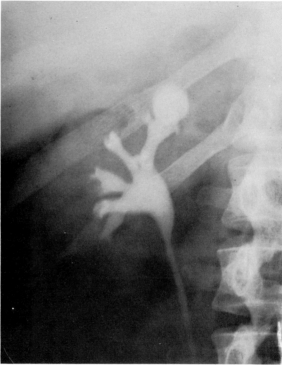

Fig. 11–43   **Fig. 11–44**

Figures 11–43 and **11–44.**   *Retrograde pyelograms.* Calyceal diverticula or pyelogenic cysts communicating with branches of upper calyces.

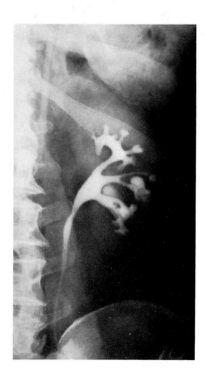

Figure 11–45.   *Left retrograde pyelogram.* Small calyceal diverticulum or pyelogenic cyst which communicates with branch of middle calyx.

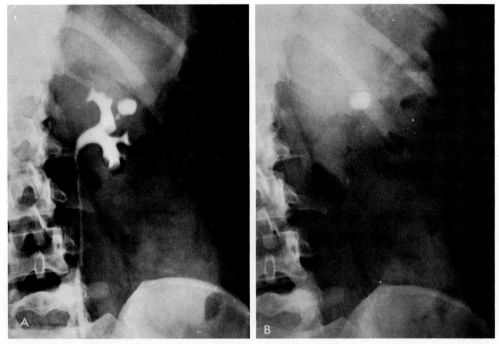

Figure 11-46.   A, *Retrograde pyelogram.* **Calyceal diverticulum or pyelogenic cyst** which communicates with branch of upper calyx. **B,** *Delayed film.* Contrast medium is retained in cyst.

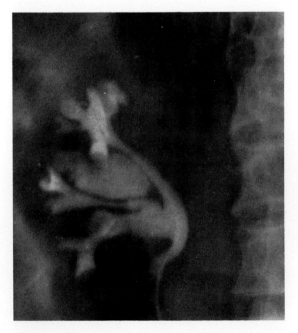

Figure 11-47. *Retrograde pyelogram.* **Rather large pyelogenic cyst or calyceal diverticulum** which communicates with infundibulum of upper calyx. (Courtesy of Dr. Hugh Rives.)

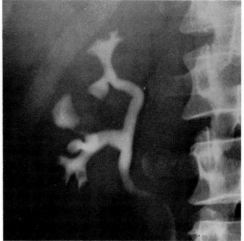

Figure 11-48. *Right retrograde pyelogram.* **Calyceal diverticulum or pyelogenic cyst** communicating with branch of lower calyx. (According to Abeshouse, this should be considered a diverticulum because of long communicating channel.)

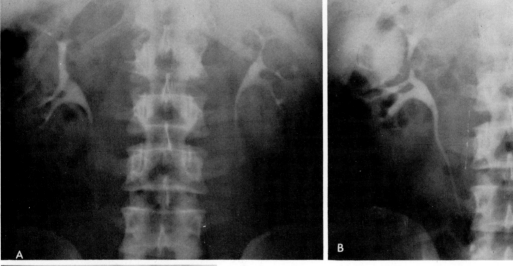

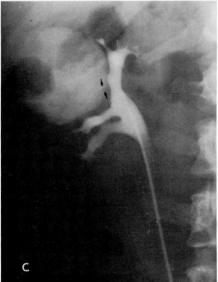

Figure 11-49. **Large calyceal diverticulum** of right kidney of 35-year-old woman. **A,** *Excretory urogram, 5-minute film.* Spreading of middle and upper calyces, but no contrast medium is visible in diverticulum. **B,** *Excretory urogram, 15-minute film.* Large diverticulum is now fairly well filled. **C,** *Retrograde pyelogram.* Diverticulum is better filled. Narrow communication (*arrows*) can be seen between upper calyx and diverticulum. (Courtesy of Dr. H. W. Calhoun.)

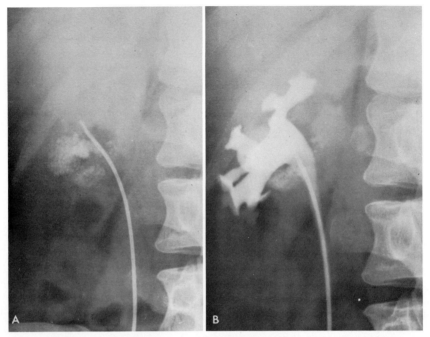

Figure 11–50. Pyelogenic cyst or calyceal diverticulum filled with many small calculi. **A,** *Plain film.* Calculi overlie midrenal area. **B,** *Retrograde pyelogram.* Diverticulum filled with stones is overlying normal appearing pelvis and calyces. (Surgical exploration showed that diverticulum communicated with branch of middle calyx in anteroposterior plane, so it is not shown in this projection.)

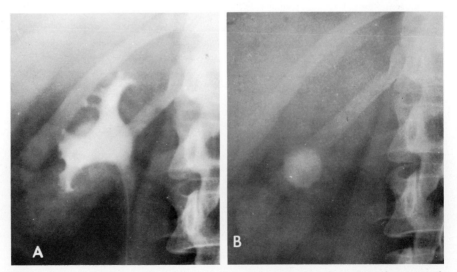

Figure 11–51. Pyelogenic cyst or calyceal diverticulum with retained medium. **A,** *Right retrograde pyelogram.* Cyst communicates with lower major calyx of right kidney and is partially obscured by this calyx. **B,** *Delayed film.* Residual contrast medium remains in cyst.

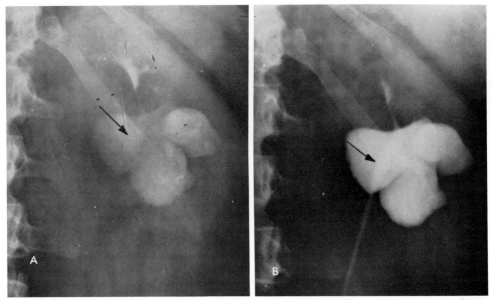

Figure 11–52. Large pyelogenic cyst, calyceal diverticulum, or hydrocalyx. **A,** *Excretory urogram.* Large irregular collection of contrast medium overlies and partially obscures pelvis and middle and lower calyces of left kidney. Pelvis, however, can be seen through the medium (*arrow*). **B,** *Left retrograde pyelogram.* Better visualization of large pyelogenic cyst. Outline of normal pelvis can be seen through medium. (On exploration, large pyelogenic cyst was found, which apparently arose from middle calyx. Calyx was obliterated and midportion of kidney was almost destroyed. This might be more accurately described as hydrocalyx.) (Courtesy of Dr. David Cristol.)

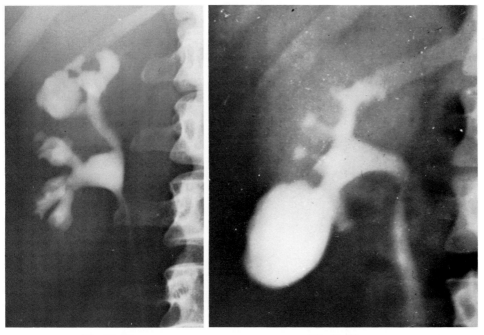

Fig. 11–53   Fig. 11–54

Figure 11–53. *Right retrograde pyelogram.* Calyceal diverticulum or pyelogenic cyst communicates with branch of upper calyx of right kidney.

Figure 11–54. *Retrograde pyelogram.* Large calyceal diverticulum or hydrocalyx communicating with lower calyces.

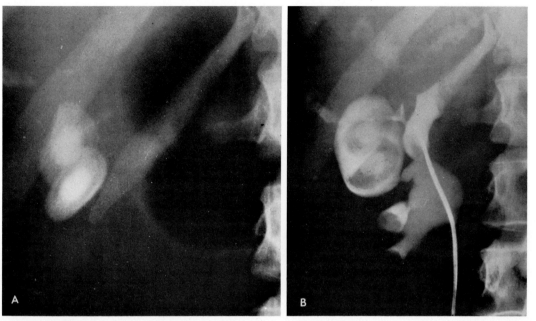

Figure 11–55.   Calculi in calyceal diverticulum. A, *Plain film.* Laminated stones overlying right kidney. **B,** *Right retrograde pyelogram.* Stones are seen to be included in diverticulum, which apparently communicates with branch of upper calyx. (Courtesy of Dr. Edwin Davis.)

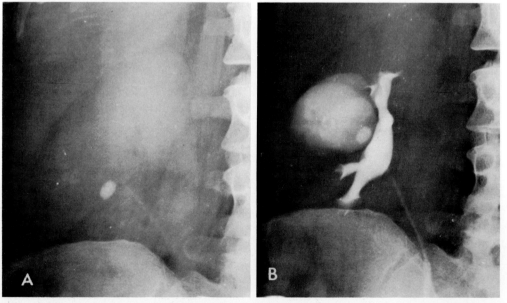

Figure 11–56.   Stone in large calyceal diverticulum, pyelogenic cyst, or simple cyst which had ruptured into renal pelvis. A, *Plain film.* Multiple shadows over midportion of right kidney. **B,** *Right retrograde pyelogram.* Large pyelogenic cyst that apparently communicates with middle calyx and extends to periphery of kidney. Calculi included in cyst. (At operation, there appeared to be large simple cortical cyst that had ruptured into pelvis, but it could not be differentiated from pyelogenic cyst.)

and that the communication is directly into the pelvis rather than into another part of the calyx. The terms *calyceal diverticulum* and *pyelogenic cyst* indicate that there is a communication between the cavity and the calyx. Abeshouse tried to distinguish these two entities on the basis of the length of the narrow communicating channel. In his opinion, a long, narrow channel indicated a calyceal diverticulum, whereas a short one suggested a pyelogenic cyst. Calyceal diverticula and pyelogenic cysts are usually small or of only moderate size in contrast to a hydrocalyx, which may be large, or to hydrocalycosis, in which the cyst may reach extreme proportions. It should be appreciated that accurate distinction may be impossible even at operation or at the time of gross and microscopic examination of a kidney. In most cases, especially if the lesion is of small or only moderate size, calyceal cysts are of no clinical importance; diagnosis is made accidentally when an excretory urogram is made for some unrelated problem. In some cases, however, infection or stones may complicate the situation and require surgical excision.

Hydrocalycosis

An extreme degree of hydrocalyx in which the calyx becomes so large that it may present as a palpable abdominal tumor has been described as a distinct clinical entity and given the name *hydrocalycosis*. Williams and Mininberg reported three cases in children, which they state comprised the third, fourth, and fifth pediatric cases reported in the literature. They found 12 well-documented cases in adults in the literature. They define this condition as a cystic dilatation of a major calyx with no obvious obstructive etiology; there must be a demonstrable connection with the renal pelvis, and the cyst wall must be lined with uroepithelium. Urographic diagnosis may be difficult, as findings are not pathognomonic. In their three pediatric cases, the problem was essentially that of a mass in the upper pole of the kidney with absent or very poor visualization of the involved calyx on excretory urog-

raphy and little or no filling during retrograde pyelography. Two of their patients also had posterior urethral valves. Theoretical considerations of the etiology of this condition suggest the possibility of a ring of muscle at the juncture of the calyceal infundibulum and renal pelvis (Moore; Watkins).

Vascular Obstruction of the Infundibulum of the Upper Calyx

Vascular impressions on the pelviocalyceal system have been a well-recognized entity since the correlation of excretory urography with renal arteriography (Baum and Gillenwater; Kreel and Pyle). In a review of 1,100 renal arteriograms, Michel and Barsamian discovered 52 arterial, 35 venous, and 12 mixed pyelocalyceal vascular impressions. In 40 of their cases, the impression involved the infundibulum of the upper calyx of the right kidney and was usually due to an artery. (Wide impressions with poorly defined borders corresponded to the passage of a vein, and a narrow impression with distinct borders generally corresponded to an artery.)

Usually the occurrence of such vascular impressions is not associated with any clinical or therapeutic implication. Fraley has pointed out, however, that in some patients vascular obstruction of the upper infundibulum will create significant caliectasis with retention of contrast medium in urographic studies. Vague abdominal pain or chronic nephralgia in these patients has disappeared after infundibulopyelostomy. (See additional discussion of this problem in Chapter 8.)

In cases of vascular obstruction of the superior infundibulum, a persistent, well-marginated, transversely oriented filling defect of the infundibulum is evident on the excretory urogram. Usually, the remaining calyces of the obstructed kidney and the collecting system of the contralateral kidney are normal. Proximal to the filling defect is marked caliectasis (Fig. 11–57A). The delayed drainage radiographs of the retrograde pyelogram show selective entrapment of contrast medium in the su-

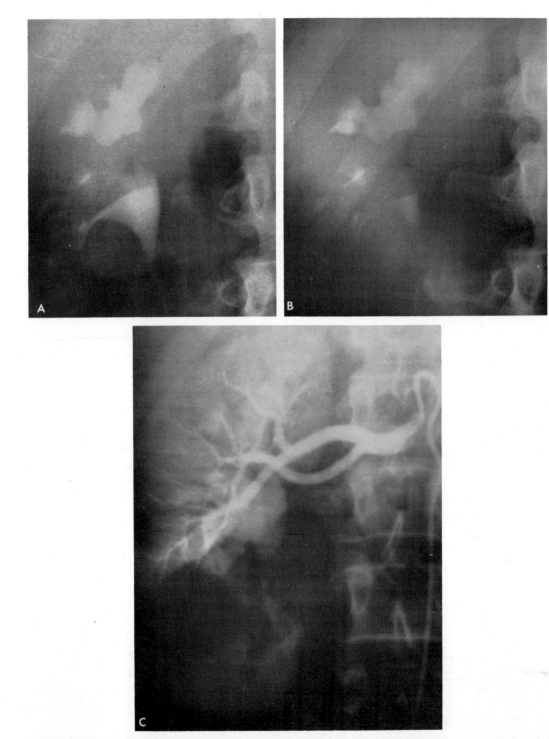

Figure 11–57. Vascular obstruction of superior infundibulum. **A,** *Excretory urogram.* Persistent filling defect in infundibulum and marked superior caliectasis. **B,** *Retrograde pyelogram, delayed film.* Selective entrapment of contrast medium proximal to point of infundibular obstruction. **C,** *Selective renal angiogram.* Large artery crosses infundibulum in area of filling defect seen on excretory urogram (**A**). Dilated calyx can be seen in background.

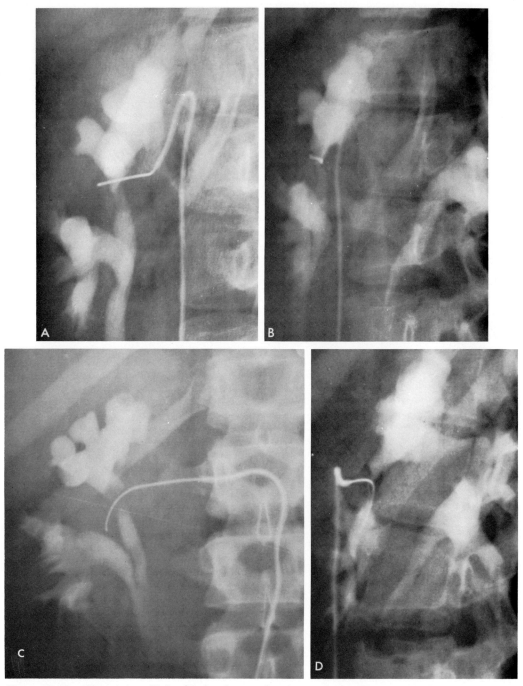

Figure 11–58. Obstruction of infundibulum by vascular vise consisting of two arteries. *Excretory urograms.* **A,** *Anteroposterior view.* Guide wire in what appeared to be obstructing artery on selective angiogram. **B,** *Oblique view.* Artery supplying middle vascular segment can be seen to pass ventral to infundibulum. **C,** *Anteroposterior view.* Wire now positioned in vessel to posterior vascular segment. **D,** *Oblique view.* This vessel is dorsal to infundibulum; thus it forms obstructive vascular vise with artery to middle segment.

perior calyx (Fig. 11–57B), and selective angiography usually demonstrates a vessel, artery or vein, crossing the infundibulum in the region of the filling defect (Fig. 11–57C).

If wires are placed in the offending vessels through the angiogram catheters, the precise anatomic relations between the vessels and the infundibulum can be studied by radiographs taken in multiple projections (Doppman and Fraley) (Fig. 11–58). Angiograms are also useful in these cases to rule out mass lesions of the kidney, which either can compress the infundibulum extrinsically or, as with renal tumors, produce infundibular obstruction by direct invasion.

OBSTRUCTION AT THE URETEROPELVIC JUNCTURE

Ureteropelvic obstruction or dysfunction with pyelocaliectasis is the most common congenital anomaly of the urinary tract. Excretory urography finds one of its most useful applications in the diagnosis and evaluation of this condition. Severe degrees of obstruction at the ureteropelvic juncture usually give rise to symptoms and findings early in life, whereas milder de-

grees may not become clinically apparent until adult life.

Tendency to Bilaterality

Although there is an unexplained predilection for the left side, some degree of bilateral involvement is usually evident (Kelalis and associates, 1971). Fortunately, however, in most cases the dilatation is less on one side than on the other, so that surgical intervention on one side may be all that is required (Figs. 11–59, 11–60, and 11–61). It is usually wise to examine the nonoperated kidney periodically by means of excretory urography for a period of years to determine whether the pyelectasis is progressive.

Occurrence in Infants and Children

The commonest cause of an upper abdominal mass in a child is not a renal tumor (Wilms' tumor or neuroblastoma; see Chapter 14) but rather a hydronephrotic kidney due to obstruction of the ureteropelvic juncture. This is true even though the mass may feel firm and solid. It is axiomatic that an abdominal mass in a child should be considered hydronephrosis until proved otherwise. Exploratory surgery

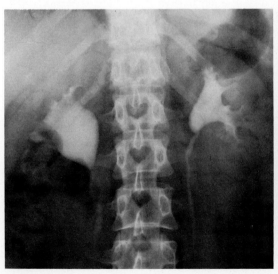
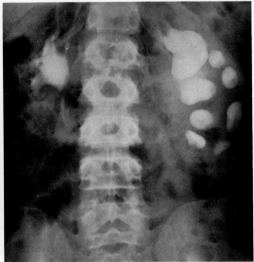

Fig. 11–59   Fig. 11–60

Figure 11–59. *Excretory urogram.* **Obstruction of both ureteropelvic junctures, greater on right than on left.**
Figure 11–60. *Excretory urogram.* **Obstruction of both ureteropelvic junctures of boy age 12 years, greater on left than on right.** (Left nephrectomy.)

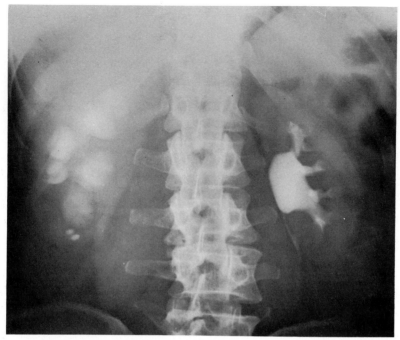

Figure 11–61. *Excretory urogram.* **Bilateral pyelocaliectasis in adult; more advanced on right than on left.** (At operation, **anomalous vessels** and **intrinsic ureteropelvic juncture obstruction** were found. **Two stones** measured 3 mm in diameter.)

should not be carried out for a suspected renal tumor on an infant or child until an excretory urogram has excluded hydronephrosis.

As has been mentioned previously, the degree of obstruction of the ureteropelvic juncture varies greatly. In cases of minimal obstruction, it may be necessary to compare the involved kidney with the contralateral kidney to determine if pyelectasis is really present. Such minimal degrees of pyelectasis usually are of no clinical importance, are not a factor in recurrent infection, and can simply be observed. (Examples of various degrees of obstruction at the ureteropelvic juncture in infants and children are shown in Figures 11–62 through 11–68).

Pathogenesis of Ureteropelvic Juncture Obstruction

There are a variety of causes of ureteropelvic juncture obstruction, and most of them are congenital. Opinions differ regarding the precise participation of each factor in a specific instance, but basically impedance at the juncture is created by either an intrinsic or an extrinsic abnormality.

Intrinsic obstruction may be mechanically related to excessive replacement of the muscle layer by collagen (Notley) or by fibroblasts (Allen). In rare instances, valvular mucosal infoldings or minute polyps may be present. Dysfunction at the ureteropelvic juncture also produces hydronephrosis. Murnaghan has described replacement of the circular muscle fibers by longitudinal muscle bundles, creating a narrow aperistaltic segment and thereby interrupting the peristaltic wave. Resulting distention of the renal transport system causes elongation of the longitudinal fibers without increasing their girth. This in turn develops narrowing instead of expansion of the ureteropelvic lumen. The dyskinetic activity of this segment will produce retrograde peristalsis, which propels the urinary

Fig. 11–62

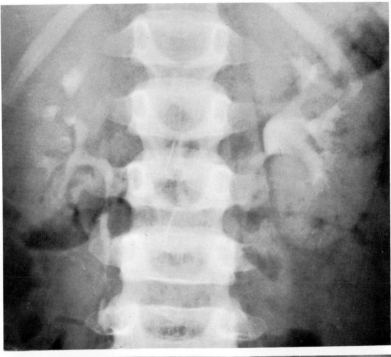

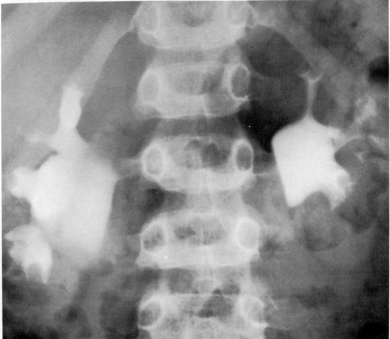

Fig. 11–63

Figure 11–62. *Excretory urogram* of 6-year-old girl. **Minimal obstruction of ureteropelvic juncture on left. Normal pelvis on right.**

Figure 11–63. *Excretory urogram* of 4-year-old boy. **Obstruction of both ureteropelvic junctures. Obstruction greater on right than on left.**

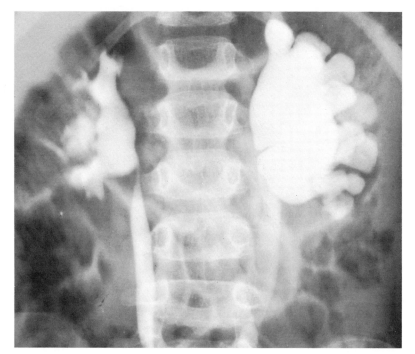

Figure 11-64. *Retrograde pyelogram.* **Obstruction of both ureteropelvic junctures** of girl, 4 years of age. **Right, pyelectasis, grade 1; left, grade 3.** (Y-V ureteropelvioplasty performed on left.)

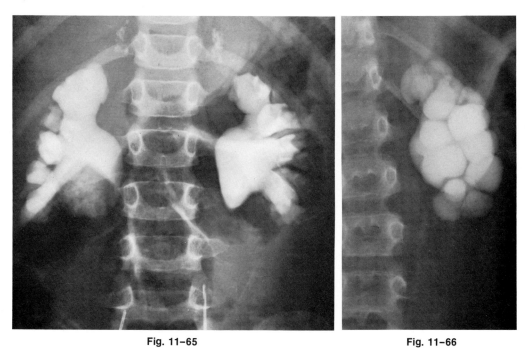

Fig. 11-65   Fig. 11-66

Figure 11-65. *Retrograde pyelogram.* **Obstruction of both ureteropelvic junctures** of boy, 6 years of age. **Bilateral pyelectasis, grade 2.** (Culp ureteropelvioplasty done on right.)

Figure 11-66. *Left retrograde pyelogram.* **Obstruction at ureteropelvic juncture with pyelocaliectasis, grade 4,** in boy, 9 years of age. (Almost all of kidney was destroyed, so nephrectomy was performed. Preoperative excretory urogram showed right pyelectasis, grade 1.)

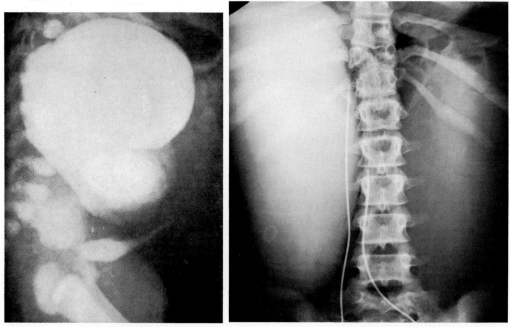

Fig. 11-67   Fig. 11-68

Figure 11-67. *Antegrade pyelogram.* Contrast medium injected with needle introduced through lumbar region. **Huge left hydronephrosis and hydroureter** in newborn male infant. Right kidney was normal on excretory urogram, but left kidney showed no function. (Courtesy of Dr. S. A. Vest.)

Figure 11-68. *Retrograde pyelogram.* **Bilateral pyelectasis, grade 4,** in girl, 13 years of age, from **obstruction of ureteropelvic junctures.** No visualization on excretory urogram. (Y-V ureteropelvioplasty was done on right, nephrectomy on left.)

bolus into the calyces. These peristaltic aberrations are clearly visible on cine-fluoroscopic study of the affected side.

Extrinsic abnormalities may coexist with an intrinsic lesion, but they are rarely the primary cause of obstruction and ordinarily are not treated independently. In about one third of cases of ureteropelvic juncture obstruction, aberrant or accessory vessels are discovered in close proximity to the juncture. This intimate relationship may appear to create obstruction by mechanical pressure against the juncture or by angulation as the ureter drapes over the vessel ("clothesline" effect) (Figs. 11-69 through 11-74).

Adventitial bands or curtains of filamentous tissue that obscure the ureteropelvic juncture and angulate the ureter or the dilated pelvis are frequently observed at surgery. As the pyelectasis progresses, the ureter is moved proximally so that it becomes nondependent. High insertion

of the ureter into the renal pelvis, therefore, is a secondary phenomenon (Figs. 11-75 through 11-79).

Vesicoureteral reflux will create, in some instances, dysfunction of the ureteropelvic juncture and ultimately an obstructive process. The regurgitation of urine from the bladder into the renal pelvis via a decompensated ureterovesical juncture and ureter exceeds the emptying capacity of the pelvis. The normal resting pressure of the renal pelvis is only about 5 cm of water. The rhythmic contractures of its muscle wall, unlike those of the ureter or detrusor, produce only a modest increase in this pressure and usually to not more than 25 cm of water. The excessive urine load from vesicoureteral reflux chronically overdistends the pelvis and retards peristalsis. Resulting stasis and infection, in turn, promote fibrosis of the ureteropelvic juncture, and the obstructive component augments the functional one (Fig. 11-80).

Text continued on page 994

Fig. 11-69

Fig. 11-70

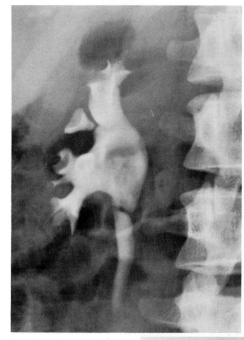

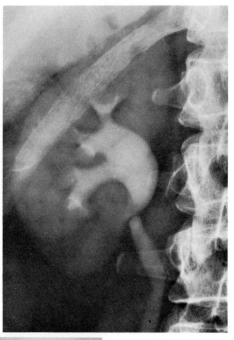

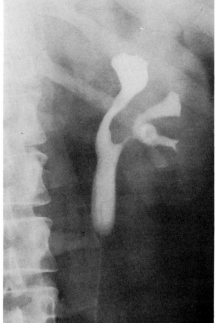

Fig. 11-71

Figure 11-69. *Retrograde pyelogram, right.* Filling defect apparently from **anomalous vessel crossing uretero-pelvic juncture. Pyelectasis, grade 1.**

Figure 11-70. *Excretory urogram.* Filling defect from **vessel crossing ureteropelvic juncture** of right kidney. **Pyelectasis, grade 1.**

Figure 11-71. *Retrograde pyelogram.* **Partial obstruction of ureter** 4 cm below ureteropelvic juncture. **Stone 1** cm in diameter in anterior projection of middle calyx. (At operation, obstruction was found to be caused by plexus of veins which crossed ureter at point of obstruction. They were excised, and stone was removed.)

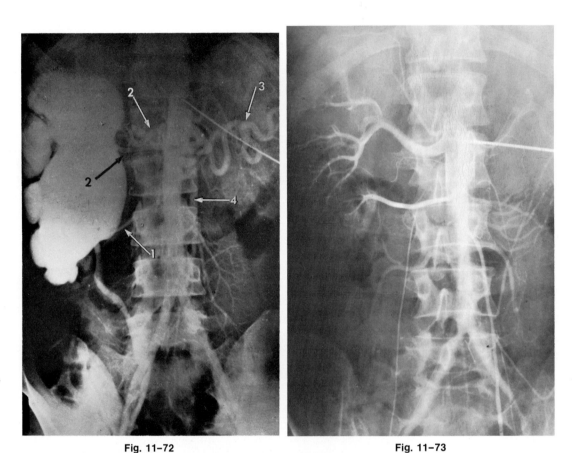

Fig. 11-72   Fig. 11-73

Figure 11-72. *Right retrograde pyelogram* of 27-year-old man, *with aortogram superimposed.* **Marked pyelectasis with aberrant artery** (*1*) **seen to be obstructing ureteropelvic juncture.** Right renal artery (*2*), splenic artery (*3*), and superior mesenteric artery (*4*) are well outlined. (Courtesy of Dr. A. K. Doss.)

Figure 11-73. *Aortogram.* **Aberrant artery** of type often found crossing ureteropelvic juncture serves lower pole of right kidney. (Courtesy of Dr. C. K. Pearlman.)

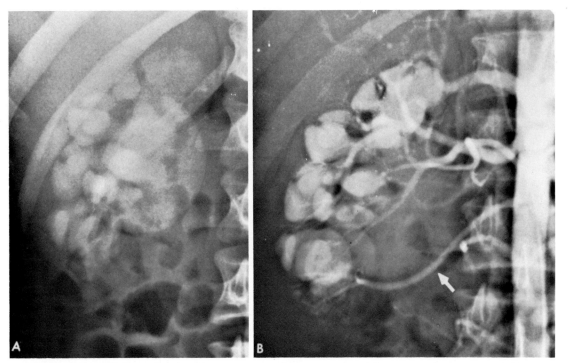

Figure 11-74. Hydronephrosis with accessory renal artery crossing right ureteropelvic juncture. A, *Excretory urogram.* **B,** *Arteriogram.* Accessory renal artery to lower pole of kidney passes across ureteropelvic juncture (*arrow*). (From Siegelman, S. S., and Bosniak, M. A.)

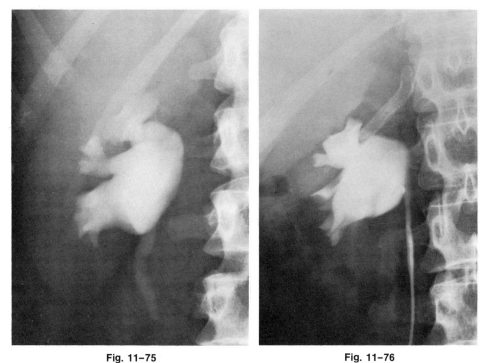

Fig. 11-75   **Fig. 11-76**

Figure 11-75. *Excretory urogram.* Obstruction of right ureteropelvic juncture from high insertion of ureter.

Figure 11-76. *Retrograde pyelogram,* right. Obstruction of ureteropelvic juncture from high insertion of ureter.

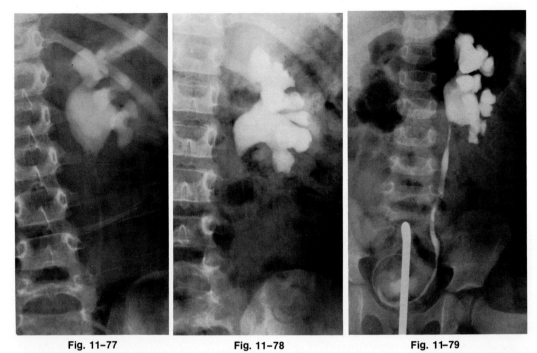

Fig. 11–77   Fig. 11–78   Fig. 11–79

Figure 11–77. *Retrograde pyelogram, left.* **Stricture of upper part of left ureter causing moderate pyelocaliectasis in girl, 5 years of age.** (At operation, stricture was found to be about 2.5 cm long and situated immediately below ureteropelvic juncture. It was treated as obstruction of ureteropelvic juncture. Flap turned down to replace entire area of narrowing.)

Figure 11–78. *Excretory urogram.* **Unilateral (left) pyelectasis in boy, 5 years of age, secondary to obstruction of ureteropelvic juncture.** Ureteropelvic juncture is in normal dependent position, but it and adjacent ureter are narrowed.

Figure 11–79. **Obstruction of ureteropelvic juncture** of child, age 5 years. Note long segment of narrow ureter adjacent to dilated renal pelvis. (Culp spiral-flap pyeloplasty was performed.) (Courtesy of Dr. Jerry D. Giesy.)

As the process continues, the ureter will dilate, elongate, and become tortuous. This occurs first at the juncture of mobile and fixed portions of the ureter such as the ureterovesical juncture and the pelvic brim. Periureteritis with exudation and necrosis results in stenosis and adhesion between adjacent and parallel segments of the tortuous ureter. Ureteral dilatation below the level of obstruction and vesicoureteral reflux are considered specific signs that stasis and dilatation are acquired, that is, secondary to infection (Shopfner, 1966b).

INTERMITTENT HYDRONEPHROSIS

The syndrome of intermittent hydronephrosis has added considerably to our knowledge of obstruction of the ureteropelvic juncture. This entity was first described in 1956 by Nesbit, who studied patients with intermittent attacks of flank pain. Excretory urograms made between attacks of pain were normal; during an attack, pyelectasis was demonstrated on the painful side. Bourne; Falk; and Ansell and Paterson have confirmed this syndrome.

Hanley in 1959 and 1960 observed that the bifid funnel-type pelvis (Fig. 11–81A) was almost never involved in this condition; it was the closed type or ampullary pelvis that was usually noted (Fig. 11–81 B). This type of pelvis tends to be large and extrarenal and to have short infundibula to the calyces. Cinepyelographic studies with overhydration showed that the bifid funnel type of pelvis could transport the increased fluid load easily without pelvic dilatation,

Figure 11–80. A, *Excretory urogram.* Undilated collecting system. B, *Cystogram.* **Vesicoureteral reflux.** Apparent obstruction of ureteropelvic juncture.

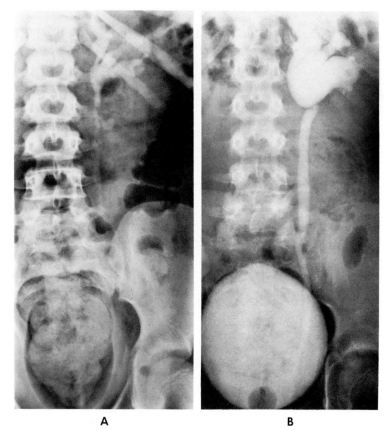

A   B

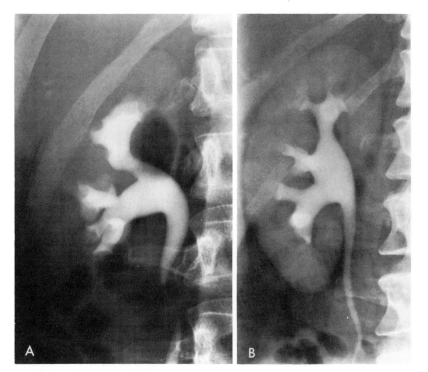

Figure 11–81. *Excretory urogram.* A, Ampullary type of pelvis. B, Funnel type of pelvis.

whereas the ampullary type of pelvis appeared to be ineffective with the increased flow of urine. The limitation, which appeared to be at the ureteropelvic juncture, resulted in temporary pyelectasis until the urine flow normalized. Hanley further commented that at least 90 per cent of all ureteropelvic obstruction occurred with the ampullary type of pelvis.

Conditions that may produce intermittent hydronephrosis are excessive fluid intake (Figs. 11–82 through 11–85), diabetes

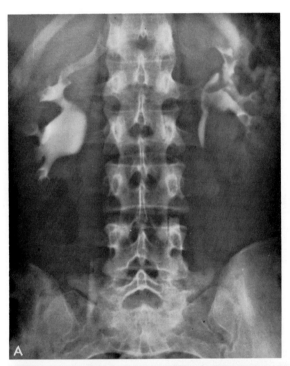

Figure 11–82. Intermittent right hydronephrosis in 22-year-old woman. **A,** *Excretory urogram* made during asymptomatic period. **Mild right pyelectasis** but normal calyces. **B,** *Excretory urogram.* Film made during flank pain induced by hydration. **Moderate hydronephrosis. C,** Film made after pain had subsided. Pelvis has returned to original size. (From Kendall, A. R., and Karafin, L.)

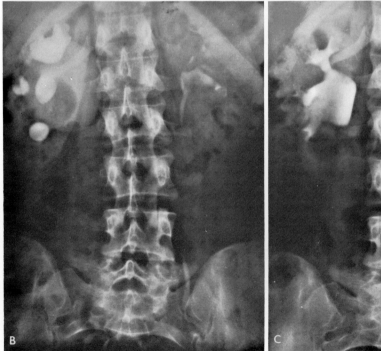

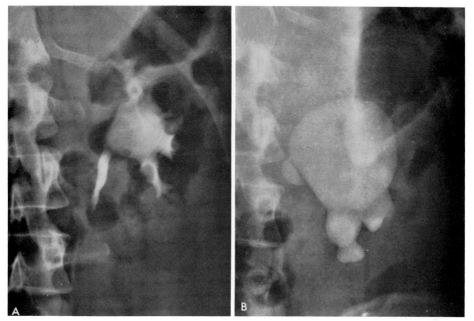

Figure 11–83. Intermittent left hydronephrosis. **A,** *Excretory urogram* made during asymptomatic period. **Mild pyelectasis** but normal calyces. **B,** *Hydration excretory urogram* (patient having mild flank pain). **Moderate hydronephrosis.** (From Kendall, A. R., and Karafin, L.)

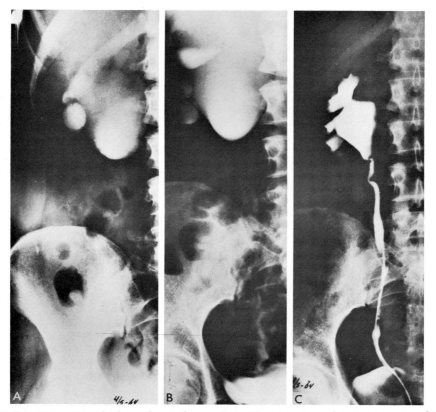

Figure 11–84. Intermittent hydronephrosis due to obstruction at ureteropelvic juncture. **A** and **B,** *Excretory urograms* during attack of right flank pain. **C,** *Retrograde pyelogram* made only 4 days later, during absence of pain, showing almost complete reduction of hydronephrosis and well-delineated area of obstruction in ureteropelvic juncture. (Courtesy of Dr. H. W. ten Cate.)

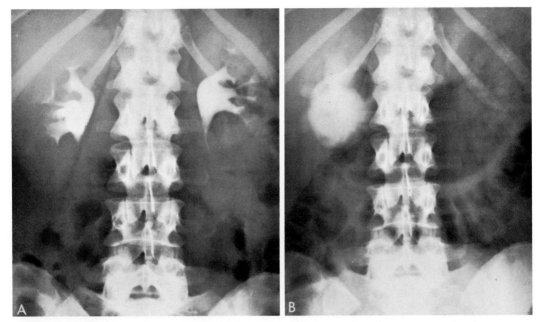

Figure 11–85.   Intermittent hydronephrosis in woman aged 33. **A,** *Excretory urogram* made when patient was free of pain. Normal. **B,** *Excretory urogram* made during acute pain after drinking three glasses of beer. Note definite right hydronephrosis. (Medium has been almost entirely evacuated from left kidney.) (From Bourne, R. B.)

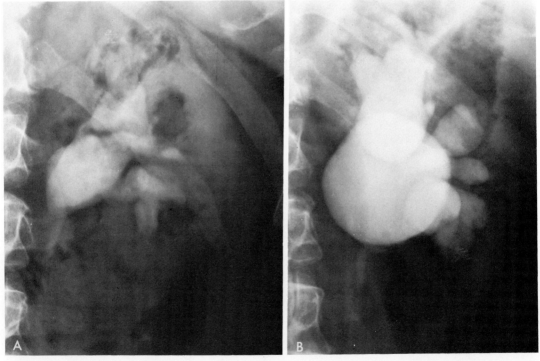

Figure 11–86.   Patient with diabetes insipidus. *Excretory urograms.* **A,** *20-minute film* with patient on water deprivation shows mild **pyelocaliectasis secondary to slight ureteropelvic juncture obstruction. B,** *20-minute film* with patient on normal diet and access to fluids indicates **decompensation of ureteropelvic juncture** due to excessive urine volume.

insipidus (Fig. 11–86), increased output of one kidney after removal of the other, and vesicoureteral reflux (see Figure 11–80).

Urographic Diagnosis of Ureteropelvic Juncture Obstruction

CLINICAL FEATURES

In infants, a palpable renal mass is the most common sign. Vomiting, failure to thrive (as a result of renal insufficiency), and attacks of abdominal pain are present in some cases.

In children and adults, ureteropelvic juncture obstruction commonly is manifested by a perverse, cramping abdominal pain that may be paraumbilical or epigastric and not localized to the involved side. The discomfort can be promptly relieved by an indwelling ureteral catheter. Nausea

or vomiting with these attacks of pain suggests a gastrointestinal disorder rather than hydronephrosis. This may account for the fact that surgical correction of this congenital disorder is most frequent during the third and fourth decades of life (Culp, 1961). Gross hematuria either from acute distention of the renal collecting system or infection is a frequent occurrence. Contrary to clinical impression and the usual association with stasis, urinary infection was present in only 17 of 109 cases reported by Kelalis and associates (1971). Fortunately, the ureteropelvic juncture obstruction is usually discovered before the patient is azotemic; nevertheless, in instances of bilateral involvement or solitary kidney, the patient may be in a severe uremic state when first seen.

The roentgenographic appearance of

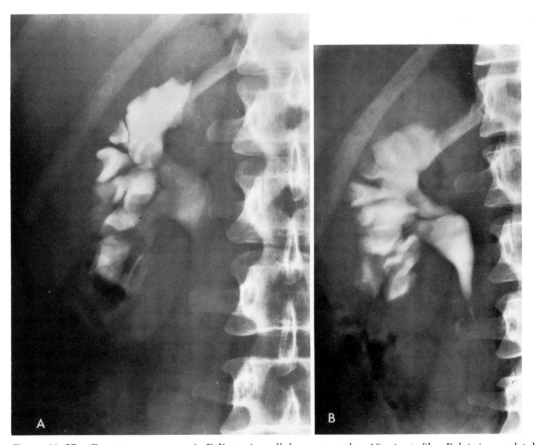

Figure 11–87.   *Excretory urograms.* **A, Caliectasis** well demonstrated on 10-minute film. Pelvis incompletely visualized. **B,** Patient was promptly turned to a prone position, which facilitated filling of the pelvis.

the hydronephrotic kidney secondary to ureteropelvic juncture obstruction corresponds to the description of hydronephrosis on pages 956 to 969. A few additional comments are pertinent to this congenital lesion.

An excretory urogram will usually demonstrate the distinctive ampullar or rectangular dilated pelvis without a visible ureteropelvic juncture. Routine dehydration prior to x-ray may obscure the diagnosis, but an infusion or hydration study (mannitol 25 g or furosemide 40 mg i.v.) with 1-hour or 2-hour postinjection exposures will intensify the deformity. This technique is also very useful if the patient is azotemic. Furthermore, exposures taken with the patient in the prone position will often display the renal pelvis and even the juncture better than exposures taken with the patient supine, because the renal pelvis projects anteriorly (Fig. 11-87). It is prudent to obtain a retrograde cystogram for patients with suspected ureteropelvic juncture obstruction to evaluate for complete vesicoureteral reflux, because these conditions may have a similar urographic appearance. It is always necessary to visualize the ureter to exclude obstruction distal to the juncture. If a retrograde pyeloureterogram is required, this is best done just prior to surgery in order to minimize the risk of infection.

SURGICAL CONSIDERATIONS IN URETEROPELVIC JUNCTURE OBSTRUCTION

The management of ureteropelvic juncture obstruction involves an analysis of a number of factors that are fundamental to a successful experience for the patient. Of special significance is the question of when surgical intervention is indicated. In the absence of pain, pyuria, or calculi, and if the calyces are well preserved and renal function is good, surgical intervention merely to reduce pyelectasis is not justified. If doubt exists about the surgical indication, it is better to observe the patient with periodic urographic, bacteriologic, and renal function studies. A moderately dilated renal pelvis may remain stabilized and asymptomatic for years. On the other hand, if the patient is symptomatic and there is any evidence of progressive hydronephrosis, procrastination may preclude reconstruction.

Deciding whether to perform a nephrectomy or a ureteropelvioplasty can be difficult. In the child, the recovery of a seemingly hopeless hydronephrotic kidney after repair can exceed all expectations. Furthermore, a nephrectomy may precipitate a subclinical or marginal juncture obstruction on the contralateral side by increasing the urine flow beyond the capability of the juncture. If pyonephrosis is present, with or without calculous development, and the margin of renal parenchyma is a centimeter or less, nephrectomy is indicated if the other kidney will provide adequate renal function. Sometimes the very difficult situation can be improved for more definitive surgery by employing a preliminary nephrostomy.

In instances of bilateral obstruction, repair should be done first on the more symptomatic side or, if a nephrectomy is planned for the contralateral side, on the side on which a pyeloplasty can be performed.

Culp (1961) has stressed that the choice of operations can never be based on arbitrary rules, rigid prerequisites, or didactic formulas. Too many earlier procedures were performed solely to remove a stone, to do a nephropexy, or to divide an aberrant vessel, while the intrinsic juncture obstruction was ignored. Anatomic variations in ureteropelvic juncture obstruction are responsible for such dissimilarities in therapeutic problems that no single operation will suffice for all situations. The basic objectives of any operation are to provide dependent drainage and a juncture of excellent caliber so that there is no discernible transition between pelvis and ureter (Figs. 11-88 through 11-91).

Conventional types of surgical procedures employed at the Mayo Clinic for repair of varieties of ureteropelvic juncture obstruction are shown in Figures 11-92 through 11-97.

Text continued on page 1005

Fig. 11–88

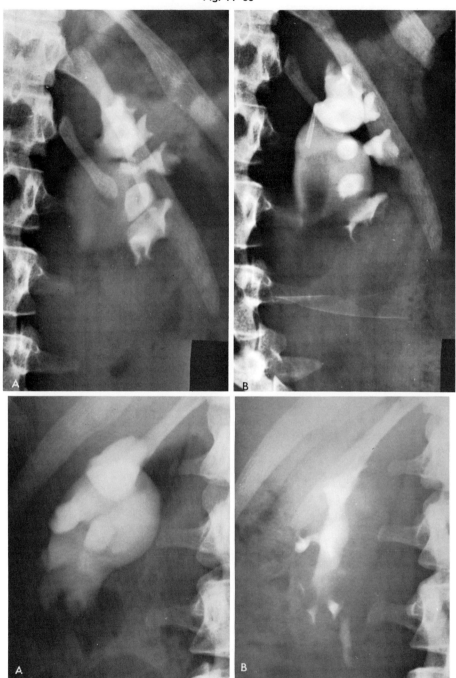

Fig. 11–89

Figure 11–88.   Fair to poor result of operation for obstruction. **A,** *Preoperative excretory urogram.* Pyelectasis, grade 2. **B,** *Postoperative film,* almost 6 months after severing anomalous vessels and performing Y-V ureteropelvioplasty on ureteropelvic juncture. Urographic change is not spectacular. **Moderate pyelectasis persists.**

Figure 11–89.   Good result of operation for obstruction. **A,** *Retrograde pyelogram, 25-minute delayed exposure.* **Grade 2 pyelectasis and caliectasis.** Marked retention of medium due to obstruction at ureteropelvic juncture. **B,** *Excretory urogram,* after plastic operation on ureteropelvic juncture. **Anomalous artery and vein at lower pole** cross ureter and produce partial obstruction. Pelvis and calyces have returned almost to normal. Some malrotation of kidney.

Fig. 11–90

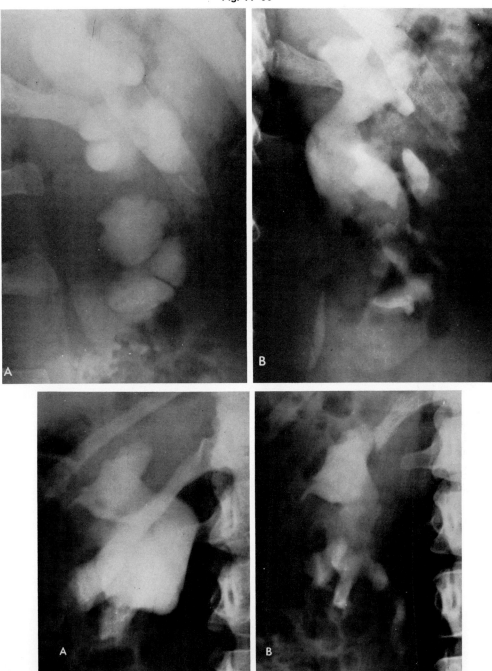

Fig. 11–91

Figure 11–90.   Good result of plastic operation on renal pelvis for hydronephrosis. **A,** *Preoperative excretory urogram.* **Marked left hydronephrosis,** showing huge dilated calyces. Pelvis not filled. Reduced function of kidney. (Left retrograde pyelogram showed **obstruction at ureteropelvic juncture** from pressure of large dilated renal pelvis. Contrast medium would not enter pelvis.) **B,** *Excretory urogram,* 13 months after operation. Improvement in function of kidney. Reduction in dilatation of pelvis and calyces.

Figure 11–91.   Good result of operation for obstruction. **A,** *Preoperative excretory urogram.* **Moderate right pyelectasis caused by obstruction at ureteropelvic juncture. B,** *Postoperative excretory urogram.* **Marked reduction in degree of dilatation of pelvis and calyces** after plastic operation on ureteropelvic juncture. Ureteropelvic juncture now patent, and medium freely enters ureter.

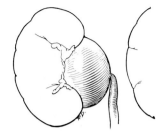

Figure 11–92. High insertion of ureter on renal pelvis. (From Culp, O. S., 1955.)

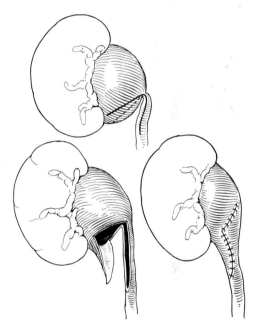

Figure 11–93. Technique of **Y-V** ureteropelvioplasty in cases of high insertion of ureter. Incisions are made on anterior and posterior surfaces of dilated pelvis and along medial aspect of ureter, thereby creating flap of pelvic tissue which is sutured to incised ureter in form of **V**. (From Culp, O. S., 1961.)

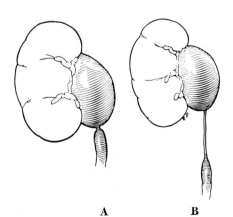

Figure 11–94. Obstructed ureteropelvic juncture that already has **dependent position. Constriction** may be located as shown in **A,** or it may be much longer as in **B.** (From Culp, O. S., and DeWeerd, J. H.)

A   B

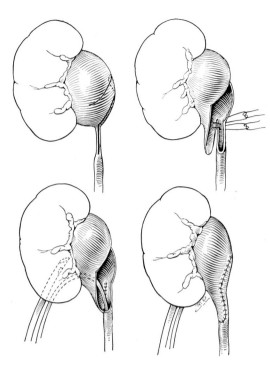

Figure 11-95. Technique of spiral-flap operation in cases in which ureteropelvic juncture is already in dependent position. Converging incisions from broad, slightly oblique base adjacent to original juncture are joined after following spherical contour of dilated renal pelvis for sufficient distance to assure flap longer than constricted segment of the ureter. This flap is interposed between edges of split ureter, and defect in pelvis is closed. (From Culp, O. S., and DeWeerd, J. H.)

Figure 11-96. Unusually long constriction of ureter. (From Culp, O. S., 1955.)

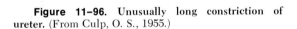

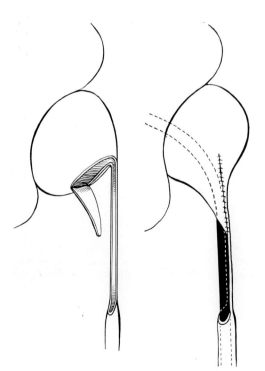

Figure 11-97. Technique of Davis, intubated ureterotomy combined with **Y-V ureteropelvioplasty** used in patients who have long segment of ureteral constriction. (From Culp, O. S., 1955.)

URETERECTASIS AND URETEROPYELECTASIS

GENERAL PRINCIPLES AND CONSIDERATIONS

It may be difficult to distinguish minimal degrees of ureterectasis from the normal because of the considerable variation in the size of normal ureters and the completeness with which the ureter is filled with contrast medium. Unless ureterectasis is definite, it should be considered of doubtful clinical significance.

Widening of the ureter is the first sign of dilatation (Fig. 11–98). As the process continues, the ureter also may lengthen and become tortuous (Figs. 11–99 and 11–100). If ureterectasis results from obstruction, the dilatation usually is confined to

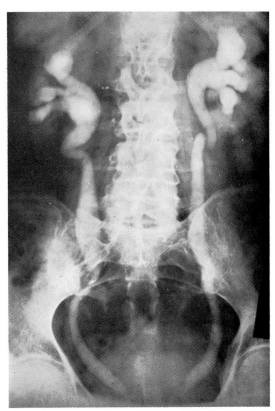

Figure 11–99. *Excretory urogram.* **Bilateral ureteropyelectasis** caused by obstruction from carcinoma of cervix.

the part of the ureter above the point of obstruction (Fig. 11–101). If infection is present, however, there also may be dilatation below. Dilatation of the lower third of the ureter is a fairly common result of urinary infection, especially of recurring cystitis (Fig. 11–102). It also may be the first manifestation of obstruction of the vesical neck or urethra.

Diagnostic Errors From Incomplete Filling

As mentioned previously, serious diagnostic errors may occur with either the excretory urogram or retrograde pyelogram if complete filling of the pelvis and ureter is not obtained. Examples of such possibilities are seen in Figures 11–103, 11–104, and 11–105. Attention has already been called to the propensity of pelves and ureters that have been previously infected and dilated (or are involved with vesi-

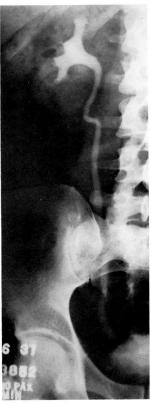

Figure 11–98. *Excretory urogram.* **Right ureteropyelectasis, grade 1,** with filling defect in region of ureterovesical juncture due to edema secondary to recently passed stone.

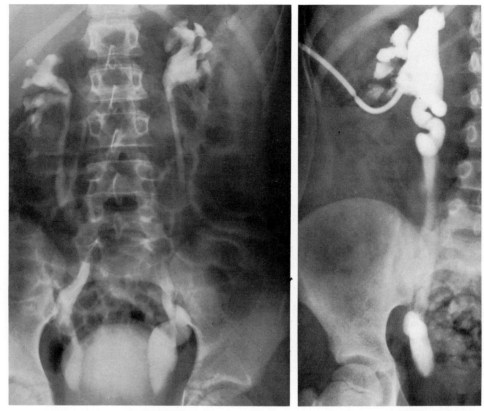

Fig. 11–100   Fig. 11–101

Figure 11–100. *Excretory urogram.* **Marked dilatation of lower third of each ureter, with lesser degree of ureterectasis above.** Cicatricial and inflammatory changes in both pelves and calyces from long-standing infection. Patient had **urinary obstruction due to stenosis of urethral meatus.** Cystogram in this case showed reflux up both ureters. Cystoscopy showed bladder trabeculation, grade 1.

Figure 11–101. *Pyelogram made through nephrostomy tube.* Boy, aged 12 years, had **long-standing congenital obstruction of vesical neck. There are marked tortuosity and dilatation of ureter, with associated pyelocaliectasis.**

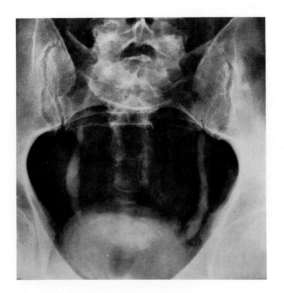

Figure 11–102. *Excretory urogram.* **Dilatation of lower third of each ureter.** Apparently result of ascending infection.

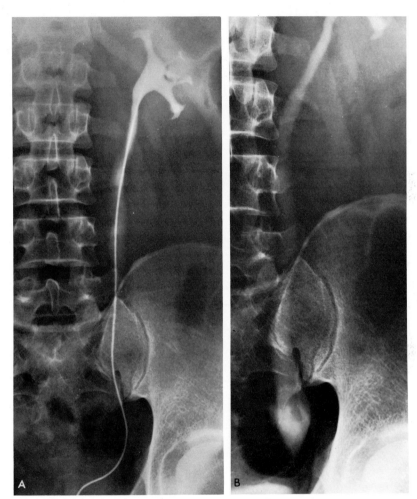

Figure 11-103. Possible diagnostic error from incomplete filling with contrast medium. *Left retrograde pyelograms.* **A,** *First pyelogram, made with only upper half of ureter filled.* Pelvis and calyces normal. Suggestion of **mild ureterectasis in middle third. B,** *Second pyelogram, made with ureter completely filled.* **Marked dilatation in lower third of left ureter,** which could be missed because of incomplete filling in first pyelogram. Note that ureter narrows to normal size at its intramural site. No reflux.

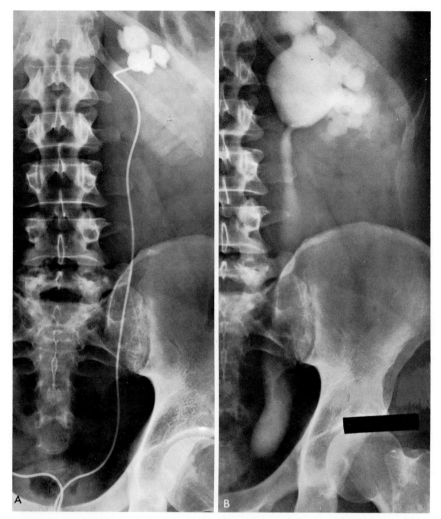

Figure 11–104.   Possible diagnostic error from incomplete filling with contrast medium. *Left retrograde pyelograms.* **A,** Only group of calyces in upper half of left kidney outlined. Calyces irregularly dilated, suggesting possibility of renal tuberculosis. **B,** *Pelvis and ureter completely filled.* Lesion shown to be marked hydronephrosis and hydroureter, with marked dilatation of lower third of left ureter. Note that ureter narrows to normal size at its intramural site. No reflux. (At operation, no evidence of obstruction to ureter was found.)

coureteral reflux) to dilate readily from retrograde injection of contrast medium or from ureteral compression during excretory urography.

Segmental Ureterectasis

Dilatation of isolated segments of the ureter provides interesting urograms. Usually, the explanation of the dilatation is not clear. It is most likely the result of some congenital error in development. The most common site is the lower third of the ureter (Figs. 11–106, 11–107, and 11–108), although other parts of the ureter may be involved (Figs. 11–109 and 11–110). Abnormalities of the intramural ureter (both physiologic and pathologic) as causes of dilatation of the terminal ureter are discussed further on in this chapter.

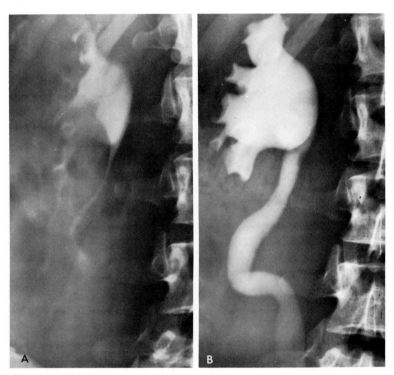

Figure 11–105.   Pelvis and ureter appear normal in excretory urogram but definite pyeloureterectasis demonstrated in retrograde pyelogram. A, *Excretory urogram.* Pyelectasis, grade 1. B, *Right retrograde pyelogram* few days later. Pelvis and ureter completely filled and dilated – **pyeloureterectasis, grade 2.** (No surgical exploration.)

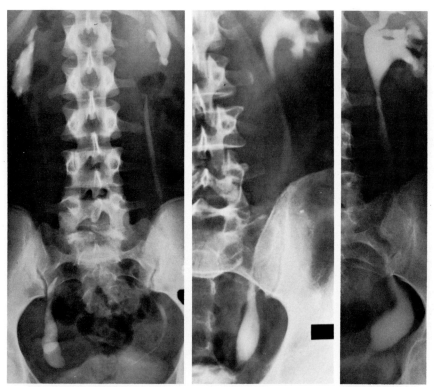

Fig. 11–106   Fig. 11–107   Fig. 11–108

Figure 11–106.   *Excretory urogram.* Localized dilatation of lower third of right ureter with apparently normal intramural ureter. Bilateral malrotation of kidneys.

Figures 11–107 and **11–108.**   *Left retrograde pyelogram.* Localized, apparently congenital, dilatation of lower third of left ureter with little or no dilatation above. Ureter narrows to normal size before entering bladder. No reflux.

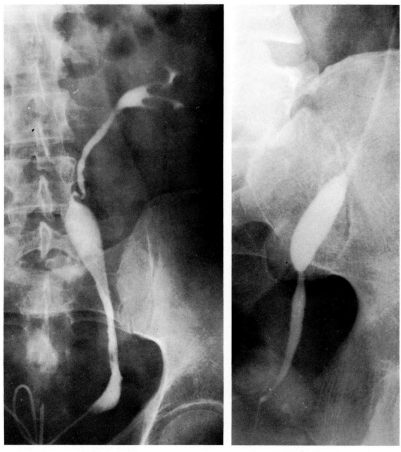

Fig. 11–109   **Fig. 11–110**

Figure 11–109. *Left retrograde pyelogram.* **Dilatation of lower two thirds of ureter** with no dilatation above. Marked angulation at juncture of normal upper third and dilated lower two thirds of ureter.

Figure 11–110. *Left retrograde pyelogram.* **Unusually localized dilatation of ureter over promontory of sacrum.** Could be regarded as exaggerated spindle.

Obstructive Ureterectasis: Obstruction at or Above the Ureterovesical Juncture

INTRINSIC OBSTRUCTION

Obstructive ureterectasis may result from intrinsic or extrinsic obstruction. The common causes of obstruction within the ureter are stone, tumor, stricture, stenosis of the ureteral meatus, and ureterocele. Ureterectasis caused by stone is discussed in Chapter 12; by tumor, in Chapter 14; and by ureterocele, in Chapter 9.

Stricture of the Ureter

Strictures may be of inflammatory, traumatic, or congenital origin. *Stricture of inflammatory origin* may result from infection within the urinary tract or from infection of nearby structures such as an appendiceal abscess (see Chapter 7). *Congenital stricture* is seen most frequently in the upper third of the ureter and is considered under the subject of obstruction of the ureteropelvic juncture (see also Figs. 11–77 through 11–79, 11–88 through 11–91, and 11–94 through 11–97). The next most common site is the ureteral meatus or intramural portion of the ureter or both. The accuracy of the diagnosis of many reported cases of so-called congenital stenosis of the ureteral orifice, however, may be questioned, because of the controversy regarding what constitutes an abnormal ureterovesical juncture. If a size 5-F catheter will pass unobstructed through the meatus and intramural portion of the ureter, the diagnosis of obstruction is questionable. This subject is discussed more fully later in this chapter under the subject of nonobstructive ureterectasis.

Iatrogenic Stricture of the Ureteral Meatus and of the Intramural Ureter. Postoperative stricture of the ureteral meatus and intramural portion of the ureter is a definite and not infrequently encountered entity. Usually it is the result of transurethral prostatic resection, although it also may result from open or transurethral resection of the bladder for cancer, open prostatectomy, or other surgical procedures on the bladder. When it occurs after transurethral prostatic resection, the operation usually has been carried a little too far

cephalad so that either the ureteral orifice was damaged or the adjacent bladder was resected so near the orifice that in healing the scar tissue involved the ureteral orifice. Cystoscopically, the orifice then is visualized as retracted into the scarred vesical neck, and it may or may not be identified. This situation is a common complication of postoperative contracture of the vesical neck. The degree of obstruction may vary from minimal to advanced with complete occlusion (Figs. 11–111 and 11–112).

A less common type of iatrogenic ureteral stricture is that resulting from implantation of radon seeds near the ureteral orifice or near the intramural ureter in cases of bladder cancer (Fig. 11–113). Ureteral stricture may also result from manipulation of ureteral calculi (Figs. 11–114 and 11–115).

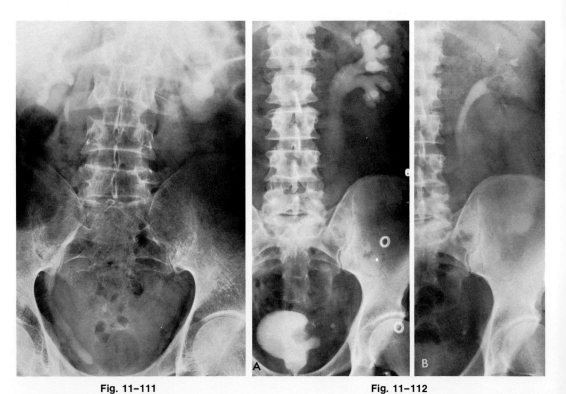

Fig. 11–111   **Fig. 11–112**

Figure 11–111. *Excretory urogram.* **Bilateral obstruction of ureteral orifices secondary to repeated transurethral resection of bladder and vesical neck.** Obstruction most marked on left, with **pyelectasis, grade 3,** and ureter not filled. On right, entire ureter outlined, showing mild obstruction at ureteral orifice.

Figure 11–112. **Stenosis of left ureteral orifice after transurethral resection.** No function on left. Normal kidney and ureter on right. *Excretory urograms.* **A,** Two weeks after left ureteroneocystostomy. Function has returned. **Pyeloureterectasis, grade 2.** Note negative filling defect from cuff of ureter in bladder. **B,** Fourteen months after operation. Kidney and ureter have returned almost to normal.

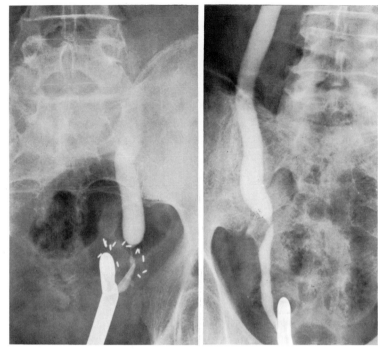

Figure 11–113. *Retrograde pyelogram made with bulb catheter inserted just inside ureteral meatus.* Ureteral stricture resulting from radon seeds implanted into bladder tumor. (Tumor was eradicated.) Ureter is kept open and kidney function maintained by ureteral dilation every 4 months.

Figure 11–114. *Retrograde pyelogram.* Stricture of right ureter following transurethral manipulation of ureteral stone. (Excision and end-to-end anastomosis.)

Fig. 11–113   Fig. 11–114

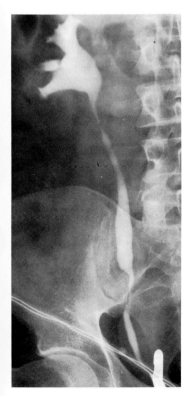

Figure 11–115. *Retrograde pyelogram.* Stricture and deformity of lower third of right ureter after traumatic manipulation of ureteral stone.

*EXTRINSIC (EXTRAURETERAL)
OBSTRUCTION*

A seemingly endless variety of neo-plastic or inflammatory intra-abdominal or retroperitoneal lesions may obstruct the ureter by pressure, constriction, or direct invasion.

Neoplastic Obstruction. Among the neoplasms that may involve the ureter is *carcinoma of the colon*, especially of the rectosigmoid (Figs. 11–116, 11–117, and 11–118). All pelvic tumors in women, in-cluding carcinoma of the cervix, are poten-tial causes of obstruction (see Chapter 19). *Retroperitoneal tumors* such as sarcoma, lymphoma, and carcinoma of the pancreas may obstruct the ureters (Fig. 11–119; see also Chapter 14). Of course, any malignant tumor can metastasize and compromise the ureter at some level. Extravesical extension of *carcinoma of the prostate* is a frequent cause of obstruction of the lower part of the ureter (Fig. 11–120). Ureteral obstruction from carcinoma of the bladder is shown in Figure 11–121.

Endometriosis is discussed separately in Chapter 19.

Inflammatory Obstruction. Probably the inflammatory lesion that most fre-quently causes ureteral obstruction is *pel-vic inflammatory disease in women* (see Chapter 19, Figures 19–82 and 19–83).

Ureteral obstruction from *retroperito-neal fibrosis* is discussed in Chapter 20.

Vascular Obstruction. Aneurysms of the abdominal aorta will frequently cause ureteral obstruction (see Chapter 19). Ob-

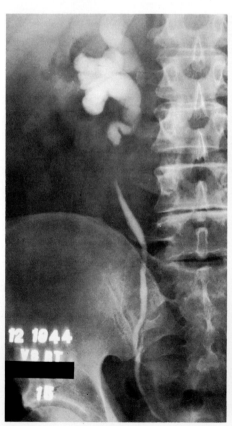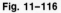

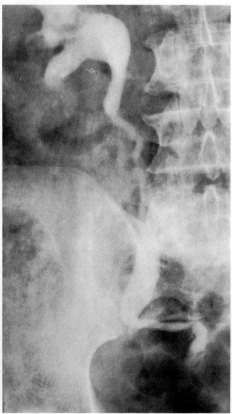

Fig. 11–116   Fig. 11–117

Figure 11–116. *Right retrograde pyelogram.* **Obstruction in upper third of right ureter caused by extension of carcinoma of hepatic flexure of colon.**

Figure 11–117. *Retrograde pyelogram.* **Postoperative recurrence of carcinoma of rectosigmoid. Obstruction of right ureter.** Later, left ureter also became obstructed. (Palliative left nephrostomy was done.)

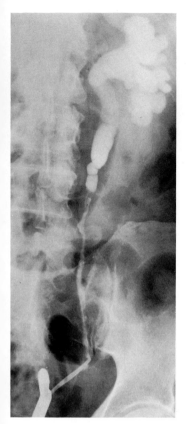

Figure 11–118. *Retrograde pyelogram.* **Ureteral obstruction from recurring carcinoma of lower part of sigmoid.** Narrowing of lower two thirds of ureter. Kidney showed no function on excretory urography.

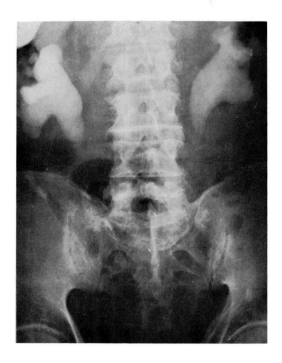

Figure 11–119. *Excretory urogram.* **Bilateral ureteral obstruction caused by carcinoma of pancreas.** (Courtesy of Dr. R. O. Pearman.)

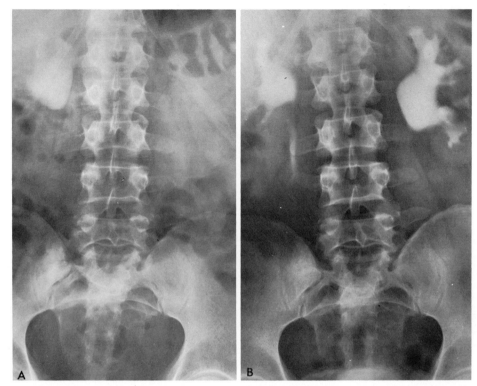

Figure 11–120. Lower ureteral obstruction from cephalad extravesical extension of carcinoma of prostate. A, *Excretory urogram.* **Nonfunctioning left kidney. Pyelectasis on right. B,** *Excretory urogram* made 14 months after bilateral orchiectomy. Regression in growth. Left kidney now functioning, although pyelectasis persists. Reduction in degree of pyelectasis on right.

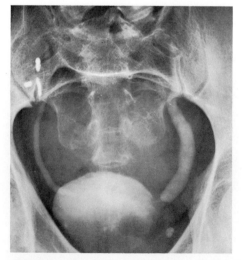

Figure 11–121. *Excretory urogram.* Obstruction of left ureter from infiltrating carcinoma of bladder.

struction of the ureteropelvic juncture and upper part of the ureter by anomalous blood vessels may accompany intrinsic lesions. Obstruction of the lower part of the ureter from this cause is less common. Relatively few such cases have been reported. In the majority of these, the primary obstruction was near the ureterovesical juncture, and the vessel compromised the ureter only after the ureter had become dilated. In a few cases, however, anomalous vessels are the primary cause of obstruction low in the ureter (Greene and associates, 1954) (see Chapter 17, Figs. 17–69 and 17–70).

Miscellaneous Obstructions. *Vesical diverticula* may cause ureteral obstruction. The ureter may be compressed and dis-

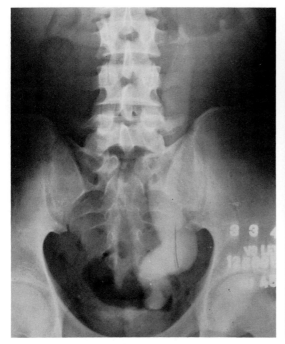
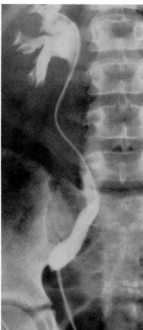

Fig. 11–122   Fig. 11–123

Figure 11–122. *Forty-five-minute excretory urogram.* **Huge dilatation of left ureter, resulting from obstruction by vesical diverticulum and congenital obstruction of vesical neck** in man aged 19 years. Right kidney urographically normal, as was shown in 15- and 20-minute urograms. In this urogram most of the medium had exited from right kidney.

Figure 11–123. *Retrograde pyelogram.* **Ureteral obstruction from fixation by band of periureteral tissue** (in boy, age 12). (Operation showed abrupt transition between dilated flabby portion of ureter and normal ureter below. There appeared to be angulation at this point. Sheath of ureter and adjacent tissues were divided and ureter became perfectly straight.) Subsequent excretory urogram showed that ureter had returned to normal.

placed by the diverticulum (Fig. 11–122).

Pregnancy results in ureteral obstruction and infection that is called either *pyelitis* or *pyeloureterectasis of pregnancy.* This is discussed in Chapter 19.

Congenital bands and *adhesions* may occasionally be responsible for ureteral obstruction (Fig. 11–123).

VESICOURETERAL REFLUX

by Panayotis P. Kelalis

Vesicoureteral reflux was demonstrated in animals toward the end of the last century (Lewin and Goldschmidt), and soon thereafter its importance in urinary infection was recognized by several authors who tried, unsuccessfully, to focus attention on the problem (Graves and Davidoff,

1923, 1924; Gruber, 1929a, 1929b; Sampson). Hutch's description of reflux in the neurogenic bladder in 1952 rekindled interest in the disorder, and this soon multiplied in a geometric fashion. As a result, reflux has been subjected to more detailed analysis and scrutiny than any other urinary tract disorder of childhood.

Irrefutable evidence accumulated to date, and contrary to convictions previously held by some, suggests that in the majority of cases reflux is a congenital disorder and may be familial. It is in the area of treatment, however, that much of the debate has continued. There has been considerable meeting of minds, and yet as one reviews the subject, one soon realizes that separation of reliable data from clinical impressions is difficult; a certain individualistic approach is evident, based mostly on personal experiences rather than applied scientific data.

General Considerations

Several well-conducted studies in asymptomatic normal children and adults have established conclusively that vesicoureteral reflux does not occur in the normal urinary tract (Iannaccone and Panzironi; Jones and Headstream; Leadbetter and associates) and that in a significant number of cases it may have a familial incidence involving several generations (Burger; Mulcahy and associates; Tobenkin; Zel and Retik), siblings, or even twins (Stephens and associates).

Epidemiologic studies of the true incidence of reflux in the general population are lacking, but the disorder is known to be rare in blacks (King, Kazmi, and Belman). The more frequent occurrence in female children noted in clinical studies is probably related to the ease with which girls acquire urinary infections that lead to investigation and the subsequent diagnosis of reflux (Kelalis, 1971).

Children who have reflux appear to experience urinary tract infection at an earlier age than their anatomically normal counterparts (Govan and Palmer). Even though the clinical picture nearly always suggests urinary infection, it is not always possible from the symptoms alone to predict which patients will have significant anatomic abnormalities or vesicoureteral reflux (Segura and associates). When both urinary infection and reflux are present, however, the morbidity is increased. Pain in the renal region when the bladder is full or during voiding is almost diagnostic of reflux, but this symptom is infrequent in children and, in the adult, is usually related to an undilated urinary collecting system. Hypertension and progressive renal failure, with polyuria but without urographic evidence of urinary infection, interstitial changes in the kidneys, or vesicoureteral reflux, have been described in association with reflux (Stickler and associates).

Between 30 per cent and 55 per cent of children with urinary infective symptoms have reflux. Differences in the recorded rate of incidence mainly reflect variations in patient age, the indications for and technique of cystography used, and such variables as the dye, its concentration, and the mode of its introduction, the presence or absence of infection, the use of anesthesia, and the origin and nature of the population studied. For example, black children, especially girls, have a much lower incidence of reflux than whites. Furthermore, the problem of calculating prevalence is further complicated by the spontaneous cure of reflux. Nevertheless, over 40 per cent of children who have urinary infection in the first two years of life will have significant renal disease related to reflux.

Clearly the search for reflux is closely linked to the investigation of urinary infection. Usually such investigation is pursued upon the first attack in boys, but it is frequently deferred until the second or third infection in girls. The rationale for delaying investigation in girls is not supported by objective data; reflux associated with significant anomalies occurs equally in both sexes, and children with their first attack of urinary infection are as likely to have renal cortical changes from reflux as are those with multiple infections. Therefore, if urinary infection is present, radiologic studies should be performed without delay, except in acute cases, as the clinical pattern alone does not allow one to confirm the presence or establish the severity of vesicoureteral reflux, and there is no other method of assessing the extent of the disease (Bailey).

Such an investigation should include cine cystourethrography and excretory urography; the two tests are complementary and by no means supplant each other. Cystoscopy is necessary for accurate classification of the etiology of reflux for purposes of treatment.

Roentgen Findings in Vesicoureteral Reflux

The methods available for investigating reflux are at best crude, and they frequently fail to demonstrate it even though positive features suggest its presence.

Nonradiologic techniques such as chromatocystoscopy (Motzkin) have not gained popular acceptance. Direct radionuclide cystography using short half-life radiopharmaceuticals (99m Tc pertechnetate) is considered by some to be more reliable for detecting vesicoureteral reflux than conventional roentgenographic techniques (Conway and associates). In addition to the presence of reflux, parameters that simultaneously can be determined by this method include the bladder volume when reflux occurs, calculation of the volume of fluid that has refluxed, accurate calculation of residual urine volume, and estimation of reflux drainage time. The main disadvantage at this time is poor resolution. The major advantage of nuclear cystography is of course the small radiation dose, which is estimated to be 1 per cent of that incurred in a single urographic study.

Bartrina in 1935 introduced cystography for the study of reflux, and at present *cystourethrography* and *standard cystography* are almost universally used. They should be deferred until the child has recovered from any episode of active urinary infection, because it is probable that the reflux is secondary to the infection. However, bacteriuria in itself is not considered a contraindication to such evaluation. The great advantage of performing the investigation without anesthesia is that the child can inform the examiner when his bladder is full (or else this will become evident from the patient's expressions of discomfort), providing valid guidance regarding the functional capacity of the bladder and a physiologic measure of the extent of reflux.

Cystourethrography combined with fluoroscopy has the advantage of monitored filling, controlled continuous visualization of the bladder, and the opportunity to take spot films as necessary to depict a momentary incident in the act of voiding. At the same time, the functional state of the urinary tract, specifically the peristaltic activity of the refluxing unit and the ability of the bladder to empty, can be ascertained, thus excluding significant vesical neck obstruction or dysfunction.

Reports of the relative effectiveness of both methods are available (Gross and Sanderson; Smith; Stewart), though the fleeting nature of the reflux per se would naturally raise questions about the value of the negative retrograde cystogram. Clearly, the cystogram provides information about the state of the urinary tract at only one particular moment and therefore does not represent the events that take place before or after (Fig. 11–124). Indeed, it is likely that the two methods are neither comparable nor complementary, except in patients in whom advanced ureteral dilatation from reflux is present (Vlahakis and associates).

Grading of Vesicoureteral Reflux

Various attempts have been made to grade vesicoureteral reflux according to severity, in the hope that comparison among series cases would be facilitated. Some studies classify vesicoureteral reflux according to degree (partial or complete), some according to timing—occurring during filling or voiding (low or high pressure reflux)—and some according to the degree of associated ureterectasis. Unfortunately, there is no uniformity of opinion among the various authors about basic premises or about the criteria upon which the grading should be based. Most authors use grading schemes based solely on radiologic findings. In all these attempts at categorization, emphasis is laid on the extent to which reflux fills the ureters and the degree of ureteral dilatation it produces on the cystographic study (Winberg and associates). Certainly the volume of urine refluxed is important in planning therapy. Large volumes comprise pools of residual urine that clearly predispose to infection. However, such grading carries the implication that there is a difference with respect to the potential for kidney damage—for example, between complete and incomplete ureteral filling. In this regard, Duffy found parenchymal scarring of the kidneys irrespective

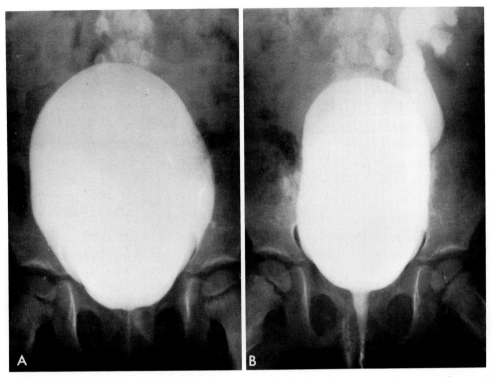

Figure 11–124. Demonstration of reflux. **A,** *Cystogram* of girl, aged 3½. No evidence of reflux. **B,** *Voiding cystourethrogram.* **Marked reflux up dilated left ureter.** Bladder neck and urethra appear as normal. (From Gould, H. R., and Peterson, C. G., Jr.)

of whether reflux was partial or complete. Complete but transitory ureteral filling should not be considered any less dangerous than partial filling that persists throughout the cystographic examination — and vice versa.

Others employ intravesical pressure measurements at cineradiography in addition, and subdivide the cases into groups depending on the pressure and bladder volume at which reflux first appears (Lattimer and associates, 1963; Melick and associates). The problem here, of course, is the variation of normal bladder volumes and pressures, not only in different individuals but also in the same individual at different times — which can produce misleading interpretations.

Again, because the urethra is blocked by the catheter during the filling phase of the cystogram, the intravesical pressure generated during this stage may be greater than the normal voiding pressure, especially when the child is straining or crying. Thus the filling phase of the cystogram is not always the low-pressure phase of the examination, and therefore the distinction between low-pressure reflux occurring during the filling stages of the cystogram and high-pressure reflux occurring during the voiding stages is probably meaningless. Again, reflux may be present early during filling at one examination and during a later phase in another, and may be absent during the third. Conway and associates, using nuclear techniques to monitor the bladder during the entire examination, have found that reflux occurs during the filling phase but not during the voiding phase much more frequently than the other way around.

Posture appears at times to influence the function of the ureterovesical juncture. Reflux may not be apparent when the patient is in the supine position, but when the table is tilted into the erect position, reflux often appears. This may be caused by an increase in the intravesical pressure produced by the weight of the abdominal contents or by the posterior displacement

Pyelotubular Backflow

of the bladder, leading to shortening of the intramural ureter (Cass and Lenaghan).

Despite the deficiencies of any classification mentioned, some form of "grading" is essential for purposes of comparison and meaningful therapeutic data. Grading the reflux according to the maximum degree seen during the cystographic study is quite logical because the proportion of patients with renal changes generally increases with the grade of reflux (Willscher and associates). Such schemes should be used with the full realization that the vagaries of reflux are endless and that there has been no study in which a group of children has been evaluated on consecutive days to demonstrate variations of the patterns of reflux.

Ureteral reflux has been described as an evanescent condition, sometimes present, sometimes absent, sometimes unilateral and at other times bilateral. It may also be an intermittent phenomenon.

Dwoskin and Perlmutter have proposed the following scheme of grading reflux (Fig. 11–125):

Grade I: Lower ureteral filling.
Grade II A: Ureteral and pelviocalyceal filling without other changes.
Grade II B: Ureteral and pelviocalyceal filling with mild calyceal blunting but without clubbing and without dilatation of the pelvis or tortuosity of the ureter.
Grade III: Ureteral and pelviocalyceal filling, calyceal clubbing, and minimum to moderate pelvic dilatation with slight tortuosity of the ureter.
Grade IV: Massive hydronephrosis and hydroureter—refluxing mega-ureter.

Winberg and associates similarly classify reflux into four grades but do not subdivide Group II. This system of classification is also employed at the Mayo Clinic (Figs. 11–126 through 11–129).

Pyelotubular backflow during reflux may be an important route of infection into the papillary ducts (Fig. 11–130) (Hodson and associates; Rolleston, Shannon, and Utley, 1970a, 1970b). In the experience of this author it is most often seen in infants

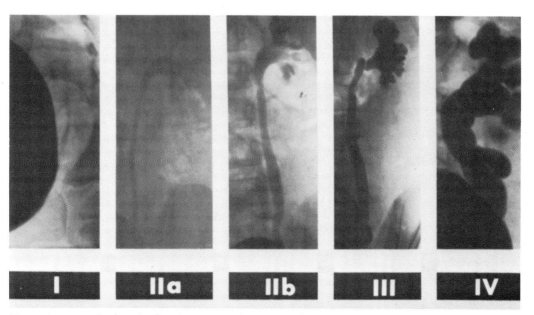

Figure 11–125. Grades of reflux. (From Dwoskin, J. Y., and Perlmutter, A. D.: Vesicoureteral Reflux in Children: A Computerized Review. J. Urol. *109*:888–890, 1973.)

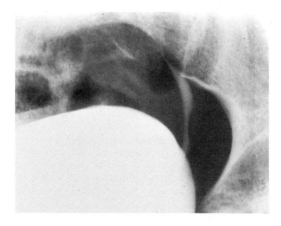

Figure 11-126. *Cystogram.* Vesicoureteral reflux, grade 1.

during phases of the cystogram corresponding to high intravesical pressures. When these children are followed into childhood, some exhibit parenchymal scars, at times in the absence of obstructive uropathy or urinary infection. Rolleston, Maling, and Hodson discussed 386 children with vesicoureteral reflux and indicated that intrarenal reflux occurred in 16, all under 4 years old, each of whom had rather marked degrees of reflux. Renal scarring later developed in 13 of the 20 kidneys showing intrarenal reflux, and in 12 of those 13 renal scarring corresponded to the part of the kidney with intrarenal reflux. However, 7 of the 20 kidneys with intrarenal reflux remained normal, and 45 ad-

ditional kidneys in which renal clubbing and scarring developed had no evidence of intrarenal reflux.

Probably one of the most paradoxic situations in urology is the occasional tremendous difference in appearance of the excretory urogram and the retrograde cystogram; in this regard the excretory urogram may be misleading because minimal degrees of ureterectasis, a common urographic finding, may convert to gross dilatation during retrograde flow of urine to the kidneys (Figs. 11-131 and 11-132) (Stephens and Lenaghan). Because the regurgitated column of urine is added to the contents of the renal pelvis, distention of the pelvis may simulate apparent ureteropelvic obstruc-

Text continued on page 1027

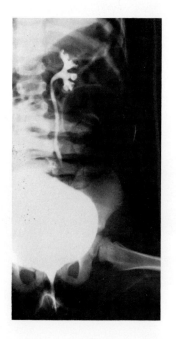

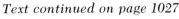

Figure 11-127. *Cystogram.* Unilateral vesicoureteral reflux, grade 2.

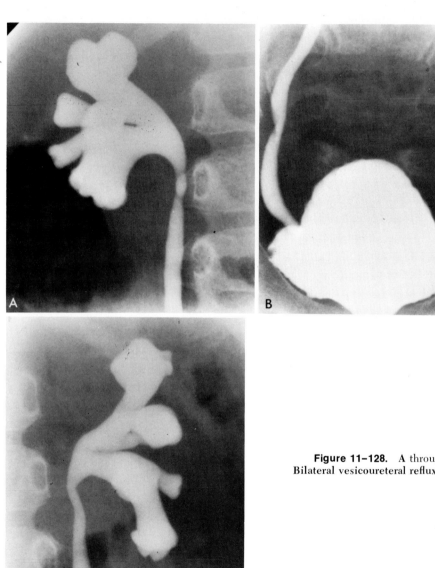

Figure 11–128. A through C. *Cystograms.* Bilateral vesicoureteral reflux, grade 3.

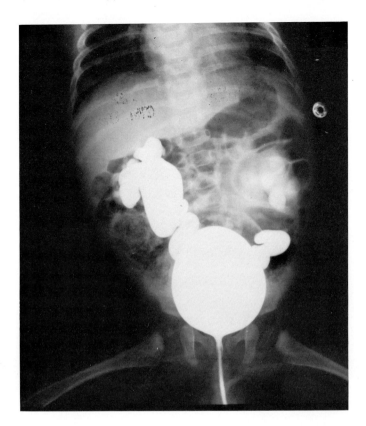

Figure 11–129. *Cystogram.* Massive bilateral vesicoureteral reflux, grade 4, in newborn infant.

Figure 11–130. *Cystogram.* Bilateral vesicoureteral reflux. Paraureteral diverticula. Intrarenal reflux on right.

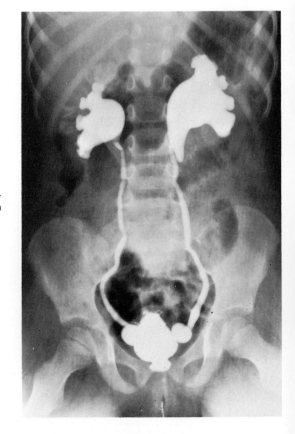

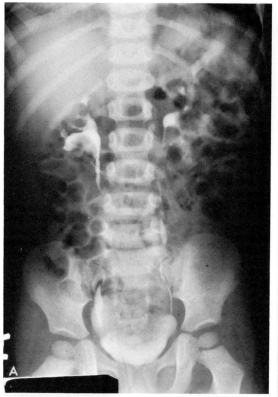

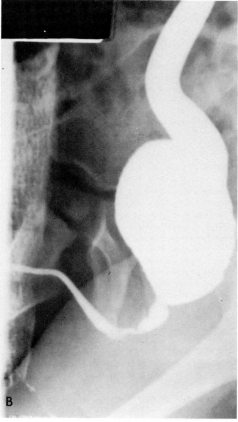

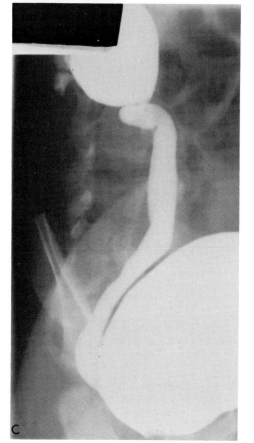

Figure 11-131. A, *Excretory urogram.* B and C, *Voiding cystourethrograms.* **Dilatation of upper urinary tract** apparent only at cystourethrography.

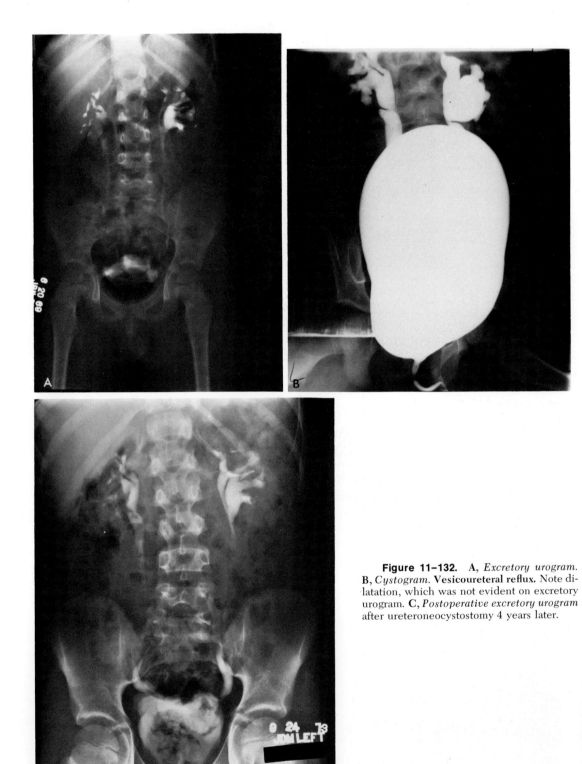

Figure 11–132. A, *Excretory urogram.* B, *Cystogram.* **Vesicoureteral reflux.** Note dilatation, which was not evident on excretory urogram. **C,** *Postoperative excretory urogram* after ureteroneocystostomy 4 years later.

tion, a common diagnostic pitfall (Figs. 11–133, 11–134, and 11–135) (Kelalis and associates, 1971).

Reflux and ureterovesical juncture obstruction may coexist. Weiss and Lytton found that 15 per cent of refluxing ureters showed evidence of such an obstruction, judged by delayed ureteral drainage and the characteristic rounded appearance of the dilated distal ureter, which seemed separate from the bladder (Figs. 11–136 and 11–137). This is an important observation, for relief of obstruction in such cases should take precedence over the management of reflux.

The excretory urogram accurately depicts anatomic derangement of the renal parenchyma consisting of either generalized or focal atrophy, which in turn at times is secondary to pyramidal retraction or destruction of the papilla from infection (Figs. 11–138 through 11–144).

Other indications of the presence of reflux include generalized caliectasis with marked narrowing of the cortical substance and an irregular renal outline (Fig. 11–145), generalized dilatation of the entire ureter or its lower third (Figs. 11–146 and 11–147), and striations in the pelvis or ureter suggesting temporary collapse of a dilated system (Figs. 11–148 and 11–149) (Silber and McAlister). The sudden appearance of contrast medium in a previously functionless or poorly visualized collecting system during excretory urography suggests reflux (Figs. 11–150 and 11–151). Occasionally, the bizarre shape of the kidney with reflux, caused by selective growth of normal areas, may lead to a misdiagnosis of renal tumor (Figs. 11–152 and 11–153).

Depending on the population studied, between one third and three fifths of children with reflux and the majority of adults will demonstrate scarring of the kidney on

Text continued on page 1038

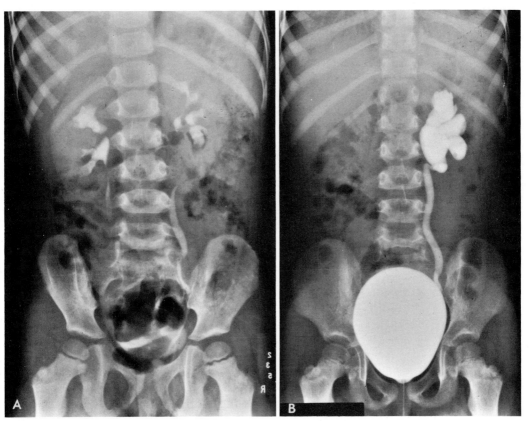

Figure 11–133. **A,** *Excretory urogram.* Collecting system essentially normal. **B,** *Cystogram.* **Vesicoureteral reflux** on left. Incipient obstruction of the ureteropelvic juncture.

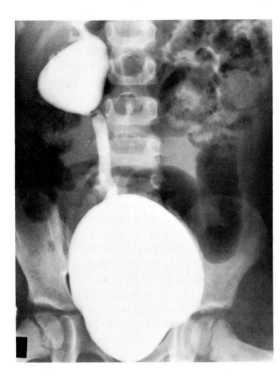

Figure 11-134. *Cystogram.* **Right vesicoureteral reflux** with apparent obstruction of ureteropelvic juncture. Excretory urogram was normal.

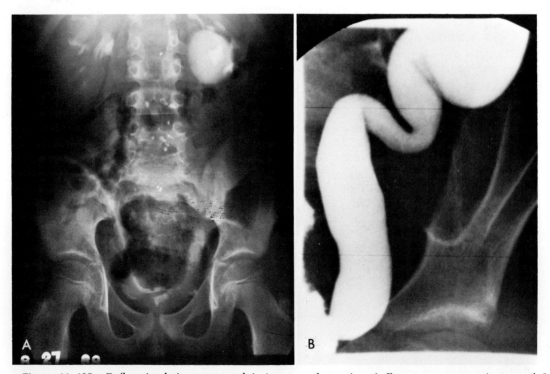

Figure 11-135. Reflux simulating ureteropelvic juncture obstruction. **A,** *Excretory urogram.* Apparent left ureteropelvic juncture obstruction. Note distal ureterectasis suggesting reflux. **B,** *Cystogram.* **Massive left vesico-ureteral reflux.**

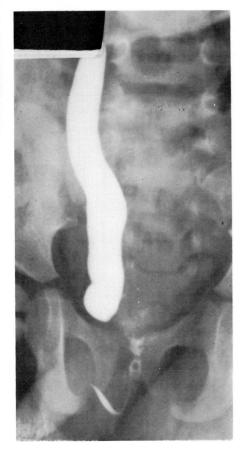

Figure 11–136. *Urethrogram.* **Obstructive refluxing megaureter.** Delayed emptying of refluxed contrast medium at cystography after completion of voiding.

Figure 11–137. *Voiding cinecystourethrogram.* **Bilateral vesicoureteral reflux.** Obstructive megaureter on left side.

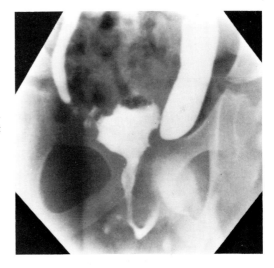

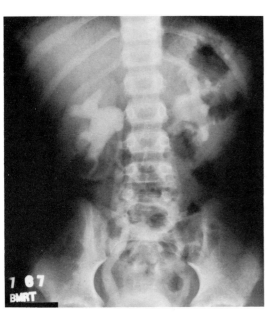

Figure 11–138. *Excretory urogram.* "Reflux" kidney. Localized retraction of cortex.

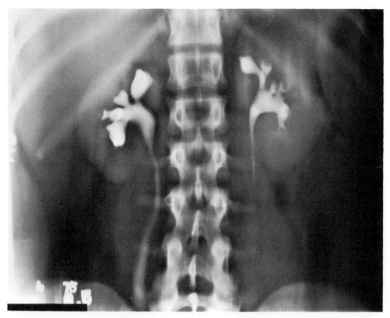

Figure 11–139. *Excretory urogram.* **Bilateral vesicoureteral reflux.** Excretory urographic changes confined to upper poles.

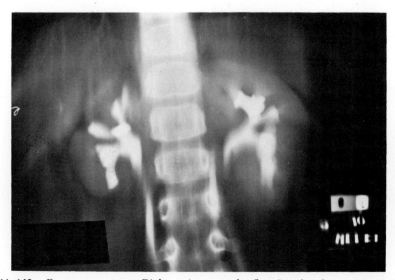

Figure 11–140. *Excretory urogram.* **Right vesicoureteral reflux.** Localized scars in right kidney.

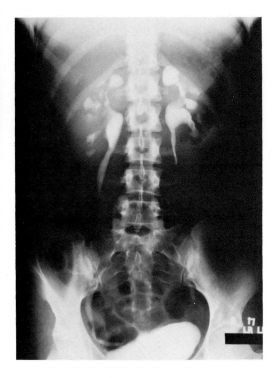

Figure 11–141. *Excretory urogram.* Bilateral "reflux" kidneys.

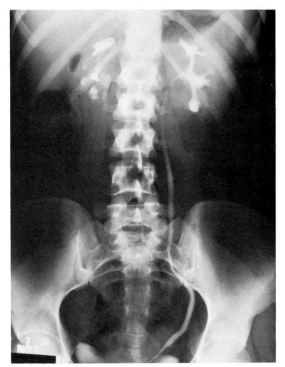

Figure 11–142. *Excretory urogram.* Bizarre changes in both kidneys. **Bilateral vesicoureteral reflux.**

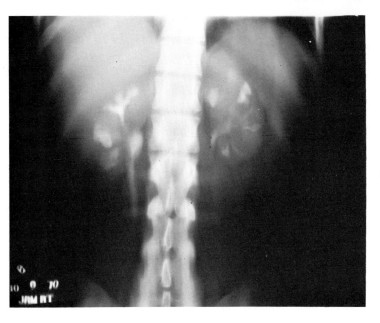

Figure 11–143. *Excretory urogram.* Bilateral "reflux" kidneys.

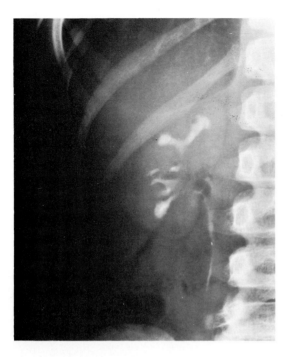

Figure 11–144. *Excretory urogram.* "Reflux" kidney. Diffuse but not uniform atrophy of renal cortex.

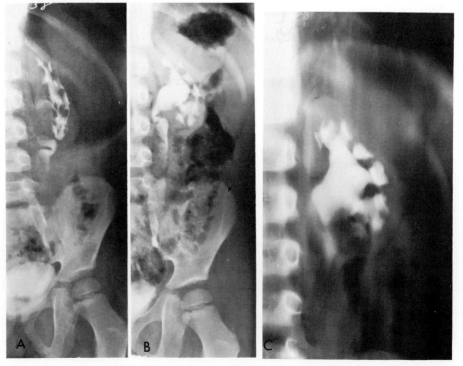

Figure 11–145. A through C, *Excretory urograms.* **Massive vesicoureteral reflux.** Diffuse loss of cortex.

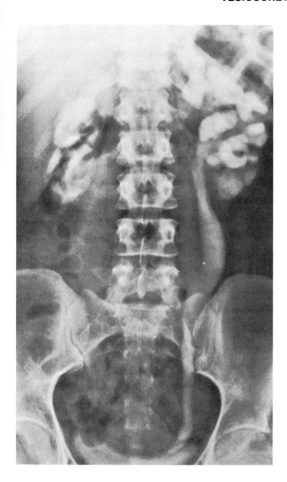

Figure 11–146. *Excretory urogram.* **Dilatation of entire left ureter and collecting system,** with diffuse parenchymal atrophy in involved kidney. (From Berquist, T. H., Hattery, R. R., Hartman, G. W., Kelalis, P. P., and DeWeerd, J. H.)

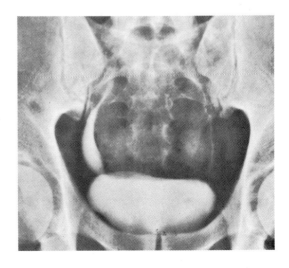

Figure 11–147. *Excretory urogram.* **Vesicoureteral reflux.** Bladder and lower ureters, showing dilatation of lower right ureter. (From Berquist, T. H., Hattery, R. R., Hartman, G. W., Kelalis, P. P., and DeWeerd, J. H.)

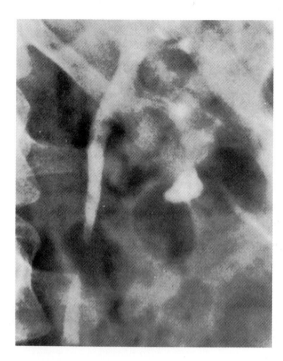

Figure 11–148. *Excretory urogram.* **Mucosal striations in upper ureter and pelvis,** more marked in renal pelvis. (From Berquist, T. H., Hattery, R. R., Hartman, G. W., Kelalis, P. P., and DeWeerd, J. H.)

Figure 11–149. *Excretory urogram.* Prominent **mucosal striations in upper ureter** and, to a lesser degree, in dilated midureter. (From Berquist, T. H., Hattery, R. R., Hartman, G. W., Kelalis, P. P., and DeWeerd, J. H.)

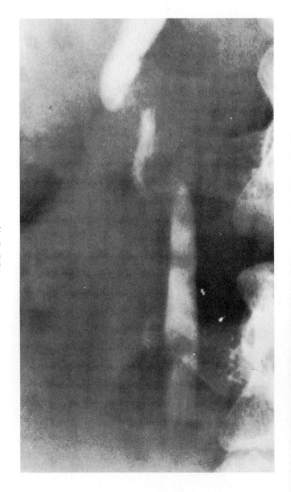

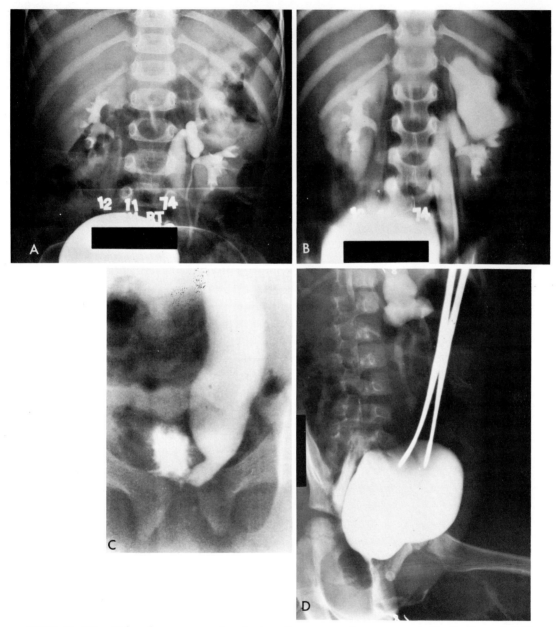

Figure 11–150.   Delayed appearance of contrast medium on excretory urogram. **A,** Duplication on left. Upper left segment functioning poorly. **B,** Upper segment and ureter outlined later in study from reflux of contrast medium into ectopic ureter. **C,** Reflux into ectopic ureter after voiding. **D,** *Cystogram under anesthesia* demonstrates reflux into upper segment on left and lower ureter on right.

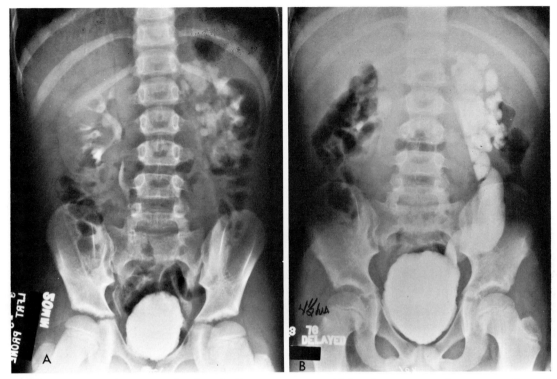

Figure 11–151. Vesicoureteral reflux. **A,** *Excretory urogram.* Delayed appearance of contrast medium. **B,** Delayed film, 4½ hours. Collecting system filled with contrast medium in a retrograde fashion from bladder.

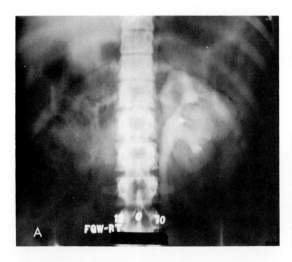

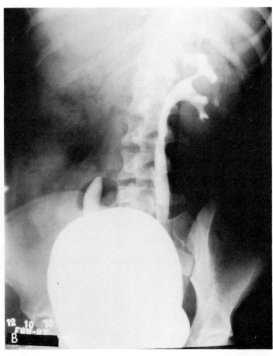

Figure 11–152. A, "Pseudotumor" of reflux kidney due to irregular growth next to scar. Previous right nephrectomy for "tumor." **B,** Reflux into right ureteral stump and left collecting system.

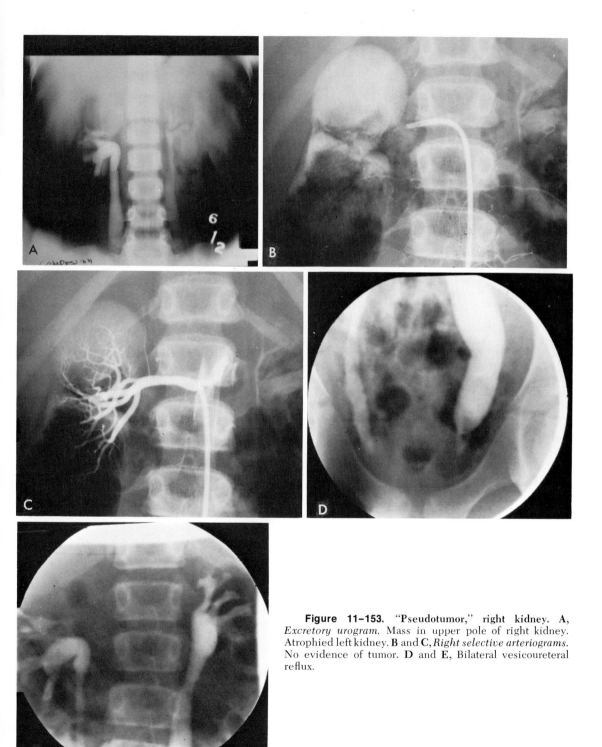

Figure 11–153. "Pseudotumor," right kidney. **A,** *Excretory urogram.* Mass in upper pole of right kidney. Atrophied left kidney. **B** and **C,** *Right selective arteriograms.* No evidence of tumor. **D** and **E,** Bilateral vesicoureteral reflux.

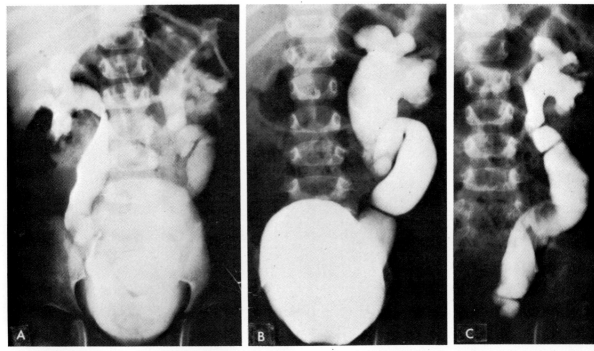

Figure 11–154. **A**, *Excretory urogram* shows **bilateral hydroureteronephrosis. B**, *Voiding cystourethrogram* shows **left vesicoureteral reflux** with bladder filling. **C**, Film taken after voiding shows complete bladder emptying and retention of contrast material in the dilated left upper collecting system, indicative of an associated obstructive factor at the ureterovesical juncture.

the initial excretory urogram (Dwoskin and Perlmutter). Between 80 and 85 per cent of scarred kidneys will demonstrate reflux at one time or another (Hodson and Wilson; Scott and Stansfeld, 1968b), but reflux is seen only in 22 per cent of normal renal units. In fact, in children, reflux is nearly always present when chronic pyelonephritic scarring is identified.

✱ A normal excretory urogram is not sufficient evidence of a normal urinary tract in a child. In fact, cystourethrography with fluoroscopy is the single most important investigation of the urinary tract with infection. Nonetheless, neither this nor the excretory urogram can accurately depict associated obstruction, either at the vesical neck or the distal urethra (Shopfner, 1967a).

REFLUXING MEGAURETER

The grossly dilated ureter in which reflux is demonstrated by cystography is referred to as a refluxing megaureter. This condition differs from primary megaureter in that no specific point of obstruction such as a narrowed distal segment can be incriminated as being responsible for the gross dilatation produced.

The mere presence of reflux does not, however, rule out an area of physiologic obstruction. As illustrated in Figure 11–137, reflux with gross ureteral dilatation may combine with an element of juxtavesical obstruction to form the serious combination of severe stasis with reflux, permitting gross bacterial contamination of the obstructed kidney (see Figure 11–154).

Etiology of Vesicoureteral Reflux

Even now, too much emphasis is given to making the diagnosis of reflux and too little effort to defining the etiology—that is, defining the mechanism that permits reflux to occur in a child undergoing evaluation.

There is no doubt that reflux reflects a variety of clinical states with a common characteristic: incompetence of the uretero-vesical juncture. The term *primary reflux* denotes intrinsic maldevelopment of the ureterovesical juncture, whereas the term *secondary reflux* implies an acquired disorder or one secondary to disorders elsewhere in the urinary tract or in other parts of the body.

THE URETEROVESICAL JUNCTURE

Many anatomic and physiologic studies have attempted to elucidate the delicate mechanism of the ureterovesical juncture by defining both its structural features and its functional characteristics. The conclusions of the many observers who have studied this problem are often conflicting and diverging. There is, however, enough uniformity of opinion, at least as to the major features that play a role in the competence of the ureterovesical angle, to allow some valid conclusions (Gruber, 1929a, 1929b; Hutch and associates; Tanagho and Pugh; Tanagho and associates, 1965, 1969).

All agree that there exists a ureterotrigonal continuity that acts as a single functional unit. This is the result of longitudinal ureteral muscle fibers in the roof of the intramural ureter that diverge and sweep around to become continuous with the fibers in the floor, which then pass distally on the superficial trigonal muscle to be firmly attached near the verumontanum (Tanagho, Meyers, and Smith). This prevents excessive mobility of the orifice by fixing it in position and allowing a submucosal tunnel to persist or enlarge with progressive filling of the bladder and thereby maintains or enhances the valve-like action of the structure. At the beginning of micturition, further stress is put on the region of the ureterovesical juncture because of contraction of the bladder detrusor and subsequent increase in intravesical pressure, which tends to herniate the ureteral orifice through the wall of the blad-der. Such herniation is likely to occur when the ureterotrigonal continuity is deficient or compromised by maldevelopment of the trigonal region and lateral placement of the ureteral orifice. In the normal state, because of the firm attachment of the ureter, this cannot occur.

Theoretically, the significant contribution to the one-way characteristic of the ureterovesical juncture is the occlusion of the ureteral lumen as the increase in intravesical pressure presses it against the detrusor muscle—the flap valve mechanism. For this to occur, both immobility of the orifice (to allow persistence of the sub-mucosal tunnel) and a good detrusor support are essential. Paraureteral diverticula clearly demonstrate the dynamics of the ureterovesical angle because they tend to enlarge with filling of the bladder and obliterate the tunnel by displacing the intramural ureter and at times the orifice extravesically (see Figures 11–158 and 11–160).

Other factors also may have a bearing on the competence of the angle. For example, the longitudinal fibers of the ureter may contract, acting as a ureteric sphincter that occludes the ureteral lumen and thus prevents or reduces retrograde flow of urine (Tanagho, Guthrie, and Lyon). This phenomenon is often seen roentgenographically when the peristaltic activity of the ureter empties the refluxing column of urine back into the bladder. This sphincter-like action may play a part in the early stages of the development of reflux, but it is unlikely that it can prevent reflux for prolonged periods in the presence of a deranged ureterovesical angle (Scott and De Luca).

From this oversimplified description of the function of the ureterovesical juncture, it would appear that the absence of reflux requires a well-developed trigone, a good detrusor support, and a long intravesical ureter. Trigonal weakness or deficiency of the musculature of the terminal ureter is the most common cause of incompetence of the ureterovesical junction and will result in reflux that is termed primary.

PRIMARY REFLUX

Congenital Malformations of the Ureterovesical Angle

Abnormalities in the morphology of the ureteral orifice are indicated by lateral placement (ectopia lateralis), abnormal configuration (golfhole, stadium, or horseshoe shape), and association with an absent or poorly developed trigone (Lyon and associates). The extent of such abnormalities correlates well with the associated degree of reflux (Fig. 11–155).

When there is complete duplication of the upper urinary tract, the ureter of the lower renal segment (orthotopic) enters the bladder at a higher level than the ureter from the upper one. It is in the ureter to the lower pole that reflux nearly always takes place (Ambrose and Nicolson). Such reflux is unlikely to abate with growth and usually persists into adulthood (Amar and Chabra) (Fig. 11–156). Reflux is the most frequent abnormality seen with complete ureteral duplication; three of four children who have urinary infection and complete duplication will demonstrate reflux into the lower renal segment, which is often severely damaged (Fehrenbaker and

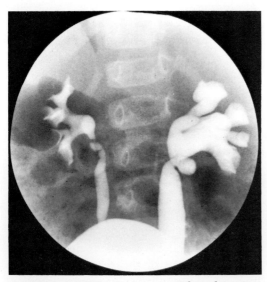

Figure 11–155. *Cystogram.* **Bilateral vesicoureteral reflux.** Right, grade 2; left, grade 3. At cystoscopy, right ureteral orifice was found to be "stadium"-shaped with fair submucosal tunnel, and left was "golf-hole" orifice lacking submucosal tunnel almost completely.

associates). In about 10 per cent of cases, reflux into both components of the duplication takes place (Fig. 11–157).

Because the point of the insertion of the ureter in the bladder wall is a weak spot in the detrusor, this area is a common site of a diverticulum formation when bladder outlet obstruction is present and also in spastic neurogenic bladders. In children, however, paraureteral diverticula are frequently congenital and are rarely secondary to or associated with outlet obstruction (Amar). Such diverticula may be small or subtle and may be missed at the beginning of the examination. With the bladder full or slightly overdistended, a typical diverticulum develops, which shortens the intravesical ureter and impairs its posterior detrusor support, rendering the ureterovesical angle incompetent (Figs. 11–158, 11–159, and 11–160) (Hutch, 1958). Urographic demonstration of Hutch's theory is shown in Fig. 11–161.

The hypothesis that intrinsic incompetence of the ureterovesical juncture is caused by a developmental defect in the renal and ureteral unit is increasingly attractive. According to this theory, a genetic abnormality of the ureteral bud produces an abnormal ureterovesical juncture, ureteral dilatation, and, at least focally, metanephric induction and differentiation. Interestingly, the rate of incidence of reflux rises sharply when congenital anomalies of the kidney, either of shape (horseshoe kidney) or position (pelvic kidney) are found (Figs. 11–162 and 11–163) (Bialestock; Kelalis, Malek and Segura).

According to Stephens, the site of the ureteral orifice correlates with the degree of hydronephrosis or renal hypoplasia or dysplasia found on careful microscopic and macroscopic evaluation of the kidney. In brief, the more lateral the position of the refluxing orifice, the more likely the ectopia is to be associated with congenital hydronephrosis and renal hypoplasia. In other words, the urogram provides a guide to the orifice location that is correct in a high proportion of instances. When the urogram looks normal, the orifice will be in a normal or nearly normal position.

Text continued on page 1046

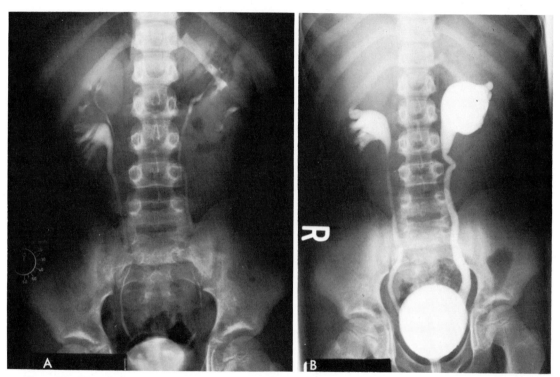

Figure 11–156. *Excretory urogram.* Bilateral complete ureteral duplication with pyelectasis and ureterectasis of lower segment on right and atrophic lower segment on left. **B,** *Retrograde cystogram.* Bilateral vesicoureteral reflux into both lower segments. Degree of reflux correlates with renal changes on two sides. (From Kelalis, P. P., 1971.)

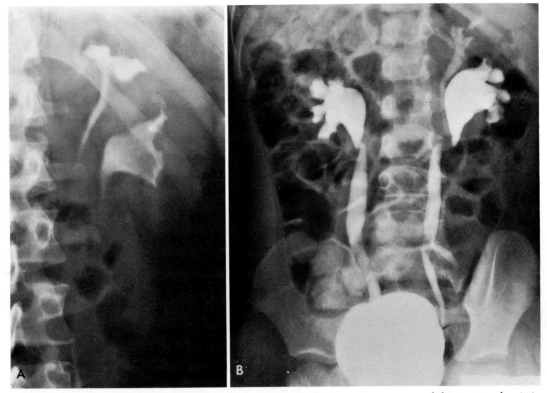

Figure 11–157. Duplication and reflux. **A,** *Excretory urogram.* Lower segment exhibits mucosal striations due to vesicoureteral reflux. **B,** *Cystogram* of different patient. Reflux into lower segment of complete duplication on right side and both segments on left (orifices on left enter bladder side by side via a common canal).

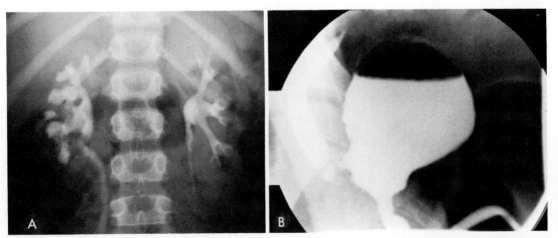

Figure 11–158. Six-year-old boy with urinary infection. **A,** *Excretory urogram.* Smaller right kidney with thin cortex and abnormal calyces. **B,** *Voiding cystourethrogram.* **Right vesicoureteral reflux. Small diverticulum** producing complete dissociation of ureter and bladder.

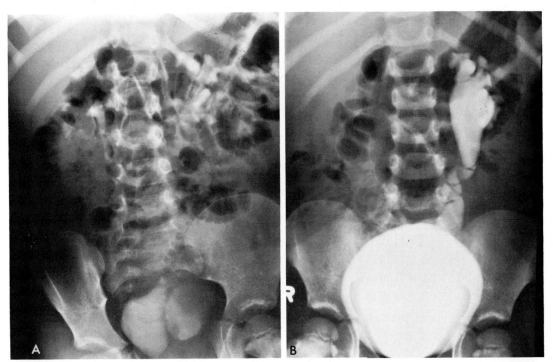

Figure 11–159. Paraureteral diverticulum. **A,** *Excretory urogram.* Diverticulum on left side of bladder. **B,** *Cystogram, anteroposterior view. Vesicoureteral reflux on left.* Observe **diverticulum.**

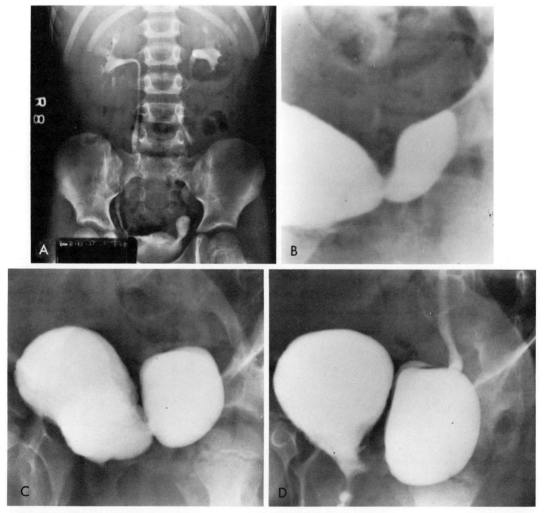

Figure 11–160. Vesical diverticulum and reflux. **A,** *Excretory urogram.* **B, C,** and **D,** *Cystograms.* Progressive distention of diverticulum and appearance of reflux.

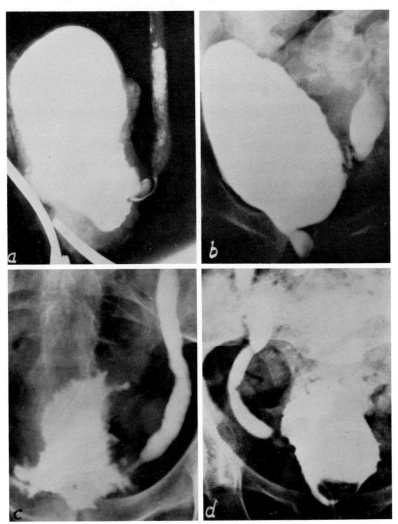

Figure 11–161. Extravesical position of normally intravesical part of ureter associated with neurologic disease. *Cystograms.* **A, Paraplegia.** Patient died of progressive renal failure. At necropsy, urinary tract was removed intact, and this cystogram was made. Lateral exposure clearly shows saccule lying above intravesical ureter. Intravesical ureter can be seen passing along floor of saccule. Note that dilatation begins at juncture of intravesical and extravesical segments of ureter. **B, Meningomyelocele,** in child. In complete x-ray series, peristaltic wave was seen passing down ureter and forcing contrast medium into dilated lower portion of ureter. Note tortuous, undilated intravesical ureter in extravesical position. **C, Paraplegia and spastic bladder.** Intravesical ureter on left is clearly visible in extravesical position. **D, Paraplegia.** Intravesical ureter in extravesical position. (From Hutch, J. A., 1958.)

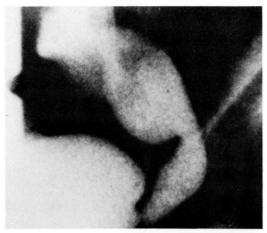

Figure 11–162. *Cystogram.* **Reflux into pelvic kidney.**

When reflux produces hydronephrosis, the orifice will be found in quite a lateral position or even in a diverticulum (Mackie and associates). In such extreme instances, the kidney may exhibit dysplasia. This theory sheds considerable light on the serious clinical problem of the relation of reflux and renal changes and confirms that what has been termed "chronic pyelonephritis" is neither chronic nor pyelonephritic, and therefore diagnosis of pyelonephritis should not be made on the basis of excretory urographic data alone (Heptinstall; Stickler and associates) (see also section on pyelonephritis).

SECONDARY REFLUX

Any irritation in the region of the ureterovesical angle may produce reflux. Infection and inflammation are no exception (Bumpus; Graves and Davidoff, 1923, 1924). Indeed, in 1924 Bumpus wrote, solely on the basis of his clinical experience, "The intravesical portion of the ureter, if it is involved in an inflammatory process in the bladder, becomes a more or less rigid tube and being unaffected by various contractions of the bladder, ceases to function as a valve."

Infection may initiate reflux, particularly when the ureterovesical juncture is of marginal competence, because the tissues comprising the roof of the intravesical ureter become rigid as a result of edema and cellular infiltrate, and the flap valve mechanism is therefore lost.

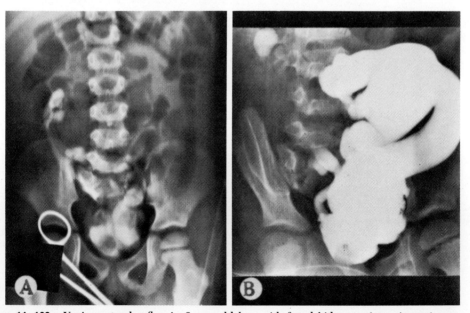

Figure 11–163. **Vesicoureteral reflux in 6-year-old boy with fused kidney, urinary incontinence, and imperforate anus. A,** *Excretory urogram* shows "pancake" kidney and dilatation of left ureter, probably from reflux of medium from bladder. **B,** *Retrograde cystogram. Bilateral vesicoureteral reflux,* massive into left collecting system. (From Kelalis, P. P., Malek, R. S., and Segura, J. W.)

Reflux present on cystography performed during or soon after an infection tends to be mild in degree with little if any ureterectasis, and the excretory urogram is usually normal (Figs. 11–164 and 11–165). Although infection is a fairly common cause of reflux, it is not a very important one, since the volume of residual urine associated is slight and infection is usually easily eradicated. In such instances, the reflux stops a few weeks after the infection subsides. It is now clear that the role of infection in the etiology of reflux has been overestimated in the past. In most children reflux persists long after the infection has been eradicated because congenital incompetency of the ureterovesical angle is also present.

Vesicoureteral reflux is a frequent accompaniment of the neurogenic bladder, both in its congenital and its acquired form (Fig. 11–166) (Emmett, Simon, and Mills). Experiments indicate that the competence of the ureterovesical juncture is closely linked to neuromuscular activity, but the extent of such activity is open to question (Langworthy and Kolb; Zinner and Paquin). Reflux is present at birth in about 20 per cent of infants with myelomeningocele, but the overall incidence of reflux in children with myelomeningocele is around 60 per cent (Magnus; Levitt and Sandler) (see section on neurogenic bladder).

A belief that reflux is seen only in conjunction with bladder outlet obstruction, possibly a rough analogy to the occasional reflux found in the adult with prostatism, existed until the 1960s (Fig. 11–167). The widespread use of voiding cystourethrography further supported this impression because in children, particularly girls, the bladder neck tends to look narrow in respect to the proximal urethra on voiding films. The general consensus now is that obstruction and reflux, though sometimes occurring in the same patient, are rarely a cause and effect (Lenaghan and Cussen). Reflux, of course, is sometimes found in children with obstructive conditions such as ectopic ureterocele, posterior urethral valves, and urethral stricture, but according to Stephens and Lenaghan, the combina-

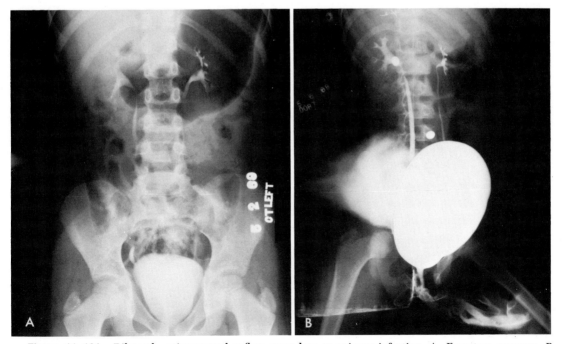

Figure 11–164. Bilateral vesicoureteral reflux secondary to urinary infection. **A,** *Excretory urogram.* **B,** *Retrograde cystogram.* Ureterovesical juncture fairly normal cystoscopically.

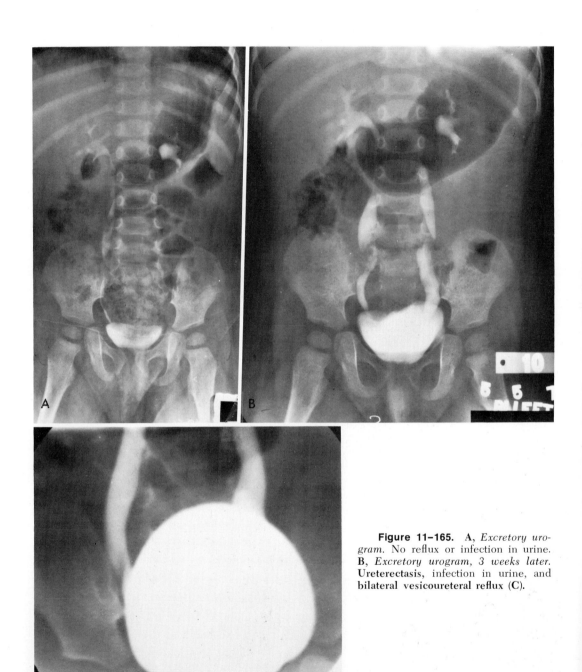

Figure 11–165. A, *Excretory urogram.* No reflux or infection in urine. **B,** *Excretory urogram, 3 weeks later.* **Ureterectasis,** infection in urine, and bilateral vesicoureteral reflux (**C**).

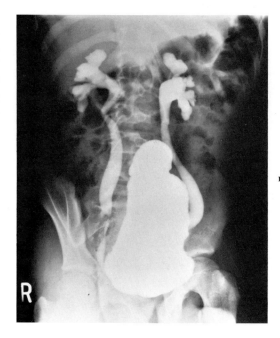

Figure 11–166. *Cystogram.* Bilateral vesicoureteral reflux; (?) neurogenic bladder.

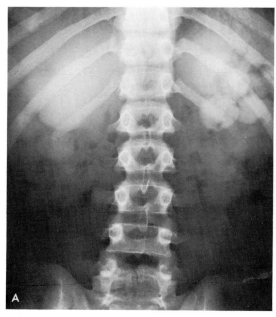

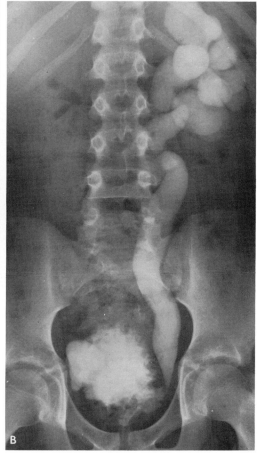

Figure 11–167. Congenital obstruction of vesical neck of boy, aged 13 years. **A,** *Excretory urogram.* Bilateral hydronephrosis. Poor renal function. **B,** *Retrograde cystogram.* Markedly trabeculated bladder with left ureteropyelectasis and reflux. (From Emmett, J. L., and Simon, H. B.)

tion of obstruction and reflux is a coincidental association and not a causal one in most cases.

Distal urethral stenosis is a term used by Lyon and Smith to describe a narrowed area normally present in girls, as evidenced by the similarity of the urethral caliber in normal children and those with infection (Graham and associates). Its relative significance in urinary infection and therefore reflux continues to be controversial.

Reflux is frequently found in patients with the prune-belly syndrome (Figs. 11–168 and 11–169) (Burke and associates; Williams and Burkholder) and in cases of exstrophy of the bladder after primary closure (Fig. 11–170) (Lattimer and associates, 1960). Occasionally, it occurs in the ectopic ureter, with or without ureterocele, that opens between the vesical neck and the external urethral sphincter; such incompetence is probably related to the deficiency of the musculature in the terminal portion of the ureter, which therefore lacks sphincteric action (Figs. 11–171 through 11–174) (Malek and associates).

Iatrogenic reflux is not uncommon, particularly after unroofing or incision of a ureterocele or after ureteral reimplantation done for any reason. Surgical procedures involving the ureterovesical angle may lead to reflux. Simple ureteral meatotomy

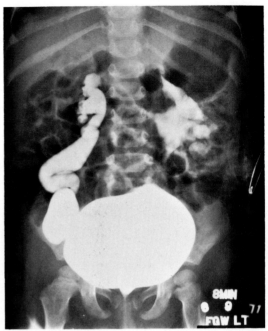

Figure 11–169. **Prune-belly syndrome.** *Cystogram* shows bilateral vesicoureteral reflux with tortuosity and dilatation of right ureter.

to facilitate removal of stone and incision of a ureterocele are the procedures that most frequently, but not always, cause reflux (Figs. 11–175 through 11–179) (Roper and Smith).

Factors Affecting the Course and Prognosis of Vesicoureteral Reflux

Because the percentage of children with infection who exhibit reflux (up to 50 per cent) greatly exceeds the percentage of adults (less than 10 per cent), one must conclude that there is a progressive decline in its rate of incidence with age (Estes and Brooks; Servadio and Shachner). Actually, the incidence of primary reflux is high in the first five years of life, then drops precipitously. Thus, reflux is not a permanent phenomenon in all instances, and there is good evidence that such temporary reflux early in life is caused by delayed maturation of the ureterovesical angle.

The pathologic significance of reflux was recognized by Sampson, who sug-

Text continued on page 1055

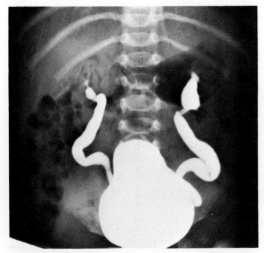

Figure 11–168. *Cystogram* of patient with prune-belly syndrome. **Bilateral vesicoureteral reflux.** Dysplastic kidneys.

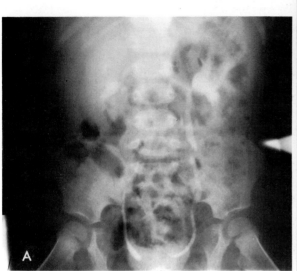

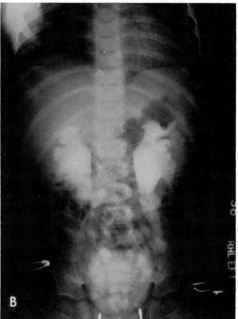

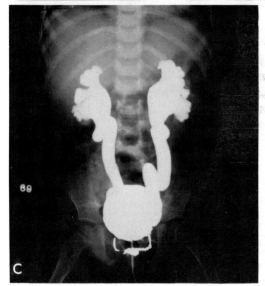

Figure 11–170. Exstrophy of bladder. A, *Preoperative excretory urogram.* B, *Excretory urogram* after primary closure. **Bilateral hydroureteronephrosis.** C, *Cystogram.* Massive **bilateral vesicoureteral reflux.**

Figure 11–171. *Voiding cystourethrogram.* Reflux into **ectopic ureter** draining into proximal urethra.

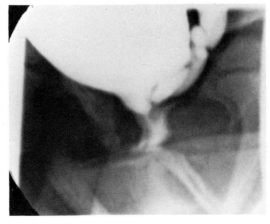

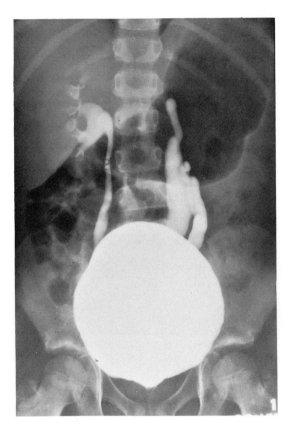

Figure 11–172. *Cystogram.* Bilateral vesicoureteral reflux. Duplex ureters; left upper-segment ureter is ectopic. Previous nephrectomy.

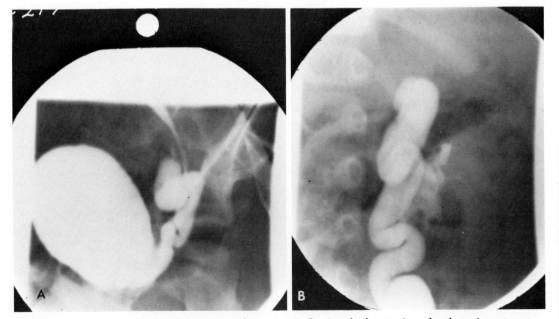

Figure 11–173. A and B, *Voiding cystourethrograms.* Reflux into both ectopic and orthotopic ureters.

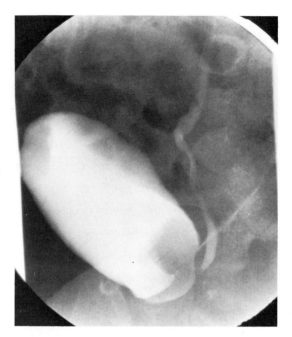

Figure 11–174. *Voiding cystourethrogram.* Negative shadow due to **ectopic ureterocele.** Reflux into orthotopic ureter.

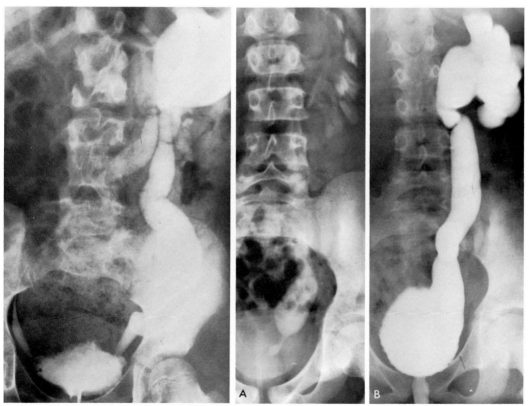

Fig. 11–175   Fig. 11–176

Figure 11–175. *Retrograde cystogram* of boy, 8 years of age, with persistent pyuria and urinary incontinence who had been operated on for imperforate anus at the age of 3 days. Vesicorectal fistula suspected. Note **bilateral reflux showing crossed renal ectopia.** (Courtesy of Dr. H. W. ten Cate.)

Figure 11–176. **Reflux after transurethral meatotomy for ureterocele** of girl, 8 years of age. **A,** *Excretory urogram.* Dilatation of lower third of ureter which narrows down to normal size in intramural ureter, then ends in small ureterocele. **B,** *Voiding cystourethrogram* made 8 months after transurethral meatotomy. **Vesicoureteral reflux with advanced ureteropyelectasis.**

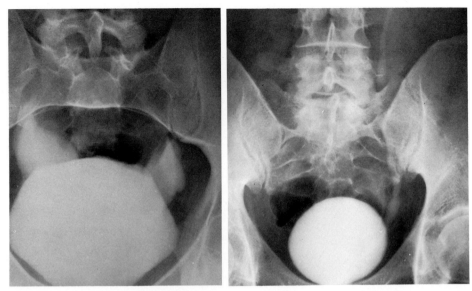

Fig. 11–177   **Fig. 11–178**

Figure 11–177. *Retrograde cystogram.* Reflux up hugely dilated ureters resulting from bilateral (suprapubic) ureteral meatotomy to relieve bilateral congenital hydroureter without reflux.

Figure 11–178. *Retrograde cystogram.* Reflux up left ureter resulting from transurethral fulguration of inflammatory lesion in vicinity of left ureteral orifice.

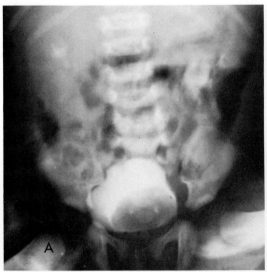

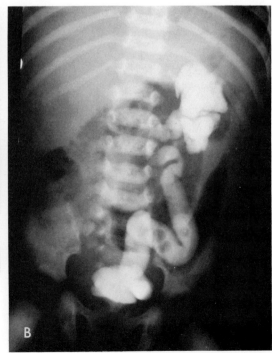

Figure 11–179. Iatrogenic reflux. A, *Excretory cystogram* shows **ureterocele.** B, *Cystogram* after transurethral incision of ureterocele. Massive **vesicoureteral reflux.**

gested that it might be one of the mechanisms by which infection reaches the kidneys. Bumpus and also Helmholz found that a high proportion of patients with urinary infection and pyelonephritis had reflux. In 1960, Hodson and Edwards pointed out that reflux was not only associated with urinary infection but was also associated with radiographic evidence of chronic pyelonephritis.

Irrespective of the sequence of events, reflux and infection together lead to renal involvement. Cortical scarring is seen at least eight times more frequently when reflux is associated with infection than when infection is present alone (Scott and Stansfeld, 1968a). Measurement of kidney growth, or lack of it, is a good indication of whether renal involvement is present. Infection of the kidney will retard such growth, which resumes after infection has been eliminated (Hodson and Edwards; Scott and Stansfeld, 1968a, 1968b).

Despite this definite association of reflux and renal damage, the cause and effect relationship is not clear in all cases. In the majority, the refluxing column of infected urine, together with the diffuse pressure within the collecting system, may lead to generalized renal atrophy. It is difficult, however, to explain on this basis the focal atrophy that occurs in some kidneys with reflux. The possibility that intrarenal reflux is selectively responsible in some cases should be at least considered, but it is also likely that such changes may be present on a congenital basis.

Another question that requires further clarification is whether so-called progressive renal damage is really progressive or is merely a radiologic appearance produced by differential renal growth (Filly and associates). At the time when a child's kidney is affected by pyelonephritis associated with reflux, it may be normal radiographically. During the years that follow, healthy areas of renal parenchyma continue to grow normally but the scarred areas do not, and this leads to an outline that appears far from normal and that has the appearance of progressive damage. This should not necessarily be interpreted as a continuation of the inflammatory process. According to Govan and Palmer, renal scarring may take up to two years to develop after an acute episode of clinical pyelonephritis. This continued retraction of an established scar is sometimes seen on serial excretory urograms covering a period of several years, even though there is no clinical evidence of infection.

Nonetheless, the most striking feature of scarring is how seldom it actually is seen to develop or progress, particularly in a previously normal kidney (Smellie and associates). This observation is of the utmost importance because, if it is valid, it suggests either that the scar is present from birth or that it develops in early childhood. It would appear that the majority of children with reflux have renal scarring when they are first seen by the physician, and with few exceptions the extent of scarring does not change during follow-up even if reflux persists (Figs. 11–180 through 11–184).

The hydrodynamic effect of reflux (without infection) upon the kidney is also a matter of continuing debate, and whether this alone can lead to renal changes (at least in some situations) has not been totally resolved.

Experimental evidence to date suggests that unless infection or obstruction is present, reflux is unlikely to produce any significant renal change, either anatomic or functional. Furthermore, there has been no convincing clinical evidence that reflux without infection, followed over a sufficient period, has induced significant renal damage or interference with renal growth. Accumulating clinical and experimental data suggest that in the absence of infection or obstruction, reflux is a benign phenomenon that produces neither anatomic nor permanent functional derangement of the involved kidney, at least for several years (King and associates, 1972). Walker and associates and Uehling have found that unless severe hydronephrosis exists in conjunction with reflux, the creatinine clearance remains normal. How-

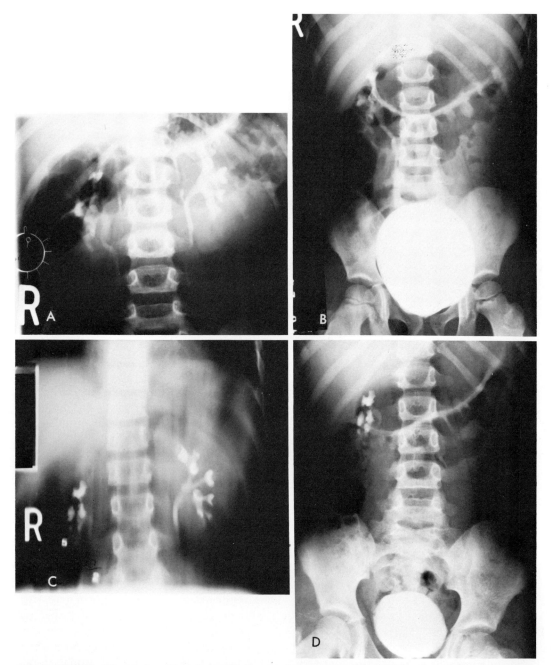

Figure 11–180.　Progression of renal atrophy from vesicoureteral reflux and infection. **A,** *Excretory urogram.* Reflux on right side, left kidney normal. **B,** *Cystogram.* Total vesicoureteral reflux on right. **C,** *Excretory urogram* and **D,** *cystogram* made 4 years later. Note progression of atrophy of right kidney (**C**) and presence of reflux (**D**).

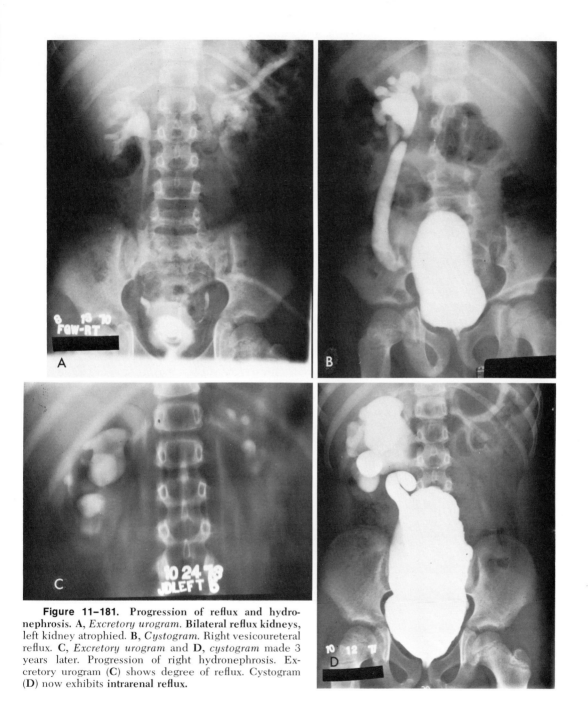

Figure 11–181. Progression of reflux and hydronephrosis. **A**, *Excretory urogram.* Bilateral reflux kidneys, left kidney atrophied. **B**, *Cystogram.* Right vesicoureteral reflux. **C**, *Excretory urogram* and **D**, *cystogram* made 3 years later. Progression of right hydronephrosis. Excretory urogram (**C**) shows degree of reflux. Cystogram (**D**) now exhibits **intrarenal reflux.**

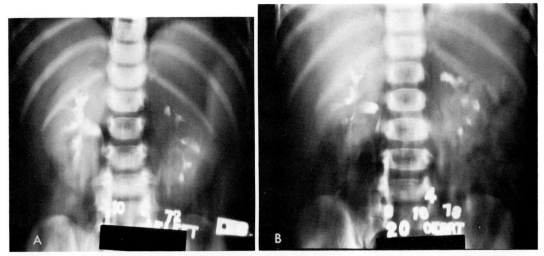

Figure 11–182. **A** and **B**, *Excretory urograms, 8 months apart,* showing changes in left kidney from vesicoureteral reflux and infection.

ever, concentrating ability is decreased in patients with sterile reflux when caliectasis or even mild calyceal blunting is present, which is reversible once the reflux is corrected.

Stickler and associates described a group of children who had reflux but no evidence of urinary infection and who had progressive renal deterioration. Admittedly, this small fraction of the large number of children with vesicoureteral reflux—they are said to have interstitial nephritis rather than chronic pyelonephritis—can hardly be used as evidence of the effect of sterile reflux on the kidney, especially when the cause-and-effect relationship between the

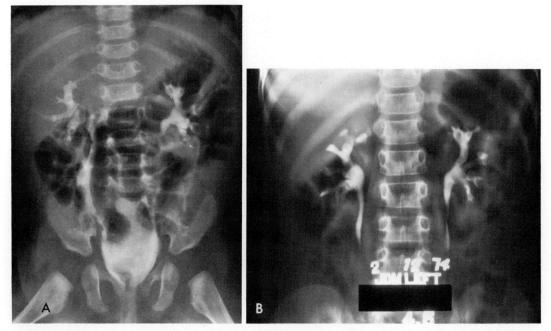

Figure 11–183. *Excretory urograms, 3½ years apart.* **A,** Note normal right kidney. **B,** Cortical atrophy and calyceal distortion from vesicoureteral reflux and urinary infection, years later.

reflux and the changes in the kidney has not been conclusively demonstrated and the probability exists that other factors may be involved. Also, progressive lesions were demonstrated in some children having gross vesicoureteral reflux in the continued absence of infection, but these patients initially came to attention because of urinary tract infection, and the possibility that the renal changes are at least related to this should be entertained (Rolleston, Shannon, and Utley 1970a, 1970b). Reports of small series of patients with sterile reflux and progressive renal damage are available (Geist and Antolak; Hutch and Smith; Penn and Breidahl; Salvatierra and associates). It is at least theoretically possible that the "progressive" damage seen was actually latent change caused by an earlier, undiagnosed, asymptomatic urinary infection or that the renal abnormalities were congenital.

Vesicoureteral Reflux in Adults

The rate of incidence of reflux is significantly lower in adults than in children. This is, of course, in accord with the gradual decreasing incidence of reflux in older children. That there is a definite group of adults with severe kidney disease apparently associated with reflux is well documented (Fig. 11–185) (Amar and associates; Ambrose; Markland and Kelly; Salvatierra and associates; Servadio and Shachner).

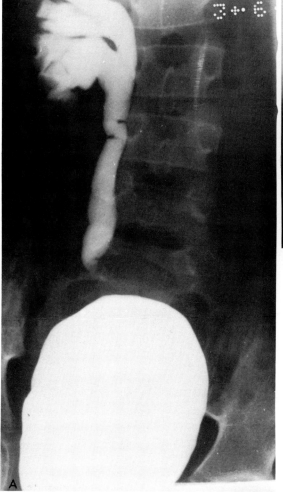

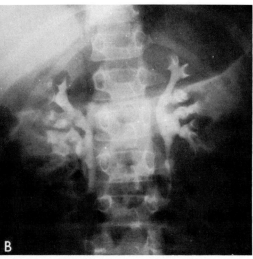

Figure 11–184. A, Grade 4 reflux in boy at age 5. B, *Intravenous urogram.*

Legend continued on following page

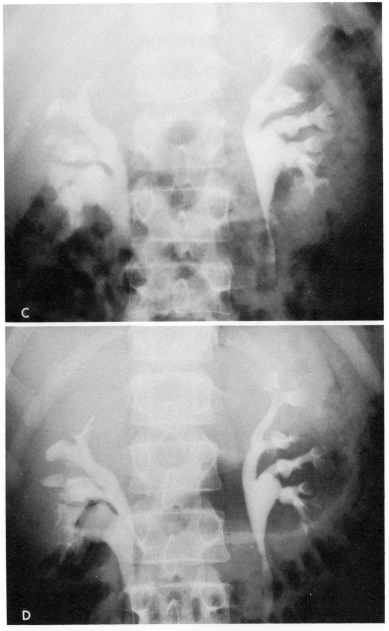

Figure 11–184 *Continued.* **C,** *Intravenous urogram* at age 10, 6 months after *Streptococcus faecalis* infection (after a known 5 years' freedom from infection), showing right midzone scar. **D,** *Intravenous urogram* at age 14, showing contraction of scar in right kidney, 4 years after reflux-stopping surgery, and with no further urinary infection. (From Smellie, J., Edwards, D., Hunter, N., Normand, I. C. S., and Prescod, N. Reprinted from Kidney International, Vol. 8, pp. S-65–S-72, 1975, with permission.)

Berquist and associates, in their study of 200 consecutive adults with vesicoureteral reflux, found the excretory urogram to be abnormal in four out of five. When a childhood history of urinary infection was noted, parenchymal scarring was present in 87 per cent, and when there was no history of urinary tract infection until adulthood, scarring was found in only 49 per cent. The most common abnormality found on the excretory urogram was localized, often solitary parenchymal scarring associated with blunting of underlying calyces (Berquist and associates) (Figs. 11–186 and 11–188).

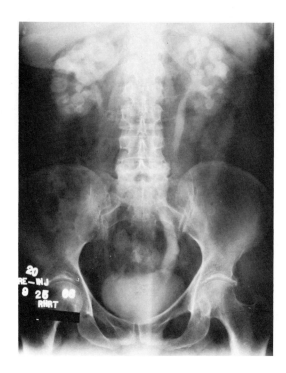

Figure 11–185. *Excretory urogram.* **Advanced bilateral renal atrophy and renal failure** in 65-year-old woman due to life-long reflux and infection.

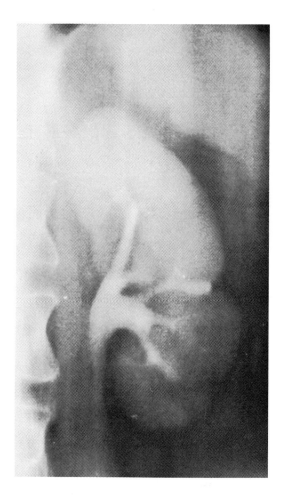

Figure 11–186. *Tomogram of left kidney,* showing **parenchymal scar** on lateral border with **blunting of underlying calyx.** (From Berquist, T. H., Hattery, R. R., Hartman, G. W., Kelalis, P. P., and DeWeerd, J. H.)

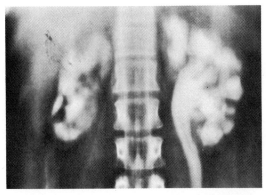

Figure 11–187. *Tomogram* of kidneys, showing **diffuse bilateral parenchymal loss** (with dilatation of collecting systems and renal asymmetry). (From Berquist, T. H., Hattery, R. R., Hartman, G. W., Kelalis, P. P., and DeWeerd, J. H.)

Duffy, also studying this problem in adults, detected reflux in 75 per cent of patients with roentgenographic evidence of pyelonephritis. He found renal parenchymal scarring in 72 per cent of the kidneys when there was reflux and dilatation, whether reflux was partial or complete. Between one- and two-thirds of adult patients with reflux also show mucosal striations.

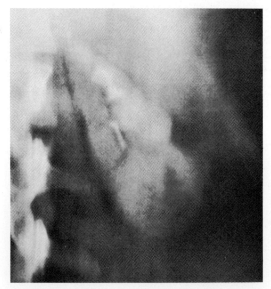

Figure 11–188. *Tomogram of left kidney,* showing **marked parenchymal atrophy involving upper pole and lateral scarring.** Calyceal system is poorly visualized, and there is compensatory hypertrophy of the lower pole. (From Berquist, T. H., Hattery, R. R., Hartman, G. W., Kelalis, P. P., and DeWeerd, J. H.)

Even a brief review of the problem of reflux in adults demonstrates its potential for renal damage and leads to the inescapable conclusion that permanent reflux (that is, reflux associated with permanent incompetence of the ureterovesical angle) places the kidney at great risk.

Management of Vesicoureteral Reflux

Basically, the management of vesicoureteral reflux is a question of conservative versus surgical treatment—or a combination of both. As emphasized previously, several causes of reflux exist. Each may be considered as a separate disease. Optimal treatment is different in each instance and must depend on the cause of the reflux.

That surgical treatment is necessary to correct some of the deformities of the ureterovesical juncture responsible for primary reflux is accepted by all. What is in question is the degree of incompetence that justifies surgery (Kelalis, 1974).

There is a degree of ureteral dilatation and/or associated incompetence of the ureterovesical juncture beyond which spontaneous disappearance of reflux is unlikely to occur even though optimal conditions are provided. One can become increasingly adept at predicting this eventual outcome on the basis of cystographic and endoscopic findings, the former relating to the grade of reflux and the latter to the morphology of the ureterovesical juncture. In this way, one can distinguish persistent (lifelong) reflux from temporary reflux. The former justifies surgical treatment, the latter a conservative approach, at least in the initial stages. Gross ureteral dilatation (grade 4) and gross incompetence of the ureterovesical juncture (the golfhole orifice) suggest permanent reflux and the need for surgery.

The possibility exists that reflux will ultimately disappear spontaneously (Blight and O'Shaughnessy; Stephens, 1970). Cystographic examination should be repeated at intervals of 1 to 2 years, depending on the progress of the treatment of the urinary infection. Although it has been suggested that those who stop refluxing do so within two years (Dwoskin and Perlmutter), there is no doubt that this change can happen over longer periods of time. As long as the urine remains sterile, it is unlikely that the kidneys will suffer from progressive damage (Figs. 11–189 through 11–192). Basically, the principle of conservative treatment rests on the premise that elimination of infection plus expectant treatment might effect improvement of the marginally competent ureterovesical juncture (King and associates, 1972).

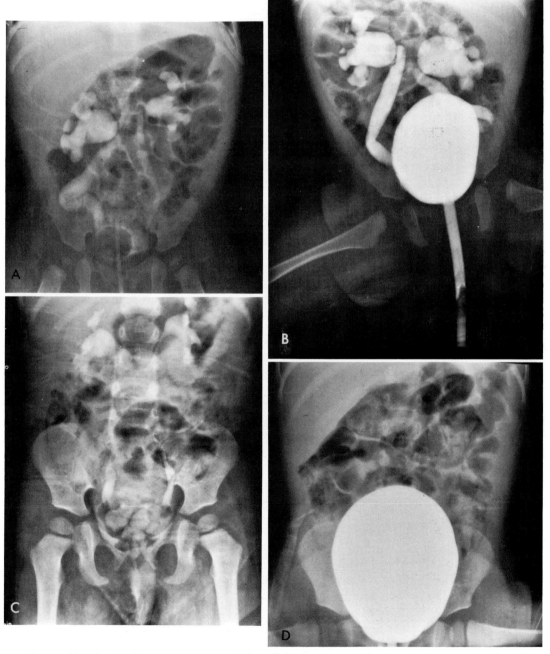

Figure 11–189. A, *Excretory urogram.* **Bilateral hydroureteronephrosis. B,** *Cystogram.* **Bilateral vesicoureteral reflux. C,** *Excretory urogram* showing regression of hydroureteronephrosis. **D,** *Cystogram* made after 18 months shows disappearance of reflux.

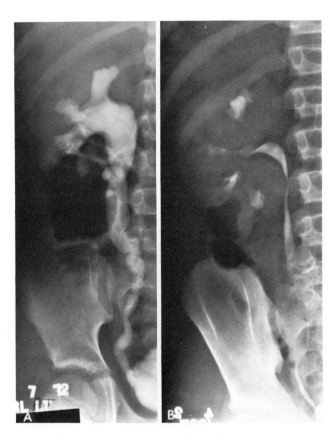

Figure 11–190. Regression of hydro-ureteronephrosis. A, Reflux and urinary infection. Dilatation of collecting system. B, One year later. Reflux has stopped and dilatation abated.

All long-term students of reflux now advocate early reimplantation when renal cortical scarring or marked ureterectasis is demonstrable. There is no longer any doubt that reflux in conjunction with obstruction or infection (or both) may result in renal scarring and a measurable decrease in renal function. On the other hand, reflux not complicated by obstruction or recurrent infection does not prevent renal growth and is benign even if gross ureterectasis is present, but in our present state of knowledge, this does not permit us to conclude that life-long reflux is not harmful. Moreover, the implications of life-long follow-up of patients with reflux are so overwhelming, in terms of cost and the patient's time as well as the physician's, that this course might be elected only rarely. Although elderly patients with good renal function despite congenital reflux have been reported, it would seem conservative to correct reflux if (1) the initial evaluation of the various parameters already

mentioned suggests a permanent situation or (2) if reflux persists after the first decade of life, despite appropriate conservative treatment. Ureteral reimplantation is, of course, performed when infection persists in the face of therapy. Early surgery also seems the more positive approach when children and their families are judged unlikely to return for adequate surveillance.

When reflux stops, it seems to do so as a function of the degree of derangement of the ureterovesical juncture and the severity of the reflux. Success, however, represents not only the elimination of infection but also the permanent disappearance of the reflux. A single negative examination for reflux should not be interpreted as a success, since reflux is likely to reappear in subsequent examinations even though there is no infection. It did so in 18 per cent of patients in the Mayo Clinic series. Failure to demonstrate reflux over a period of at least three years is necessary before expectant treatment is considered a suc-

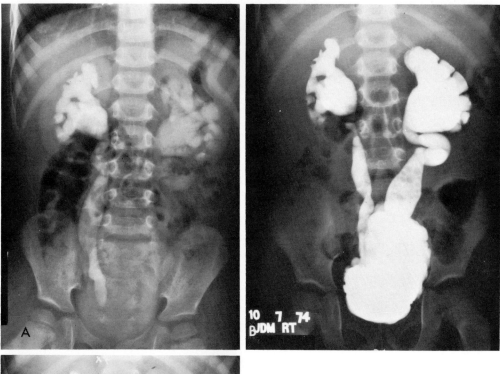

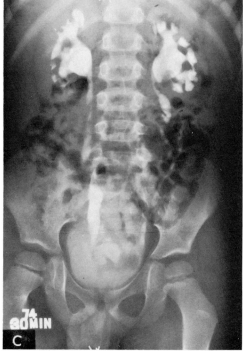

Figure 11–191. Conservative management of reflux with improvement. **A,** *Excretory urogram.* Bilateral hydroureteronephrosis more severe on left. **B,** *Cystogram.* Massive reflux bilaterally. Neurogenic bladder(?). **C,** *Excretory urogram several months later.* Improvement with conservative treatment.

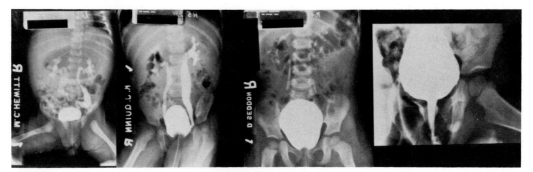

Figure 11–192. Conservative management of reflux. *Serial cystograms* depicting diminution of grade of reflux and finally cessation of reflux. Time span: 2 years.

cess (Fig. 11–193). As the grade of reflux increases, the percentage of ureters in which reflux ceases diminishes. Overall reflux should be expected to stop under conservative treatment in about 50 per cent of cases. At least two thirds of ureters stop refluxing within two years and 80 per cent in three years.

SURGICAL TREATMENT AND RESULTS

It is unfortunate that the purpose of ureteroneocystostomy has been misunderstood, and as a result the operation has been maligned. Its immediate objective should be to prevent a pathway of infection to the kidneys and to eliminate a mechanism by which infection propagates itself (Johnston, 1963; Scott; Scott and Stansfeld, 1968b). Specifically, the goal of this operation must be to protect the kidneys and not

necessarily to eliminate infection or prevent its recurrence. Many times such an operation has been classified as a failure because of a recurrence of infection, but this ignores the principle on the basis of which the operation was undertaken. One therefore should expect antireflux surgery to decrease the clinical morbidity of infection markedly by eliminating involvement of the upper urinary tract. The operation clearly achieves a great reduction in the postoperative incidence of pyelonephritis, but bacteriuria, as expected, occurs as often in children after surgery as it does in children with normal urinary tracts (Govan and Palmer; Scott and Stansfeld, 1968a).

Ureteroneocystostomy

The multiplicity of antireflux procedures and their countless individual variations reflect the intense interest in the

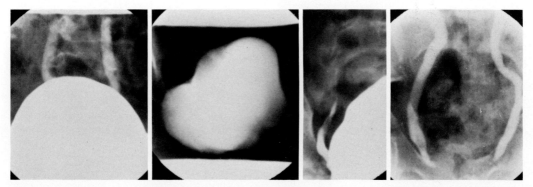

Figure 11–193. Conservative management of reflux. *Extreme left,* bilateral vesicoureteral reflux. *Middle left, cystogram made 2 years later.* No reflux. *Middle right, cystogram made 1 year later.* Reflux has appeared again at cystography and continues despite absence of infection 1 year later *(extreme right).*

problem rather than the inadequacy of any particular method. These procedures are generally concerned with intravesical or extravesical lengthening of the intramural ureter (suprahiatal repair) (Grégoir and Van Regemorter; Lich and associates, 1960, 1961b; Palken; Politano and Leadbetter) or advancing the ureteral orifice toward the vesical neck (infrahiatal repair) (Glenn and Anderson). A combination of these is ideal (Kelalis, 1974). Some procedures are more popular than others, but all are acceptable provided that they achieve comparable results in the hands of the surgeons who are using them. The technical success (eliminating the reflux without producing hydronephrosis) and the effect of the operation on the course of urinary infection are the two criteria most frequently used in evaluating postoperative results. Recent experiences in large series show that well over 90 per cent and indeed more than 95 per cent of such surgical procedures are successful technically (Figs. 11-194 through 11-198) (Garrett and Schlueter; Gonzales and associates; Hendren, 1969; Palken; Politano and Leadbetter; Woodard and Keats).

Perhaps more important is the effect that elimination of reflux has on the subsequent growth of the kidney and the development of scars. Recently, Willscher and associates, after a carefully conducted retrospective study, reported on the effect of antireflux surgery on renal growth in a series of children for whom accurate urographic data was available for purposes of comparison. When unilateral reflux without pyelonephritis was present, the refluxing kidney grew to greater length after surgery than would normally be expected. When unilateral reflux was associated with pyelonephritis, the normally expected renal length was seen, with no accentuated growth. When bilateral reflux was present in normal kidneys, there was accentuated postoperative renal growth on both sides.

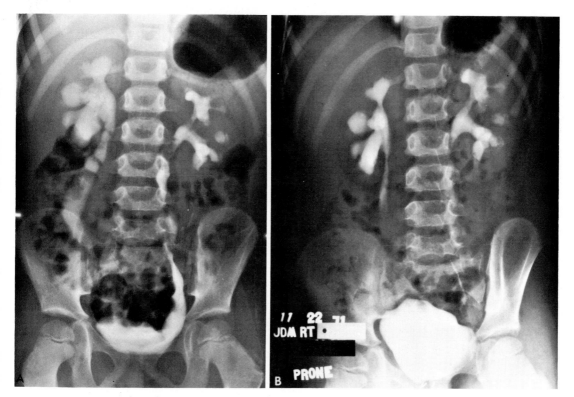

Figure 11-194. Bilateral ureteroneocystostomy. **A,** *Excretory urogram.* Bilateral hydroureteronephrosis due to reflux. **B,** *Same study,* made *3 months after operation,* shows regression of dilatation. No reflux.

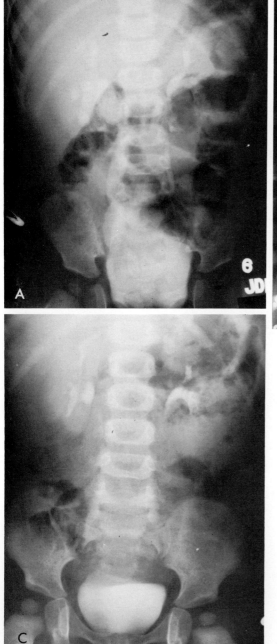
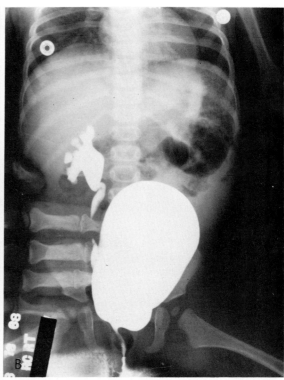

Figure 11–195. Ureteroneocystostomy. **A,** *Preoperative excretory urogram.* **B,** *Preoperative cystogram.* Right vesicoureteral reflux. Right ureteroneocystostomy was performed. **C,** *Excretory urogram.* Postoperative regression of hydronephrosis.

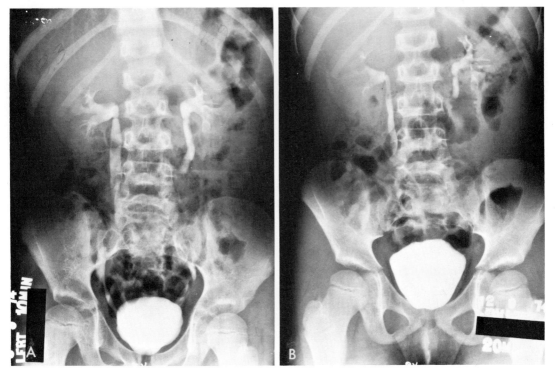

Figure 11–196. Bilateral ureteroneocystostomy for vesicoureteral reflux. *Excretory urograms* (A) *preoperative,* and (B) *postoperative (4 months),* showing regression of ureterectasis.

Figure 11–197. Successful surgical correction of vesicoureteral reflux. Patient, 3¹/₂-year-old girl, had 1-year history of urinary tract infections. A, *Excretory urogram* obtained in course of workup. Ureterectasis of lower half of right ureter. (Cinecystourethrogram demonstrated right vesicoureteral reflux.) B, *Excretory urogram* made 7 months after right ureteroneocystostomy. Normal.

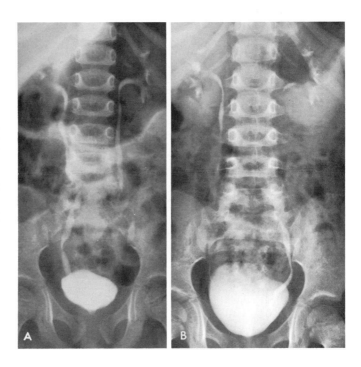

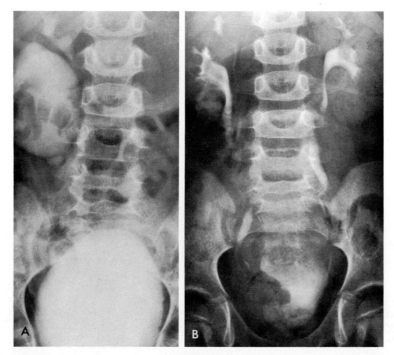

Figure 11–198. Reflux associated with ureteral duplication. **A,** *Retrograde cystogram.* Duplicated ureter on right (juncture within intramural ureter) with reflux up both limbs. Hydronephrosis of lower segment only. (At ureteroneocystostomy orifices not separated, but entire ureter brought through tunnel under vesical mucosa.) **B,** *Postoperative excretory urogram.* Normal. Note negative filling defect from "turned back" cuff of ureter projecting into bladder.

Finally, when bilateral reflux was associated with bilateral pyelonephritis, the growth of both kidneys was accelerated after surgery. In other words, all refluxing kidneys in which there was no radiologic evidence of pyelonephritis demonstrated accelerated growth postoperatively, but the "pyelonephritic" kidney showed accelerated growth postoperatively only when radiographic changes were seen bilaterally.

McRae, Shannon, and Utley suggest that successful surgical correction of the grossly dilated refluxing unit may have a beneficial effect on renal growth; in lesser degrees of dilatation, surgery is not likely to change events because the kidneys will grow irrespective of the presence or absence of reflux. A strictly controlled series including both medical and surgical treatments reported by Scott and Stansfeld (1968b) was quite small and probably reflected a selective population; however, they found that surgical treatment affords a small but significant overall beneficial effect on renal growth.

Complications of Ureteroneocystostomy. It is clear that surgical treatment offers a good chance of eliminating reflux, but it is not entirely free of risk. In a small but significant number of patients, reflux may persist (although sometimes to a lesser degree than preoperatively), or obstruction with hydronephrosis may ensue. Minimal degrees of obstruction regress with time (Figs. 11–199 and 11–200). Although injudicious dissection may lead to devascularization of the lower ureter with subsequent stricture, most often the obstruction or angulation appears to be at the new entrance of the ureter into the bladder. It may be temporary or intermittent, and it results from variations of tension at this level when the bladder fills. In such instances, a film taken with the bladder empty will show regression of the hydroureteronephrosis (Figs. 11–201 through 11–204).

Text continued on page 1076

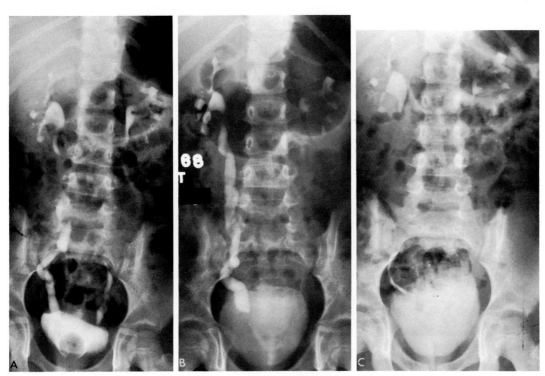

Figure 11–199. Temporary ureteral obstruction from edema after ureteroneocystostomy to correct reflux. Patient, 6-year-old girl, had 2-year history of recurring urinary tract infections caused by bilateral vesicoureteral reflux. **A,** *Preoperative excretory urogram.* **Bilateral parenchymal thinning and ureterectasis.** Note balloon of Foley catheter in bladder. Patient had been on catheter drainage because of bilateral vesicoureteral reflux. (At cystoscopy, large, thin-walled, nontrabeculated bladder was seen. Ureteral orifices were gaping, and intramural ureters were entirely absent while bladder was full.) **B,** *Excretory urogram,* 9 months after bilateral ureteroneocystostomy. **Ureteropyelocaliectasis on right, secondary to residual postoperative edema.** Patient was asymptomatic and free of reflux. **C,** *Excretory urogram,* 14 months after operation. Essentially normal.

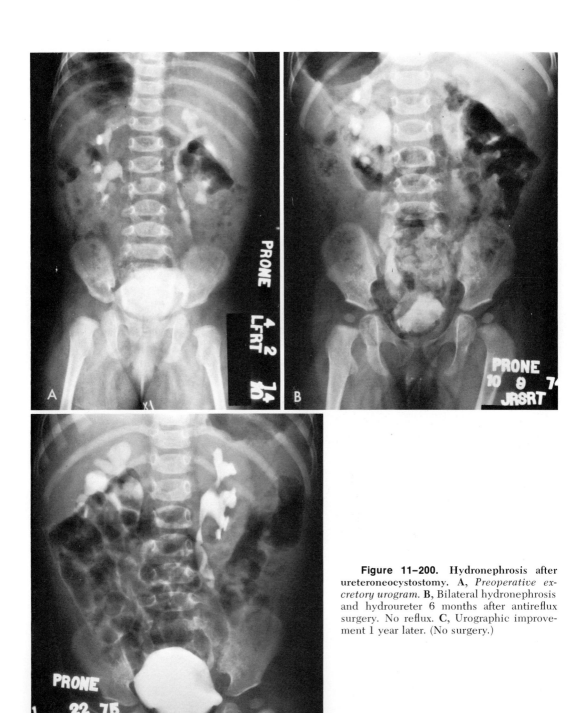

Figure 11–200. Hydronephrosis after ureteroneocystostomy. **A,** *Preoperative excretory urogram.* **B,** Bilateral hydronephrosis and hydroureter 6 months after antireflux surgery. No reflux. **C,** Urographic improvement 1 year later. (No surgery.)

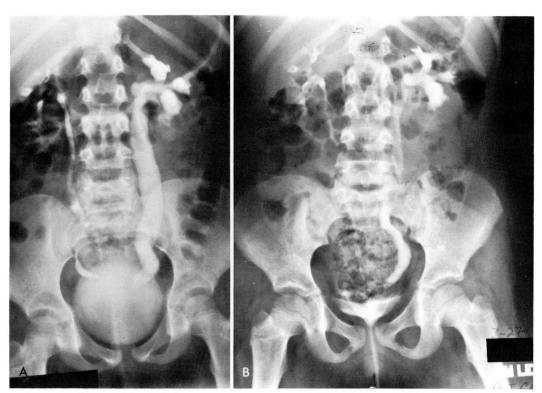

Figure 11–201. Ureteroneocystostomy. **A,** *Excretory urogram.* Bladder full. Left hydroureteronephrosis. **B,** *Excretory urogram.* Bladder empty. Regression of hydroureteronephrosis.

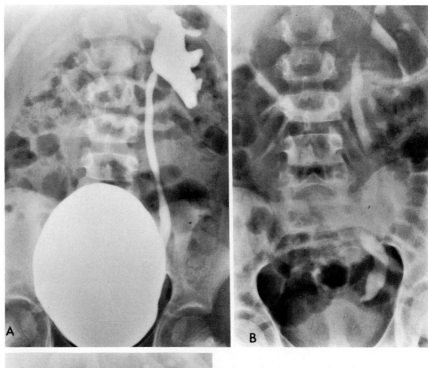

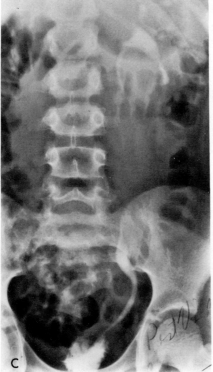

Figure 11–202. Complications of ureteroneocystostomy. **A,** *Cystogram.* Reflux into solitary left ureter and pelvis. **B,** *Excretory urogram* made 9 months after surgery. **Ureterectasis. C,** *Same study with bladder empty.* Regression of ureterectasis.

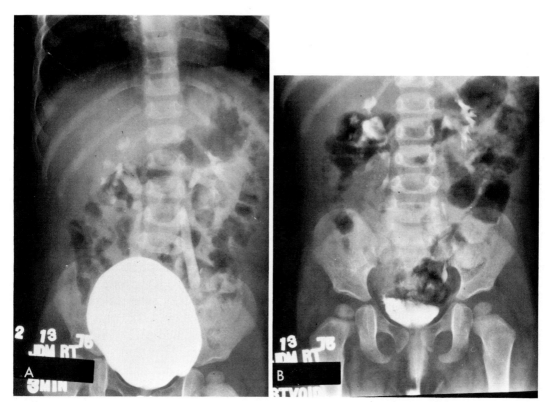

Figure 11–203. Ureteroneocystostomy. *Excretory urograms* taken (**A**) with bladder full and (**B**) with bladder empty. Note difference in ureteral caliber.

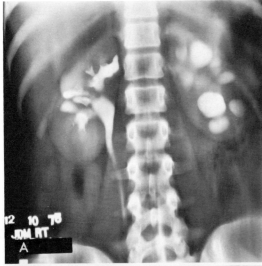

Figure 11–204.   Left ureteroneocystostomy. *Excretory urograms.* **A, Left hydroureteronephrosis** 3 months after antireflux surgery. **B,** Three months later. Left hydroureteronephrosis. **C,** Three months later (without surgery). Regression of hydronephrosis. Probably was caused by intermittent obstruction.

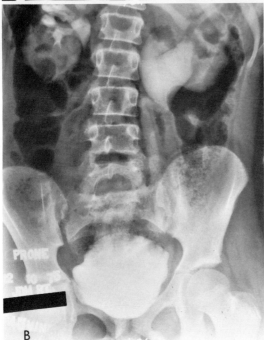

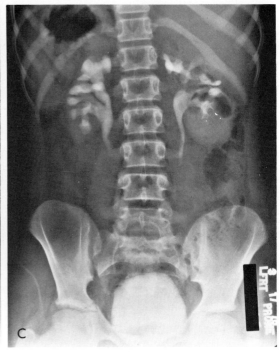

Rarely, obstruction can first appear several years after ureteroneocystostomy (Weiss and associates). This probably is the effect of growth on the ureterovesical angle and clearly stresses the need for careful follow-up of the kidneys through periods of growth (Fig. 11–205) (Filly and associates). Certainly, with the present refinement in surgical techniques, the general incidence of postoperative obstruction should not exceed 5 per cent.

It must be stressed that hydronephrosis after obstruction from antireflux surgery can be severe and alarmingly progressive, especially in the presence of infection. An excretory urogram should be obtained just before the patient is discharged to make sure that both kidneys are draining well. Further evaluation of the efficacy of the surgical treatment is performed at three months and then one to two years thereafter.

In some children, progressive ureteral

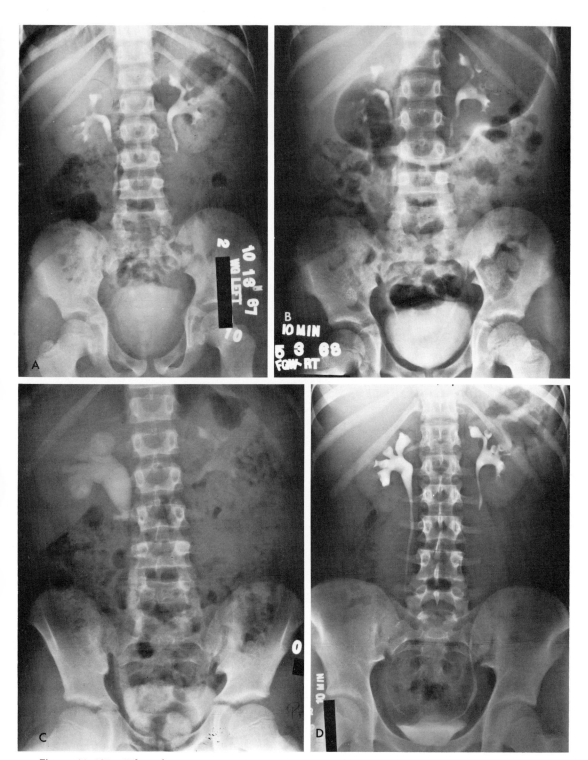

Figure 11–205. Bilateral ureteroneocystostomy. **A,** *Preoperative excretory urogram.* **B,** *Postoperative excretory urogram.* **C,** *Excretory urogram.* Development of **hydroureteronephrosis** 3 years later. Transurethral meatotomy leading to recurrence of reflux. **D,** *Excretory urogram,* 6 years later. Good growth of kidney despite persisting reflux.

dilatation takes place after antireflux surgery, but obstruction cannot be demonstrated in either a retrograde or an antegrade fashion; in these children, reflux is also absent. A possible explanation in these instances is that one is dealing with a form of ureterovesical incoordination resulting in a functional type of obstruction. It is unlikely that a secondary procedure would be of benefit. When the disorder is unilateral, anastomosis of the dilated ureter to the normal ureter (transureteroureterostomy)

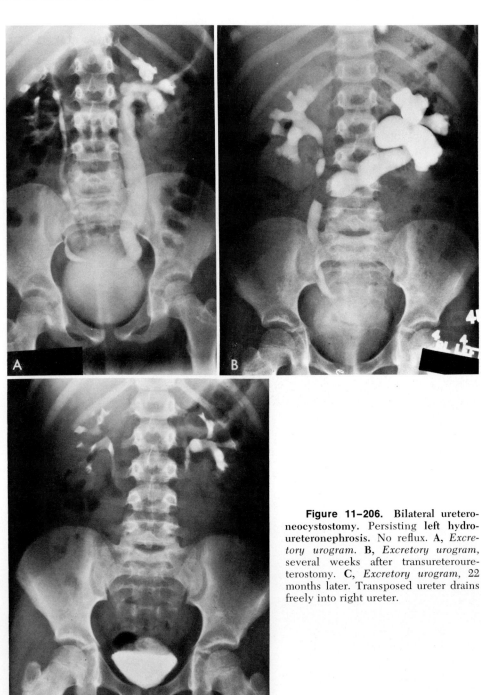

Figure 11–206. Bilateral ureteroneocystostomy. Persisting **left** hydroureteronephrosis. No reflux. **A,** *Excretory urogram.* **B,** *Excretory urogram,* several weeks after transureteroureterostomy. **C,** *Excretory urogram,* 22 months later. Transposed ureter drains freely into right ureter.

should be given at least equal, if not preferential, consideration to secondary ureteroneocystostomy (Fig. 11–206).

Persistence of reflux in the reimplanted ureterovesical angle is perhaps slightly more common than obstruction. It is probably related to an inadequate tunnel, especially with ureteral dilatation or reimplantation of the ureter into a bladder affected by neurogenic dysfunction. Such reflux on the operated or ipsilateral side subsides spontaneously in the majority of cases. When unilateral ureteroneocystostomy is performed, contralateral reflux may appear subsequently in 15 to 20 per cent of children. Elimination of the safety valve and readjustment of bladder pressure precipitates reflux in the marginally incompetent ureterovesical juncture on the contralateral side, or this may simply be the result of failure to demonstrate reflux on that side preoperatively. In the former instances (the majority of cases), such contralateral reflux is likely to abate on conservative treatment; in the latter instance, in which the orifice is most likely to be distinctly abnormal—and especially when associated with changes on the excretory urogram suggesting reflux, such as ureterectasis or renal changes—prophylactic reimplantation of the nonrefluxing contralateral ureter must then be considered (Warren and associates).

Surgical Treatment of Megaureter (Reductive Ureteroplasty; Ureteral Caliber Reduction-Modelage)

Revision of the ureterovesical juncture in the refluxing megaureter entails reduction of the ureteral caliber in addition to reimplantation (Fig. 11–207). It should be stressed that, although spectacular results have been achieved, great problems and disastrous consequences have also been encountered. When the problem is bilateral with severe upper tract damage and the bladder is very abnormal, it is a very

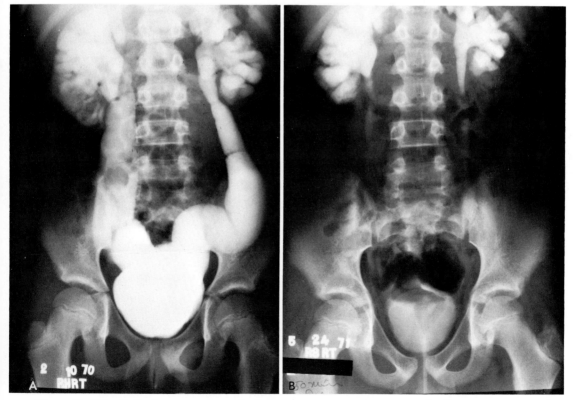

Figure 11–207. Refluxing megaureter. **A**, *Excretory urogram,* preoperative. **B**, *Excretory urogram* after ureteral caliber reduction.

difficult procedure indeed (Hendren, 1969).

Bischoff (1961), Johnston (1967), and Hendren (1968) all have advocated segmental management of the dilated upper urinary tract, and it would appear that the response to this approach is good.

The results of the operation should not be evaluated solely on the basis of urographic improvement; one must also consider renal growth and function (information frequently lacking in evaluations of such results).

Even though the results of such procedures have varied widely, technical success can be expected in at least two thirds of patients overall. However, a controlled comparison of this aggressive but delicate surgical approach with multistage procedures, including preliminary diversion with later reconstruction, or indeed simple expectant treatment, is necessary in each category before specific conclusions can be reached.

STASIS INVOLVING THE LOWER PART OF THE URINARY TRACT

by David C. Utz and David M. Barrett

Neurogenic Bladder

ACQUIRED NEUROGENIC BLADDER

As Ney and Duff pointed out, several abnormalities are seen in cystourethrograms of patients with neurogenic bladder; yet none of them is pathognomonic of the disease, and almost all can be seen in cystourethrograms of patients who do not have neurologic disease. Furthermore, there is no common agreement on the clinical significance of these abnormal findings. The following are among the cystographic variations: trabeculated bladder of either circular or pyramidal ("pine tree") contour; hourglass bladder with pseudosphincteric formations; normal-sized or small hypertonic trabeculated bladder; large, dilated hypotonic bladder without trabeculation; vesicoureteral reflux; variations in the contour of the vesical neck and prostatic urethra, such as the dilated funnel shape, saccular dilatation, and contracted spastic vesical neck; and spastic or relaxed external striated muscle sphincter.

The plain film should be examined carefully, especially if the patient is an infant or child with vesical and rectal dysfunction, for evidence of deformity or agenesis (partial or complete) of the sacrum.

Trabeculation of the Bladder

Except in disorders in which only the sensory pathways are comprised, such as tabes dorsalis, syringomyelia, and diabetes mellitus, almost all neurogenic bladders have some degree of trabeculation, and many are associated with vesicoureteral reflux (Figs. 11–208 through 11–211). Some authors have tried to correlate the degree of trabeculation, and the contour, size, and tonicity of the bladder with the level of the spinal lesion (Giertz and Lindblom; McLellan). Others have concluded that these characteristics of the bladder relate more directly to the duration of the lesion, the degree of recovery, and the type of treatment applied to the bladder (Bors, 1951, 1957). It has been stated that trabeculation of the bladder is slight and the capacity of the bladder is large in the case of lower motor neuron lesions (involving the conus). In the experience of Emmett, at least 80 per cent of patients with congenital spina bifida and myelodysplasia (a lower motor neuron lesion) have trabeculated bladders (Emmett, 1947, 1954). In fact, severe degrees of trabeculation can be seen in cases with conus and cauda equina lesions. Giertz and Lindblom apparently have had similar experience. They state that the trabeculated "pine tree-shaped" bladder is seen almost exclusively in association with nuclear and infranuclear lesions. They found that in the case of upper motor neuron lesions, the bladder is circular and usually has less trabeculation.

It is generally conceded that most

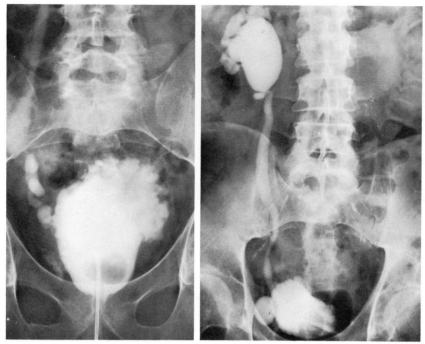

Fig. 11–208   Fig. 11–209

Figure 11–208. *Retrograde cystogram.* **Neurogenic bladder, secondary to traumatic lesion of spinal cord at C-5** in boy, 18 years of age. Marked trabeculation of bladder with cellule formation and reflux up right ureter. Prostatic urethra wide open and filled with medium as result of previous transurethral resection of vesical neck. Negative shadow in base of bladder represents bag of catheter.

Figure 11–209. *Retrograde cystogram.* **War injury (gunshot) of spinal cord at level of T-12 and L-1.** Outline of irregular, trabeculated bladder with cellules and diverticulum on right. Reflux up right ureter, which is dilated, grade 2. Renal pelvis is dilated, grade 3.

Figure 11–210. *Retrograde cystogram.* **Neurogenic bladder, resulting from transverse lesion of spinal cord secondary to surgical removal of tumor at L-1 and L-2,** in boy of 17 years; 1,200 ml of residual urine. Typical pyramid-shaped bladder with cellule formation and reflux up left ureter. **Pyeloureterectasis, grade 3.** (Urinary retention was relieved by transurethral resection of vesical neck. Patient now voids voluntarily, at regular intervals, and empties bladder completely.)

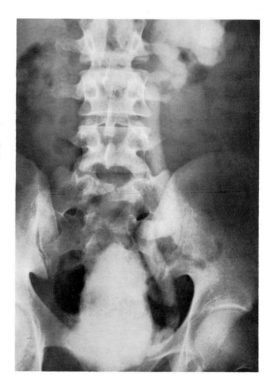

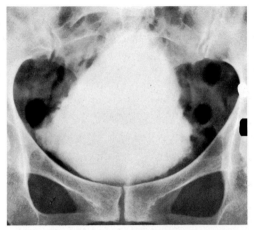

Figure 11–211. *Retrograde cystogram.* **Neurogenic bladder resulting from multiple sclerosis** in woman 46 years of age. Note trabeculation, cellule formation, and pyramidal contour.

small, spastic, trabeculated bladders are associated with upper motor neuron lesions, yet relatively efficient and balanced automatic bladders with good capacity and minimal trabeculation are encountered in association with lesions of the midthoracic cord. It should not be forgotten that almost any type or degree of trabeculated bladder, including the "pine tree" bladder, may be seen in patients with no neurologic disease who have only simple obstruction of the vesical neck.

The large, smooth, thin-walled, atonic type of bladder with little or no trabeculation is seen in tabes dorsalis, diabetes mellitus, and syringomyelia, but it is also seen in patients without demonstrable neurologic disease who have psychogenic vesical decompensation (Larson and associates). Certainly, recent advances in the methodology of urodynamics (cystometrogram, sphincter electromyography, urofluorimetry, and urethral profilometry), when combined with cystourethrography, offer an opportunity for a more complete understanding of these problems.

Characteristics of the Vesical Neck and External Urethral Sphincter

Attempts to correlate the various urographic contours of the vesical neck and prostatic urethra with the level of the spinal lesion, type of neurogenic vesical dysfunction, type of treatment indicated, and prognosis have not, generally speaking, been rewarding. An exception to this has been the demonstration of a spastic external (striated muscle) sphincter by means of cystourethrography and combined cystometrogram and sphincter electromyography. It has been shown that, in upper motor neuron lesions, spasticity of the striated muscle fibers of the external sphincter may be the obstructive factor that prevents the bladder from emptying satisfactorily (Figs. 11–212 through 11–215) (Emmett, Daut, and Dunn). Bors has contended that some of the striated muscle fibers of the external sphincter may extend upward and interdigitate with the smooth muscle fibers of the vesical neck so that the vesical neck may also become spastic (Bors, 1951, 1957). Transurethral resection of the vesical neck may eliminate the bladder-neck factor, but obstruction will persist unless external sphincterotomy is also performed (Perkash). Other procedures to eliminate external sphincter obstruction include pudendal nerve block and section (Ross and Damanski), subarachnoid alcohol block (Shelden and Bors), and selective spinal cordotomy (MacCarty) (Figs. 11–216 through 11–222).

CONGENITAL NEUROGENIC BLADDER (MYELODYSPLASIA, SPINA BIFIDA OCCULTA, SPINA BIFIDA CYSTICA, MENINGOCELE, MENINGOMYELOCELE; ANOMALIES OF THE SACRUM; AGENESIS OF THE SACRUM)

Terminology

Vertebral Defects and Associated Neural Abnormalities. *Spina bifida* means a failure of fusion of the laminae of the vertebra. If a cystic lesion appears on the surface of the body, the combination lesion is called *spina bifida cystica.* The lesion may be designated (1) *meningocele,* if the cyst includes only the spinal membranes; (2) *meningomyelocele,* if it includes portions

Text continued on page 1088

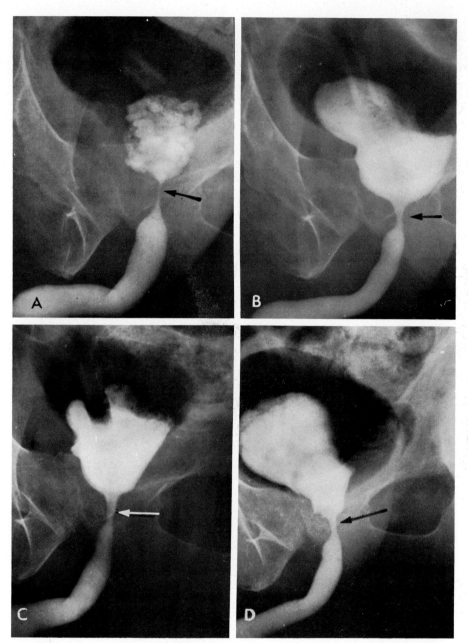

Figure 11–212. Determination of increased spasticity of external sphincter in paraplegic patient with spastic paralysis of lower extremities. **A,** *Retrograde cystourethrogram.* **Spastic external sphincter** (*arrow*). (Patient had undergone previous transurethral resection because of cord bladder and was unable to void.) **B,** *Cystourethrogram* during sacral block with procaine hydrochloride. Relaxation of external sphincter allowed patient to void easily. **C,** *Cystourethrogram* during bilateral pudendal block with procaine. Relaxation of external sphincter allowed patient to void easily. **D,** *Cystourethrogram* after surgical section of both anterior and posterior roots of fourth and fifth lumbar and all five sacral nerves. Relaxation of external sphincter allowed patient to void easily and empty bladder completely. (From Emmett, J. L., Daut, R. V., and Dunn, J. H.)

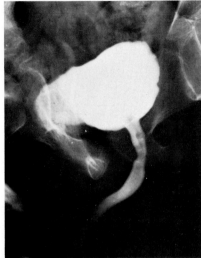

Figure 11–213. *Retrograde cystourethrogram.* Relaxation of external sphincter in paraplegic patient with flaccid paralysis of lower extremities. (From Emmett, J. L., Daut, R. V., and Dunn, J. H.)

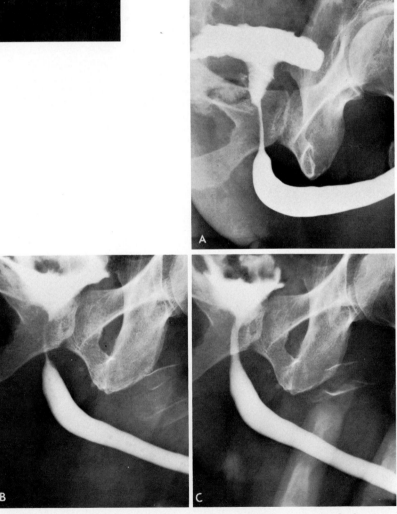

Figure 11–214. Increased spasticity of external urethral sphincter with residual urine associated with neurogenic bladder from primary lateral sclerosis of spinal cord in man, 57 years of age. (Transurethral resection of vesical neck done 3 years previously, but substantial amount of residual urine persisted.) A, *Retrograde urethrogram.* Note marked spasticity and elongation of external sphincter. (Exploratory cervical laminectomy done.) B, *Retrograde urethrogram,* 1 year after laminectomy. External sphincter still spastic, but length seems diminished. C, *Retrograde urethrogram* made immediately after caudal and transsacral procaine block. Note relaxation of external sphincter.

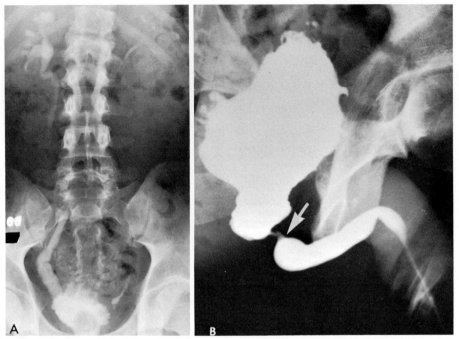

Figure 11–215.   **Neurogenic bladder with spastic external sphincter** in man, aged 21, with traumatic lesion of cauda equina. Bladder dysfunction was only residual disability from accident. Transurethral resection of vesical neck was only partially helpful. **A,** *Excretory urogram,* after transurethral resection. Dilatation of lower half of right ureter, trabeculated (incompletely filled) bladder, and wide open vesical neck. **B,** *Voiding cystourethrogram.* Marked spasticity of external sphincter *(arrow).* (Transurethral excision of lower left quadrant of external sphincter resulted in substantial improvement.)

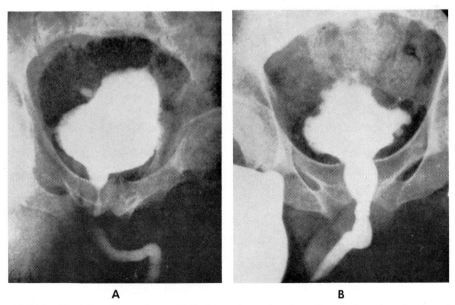

Figure 11–216.   **Partial and complete relief of spastic contraction of vesical neck and external sphincter.** *Retrograde urethrograms.* **A,** *After transurethral resection.* Residual urine of 300 ml persists. Vesical neck has been widened, but clinical result was not satisfactory. **B,** *After subarachnoid alcohol block.* Marked relaxation of vesical neck, entire prostatic urethra, and external sphincter. (From Damanski, M., and Kerr, A. S.)

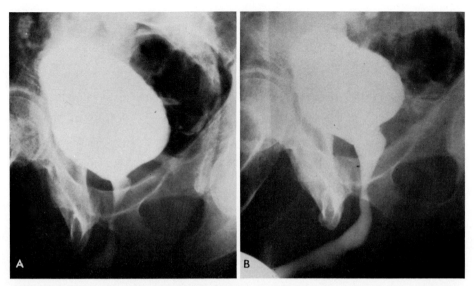

Figure 11–217. Spastic external urethral sphincter of paraplegic patient. *Retrograde urethrograms.* **A,** *Pre-operative.* Spasticity of external sphincter is evident. **B,** *After transurethral resection* of external sphincter. Note relaxation of external sphincter. (From Ross, J. C., Damanski, M., and Gibbon, N.)

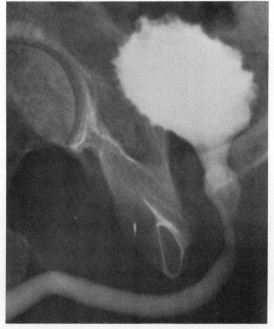

Figure 11–218. *Oblique retrograde cystourethrogram.* **Neurogenic bladder with balanced reflex type of micturition.** Paraplegic patient had upper motor neuron lesion at T-5. No residual urine. (Conservative treatment only.) Note descent of bladder neck, wide opening of prostatic urethra, and lack of spasticity of vesical neck and external sphincter. (From Damanski, M.)

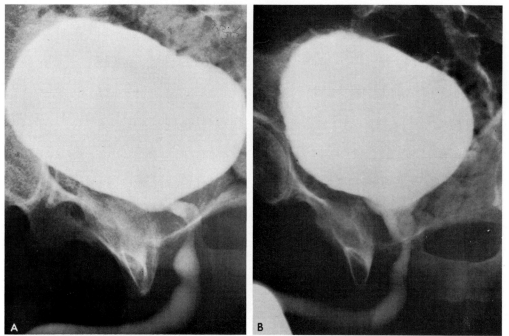

Figure 11–219. Relief of urinary retention by transurethral resection of vesical neck of quadriplegic patient with upper motor neuron lesion at C-7. *Retrograde cystourethrograms.* **A,** *Preoperative oblique view.* Anterior tilt and posterior ledge of vesical neck. (Complete retention with autonomic hyperreflexia.) **B,** *Postoperative oblique view.* Note wide opening of proximal part of prostatic urethra. (Residual urine was reduced to 350 ml and autonomic hyperreflexia disappeared. Patient had normal excretory urogram 4 years after spinal injury.) (From Damanski, M.)

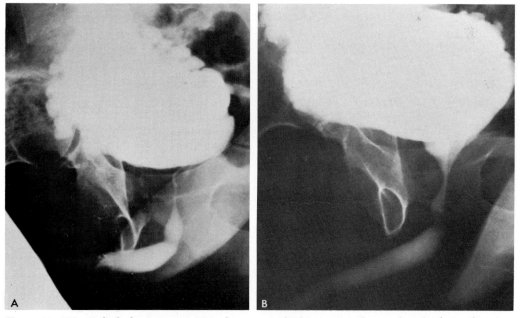

Figure 11–220. Relief of urinary retention by transurethral resection of vesical neck of paraplegic patient with upper motor neuron lesion at T-10. *Retrograde cystourethrograms.* **A,** *Preoperative oblique view.* Posterior tilt and anterior ledge. Note also **diverticulosis of bladder** resulting from urinary infection of long standing. **B,** *Postoperative oblique view.* Note funnel-shaped proximal portion of prostatic urethra. (Residual urine reduced from 480 ml to nil.) (From Damanski, M.)

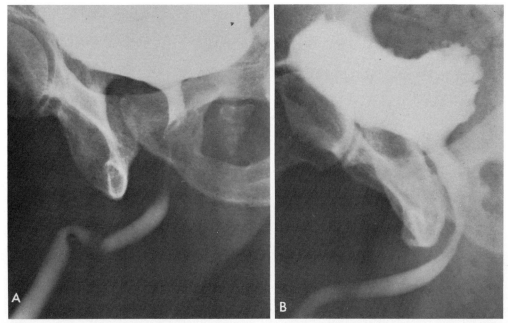

Figure 11–221. Relief, by pudendal neurectomy, of urinary retention from spastic external sphincter of paraplegic patient with upper motor neuron lesion at T-11. *Retrograde cystourethrograms.* **A,** *Preoperative oblique view.* Prostatic urethra is patent above verumontanum, and external sphincter is spastic (very narrow). (Residual urine measured 570 ml. **Hydronephrosis.** Pudendal neurectomy was performed.) **B,** *Postoperative oblique view.* Much better opening of external sphincter. (Residual urine reduced to 60 ml. Hydronephrosis reduced. (From Damanski, M.)

of the meninges and the spinal cord; and (3) *myelocele,* if the cord itself is exposed. Nerve roots also may be included.

Spina bifida occulta is the term used if there is failure of fusion of the lamina but no external swelling or "tumor" over the defect to indicate its presence. The condition may be suspected, however, from thickening or dimpling of the skin, abnormal growth of hair, abnormal pigmentation, or the presence of a lipoma or fibroma. Spina bifida may occur at any level of the spine, but it most often involves the lumbosacral levels. The laminal defect is almost always posterior and is usually filled in by a fibrofatty pad (Williams, 1958), which Campbell (1960) has described as an intramedullary lipoma. Ventral (anterior) spina bifida is rare (Fig. 11–223).

There is no correlation between the type and degree of spina bifida and the incidence or severity of the neurologic defect. For instance, it has been estimated that in routine roentgenographic examina-tions of the lumbar spine in "normal" adults, some defect in closure of the laminae is apparent in at least one-third of cases. Karlin estimated that it is encountered in more than 50 per cent of "normal" children. The defect varies from involvement of only the lower sacral segments (open neural arch) to wide separation of the laminae of all the sacral and many of the lumbar vertebrae (see Figures 11–231 through 11–234).

In the remainder of this discussion, the general term *myelodysplasia* will be used to include all congenital malformations of the sacral neural axis.

Sacral and Coccygeal Defects. Other types of congenital defects occur either alone or in association with spina bifida. These defects, sacral scoliosis ("twisted" sacrum) and agenesis of part or all of the sacrum, are often overlooked when one is reading urograms, especially of infants and children. Agenesis of the sacrum is the general term used when any or all seg-

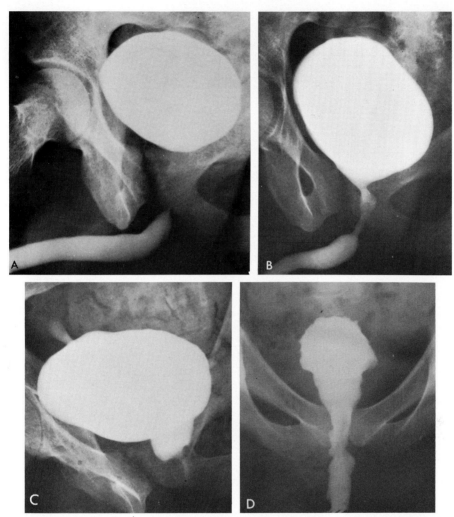

Figure 11–222.   Relief of bladder retention and dilatation of upper part of urinary tract of quadriplegic patient (C-8) after (1) subarachnoid alcohol block, (2) transurethral resection of vesical neck, and (3) division of external urethral sphincter (performed in sequence). **A,** *Retrograde cystourethrogram, oblique view.* Normal anterior urethra ends abruptly at level of external urethral sphincter. (Attempt at overcoming its resistance by forceful injection might result in extravasation. Indwelling catheter was inserted to relieve complete retention.) Subarachnoid alcohol block was performed. **B,** *Retrograde cystourethrogram, oblique view, after alcohol block* (and conversion of upper motor neuron lesion into lower one). Note difference at bladder outlet. Prostatic urethra is patent, but there remains posterior ledge. Moderate relaxation of external urethral sphincter as compared to **A.** Note descent of bladder base. Urinary retention persisted. (Transurethral resection of bladder neck was performed.) **C,** *Cystogram, oblique view,* after resection of bladder neck. Prostatic urethra is wide open but spasticity of external sphincter persists. (Note vesicoureteral reflux on right.) Urinary retention persisted. (By this time patient had acquired bilateral hydronephrosis. Division of external sphincter was performed.) **D,** *Micturition cystourethrogram, anteroposterior view, after division of external sphincter.* Patient reacted to introduction of contrast medium with immediate emptying of bladder, associated with wide opening of all structures at bladder outlet and external urethral sphincter. Note absence of reflux. (Residual urine eliminated. Hydronephrotic changes disappeared almost completely.) (From Damanski, M.)

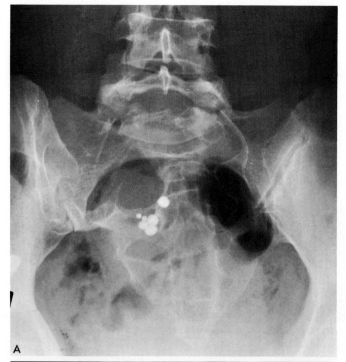

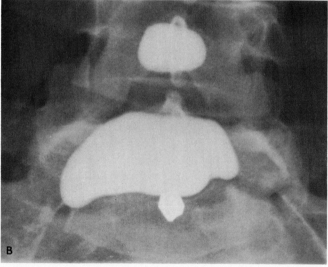

Figure 11–223. Large anterior meningocele. Woman, aged 33, had had bladder dysfunction requiring use of indwelling urethral catheter since age 20. **A,** *Plain film.* Erosion of right half of sacrum from pressure of meningocele. Residual Lipiodol from ancient myelogram. **B,** *Myelogram.* Large meningocele sac partially filled. (Patient's only disability was of bladder; she had normal bowel function and no sensory or motor impairment. Surgical exploration revealed that marked erosion had destroyed anterior wall of sacrum; posterior wall also was eroded and thin. Rectum protruded into sacral canal. Surgical repair was impossible. Note: Pressure over thin eroded portion of posterior wall of sacrum produced headache.)

ments of the sacrum are missing. For the lesion to be classified as "true" sacral agenesis, two or more sacral segments should be absent (Williams and Nixon). Sacral agenesis is often associated with anorectal anomalies, such as imperforate anus and atresia, rectourethral fistula, and so on (Williams and Nixon). In a review of 50 cases, Blumel, Evans, and Eggers found complete absence of the sacrum in 32 patients and partial absence in 18.

There is little doubt that the condition is more common than is appreciated, because roentgenologic recognition is difficult owing to poor visualization of the sacrum, especially in children. Missing segments are often interpreted simply as poor visualization, and although the radiologist may suspect presence of the lesion, exact interpretation of the x-ray films may be exceedingly difficult.

Cause of Neurologic Defects in Cases of Spina Bifida With Myelodysplasia.

The reason for the neurologic disability is the arrested ascent of the spinal cord because of fixation of the cord and its coverings at the site of the laminal defect (anchored conus medullaris). This usually is seen as a confluence of the conus medullaris and intramedullary lipoma with extension into the soft tissues overlying the spina bifida (Campbell, 1960) (Figs. 11–224 and 11–225). Because of this fixation, the cord is unable to go through the normal "shortening" process that occurs in intrauterine growth and development. The fixation continues after birth, and as the child grows taller, the traction on the cord may

increase. As a matter of fact, this is the explanation given for cases in which symptoms and signs of myelodysplasia do not appear until several years after birth (in some cases as late as puberty, or even later). Cord fixation and the so-called tight filum terminale or tethered-cord syndrome also provide the rationale for neurosurgical operations in which the bands and adhesions that are holding the cord are severed and the lipoma is removed (Figs. 11–226 and 11–227) (Campbell, 1960). In addition to cord fixation, associated anomalous malformations of the cord such as congenital hydromyelia and diastematomyelia may be present.

Degree of Disability; Clinical Findings

The degree of disability associated with spina bifida depends on the extent of the defect and the amount of damage and

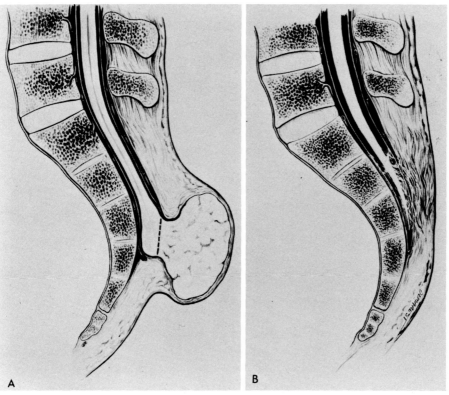

Figure 11–224. Representation of arrested ascent of spinal cord in spina bifida. **A,** Confluence of conus medullaris and intramedullary lipoma, with extension into soft tissues overlying spina bifida. (Broken line marks site of amputation of the lipoma.) **B,** Retention of the conus medullaris at a low sacral level as the result of adhesions arising in conjunction with a **meningocele.** (From Campbell, J. B., 1960.)

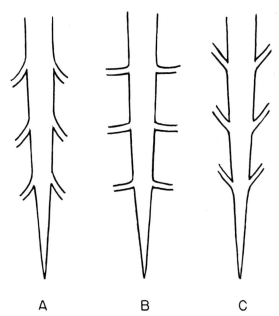

Figure 11–225. Abnormal angles that may be assumed by nerve roots in caudal portion of spinal cord when ascent of conus is prevented by fixation, by adhesions, or by intramedullary lipoma in continuity with overlying soft tissues. (From Campbell, J. B., 1960.)

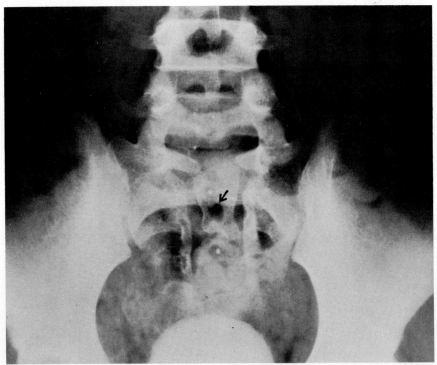

Figure 11–226. *Plain film.* **Spina bifida occulta without meningocele.** (At operation, fibrous strand containing both neural and fibrous tissue ran from conus through dura to hole [*arrow*] in bony plate which probably represents confluence of maldeveloped lamina. This probably represented "tight filum terminale" syndrome.) (From Campbell, J. B., 1960.)

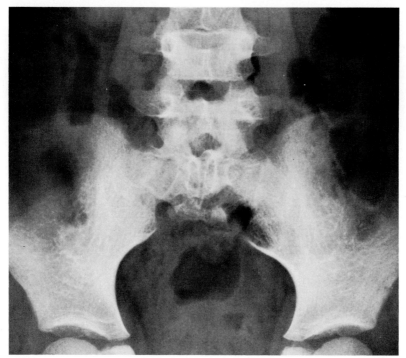

Figure 11–227. *Plain film* of little girl with dysfunction of bladder. **Absence of sacrum and coccyx, without meningocele.** Conus had ascended to level just above bony malformation, and cauda equina was funneled through small bony canal. (Decompression of bony canal and removal of abnormal amount of epidural fat restored bladder function.) (From Campbell, J. B., 1960.)

degeneration of the sacral cord and cauda equina. Symptoms and clinical findings in myelodysplasia range from minimal or nonexistent to extensive and disabling. For instance, the disorder may affect only visceral innervation, such as that of the rectum and bladder. On the other hand, the lesion may involve the somatic (sensory and motor) nerves, producing various degrees of anesthesia in the saddle area and over the lower extremities, as well as various degrees of flaccid paralysis of the muscles of the legs. In a general way, the vesical dysfunction simulates that associated with an acquired lower motor neuron lesion, except that passive dribbling incontinence from a relaxed external sphincter is common. Trabeculation of the bladder may be extreme, and ureteropyelectasis and reflux may be present. Incontinence is the most troublesome problem. Some children are totally incontinent and "leak empty," so that the upper urinary tract is protected; others

have overflow incontinence and large amounts of residual urine, which cause the threat of death from renal insufficiency.

Vesical dysfunction associated with myelodysplasia is notoriously erratic and does not conform to one pattern as does dysfunction associated with acquired lesions. For instance, although one would expect this type of case to simulate an acquired lower motor neuron lesion, it often exhibits mixed characteristics. Williams (1958) suggested three main types of vesical dysfunction as follows: (1) a flaccid, thin-walled bladder with no trabeculation in a patient who has no sensation of bladder fullness, (2) a markedly trabeculated bladder with saccules and diverticula that may be emptied by means of the manual Credé technique, and (3) a trabeculated bladder that simulates one associated with a lesion of the higher centers, such as multiple sclerosis. Patients having the last-mentioned type retain sensation of bladder fullness and do not have constant passive dribbling; rather, they have an urgency-incontinence pattern.

A study of 53 cases of myelodysplasia suggested that the crux of the situation was the degree of tonicity remaining in the external urethral sphincter (commonly called urethral resistance) (Emmett and Simon). If the sphincter was flaccid, the leakage was "passive" and constant, and the bladder tended to leak completely empty; thus, there was no residual urine, no ureteropyelectasis, and no reflux (see Figure 11–213). On the other hand, if the urethral sphincter had been partially spared, residual urine, ureteropyelectasis, and reflux could be substantial. These findings are essentially in agreement with those of Pellman, who, in discussing 61 cases of myelodysplasia, said that there was an "inverse relationship between the severity of the neuromuscular deficit and the degree of vesicoureteral reflux and residual urine." He noted reflux in 30 of his 61 cases.

Unrecognized Myelodysplasia as Cause of Vesical Dysfunction

In 1968, Cooper and also Stark employed pressure-flow measurements and sphincter electromyographic studies of patients with myelodysplasia to confirm that the function of the detrusor and the activity of the striated muscle sphincter vary considerably. Thus it is easy to comprehend the value of urographic findings in children with meningomyelocele described by Ericsson and associates.

There is currently much concern that some cases of unexplained vesical dysfunction may be the result of myelodysplasia or some involvement of the cauda equina even though typical findings of myelodysplasia are absent. For instance, it is becoming more and more apparent that visceral fibers of the cauda equina (that is, those serving the bladder and rectum) may be more susceptible to impairment than are somatic fibers. Also, it has been pointed out

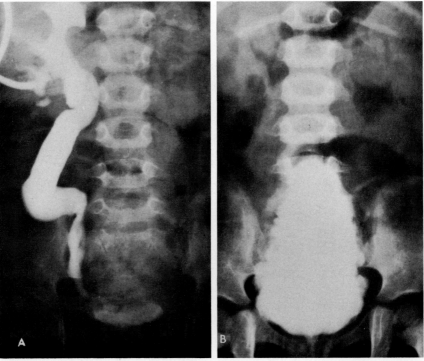

Figure 11–228. Partial absence of sacrum (S4-5 and coccyx) in girl aged 3 years. Unrecognized neurogenic vesical dysfunction. **A,** *Excretory urogram.* Absence of sacral segments 4, 5, and coccyx. Pyeloureterectasis in "solitary" right kidney. (Previous left nephrectomy for infected "hydronephrosis.") **B,** *Retrograde cystogram.* "Pine tree" shaped trabeculated bladder typical of neurogenic dysfunction. (From Koontz, W. W., Jr., and Prout, G. R., Jr.)

that deformities of the sacrum such as partial or total agenesis in many infants and children suffering from the well-known syndrome of distended bladder and extensive ureteropyelectasis have been misinterpreted as congenital obstruction of the vesical neck (Figs. 11–228, 11–229, and 11–230) (Koontz and Prout).

UROGRAPHIC DIAGNOSIS OF CONGENITAL NEUROGENIC BLADDER

Roentgenographic characteristics of the bony defects in spina bifida and agenesis of the sacrum have already been described (see Figures 11–226 through 11–230).

In congenital neurogenic bladder, the urographic findings in the bladder and upper part of the urinary tract tend to resemble those in a patient with an acquired lesion of the spinal cord, as has already been discussed. Trabeculation of the bladder and various degrees of ureteropyelectasis (often with reflux) are the most common findings, although an occasional smooth, flaccid, distended bladder may be seen (Figs. 11–231 through 11–233). The similarity of urograms of children having a presumptive diagnosis of congenital obstruction of the vesical neck and of those having myelodysplasia is shown in Figures 11–234, 11–235, and 11–236. The relaxation of the external urethral sphincter, which often can be demonstrated in the male by cystourethrography (see Figure 11–213), resembles that seen on the urethrogram of a patient with an acquired upper motor neuron lesion after subarachnoid alcohol block, pudendal neurectomy, or surgical

Text continued on page 1100

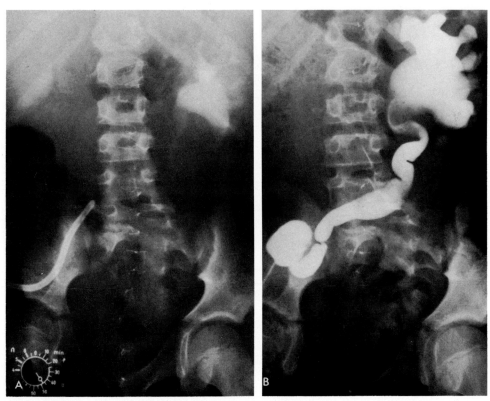

Figure 11–229.   Boy, aged 14 years, with **right renal agenesis. Absence of right half of sacrum and distortion of left half.** Neurogenic vesical dysfunction diagnosed as congenital obstruction of vesical neck. Multiple operations on vesical neck finally culminating in urinary diversion with an ileal conduit. **A,** *Excretory urogram.* Absence of right half of sacrum with distortion of left half. Solitary left kidney. **B,** *Retrograde pyelogram* made through ileal conduit. (From Koontz, W. W., Jr., and Prout, G. R., Jr.)

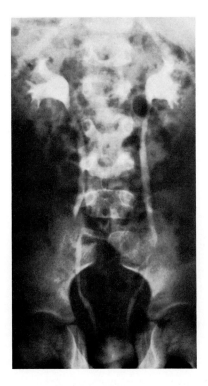

Figure 11–230. Boy, aged 4 years, with **complete absence of sacrum and coccyx except for hemivertebra of S-I.** *Excretory urogram.* Sacral defect as noted. Normal kidneys. Note: Patient has urinary and fecal incontinence, flaccid anal sphincter, and absent ankle jerks bilaterally but no other demonstrable neurologic deficits. (From Koontz, W. W., Jr., and Prout, G. R., Jr.)

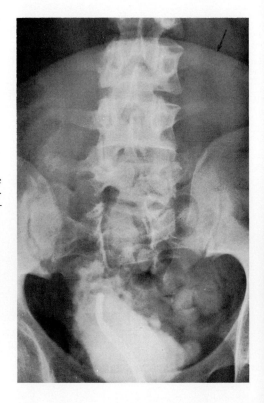

Figure 11–231. *Retrograde cystogram.* Neurogenic bladder from myelodysplasia associated with large meningomyelocele *(arrow)*. Pyramid-shaped bladder with cellule formation in boy of 19 years. Note absence of most of sacrum.

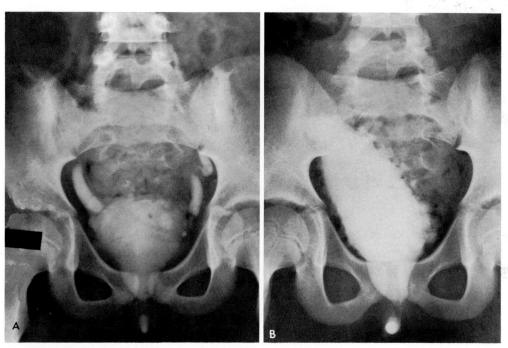

Figure 11–232. **Neurogenic bladder resulting from myelodysplasia** in boy, aged 9 years. **A,** *Excretory urogram.* Dilatation of lower portions of both ureters. Bladder is trabeculated and has multiple cellules. Prostatic urethra was dilated and filled with medium. Medium also was present in bulbous urethra, indicating urinary incontinence. **B,** *Retrograde cystogram.* Bladder better filled. Typical pyramidal bladder with multiple cellules. Medium is present in bulbous urethra.

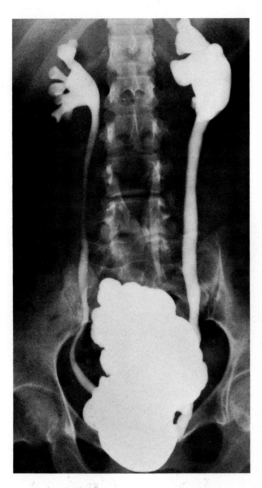

Figure 11–233. *Retrograde cystogram.* **Myelodysplasia with neurogenic bladder and bilateral ureteral reflux** in case of woman, aged 40. (Laminectomy, at age 12, had been performed to remove relatively asymptomatic meningomyelocele. Bladder dysfunction only since operation, which also resulted in somatic sensory nerve damage with trophic ulcers, finally requiring amputation of right leg above knee.)

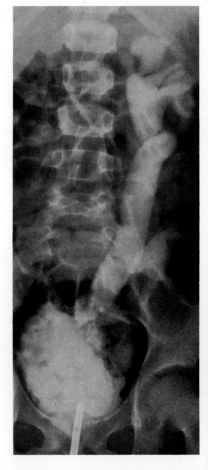

Figure 11–234. *Retrograde cystogram* of 5-year-old girl with **myelodysplasia. Marked trabeculation of bladder and left pyeloureterectasis with reflux.** (From Emmett, J. L., and Simon, H. B.)

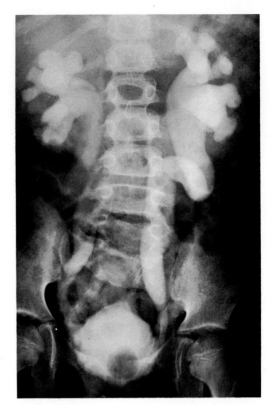

Figure 11–235. *Retrograde cystogram* of 6-year-old girl with **myelodysplasia. Minimal trabeculation of bladder with bilateral pyeloureterectasis and reflux.** (From Emmett, J. L., and Simon, H. B.)

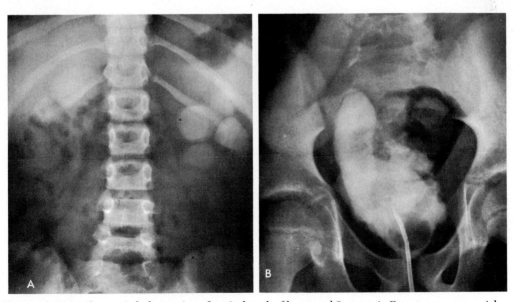

Figure 11–236. Congenital obstruction of vesical neck of boy, aged 8 years. **A,** *Excretory urogram.* Advanced **bilateral hydronephrosis. Poor renal function. B,** *Retrograde cystogram.* **Trabeculated bladder with extensive right ureteral reflux.** (From Emmett, J. L., and Simon, H. B.)

division of the external sphincter to overcome the spasticity (see Figures 11–216 through 11–222).

Congenital Obstruction of the Vesical Neck and Urethra; Distal Urethral Obstruction; Stenosis of the Urethral Meatus

These lesions constitute a clinical complex that includes a large proportion of all pediatric urologic problems. However, urographic data that were previously considered important have now been discarded.

CONGENITAL OBSTRUCTION OF THE VESICAL NECK

Because of an old notion that vesicoureteral reflux was usually secondary to obstructive uropathy, vesical neck obstruction was a common diagnosis. As the major cause of vesicoureteral reflux became apparent in the 1960s—namely, congenital deformities of the ureterovesical juncture—doubt was cast on the entity of vesical neck obstruction. In most centers, consequently, surgical revision of the vesical neck is now an unusual undertaking employed only when objective evidence of bladder outlet obstruction is present (Fig. 11–237).

In this chapter it is assumed that primary vesical neck obstruction does occur, although much more rarely than was once thought, and in male children only. Beyond question, most series presented in the literature do not deal exclusively with cases of vesical neck obstruction, because often the criteria for diagnosis are at best loose or ill-defined.

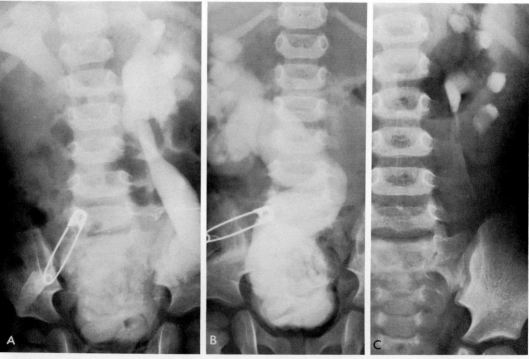

Figure 11–237. Obstruction of vesical neck in boy, 4 years of age. **A,** *Excretory urogram.* **Duplication on right with no function in lower segment. Ureteropyelectasis of upper right segment and of left kidney and ureter. B,** *Retrograde cystogram.* **Reflux up huge ureter (right) serving lower pelvis.** (On cystoscopy, upper meatus [serving lower pelvis] was found to be greatly dilated. Meatus for upper pelvis was of normal size and could be seen on lower edge of it. Right nephrectomy [ureters could not be separated] and plastic Y-V operation on vesical neck were performed.) **C,** *Excretory urogram,* 2 months after operation. Left kidney greatly improved. Patient voiding normally.

Symptoms are obstructive or infective in nature. Residual urine should be expected if the bladder is decompensated in the face of obstruction.

The diagnosis of vesical neck obstruction must be made on the basis of objective signs of bladder outlet obstruction and only after urethral obstructive lesions and neurogenic bladder have been excluded. The diagnosis is of course easier to make when severe trabeculation and residual urine are present. Flow rates and voiding pressures may allow one to make such a diagnosis on physiologic grounds, but the examiner should be aware of pitfalls and the danger of false conclusions.

Diagnosis of Congenital Obstruction of the Vesical Neck

Scandinavian roentgenologists were the first to advocate and employ *voiding cystourethrography* to study the vesical neck (Jorup and Kjellberg; Kjellberg, Ericsson, and Rudhe). Kjellberg and associates described congenital obstruction of the vesical neck as a "defective opening of the bladder neck on micturition" that may appear urographically to *encircle the bladder neck* or may present only as an *inward bulging of the posterior aspect of the vesical neck* (like a median bar in an adult) (Fig. 11–238). Waterhouse, Griesbach and associates, and Hamm and Waterhouse have questioned the validity of such urographic alterations of the vesical neck because they believe these may simply represent physiologic variations in the contractions of the trigonal region and sphincteric mechanisms during micturition which are apparent only on instantaneous roentgenograms.

In a communication regarding the roentgenographic evaluation of bladder neck obstruction, Shopfner (1967b) pointed out that the diameter of the vesical neck and of the various parts of the urethra varies in relation to the stages of voiding. He believes it axiomatic that to be considered contracted and obstructive a bladder neck must be smaller than any of the normally constricted points of the urethra; that is, it must be smaller than the urethral

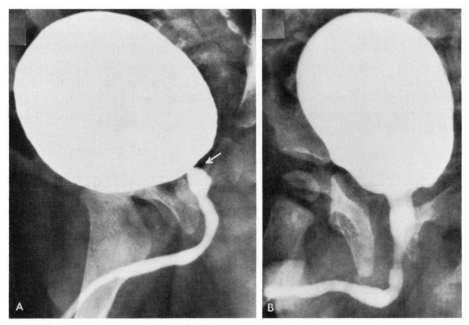

Figure 11–238. Operative relief of obstruction of vesical neck. *Voiding cystourethrograms* of boy, 7 months of age. **A,** *Preoperative.* Note inward bulging of posterior vesical lip *(arrow).* **B,** *After transurethral resection.* (From Kjellberg, S. R., Ericsson, N. D., and Rudhe, U.)

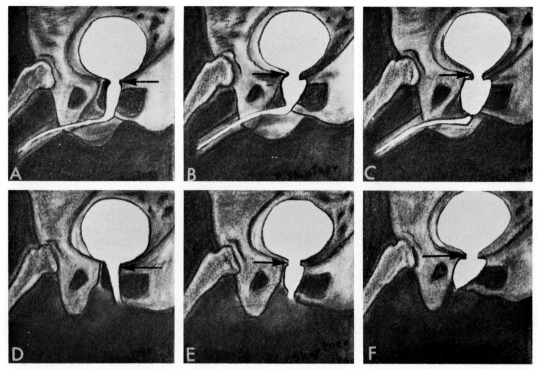

Figure 11–239. A-F, Sketches of bladder neck show relationship of so-called contracture to urethral caliber. A-C, Male urethra. D-F, Female urethra. Diameter of bladder neck is actually same in all; degree of apparent "contracture" appears to increase as urethra is distended and becomes wider. (*Arrows* indicate bladder neck.) (From Shopfner, C. E., 1967c.)

meatus, penoscrotal junction, and membranous urethra in the male and the distal urethra and urethral meatus in the female. If urethrograms are considered on the basis of these criteria, the bladder neck is almost never obstructive (Fig. 11–239).

Shopfner (1967b) also thinks that segmental irregularities seen in the bladder neck should not be interpreted as anterior or posterior "obstructive ledges," "lips," or "notches" that require surgical removal as suggested by Kjellberg and associates. He contends that these are also present in normal persons, and he considers them variations of the trigonal plates that make up the trigonal canal (Hutch, 1965; Shopfner and Hutch).

The same endoscopic features seen in the adult with vesical neck contraction should also apply to the child if such lesions are indeed congenital—that is, concentric intrusion at the bladder neck, often with some foreshortening of the prostatic urethra. Vesical trabeculation is, of course, indirect evidence of obstruction.

In conclusion, it would appear that vesical neck obstruction does not exist in girls and is exceedingly rare in the male. It can be documented with urodynamic studies, which will help rule out voiding dyssynergias and occult neuropathic bladder.

DISTAL URETHRAL STENOSIS

Lyon and Smith in 1963, and Lyon and Tanagho in 1965, published their work in which they demonstrated by anatomic dissections that the muscular components of the female urethra (inner longitudinal layer and outer circular layer, which are continuations of the detrusor muscle at the vesical neck) end sharply at the juncture of the middle and distal thirds of the urethra by inserting into dense collagenous tissue. They also found that, in little girls with persistent urinary infection, the nonmuscu-

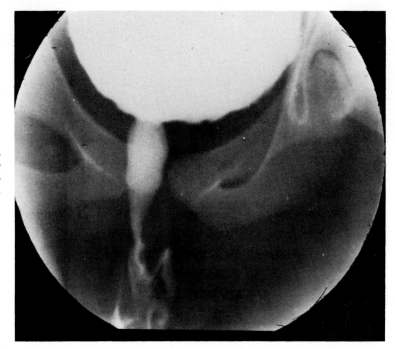

Figure 11–240. *Voiding cystourethrogram* of girl with urinary infection. Distal urethral obstruction? Normal cystourethroscopy.

lar distal segment of the urethra appeared to impede urinary flow.

Distal urethral stenosis is the lesion to which recurrent urinary tract infection in girls is probably attributed most often.

Many investigators have questioned whether distal urethral stenosis exists, whether any significance can be attached to it, and whether it indeed represents a true anomaly (Graham and associates; Immergut and Wahman).

The precise role of distal urethral stenosis in the etiology of urinary infection is uncertain. At times (but rarely) stenosis of a severe degree is accompanied by severe trabeculation, which subsides upon correction of the stenotic lesion.

Some reports indicate that procedures to reduce distal urethral resistance (meatotomy, dilation, or internal urethrotomy) reduce the recurrence of urinary infection in addition to improving the voiding pattern (Halverstadt and Leadbetter). Others have questioned this, but since it is simple to perform dilatation at the time of cystoscopy, the continued use of this procedure is justified.

The existence of distal urethral stenosis is found only by urethral calibration with bougie à boule. Radiographic demonstration of the lesion at voiding cystourethrography is at best confusing and unreliable (Figs 11–240 through 11–245). One should expect to find a distinct widening of the urethra above the stenotic ring, and, since the bladder neck remains fixed (and narrowed), one should also find the

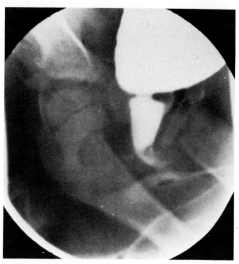

Figure 11–241. *Voiding cystourethrogram* showing "acorn" deformity of urethra in 3-year-old girl. Normal urethral calibration.

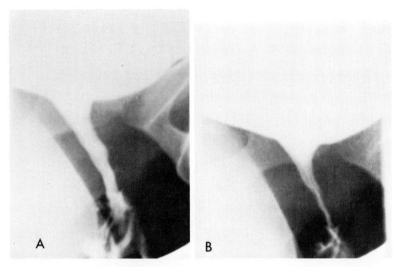

Figure 11–242. Variations in profile of female urethra (**A** and **B**) during same *voiding cystourethrogram.*

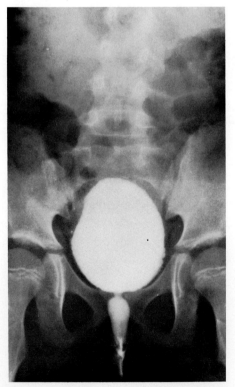

Figure 11–243. *Voiding cystourethrogram* of girl, aged 6½. "Acorn" or "spinning top" contour of bladder neck and urethra interpreted as representing contracture of bladder neck and poststenotic dilatation of urethra. (From Gould, H. R., and Peterson, C. G., Jr.)

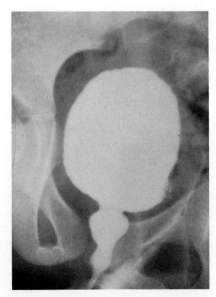

Figure 11–244. *Voiding cystourethrogram.* "Acorn" or "spinning top" deformity of vesical neck and urethra of girl, 14 years of age. No residual urine. Negative cystoscopic examination.

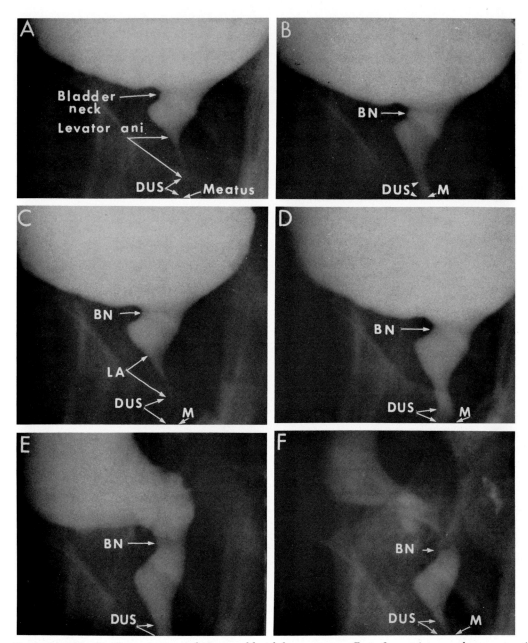

Figure 11–245.   Voiding sequence of 10-year-old girl **demonstrates effect of constrictor urethrae contraction and volume and velocity of flow on width of distal urethral segment (DUS).** **A,** Voiding has just started, and urethral flow is not fully established. **B,** Urethral flow has been fully established, and DUS is wide. **C,** Voluntary contraction of constrictor urethrae muscle has caused interruption of urethral flow and produced same appearance as in **A.** Tapering of urethra above DUS is due to simultaneous contraction of levator ani muscle (external sphincter). **D** and **E,** Voiding is again fully established with DUS maximally distended. **F,** Volume and velocity of urethral flow have decreased during late phase of voiding and have resulted in narrowing of DUS. Tapering of urethra in **A, C,** and **F** could be erroneously interpreted as stenosis without proper identification of meatus and sequential filming. (From Shopfner, C. E., 1967a.)

so-called spinning top configuration. Not infrequently, however, a urethra with this shape is normal in caliber, and conversely, urethras that appear normal at cysto-urethrography may be found at calibration to have significant stenosis. Shopfner has pointed out that such variations in diameter and contour of the urethra are simply expressions of the volume and rate of urinary flow during voiding. He contends that the urethral widening seen in the "spinning top" deformity is present in normal children and is the result of forceful passage of a large volume of urine, which distends the thin-walled urethra (Shopfner, 1967b).

There is no doubt that the diagnosis of distal urethral stenosis has been abused. A thoughtful review of available data would suggest that the urethra may indeed play a role in urinary infection in female children, but true urethral stenosis is probably rare (Keeton).

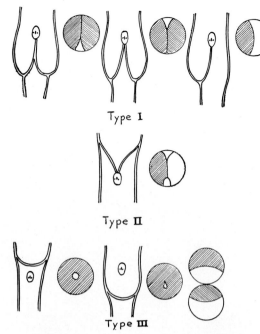

Figure 11–246. Types of congenital valves of posterior urethra with indications of cystoscopic appearances. (Modified from Young, H. H., Frontz, W. A., and Baldwin, J. C.)

Congenital Urethral Valves

CONGENITAL VALVES IN THE MALE URETHRA

Congenital urethral valves occur almost exclusively in the male.

The overall management of these children can be very complex, and the extent of surgery necessary to correct associated deformities is quite controversial. This is partly because the many series are not comparable; some deal with infants (Williams and Eckstein) and others with lesions in older children or adults (Hendren, 1971; Landes and Rall). Perhaps the lesions in infants should be referred to as obstructive urethral valves and lesions occurring later in life as urethral folds. Only the obstructive variety seen in the infant is discussed here.

In the classic paper on the subject of urethral valves published by Young, Frontz, and Baldwin in 1919, three types of valves were described, as shown in Figure 11–246.

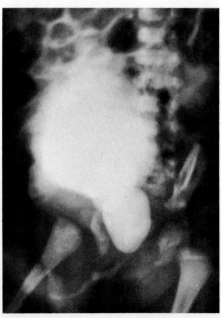

Figure 11–247. *Voiding cystourethrogram* of newborn infant boy. Huge dilatation of prostatic urethra apparently result of **congenital urethral valves.** (From Griesbach, W. A., Waterhouse, R. K., and Mellins, H. Z.)

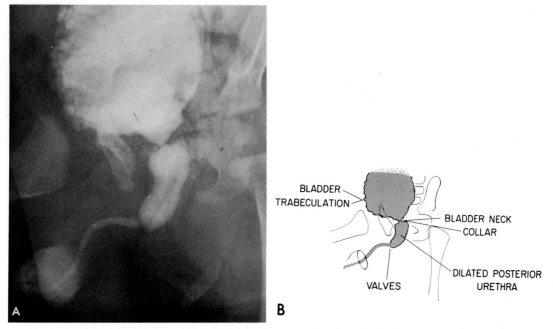

Figure 11–248. Congenital posterior urethral valves in male infant. **A,** *Voiding cystourethrogram.* **B,** Drawing, illustrating findings on cystourethrogram. (From Ellis, D. G., Fonkalsrud, E. W., and Smith, J. P.)

When valvular obstruction is present, the urethra dilates proximally and also elongates, and there is associated hypertrophy of the detrusor muscle which leads to trabeculation and sacculation. The prostatic urethra becomes fusiform in shape, with dilatation between two rigid points, the valves and vesical neck. If there is associated abnormality at the ureterovesical juncture or if a paraureteral diverticulum develops, vesicoureteral reflux is likely to occur. Hydroureteronephrosis may develop in the presence or absence of vesicoureteral reflux, and there may be renal dysplasia occurring concomitantly or as a result of valvular obstruction.

The Clinical Problem

Congenital posterior urethral valves are the cause of some of the most obstructive uropathies of infants. They are commonly encountered at birth, the kidneys being almost destroyed because of advanced hydronephrosis and hydroureter. Paradoxically, at times the infant may appear to be in good general condition at birth and may have a relatively normal level of blood urea, because during fetal life the waste products of metabolism were eliminated by the placental circulation. His condition then rapidly deteriorates and the level of urea rises.

Bladder distention or urinary ascites may develop. There may be no physical

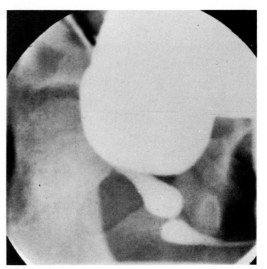

Figure 11–249. *Voiding cystourethrogram.* **Type III urethral valve.**

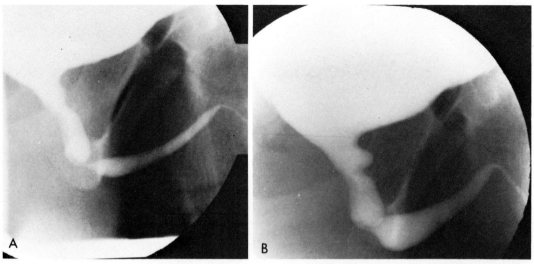

Figure 11–250. *Voiding cystourethrogram* clearly depicting **urethral valves** with **posterior urethral dilatation.**

findings, but fever, anemia, failure to thrive, jaundice, or hemorrhagic diathesis from superimposed infection or renal failure may occur. In the toddler, symptoms are likely to be those of lower urinary tract dysfunction.

Urographic Diagnosis; Voiding Cystourethrograms

Without doubt, the single most important study in the diagnosis of posterior urethral valves is the voiding cystourethrogram. Interest in voiding or expression cystourethrography to demonstrate urethral valves began with the study of Jorup and Kjellberg in 1948. Since that time, many reports of urethral valves demonstrated by this method have appeared (Fisher and Forsythe; Griesbach and associates; Hamm and Waterhouse; Raper; Williams and Sturdy). The urographic deformity consists of a bulging dilatation of the prostatic urethra, which is sharply demarcated from the narrow distal urethra; the prostatic urethra also appears to bulge forward over the bulbous urethra. The deformity is quite characteristic and is not difficult to recognize after several have been seen (Figs. 11–247 through 11–259). In addition to the characteristic "bulge," negative defects from the valves themselves may be recog-

nized. Kjellberg, Ericsson, and Rudhe have emphasized this aspect of the urethrogram, but generally it is not considered especially important (Figs. 11–260 through 11–263). Another fairly common associated finding is the apparent "ring-like" constriction of the vesical neck which is now thought to be

Text continued on page 1115

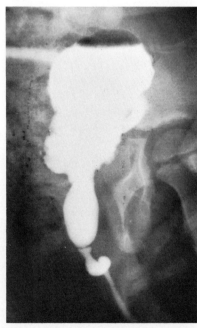

Figure 11–251. *Voiding cystourethrogram* of male infant. **Congenital posterior urethral valves.** (From Lapides, J., Anderson, E. C., and Petrone, A. F.)

Fig. 11–252   Fig. 11–253

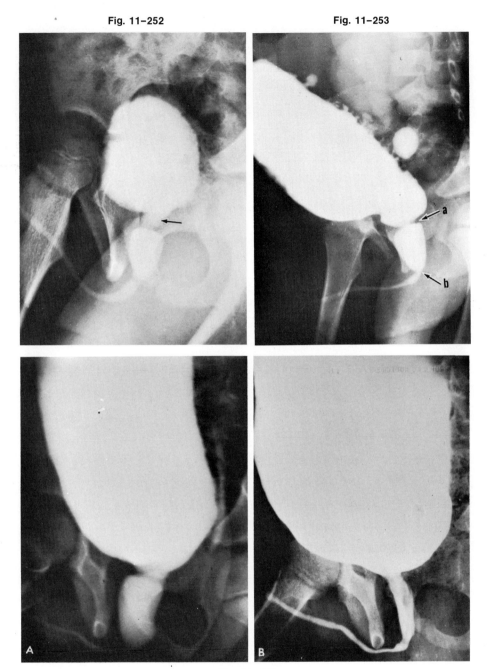

Fig. 11–254

Figure 11–252. *Voiding cystourethrogram* of boy, 7 years of age. **Congenital posterior urethral valves,** producing characteristic dilatation of prostatic urethra below grossly hypertrophied bladder neck *(arrow).* (From Griesbach, W. A., Waterhouse, R. K., and Mellins, H. Z.)

Figure 11–253. *Voiding cystourethrogram* of boy, 22 months of age. **Congenital valve** *(b)* **of posterior urethra** with typical dilatation of prostatic urethra. Note narrowing in region of vesical neck *(a).* This is apparently due to hypertrophy of vesical neck, which is part of general hypertrophy of detrusor muscle. (From Griesbach, W. A., Waterhouse, R. K., and Mellins, H. Z.)

Figure 11–254. **Congenital urethral valves.** *Voiding cystourethrograms.* **A,** *Preoperative.* Obstructive dilatation of prostatic urethra. Moderate secondary hypertrophy of vesical neck was considered to be part of generalized hypertrophy of detrusor muscle. **B,** *Seven days after transurethral removal of valve.* Prostatic urethra has returned almost to normal caliber. (From Hamm, F. C., and Waterhouse, K.)

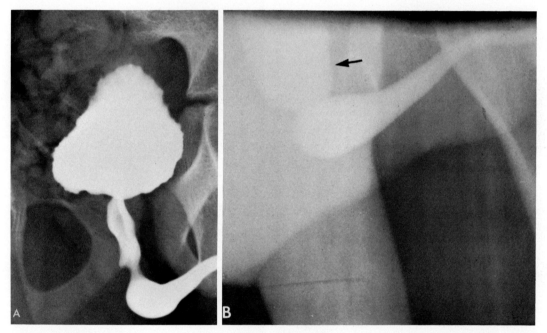

Figure 11–255.   Congenital urethral valves in boy, 10 years of age. **A,** *Retrograde urethrogram.* Rather peculiar elongated prostatic urethra with spreading. **B,** *Voiding cystourethrogram.* Greatly dilated prostatic urethra secondary to obstructive valves *(arrow).*

Fig. 11–256

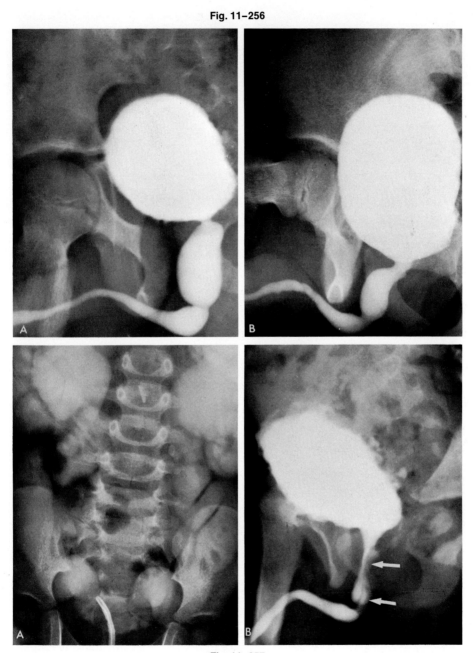

Fig. 11–257

Figure 11–256. Congenital urethral valves in boy, 7 years of age. *Voiding cystourethrograms.* **A,** *Before operation.* **B,** *Five days after transurethral fulguration of valves.*

Figure 11–257. Congenital urethral valves in boy, 21 months of age. **A,** *Excretory urogram, 4-hour film.* Bilateral advanced pyeloureterectasis. **B,** *Voiding cystourethrogram.* Verumontanum and valves visible *(arrows).*

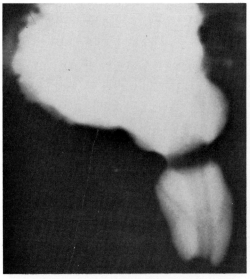 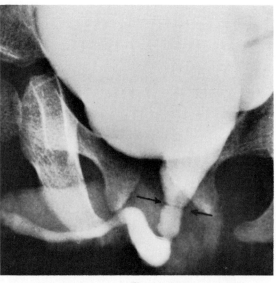

Fig. 11–258   **Fig. 11–259**

Figure 11–258. *Cystourethrogram* made with catheter in urethra of boy with **congenital urethral valves.** Radiolucent lines are considered to be valves causing great dilatation of prostatic urethra. Indentation in region of vesical neck is considered to indicate obstruction. (From Lich, R., Jr., Howerton, L. W., and Davis, L. A.)

Figure 11–259. *Voiding cystourethrogram.* **Semicircular valves** (*arrows*) at level of verumontanum in boy, 3 years of age. (From Kjellberg, S. R., Ericsson, N. D., and Rudhe, U.)

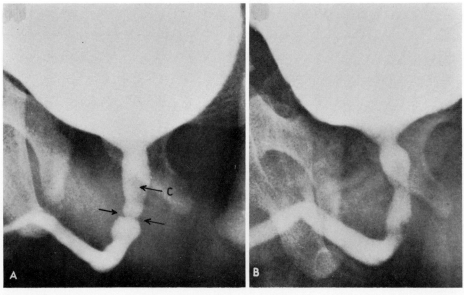

Figure 11–260. **Congenital urethral valves.** *Voiding cystourethrograms* of boy, 1½ years of age. **A,** *Preoperative film.* Negative shadows of semicircular valves (*arrows*) slightly below level of verumontanum (*c*). **B,** *Postoperative film.* (From Kjellberg, S. R., Ericsson, N. D., and Rudhe, U.)

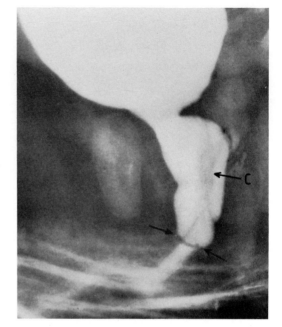

Figure 11–261. *Voiding cystourethrogram* of male infant, 6 days old. **Bicuspid type of urethral valves** *(arrows)*, well below verumontanum *(c)*, at level of urogenital diaphragm. (From Kjellberg, S. R., Ericsson, N. D., and Rudhe, U.)

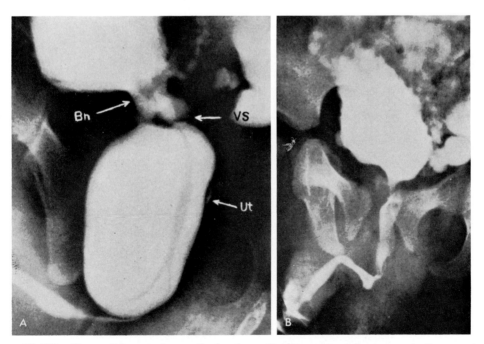

Figure 11–262. **Congenital posterior urethral valves.** *Voiding cystourethrograms.* **A,** *Preoperative film.* Posterior urethral valves at level of urogenital diaphragm, producing enormous dilatation of prostatic urethra. Utricle *(Ut)* and seminal vesicles *(VS)* also are filled with contrast medium. *Bn* = bladder neck. **B,** *Postoperative film.* Prostatic urethra is smaller. Note vesicoureteral reflux. (From Kjellberg, S. R., Ericsson, N. D., and Rudhe, U.)

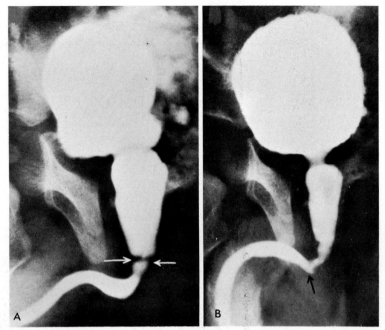

Figure 11–263. Congenital posterior urethral valves in boy, 10 months of age. *Voiding cystourethrograms.* **A,** *Preoperative film.* Valves *(arrows)* at level of urogenital diaphragm, with considerable dilatation of prostatic lumen above. **B,** *Postoperative film.* Valves are gone. Dilatation of prostatic urethra is greatly diminished. *Arrow* points to depression where external urethral incision was made. (From Kjellberg, S. R., Ericsson, N. D., and Rudhe, U.)

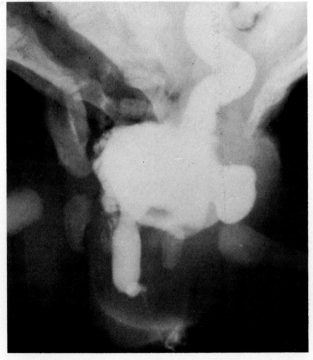

Figure 11–264. *Voiding cystourethrogram* of male infant, aged 2 days. **Congenital posterior urethral valves.** Note bilateral vesicoureteral reflux and ureterectasis. (From Ellis, D. G., Fonkalsrud, E. W., and Smith, J. P.)

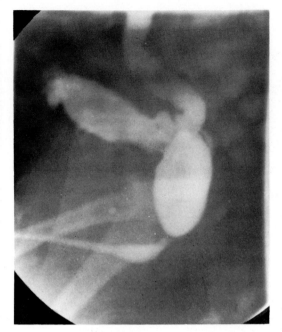

Figure 11–265. *Voiding cystourethrogram.* Infant with urethral valves and vesicoureteral reflux.

of no clinical significance. It probably represents a thickened detrusor muscle that has become hypertrophied by repeated forceful contraction to force urine past the valvular obstruction.

The consistency with which these findings can be visualized throughout the voiding sequence is important, for fleeting findings of similar nature may result from voluntary contraction at the external urethral sphincter.

The vesical neck is usually secondarily thickened and collar-like, although it can be dilated. The bladder is often trabeculated or sacculated, and vesicoureteral reflux is present at diagnosis in 30 to 45 per cent of patients (Figs. 11–264 and 11–265). Intravenous urography may show marked upper-tract dilatation with poor function. Subcapsular extravasation (the C sign) or retroperitoneal extravasation (the P sign) might alert one to severe obstruction (Fig. 11–266).

Treatment of Congenital Urethral Valves

In the infant, resuscitation is the first consideration, since many patients are azotemic, dehydrated, and infected. This effort is directed toward fluid management, appropriate electrolyte replacement, and antibiotic therapy. If resuscitation is achieved, some prefer transurethral removal of the urethral valves and expectant treatment if the infant is doing well. Recovery of ureteral function can be expected in many cases, and Johnston and Kulatilake as well as Ericsson have clearly shown that with

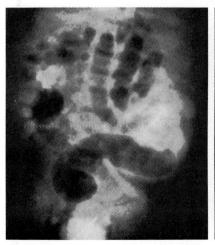 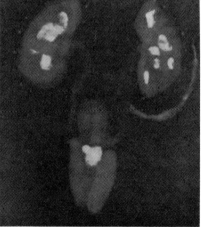

Figure 11–266. Left, *Excretory urogram* showing the **P sign of urine around left kidney and in dilated ureter.** **Right,** *Roentgenogram of autopsy specimen* with barium in calyces of normal-sized kidneys. Opaque arc below and lateral to left kidney specimen was drawn to parallel shape of perirenal extravasation as it appeared in excretory urogram. (From Dockray, K. T.)

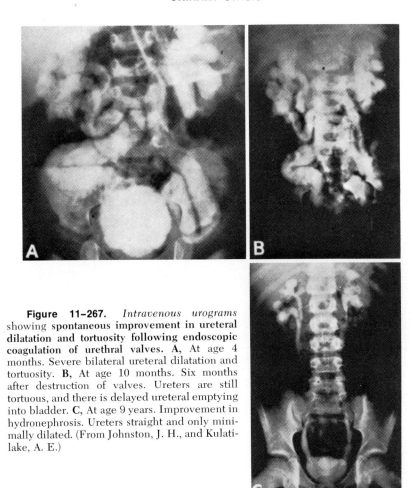

Figure 11–267. *Intravenous urograms* showing spontaneous improvement in ureteral dilatation and tortuosity following endoscopic coagulation of urethral valves. **A,** At age 4 months. Severe bilateral ureteral dilatation and tortuosity. **B,** At age 10 months. Six months after destruction of valves. Ureters are still tortuous, and there is delayed ureteral emptying into bladder. **C,** At age 9 years. Improvement in hydronephrosis. Ureters straight and only minimally dilated. (From Johnston, J. H., and Kulatilake, A. E.)

resection of the valves alone there can be dramatic recovery both anatomically and functionally (Fig. 11–267). The posterior urethra usually returns to normal configuration, and reflux abates in at least 25 per cent of patients (Fig. 11–268). Both diverticula and trabeculation of the bladder may be reduced or may disappear. If ureteral dilatation persists in the absence of reflux, an obstructive component at the uretero-vesical juncture requiring correction can be confirmed by measuring the ureteral flow rates as described by Whitaker.

Of course, drainage at either the kidney or the bladder level is necessary when azotemia or infection (or both) cannot be corrected by conservative means.

ANTERIOR URETHRAL VALVES

Anterior urethral valves are extremely rare (Chang; Daniel and associates) Symptoms are similar to those associated with posterior valves, but the degree of obstruction—as evidenced by the condition of the upper urinary tract—appears to be much less. Diagnosis is made by means of the voiding cystourethrogram (Figs. 11–269, 11–270, and 11–271). Surgical excision of an anterior valve is carried out through an external urethrotomy incision.

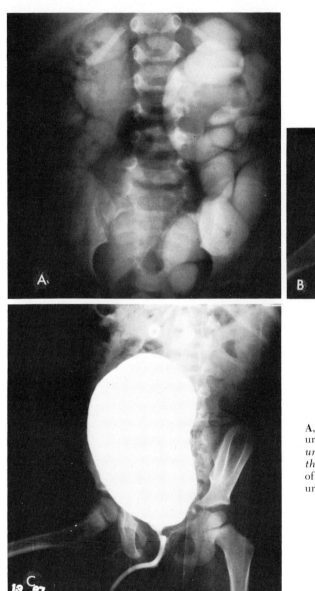

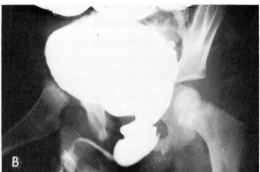

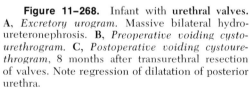

Figure 11-268. Infant with **urethral valves.** A, *Excretory urogram.* Massive bilateral hydro-ureteronephrosis. B, *Preoperative voiding cysto-urethrogram.* C, *Postoperative voiding cystoure-throgram,* 8 months after transurethral resection of valves. Note regression of dilatation of posterior urethra.

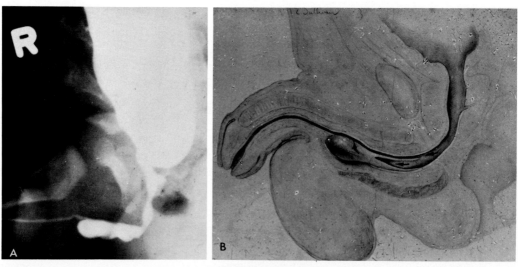

Figure 11-269. Anterior urethral valve in male infant aged 3½ months. **A,** *Cystourethrogram.* Note dilatation proximal to valve. Negative linear shadow represents valve. **B,** Position of valve and mechanism of obstruction during micturition. (From Chang, C.-Y.)

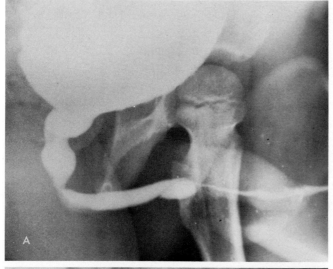

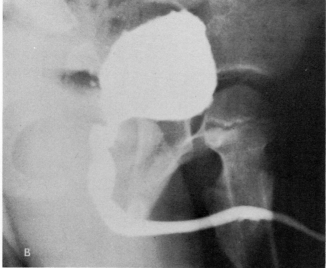

Figure 11-270. Congenital anterior urethral valve in boy, aged 6 years. *Voiding cystourethrograms.* **A,** *Preoperative film.* Note trabeculation of bladder. (At operation, thin circumferential "sail-like" valve was found and excised.) **B,** *Postoperative film.* (From Daniel, J., Stewart, A. M., and Blair, D. W.)

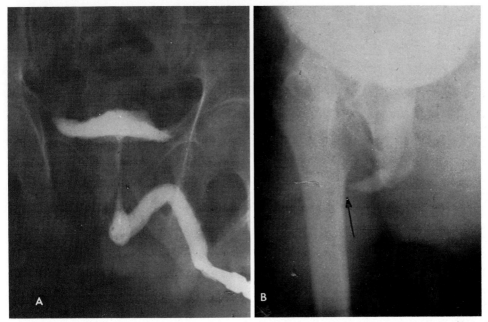

Figure 11–271. Anterior urethral valve in man, aged 25. A, *Retrograde urethrogram.* Valve not demonstrated. **B,** *Voiding cystourethrogram.* Abrupt narrowing of anterior part of urethra distal to bulb *(arrow).* Surgical exposure of urethra revealed valves, which were removed. (Upper urinary tract was normal.) (From Colabawalla, B. N.)

CONGENITAL VALVES IN THE FEMALE URETHRA

Structures resembling valves have also been encountered in girls and women (Lowsley and Kerwin; Mitchell and associates; Nesbit and associates; Stevens). In the cases reported, the valves have caused obstruction during voiding, and voiding cystourethrograms have demonstrated dilated ballooned urethras proximal to the valve and narrowing distally (Figs. 11–272 through 11–275). The valves also can be demonstrated with a blunt probe, the end of which has been bent into the shape of a buttonhook.

Valves have been encountered in both the floor and roof of the urethra; all have been close to the urethral meatus. In one of Nesbit, McDonald, and Busby's cases, the obstructing lesion proved to be a tough fibrous transverse band that "cut like cartilage" (Fig. 11–272).

In all cases reported, the obstructive symptoms have been relieved, and the cystourethrogram has returned to normal.

Urethral Polyps in Boys

A true pedunculated polyp is composed of a stalk of loose connective tissue containing blood vessels and covered with transitional epithelium. Urethral polyps occur exclusively in boys and are located in the prostatic urethra. In most cases, they are attached to the dorsal half (floor) of the prostatic urethra near the verumontanum. They are not common.

At rest, the polyp usually lies near the bladder neck; during micturition, it may prolapse into the membranous urethra. The degree of obstruction depends on the size and location, and symptoms are similar to those of any infravesical obstruction. In Meadows and Quattlebaum's four cases, the excretory urogram showed no evidence of obstruction of the upper urinary tract in any patient. On the other hand, ureteropyelectasis was present in three of Williams and Abbassian's four cases. In the cystourethrogram, the polyp appears as a negative shadow, which may be round, oval, or

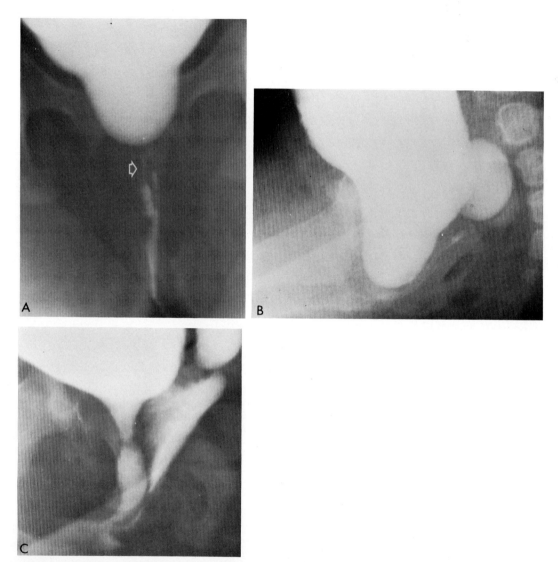

Figure 11–272. Congenital urethral valve in female. *Voiding cystourethrograms.* **A,** *Preoperative film, frontal view.* Urethra dilated proximal to valve. Tiny stream of contrast medium *(arrow)* seen in distal part of urethra. **B,** *Preoperative film, lateral view.* Note small vesical diverticulum. **C,** *Postoperative film, oblique view.* Proximal part of urethra is now of normal size and distal part is of good caliber. (From Mitchell, G. F., Makhuli, Z., and Frittelli, G.)

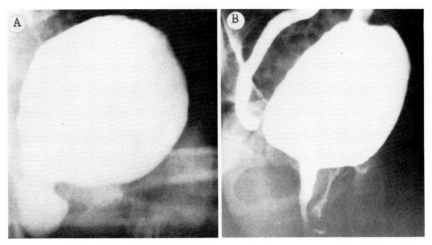

Figure 11–273. Congenital urethral valve or fibrotic band in young girl. *Voiding cystourethrograms.* **A,** *Preoperative film.* Dilatation of urethra; obstructive point appears to be near urethral meatus. (Obstructive band near meatus was demonstrated by pulling partially inflated Foley balloon catheter through urethra. Stricture was incised—"cut like cartilage."). **B,** *Postoperative film.* Urethra now appears normal. (From Nesbit, R. M., McDonald, H. P., Jr., and Busby, S.)

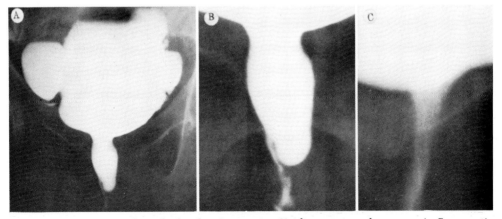

Figure 11–274. Congenital urethral valve in woman. *Voiding cystourethrograms.* **A,** *Preoperative film.* Ballooned proximal part of urethra and very narrow distal part. Note diverticula of bladder. **B,** *Close-up view of urethra.* Shadow between dilated and narrow portions of urethra has appearance of valve. (Valve was hooked with silver probe with end bent like buttonhook, pulled down through urethra, and incised.) **C,** *Postoperative film.* Obstruction relieved. (From Nesbit, R. M., McDonald, H. P., Jr., and Busby, S.)

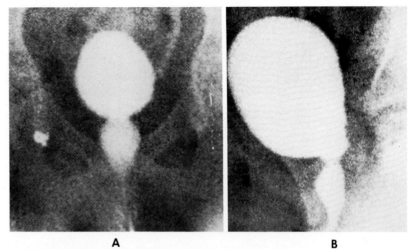

A   B

Figure 11-275. Congenital urethral valve in little girl. *Voiding cystourethrograms.* **A,** *Preoperative film.* Ballooning of urethra. (Buttonhook-shaped probe was passed into and pulled back through urethra. It hooked valve on floor of urethra near meatus. Valve was incised.) **B,** *Postoperative film.* Urethra appears normal. (From Nesbit, R. M., McDonald, H. P., Jr., and Busby, S.)

teardrop in shape. Because of its mobility, the shadow may assume different shapes and may occupy different locations in sequential films (Figs. 11-276 and 11-277).

Congenital Stenosis of the Urethral Meatus

It is important to remember that the narrowest portion of the urethra in boys and girls is the urethral meatus. In boys, there is also a second site of narrowing, namely, the penoscrotal juncture. The voiding cystourethrogram is not so important in cases of meatal stenosis as it is in cases of congenital obstruction of the vesical neck and congenital urethral valve. Nevertheless, it may be helpful and corroborative and is easily made. Kjellberg, Ericsson, and Rudhe pointed out that the actual site of the meatal narrowing may be difficult or impossible to demonstrate urographically. Dilatation of the urethra proximal to the meatus during all stages of micturition (polyview filming

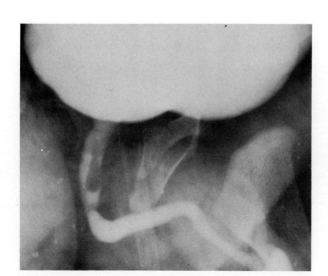

Figure 11-276. *Voiding cystourethrogram* of boy. **Polyp of prostatic urethra.** Note teardrop shape of negative shadow from polyp. (From Williams, D. I., and Abbassian, A.)

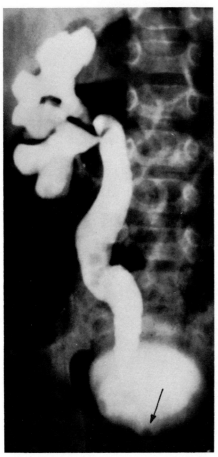

Figure 11–277. *Cystogram* of boy. Reflux up dilated ureter showing severe pyeloureterectasis caused by obstruction from **polyp of prostatic urethra,** which can be seen as small, circular negative filling defect in midline at vesical neck *(arrow).* (From Williams, D. I., and Abbassian, A.)

while the patient voids) is pathognomonic of meatal narrowing (Figs. 11–278 and 11–279).

Congenital, Iatrogenic, and Traumatic Strictures of the Urethra in Infants and Children

Bona fide congenital stricture of the urethra (excluding meatal stenosis) is rare. Kjellberg, Ericsson, and Rudhe encountered it in one case in their study—the case of a male infant who had been operated on at the age of 1 day for anal atresia with scrotal fistula. In our experience, most so-called congenital strictures are iatrogenic and have resulted from ill-advised urethral instrumentation. Many so-called congenital strictures would not occur if a cystourethrogram were made on each child needing urologic investigation before any rigid or semi-rigid instruments were introduced through the urethra. If, after a cystourethrogram and excretory urogram have been made, cystoscopy is considered necessary, it should be done under general anesthesia, and the urethra should be carefully calibrated with small Otis diagnostic bulbs before the cystoscope is introduced. Only in this way can the caliber of the meatus and penoscrotal juncture be accurately determined. Also, if areas of narrowing do exist in the urethra, their exact size and location can be charted. It is impossible to obtain this information accurately by calibration with sounds (Emmett, Kirchheim, and Greene).

Almost all congenital strictures occur in boys. These lesions are usually located at the junction of the bulbous urethra (of ectodermal origin—from the genital fold) with the prostatic and membranous urethra (of entodermal origin—from the cloaca). These are usually soft strictures that dilate quite easily, although Cobb, Wolf, and Ansell have shown that they may persist in spite of dilation and be the cause of irritative symptoms in young men which are usually diagnosed as prostatitis (Fig. 11–280 and 11–281). They found two peak ages for congenital stricture, (1) infancy and young childhood and (2) young adulthood—the early twenties.

The caliber of congenital strictures can vary in degree from complete atresia (Campbell; Engle and Schlumberger) to almost normal urethral caliber. Cobb and associates found the average caliber of the strictures to be 10 F. They defined a stricture as a narrowing of smaller caliber than the urethral meatus (based on calibration with Otis bulbs). Treatment consisted of urethral dilation with infant sounds or pediatric Kollman dilators; if this was ineffective, internal urethrotomy was performed with an infant Otis urethrotome.

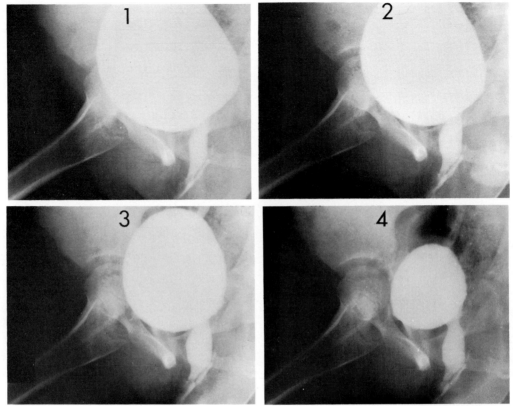

Figure 11–278. *Polyview voiding cystourethrogram* of 8-year-old girl. **Meatal stenosis.** (Films taken during several stages of voiding.) (From Thornbury, J. R.; and Immergut, M. A.)

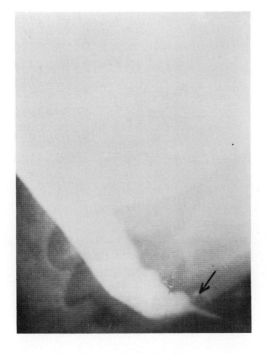

Figure 11–279. *Voiding urethrogram* of girl, 9 years of age. **Stenosis of urethral meatus** *(arrow)*, with proximal dilatation of urethra. (From Kjellberg, S. R., Ericsson, N. D., and Rudhe, U.)

meatus penoscrotal junc.

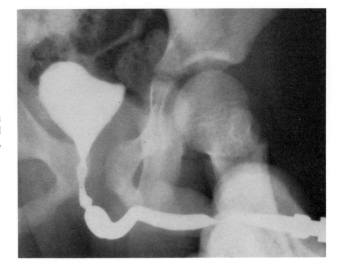

Figure 11–280. *Retrograde urethrogram* of infant. **Congenital stricture of proximal part of bulbous urethra.** (From Cobb, B. G., Wolf, J. A., Jr., and Ansell, J. S.)

In an article on urethral strictures in boys, Leadbetter and Leadbetter reported a series of cases in which dilation was ineffective, so that open operation (urethroplasty) was required (Figs. 11–282 and 11–283). In only two of these cases were the strictures regarded as congenital; in four, they resulted from trauma (straddle injury or kicks), whereas in two, they were iatrogenic (one from instrumentation and one from repair of hypospadias). Most traumatic strictures in little boys result from straddle

injuries and are located in the "proximal bulb" of the urethra (Fig. 11–284).

Iatrogenic strictures are the most common type of strictures in children. They occur most often at the penoscrotal juncture and the meatus, the two narrowest points of the male urethra, although almost any part of the pendulous urethra may be involved.

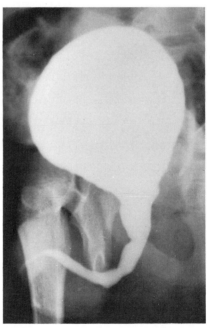

Figure 11–281. *Voiding cystourethrogram* of enuretic male child. **Congenital stricture** *(arrow)* of proximal part of bulbous urethra. (From Cobb, B. G., Wolf, J. A., Jr., and Ansell, J. S.)

Figure 11–282. *Voiding cystourethrogram* of boy. **Stricture of distal part of pendulous urethra,** causing dilatation of proximal part of urethra and of vesical neck. (From Leadbetter, G. W., and Leadbetter, W. F.)

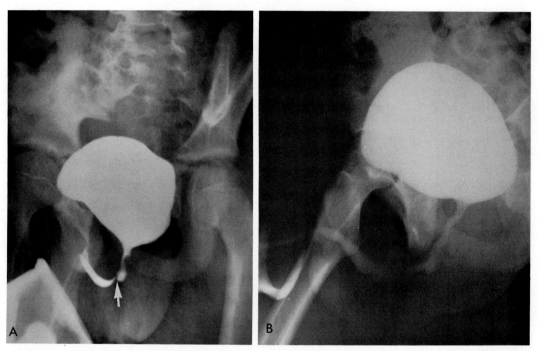

Figure 11–283. Stricture of bulbous portion of urethra of boy, age 8 years. *Voiding cystourethrograms.* **A**, *Preoperative film.* (Stricture [*arrow*] was excised, and pedicle-flap procedure was performed.) **B**, *Postoperative film.* (From Leadbetter, G. W., and Leadbetter, W. F.)

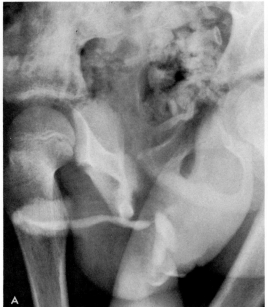

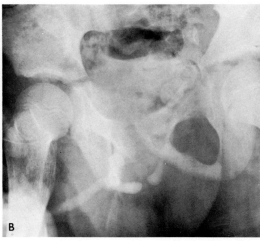

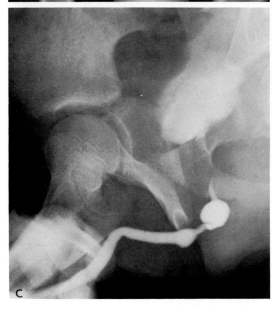

Figure 11–284. Traumatic (straddle injury) stricture of bulbous urethra in boy, 9 years of age. *Retrograde urethrograms.* **A,** *Two months after injury and rupture of urethra.* Contrast medium is running out through perineum at site of urethral defect. **B,** *One month after* **A.** Short filiform stricture in bulb. (Perineal operation with excision of stricture and end-to-end anastomosis was performed.) **C,** *Eight months postoperatively.* Recurring stricture with some dilatation of bulbous urethra proximal to stricture. (Patient responded well to periodic dilations.)

Urologists should appreciate the caliber of the normal urethra in the infant and child, since attempts to "dilate" a normal urethra usually result in traumatic avulsion, which is followed too often by disabling stricture. If instruments too large to be easily accommodated by the urethra are required, it is preferable to introduce them through an external urethrotomy incision into the bulbous urethra, which is normally the largest part of the male urethra. (Figs. 11–285 through 11–288).

Diagnosis of Urethral Stricture

In the diagnosis of urethral stricture, as in that of any obstructive problem of an infant or child, it is good judgment always to begin the investigation urographically with (1) an excretory urogram and (2) a cys-

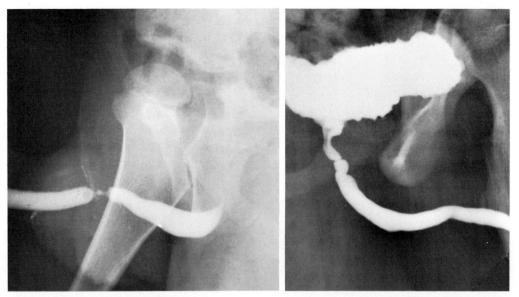

Fig. 11–285   **Fig. 11–286**

Figure 11–285. *Retrograde urethrogram* of boy, 3 years of age. **Iatrogenic (postcystoscopic) stricture of urethra at penoscrotal juncture.**

Figure 11–286. *Retrograde urethrogram* of boy, 11 years of age, with myelodysplasia. **Iatrogenic stricture of membranous urethra** from perineal transurethral resection of vesical neck at age 2 years.

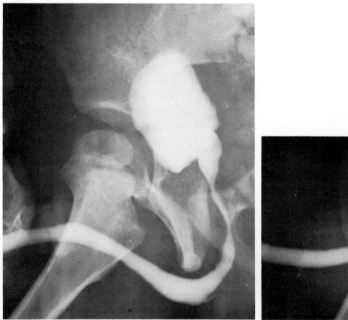
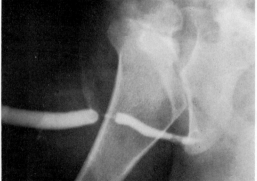

Fig. 11–287   **Fig. 11–288**

Figure 11–287. *Retrograde urethrogram* of boy, 2½ years of age. **Congenital obstruction of vesical neck with large-caliber stricture in proximal part of bulbous urethra.** Note small false passage in floor of urethra. Stricture was either congenital or result of previous cystoscopy. Instruments larger than size 14 F could not be passed. (Heineke-Mikulicz operation on vesical neck was performed with good result.)

Figure 11–288. *Retrograde urethrogram* of boy, 3 years of age. **Postoperative stricture at penoscrotal juncture** caused by previous transurethral resection of vesical neck.

tourethrogram. A voiding or expression cystourethrogram may be made in conjunction with the excretory urogram if there has been adequate excretion of concentrated contrast medium. If not, a small urethral catheter should be passed, the bladder filled with contrast medium, the catheter withdrawn, and a voiding or expression urethrogram obtained. If it is impossible to introduce a catheter, a retrograde cystourethrogram may be made to demonstrate the stricture. If it proves necessary, instrumentation can be done later, when it should be done with the child under general anesthesia to preclude his making sudden movements that might result in trauma or perforation of the urethra.

Treatment of Urethral Stricture

In the vast majority of cases, the treatment of urethral strictures in children is surgical. From the limited number of urethroplasties reported in children, it would appear that irrespective of where the strictures are located or what procedure is used, the results are highly satisfactory (Devereux and Williams).

Vesical Diverticulum

Diverticulum of the bladder may be single or multiple, large or small. Small diverticula that empty are similar to large cellules and as a general rule are of no surgical importance. Larger diverticula may assume bizarre shapes and positions and at times may reach such huge proportions that they may be larger than the bladder (Figs. 11–289 through 11–295). Although the presence of a diverticulum usually is established by cystoscopic examination, it may be easily missed if its stoma is small, unless a cystogram is made. Not only will the cystogram reveal diverticula overlooked on cystoscopy, but it will determine their capacity and the degree of retention. Diverticula that are capable of emptying are of little or no clinical significance in the absence of infection. Inability

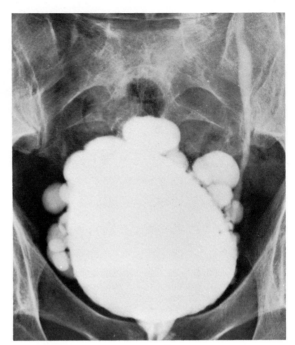

Figure 11–289. *Retrograde cystogram.* **Multiple small vesical diverticula and large cellules** associated with benign prostatic hyperplasia.

to empty results in urinary stasis and predisposes to infection and stone formation. The size of the orifice of the diverticulum may bear no relation to retention.

In many cases the orifice of the diverticulum is adjacent to a ureteral meatus. Not uncommonly, the ureteral orifice is adjacent to the stoma of the diverticulum, and in an occasional case it may open into the diverticulum itself. Ureterectasis may result from pressure of the diverticulum on the terminal portion of the ureter as it courses around the diverticulum (Fig. 11–296) or as it passes between the diverticulum and the wall of the bladder. It also may result from the disturbance of the normal ureterovesical juncture as described by Hutch (1958), allowing the intramural ureter to become extravesical and producing both obstructive ureterectasis and reflux.

Although in most cases diverticula are easily identified on the cystogram, one may encounter a large diverticulum with a small orifice that may not fill with urographic medium. In such a case the diverticulum may

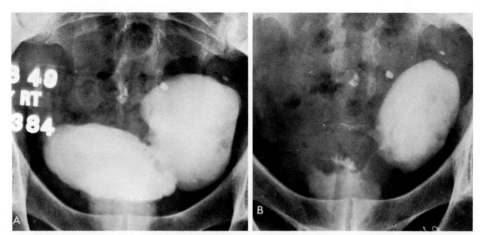

Figure 11–290. Large vesical diverticulum. *Retrograde cystograms* soon after transurethral resection of prostate gland and neck of diverticulum. **A,** *With bladder full.* Diverticulum arises from left posterior wall of bladder. Note prostatic urethra is wide open and filled with medium. **B,** *Immediately after voiding.* Bladder is empty, but there is some medium still trickling through into prostatic urethra from diverticulum.

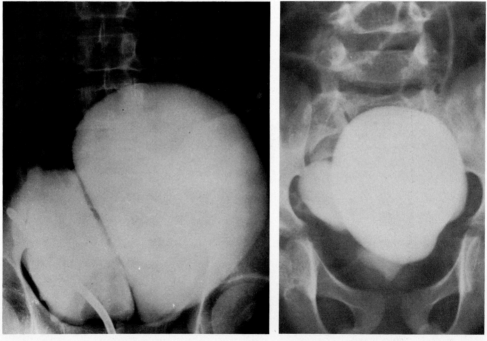

Fig. 11–291   Fig. 11–292

Figure 11–291. *Retrograde cystogram.* **Huge vesical diverticulum,** much larger than bladder, arises from left wall of bladder and displaces bladder to right of midline. Urethral catheter is in bladder.

Figure 11–292. *Cystogram made through cystostomy tube.* **Large diverticulum** arises from left side of bladder; smaller one from right. Necks of both diverticula were situated near ureteral orifices. Bladder is posterior. (Diverticulectomy and transurethral resection of vesical neck were done.)

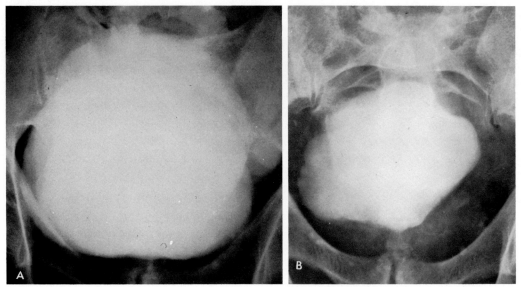

Figure 11–293. Vesical diverticulum obscured by over-filling of bladder with contrast medium. *Retrograde cystograms.* **A,** Bladder overdistended with contrast medium. Suggestion of superimposed shadows. **B,** After bladder emptied with catheter. Medium remains in large diverticulum arising from midposterior wall of bladder.

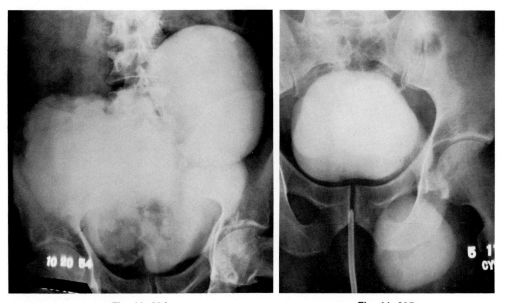

Fig. 11–294   Fig. 11–295

Figure 11–294. *Retrograde cystogram.* Multiple huge vesical diverticula in patient with hypertrophy of prostate. (Diverticulectomy and suprapubic prostatectomy were performed.)

Figure 11–295. *Retrograde cystogram.* Two moderate-sized vesical diverticula with incorporation of bladder in recurring inguinal (scrotal) hernia.

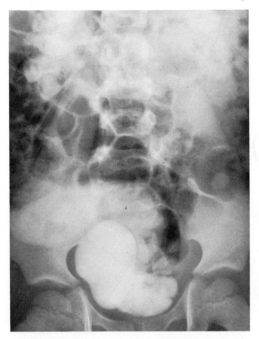

Figure 11–296. *Excretory urogram, 75-minute film,* of boy, 4 years of age. **Large vesical diverticulum on right** associated with congenital obstruction of vesical neck and **marked bilateral ureterectasis** (without reflux). Right kidney functioned better than left. Note hugely dilated right ureter curving around diverticulum to reach right ureteral orifice (which was normal in appearance and situated 1 cm medial to neck of diverticulum).

be confused with a filling defect from a tumor or nonopaque stone, or from an extravesical mass that is displacing the bladder. In some cases, error in interpretation may be avoided by observing a characteristic displacement of the ureter as it curves around the diverticulum to enter the bladder (Figs. 11–297 through 11–302).

It is important to know the degree of retention associated with a diverticulum. To obtain this information, a cystogram is made after the patient has voided the urographic medium. Another cystogram is then made after the bladder has been drained with a catheter. From these two cystograms one can estimate the degree of urinary stasis in the bladder and in the diverticulum (Fig. 11–303).

It must not be forgotten that a vesical diverticulum may be the site of a tumor or stone. Calculi usually are quite easily visualized on the plain film and cystogram. Tumors, on the other hand, may be more difficult to recognize and may require cystoscopy for accurate diagnosis. (These conditions are discussed in the chapters devoted to stone [Chapter 12] and tumor [Chapter 14]).

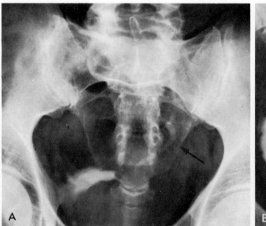
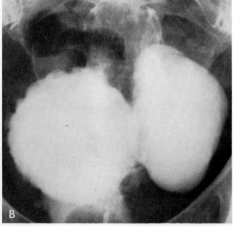

Figure 11–297. **Large vesical diverticulum. A,** *Excretory cystogram.* **Diverticulum arising from left half of bladder** does not fill with contrast medium. Small amount of medium in right side of bladder could be mistaken for deformity from large carcinoma of bladder. Pathognomonic finding here is displacement of lower portion of left ureter upward and to midline *(arrow),* denoting presence of large vesical diverticulum that does not fill with medium. **B,** *Retrograde cystogram* made after transurethral prostatic resection and excision of neck of diverticulum. Diverticulum now fills with medium. Note bag catheter in prostatic urethra, which is open wide as result of prostatic resection.

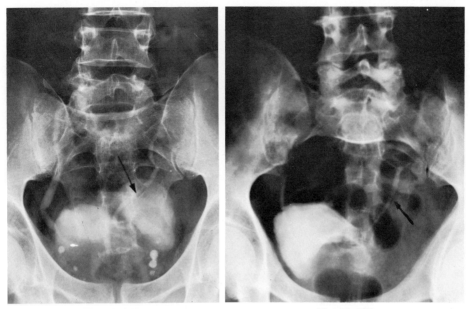

Fig. 11–298   **Fig. 11–299**

Figure 11–298. *Excretory cystogram.* **Large vesical diverticulum** arising from left wall of bladder. Note displacement of lower third of left ureter *(arrow)* as it encircles diverticulum.

Figure 11–299. *Excretory cystogram.* **Apparent filling defect of left half of bladder,** from **large unfilled vesical diverticulum,** might be mistaken for carcinoma of bladder. Displacement of lower third of left ureter *(arrow)*, however, suggests correct diagnosis.

Figure 11–300. **Ureteral obstruction from small vesical diverticulum. A,** *Right retrograde pyelogram.* Dilatation of entire ureter, especially terminal portion, with caliectasis but no pyelectasis. Note abrupt termination of ureter, suggesting stricture or obstruction. **B,** *Fifteen-minute delayed pyelogram.* Medium retained in lower third of dilated ureter. There is small vesical diverticulum adjacent to ureter at point where outline of ureter is abruptly terminated. (Cystoscopy showed small diverticulum in right base adjacent to ureteral orifice. Surgical exploration revealed ureter to lie between wall of diverticulum and wall of bladder, where it was compressed and obstructed. Reimplantation of ureter into bladder was done.)

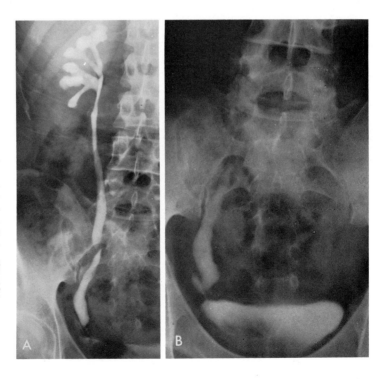

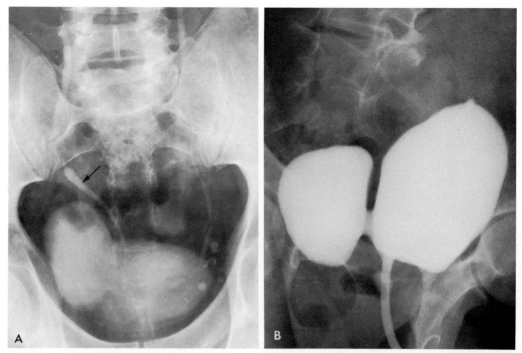

Figure 11-301. Vesical diverticulum displacing lower portion of ureter medially. **A,** *Excretory urogram.* Note displacement of right ureter to left (*arrow*). **B,** *Retrograde cystogram, oblique view.* Neck of diverticulum communicates with bladder.

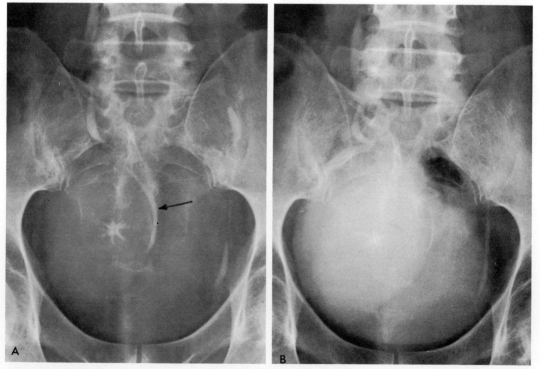

Figure 11-302. Vesical diverticulum containing jackstone. *Excretory urograms.* **A,** *Twenty-minute film.* Medial displacement of right ureter (*arrow*) around partially filled diverticulum. **B,** *One-hour film.* More complete filling of diverticulum.

Fishhook ureters

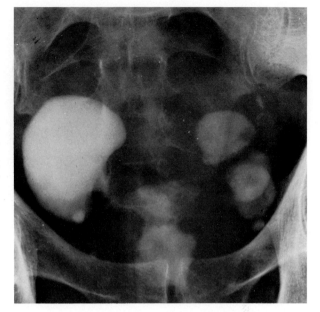

Figure 11–303. *Retrograde cystogram.* **Multiple vesical diverticula.** Cystogram had been made and bladder emptied with urethral catheter. Medium, seen running into base of bladder and prostatic urethra, was retained in large diverticulum on right and two small ones on left.

Obstruction of the Bladder Outlet in the Adult Male

BENIGN PROSTATIC HYPERPLASIA

The most common cause of obstruction of the vesical neck in adult males is benign prostatic hyperplasia. Diagnosis is usually made on the basis of symptoms, digital rectal examination, the finding of residual urine in the bladder, and cystoscopic examination. Urography is usually only a confirmatory test, but at times it can be important in diagnosis. It is impossible to determine the size of the prostate gland accurately by radiographic means (Vermooten and Schweinsberg).

Long-standing obstruction of the vesical neck with residual urine may result in dilatation of the ureters and renal pelves (Figs. 11–304 and 11–305). Even though the bladder may not be outlined with contrast medium in the excretory urogram, vesical distention may be suspected because of the abnormally wide separation of the terminal portions of the ureters (Figs. 11–306, 11–307, and 11–308). Trabeculation of the bladder is common (Figs. 11–309 and 11–310). The cystogram (either excretory or retrograde) may reveal a char-

acteristic smooth negative filling defect in the base of the bladder caused by the projection of the enlarged prostate gland into the bladder. Intravesical projections of lateral or median lobes yield typical filling defects, which may be confused at times with the negative shadows of pedunculated bladder tumors. Diagnostic errors may be made because of overlying gas in the rectum, nonopaque vesical calculi, or the inflated bag of a Foley catheter, all of which may simulate prostatic filling defects in the cystogram (Figs. 11–311 through 11–321). Enormous enlargements of the prostate gland may displace the bladder upward almost out of the pelvis (Figs. 11–322 and 11–323). When a large adenoma elevates the trigone and base of the bladder, the terminal ureters may have a "fishhook" appearance that is pathognomonic (Figs. 11–324 and 11–325).

Retrograde Cystourethrography. This urographic study offers an alternative to cystoscopic evaluation of prostatic enlargement but is not as accurate. It will, however, assist in the differentiation of urethral stricture and vesical neck contracture.

The urethrographic deformity depends on the type and position of the prostatic enlargement. Enlargement of the lateral lobes produces pressure on the urethra so that it

Text continued on page 1141

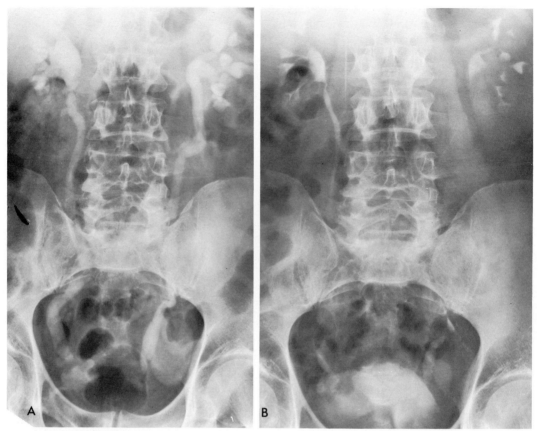

Figure 11–304. Moderate-sized vesical diverticulum associated with ureteropyelectasis secondary to urinary obstruction from benign prostatic hyperplasia. *Excretory urograms.* **A,** *Preoperative film.* **B,** *Film made 5 months after transurethral resection.* Ureteropyelectasis has almost disappeared.

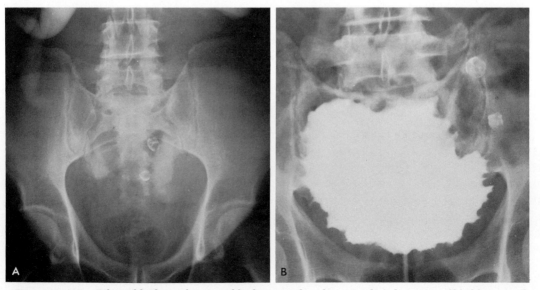

Figure 11–305. Bilateral hydronephrosis and hydroureter from long-standing distention of bladder secondary to prostatic obstruction. **A,** *Excretory urogram.* **B,** *Retrograde cystogram.*

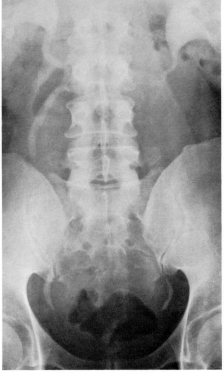

Figure 11–306. *Excretory urogram.* **Huge distended bladder** (2,000 ml of residual urine) **secondary to congenital obstruction of vesical neck** of man, aged 49. There is wide separation of terminal portions of ureters and of ureteral orifices.

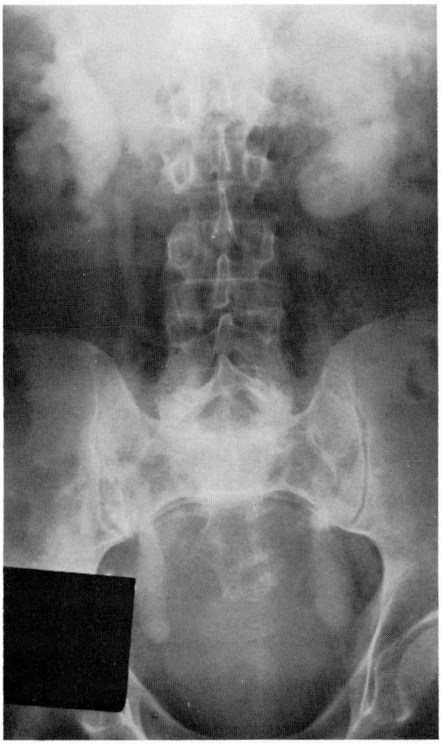

Figure 11–307. *Excretory urogram.* **Huge distended bladder secondary to prostatic obstruction.** Distance between terminal portions of ureters is increased.

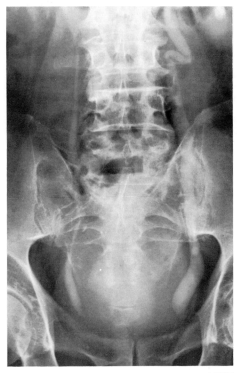

Figure 11–308. Widely separated terminal ureters from greatly distended bladder secondary to prostatic obstruction.

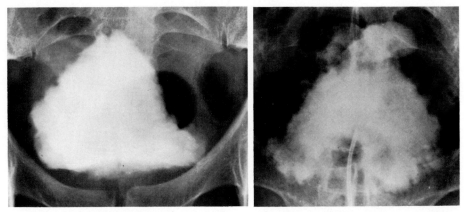

Fig. 11–309   Fig. 11–310

Figure 11–309. Moderate trabeculation of bladder associated with moderate obstruction secondary to benign prostatic hyperplasia. Pear-shaped outline of bladder commonly seen in cases of obstruction of vesical neck.

Figure 11–310. *Retrograde cystogram.* Moderate trabeculation of bladder and cellule formation caused by urinary obstruction from benign prostatic hyperplasia. Note pyramidal shape of bladder.

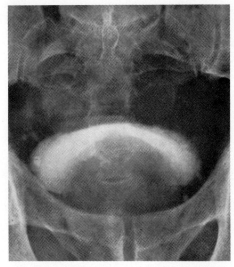

Figure 11–311. *Retrograde cystogram.* **Filling defect in base of bladder** with typical smooth outline, from benign prostatic hyperplasia.

Figure 11–314. *Excretory cystogram.* **Filling defect in bladder from intravesical trilobar benign prostatic hyperplasia.** Could be confused with filling defect from tumor.

Figure 11–315. *Excretory cystogram.* **Filling defect in base of bladder from intravesical benign hyperplasia of lateral lobes of prostate.**

Figure 11–316. *Excretory cystogram.* **Irregular filling defect in bladder from intravesical projection of benign prostatic hyperplasia.** Could be mistaken for filling defect from tumor of bladder.

Figure 11–317. *Excretory cystogram.* **Marked intravesical projection of huge benign prostatic hyperplasia,** which seems to fill bladder completely except for medium seen in periphery anteriorly.

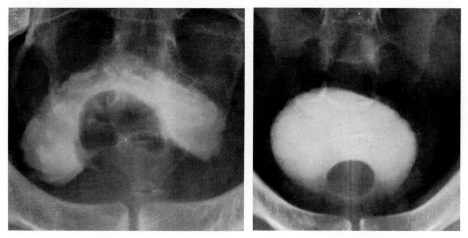

Fig. 11–312   Fig. 11–313

Figure 11–312. *Excretory cystogram.* Filling defect in base of bladder from intravesical enlargement of median lobe of prostate gland. Note trabeculation of bladder and small cellules.

Figure 11–313. *Excretory cystogram.* Unusually well-defined filling defect from small subcervical benign prostatic enlargement. Could be confused with filling defect from bag catheter.

Fig. 11–314   Fig. 11–315

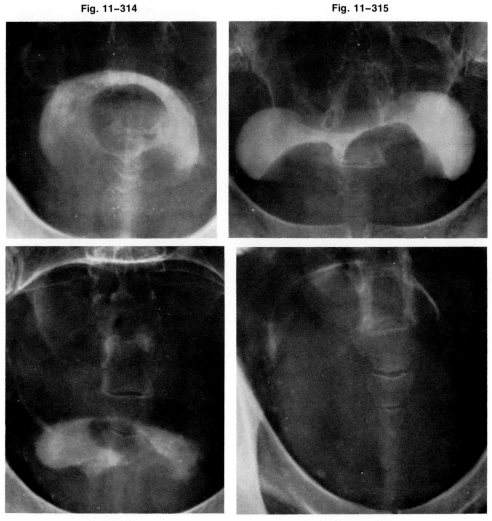

Fig. 11–316   Fig. 11–317

See legends on opposite page.

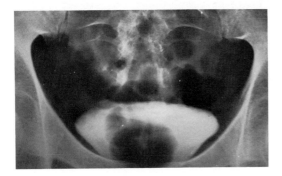

Figure 11–318. *Excretory cystogram.* Gas in rectum, which might be mistaken for filling defect from benign prostatic hyperplasia.

Figure 11–319. *Excretory cystogram.* Filling defect from benign prostatic hyperplasia and superimposed gas in rectum.

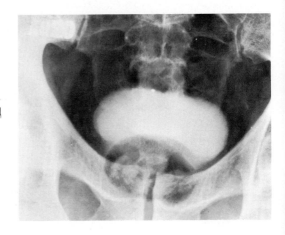

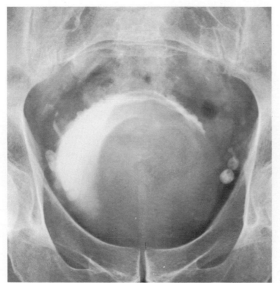

Figure 11–320. *Excretory cystogram.* Filling defect in bladder from huge intravesical hyperplasia of prostate gland.

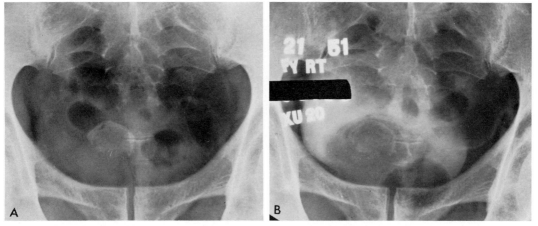

Figure 11–321.   Encrustation on residual intravesical prostatic tissue after incomplete transurethral resection. Lesion simulates encrusted bladder tumor. **A,** *Plain film.* **B,** *Excretory cystogram.*

becomes flattened in its lateral diameter but widened in its anteroposterior diameter. This urographic phenomenon is spoken of as spreading. The prostatic urethra also becomes longer. If the posterior commissure or median lobe is enlarged, a sharp anterior displacement of the urethra occurs in its proximal part where it lies against this hypertrophied lobe. This results in an angulation of the prostatic urethra with its apex directed posteriorly in the region of the verumontanum. This deformity is called anterior tilting. Inasmuch as most cases of adenofibromatous hyperplasia involve all three lobes to various degrees, many combinations of the foregoing urographic deformities are encountered (Figs. 11–326 through 11–330).

Text continued on page 1146

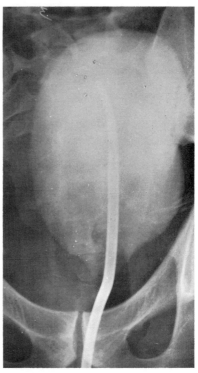

Figure 11–322.   *Retrograde cystogram.* **Marked displacement of bladder upward and to left due to enormous benign prostatic hyperplasia.** (Suprapubic prostatectomy was done; prostate gland weighed 787 g).

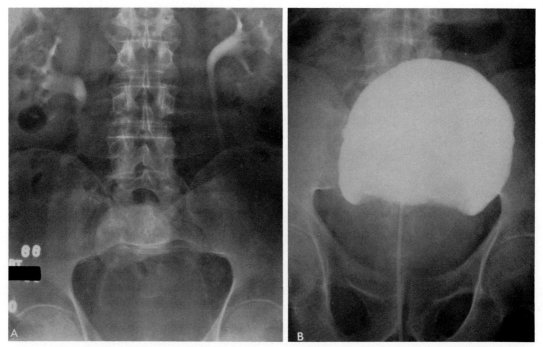

Figure 11–323. Upward displacement of bladder by large hyperplastic prostate gland (384 g). **A,** *Excretory urogram, 10-minute film.* Normal kidneys and ureters. **Large vesical calculus** overlying upper part of sacrum. Thin rim of contrast medium surrounds intravesical protrusion of prostate. **B,** *Retrograde cystogram.* Bladder pushed upward almost out of pelvis.

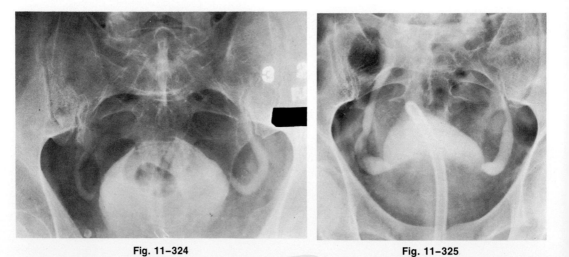

Fig. 11–324   Fig. 11–325

Figure 11–324. *Excretory urogram.* Characteristic "fish hook" contour of terminal portions of ureters caused by upward displacement of trigone and base of bladder from enlarged prostate gland.

Figure 11–325. *Excretory urogram.* "Fish hook" contour of terminal portions of ureters from hypertrophied prostate gland.

A   B

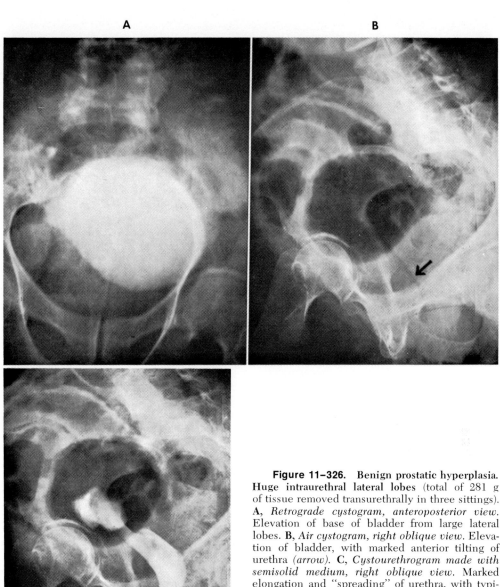

Figure 11–326. Benign prostatic hyperplasia. Huge intraurethral lateral lobes (total of 281 g of tissue removed transurethrally in three sittings). **A,** *Retrograde cystogram, anteroposterior view.* Elevation of base of bladder from large lateral lobes. **B,** *Air cystogram, right oblique view.* Elevation of bladder, with marked anterior tilting of urethra *(arrow).* **C,** *Cystourethrogram made with semisolid medium, right oblique view.* Marked elongation and "spreading" of urethra, with typical anterior tilting. (See text.) (Courtesy of Dr. R. H. Flocks.)

C

A   B

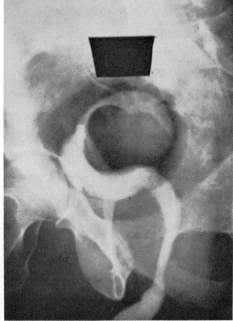

Figure 11–327. Benign prostatic hyperplasia. Very large hypertrophied subcervical gland of Albarran. **A,** *Air cystogram, anteroposterior view.* Positive filling defect of large subcervical lobe *(arrow),* surrounded by air from cystogram. **B,** *Air cystogram, right oblique view.* Positive filling defect with marked anterior tilting of urethra. **C,** *Cystourethrogram, with semisolid contrast medium, right oblique view.* Marked anterior tilting of urethra from large subcervical lobe. (See text.) (Courtesy of Dr. R. H. Flocks.)

C

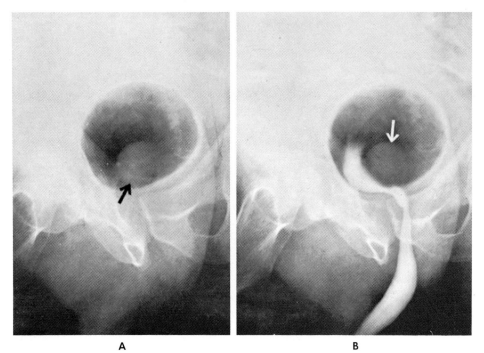

A   B

Figure 11–328.   Benign prostatic hyperplasia. Large intravesical median lobe. **A,** *Air cystogram, right oblique view.* Positive filling defect from median lobe *(arrow).* **B,** *Cystourethrogram made with semisolid medium, right oblique view.* Marked anterior tilting of urethra from enlarged median lobe, which also casts shadow of positive filling defect in air cystogram *(arrow).* (Courtesy of Dr. R. H. Flocks.)

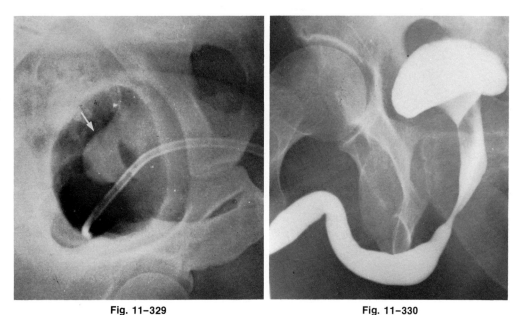

Fig. 11–329   Fig. 11–330

Figure 11–329.   *Air cystogram, right oblique view.* **Filling defect from intravesical median lobe** *(arrow).* Marked anterior tilting of urethra.

Figure 11–330.   *Retrograde urethrogram* of patient with **benign hyperplasia of prostate.** Spreading and elongation of prostatic urethra are pathognomonic of marked intraurethral enlargement of lateral lobes.

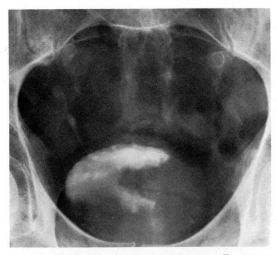

Figure 11–331. *Excretory cystogram.* **Recurrent carcinoma of prostate gland,** with irregular intravesical projection of tissue, which simulates carcinoma of bladder.

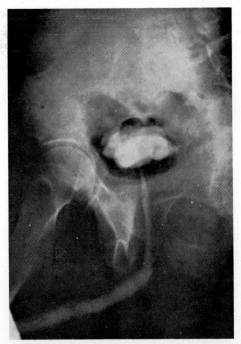

Figure 11–332. *Cystourethrogram made with semisolid medium, right oblique position.* **Carcinoma of prostate gland.** Straight, narrow prostatic urethra is typical of this disease. (Three preliminary films gave negative findings, showing no deformity of the vesical outline.) (Courtesy of Dr. R. H. Flocks.)

CARCINOMA OF THE PROSTATE

What has been said about the need for cystourethrography in the diagnosis of benign prostatic hyperplasia applies also to carcinoma of the prostate. The plain film (KUB) is important in the detection of metastasis to bone (see Chapter 7). Trabeculation of the bladder and ureterectasis may be demonstrated by excretory urography. Negative filling defects in the bladder from intravesical projection of the gland are not as commonly seen as in benign hyperplasia. When present, however, they tend to be more irregular (Fig. 11–331) and may be difficult to distinguish from those caused by infiltrating bladder tumors.

The retrograde cystourethrogram is not as impressive as it is in benign hyperplasia. There is narrowing in both the anteroposterior and lateral diameters of the prostatic urethra, so that instead of manifesting the "spreading" phenomenon, it appears as a narrow tube. It may lose its normal curve and become straight and elongated (Fig. 11–332).

POSTOPERATIVE CONTRACTURE OF THE VESICAL NECK

Postoperative contracture of the vesical neck, which consists of the formation of scar tissue at the vesical neck, may follow a suprapubic, perineal, or transurethral prostatectomy. In its mildest form, it produces an elevation of the posterior lip of the vesical neck or a slight circumferential narrowing and rigidity; in its severest form, complete or nearly complete occlusion of the vesical neck occurs. On the basis of experimental and clinical studies, Greene, Robinson, and Campbell suggested that the formation of a contracture after transurethral prostatic resection results from excessive electroexcision and electrocoagulation of the vesical neck.

A diagnosis of postoperative contracture of the vesical neck should be considered if a patient's urinary symptoms are relieved by adequate prostatic resection but return shortly thereafter. An impediment or obstruction blocking the passage of instruments in the region of the vesical neck suggests the diagnosis. Retrograde urethrography usually fails to show distinctive changes that will permit the diagnosis of a mild or moderate contracture. Severe or diaphragmatic contractures, on the other hand, may be diagnosed readily by retrograde urethrography; such contractures offer resistance to the free flow of contrast medium into the bladder, and the resulting increased intraurethral pressure causes dilatation of the distensible unscarred segments of the prostatic, bulbous, and pendulous portions of the urethra (Figs. 11–333, 11–334, and 11–335). The contracted vesical neck is visualized, and from this point the medium spreads, in a fan shape, into the bladder. If the urethrographic contrast medium is more viscid than usual, it will retain its shape as it passes through the small opening in the diaphragm and will

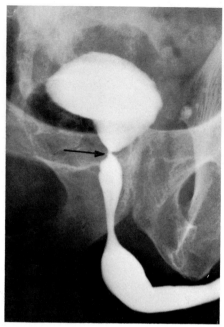

Figure 11–334. *Retrograde urethrogram.* **Severe contracture (diaphragm) of vesical neck** *(arrow)* after transurethral resection.

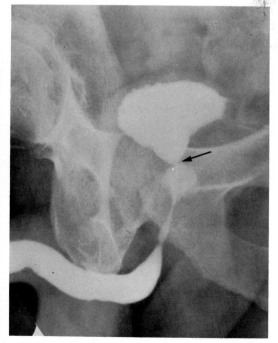

Figure 11–333. *Retrograde urethrogram.* **Severe postoperative contracture (diaphragm) of vesical neck** *(arrow)*, which occurred after transurethral prostatic resection.

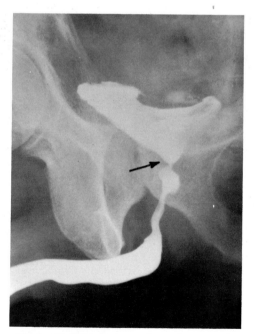

Figure 11–335. *Retrograde urethrogram.* **Severe contracture (diaphragm) of vesical neck** *(arrow)* after transurethral resection.

Fig. 11–336

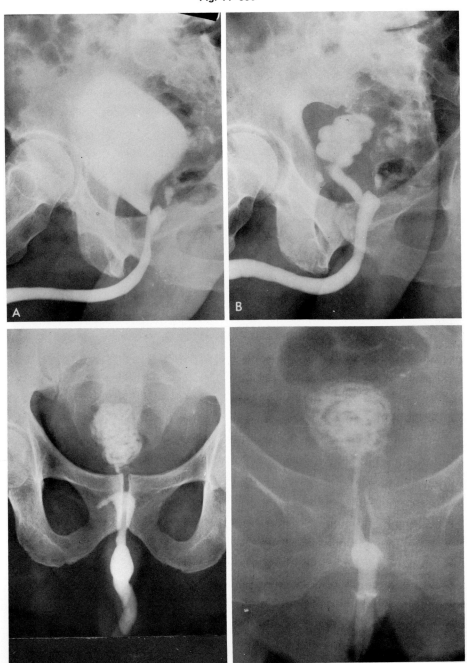

Fig. 11–337   Fig. 11–338

Figure 11–336. A, **Severe contracture of vesical neck** after transurethral prostatic resection. *Retrograde urethrograms.* **A**, *Made with usual medium.* Ventral position of small aperture of vesical neck (as seen cystoscopically in roof of prostatic urethra) is clearly shown. **B**, *Made with more viscid medium.* Medium being squeezed through contracted vesical neck layers in bladder ("toothpaste" sign).

Figure 11–337. *Retrograde urethrogram made with viscid contrast medium.* **Severe contracture of vesical neck** after transurethral prostatic resection. Note "toothpaste" sign due to medium being forced through small aperture at vesical neck and layering out in bladder.

Figure 11–338. *Retrograde urethrogram made with viscid contrast medium.* **Severe contracture of vesical neck of woman,** which occurred after repeated resections of vesical neck. Note "toothpaste" sign.

form coils or layers in the bladder. Greene and Robinson (1965, 1966) called this appearance of the medium in the roentgenogram the *toothpaste sign of diaphragmatic contracture* (Figs. 11–336, 11–337, and 11–338). Ureteral obstruction from inclusion of the ureteral orifices in the scar tissue is a not uncommon complication (Fig. 11–339).

Finally, the diagnosis may be established by using urethroscopy to visualize the contracture. For this purpose a cystourethroscope with either a Foroblique or a direct-vision telescope is the instrument of choice. The instrument is passed under vision to the contracture, and the various degrees of circumferential narrowing of the vesical neck are appreciated. When the ureteral orifices are "caught" in the scar tissue and pulled down into the region of the vesical neck, they may be very difficult to see.

Prophylaxis against postoperative contractures consists in recognizing the prostatic configuration in which trauma to the

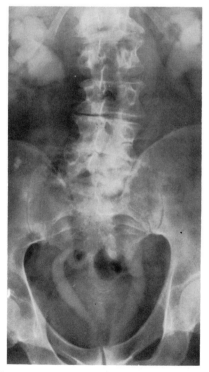

Figure 11–339.   Bilateral ureteropyelectasis from ureteral obstruction from postoperative contracture of vesical neck.

vesical neck is likely to occur during resection and modifying the operation accordingly. In such cases, the resection should be limited to the adenoma, thereby preventing trauma to the vesical neck and adjacent structures.

Conservative treatment is advisable not only for patients with mild or moderate postoperative contractures but also for selected patients with severe or even diaphragmatic contractures; occasionally, the latter type of disorder will disappear, not to reappear, after one dilation with sounds. Unfortunately, in most instances, dilation affords only temporary relief, and the contracture and associated symptoms soon recur. Nevertheless, patients whose symptoms can be controlled by the infrequent passage of sounds should follow such a regimen. If this type of therapy is unsuccessful, resection of the contracture, repeated if necessary, can be undertaken. The adjunctive injection of corticosteroids into the scarred area has been shown to prevent recontractures (Malek and Greene). However, a decision to treat a contracture by transurethral incision or excision should not be arrived at lightly, because in an appreciable number of cases, the severity of the contracture and of the associated symptoms will be increased by such procedures. Finally, if these measures fail, an open, surgical revision of the vesical neck may be necessary. In the case of marked stenosis of one or both ureteral orifices, transvesical meatotomy or ureteroneocystostomy may be necessary.

Urethral Diverticulum in the Male*

Congenital (primary) urethral diverticulum in the male is a relatively rare condition. Acquired (secondary) diverticulum is more common and usually results from trauma and infection of the urethra secondary to transurethral resection or urethral catheterization. In a review of the literature

---

*Diverticulum in the female is considered in Chapter 19.

in 1955, Warren found 236 cases, of which 96 were considered to be congenital. Primary or congenital diverticula are lined by normal urethral epithelium, whereas acquired diverticula are not. Lesions of either type may be located in the pendulous or bulbous portions of the urethra.

CONGENITAL (PRIMARY) DIVERTICULUM

Mandler and Pool found three cases of congenital diverticulum that had been treated at the Mayo Clinic during 21 years, 1945 through 1965. One patient was a boy, age 3½ years; the other two were adults.

Abeshouse stated that congenital diverticula become symptomatic during the first 20 years of the patient's life. In Mandler and Pool's cases, one presented in childhood; the other two patients were adults who had not developed symptoms until adolescence or adulthood.

Symptoms consist primarily of incontinence characterized by prolonged terminal dribbling of urine after voiding, as the diverticulum gradually empties itself. If the diverticulum is fairly large with considerable stasis from poor emptying, urinary infection will supervene.

Diagnosis is made by means of retrograde urethrography (Figs. 11–340, 11–341, and 11–342) and confirmed by urethroscopic examination.

Treatment consists of surgical excision and urethral reconstruction. Because of the high incidence of fistula formation after reconstruction of the pendulous urethra, a Cecil urethroplasty as modified by Culp (1959) is preferable.

ACQUIRED (SECONDARY) DIVERTICULUM

Acquired diverticula are usually the result of trauma or periurethral abscess. The penoscrotal juncture is the most common location for those secondary to transurethral resection or prolonged drainage with indwelling urethral catheters, as in cases of paraplegia (Figs. 11–343, 11–344, and 11–345).

Urethral Stricture in Adult Males*

Cystourethrography is of distinct value in the diagnosis of urethral stricture be-

---

*Urethral stricture in children has been discussed previously (pages 1123 to 1129).

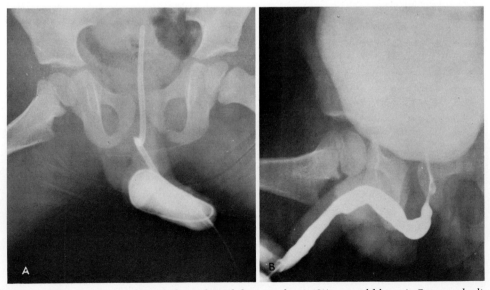

Figure 11–340.   Congenital diverticulum of pendulous urethra in 3½-year-old boy. **A,** *Retrograde diverticulogram.* Urethral catheter in bladder. Ureteral catheter was passed alongside and into diverticulum and injected with contrast medium, filling diverticulum. (Surgical excision was done.) **B,** *Postoperative retrograde urethrogram.* (From Mandler, J. I., and Pool, T. L.)

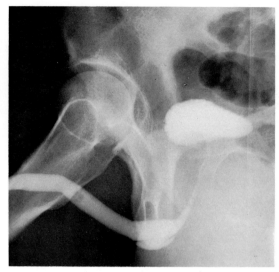

Figure 11–341. *Retrograde urethrogram.* **Congenital (?) diverticulum of bulbous urethra** in man, aged 31 (patient had had postmicturition dribbling since age 16). (With panendoscope, 3-mm opening into diverticulum could be seen in floor of urethra. Surgical excision was performed.) (From Mandler, J. I., and Pool, T. L.)

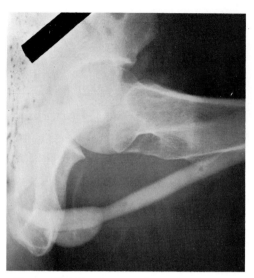

Figure 11–342. *Retrograde urethrogram.* **Diverticulum of bulbous urethra** of man, aged 44. Etiology unknown. Patient had had postmicturition dribbling for 1 year. Cystoscopy (panendoscope) showed 1.5-mm opening into diverticulum in floor of urethra. Surgical excision was performed. (From Mandler, J. I., and Pool, T. L.)

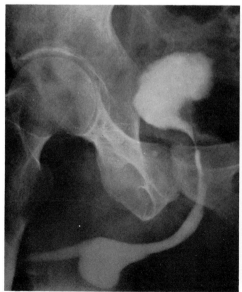

Fig. 11–343

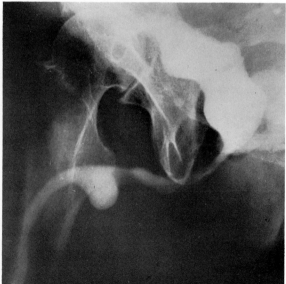

Fig. 11–344

Figure 11–343. *Retrograde cystourethrogram.* **Acquired diverticulum** (result of periurethral abscess) in anterior urethra of male patient.

Figure 11–344. *Micturition cystourethrogram* of man, 72 years of age. Urethral diverticulum, probably secondary to periurethral abscess. Note wide prostatic fossa. (Patient had had retropubic prostatectomy 1 year previously.) (Courtesy of Dr. H. W. ten Cate.)

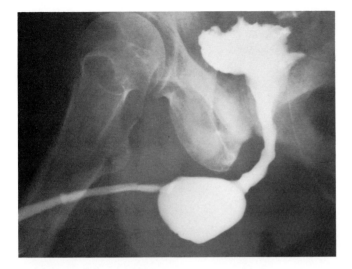

Figure 11–345. *Retrograde cystoure-throgram.* **Acquired (post-transurethral re-section) urethral diverticulum.** (Diverticulum resulted from postoperative periurethritis and periurethral abscess.)

cause it accurately localizes the site of the stricture and outlines irregularities, old false passages (from previous instrumentation), abscesses, and fistulas. The smaller the caliber of the stricture, the easier it is to demonstrate. Lapides and Stone's study indicates that strictures of 20-F caliber and smaller are more easily identified with the urethrogram than those of larger caliber.

INFLAMMATORY STRICTURE

Inflammatory strictures (chiefly from previous Neisserian urethritis) are becoming less common. The majority of these strictures are located in the bulbous urethra, although the anterior urethra may be involved. A characteristic finding in inflammatory strictures is that, although the

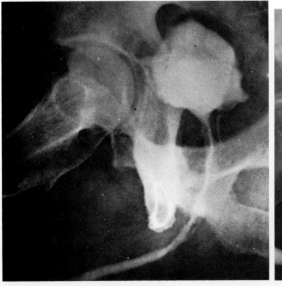

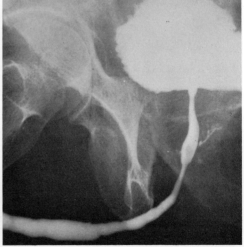

Fig. 11–346   Fig. 11–347

Figure 11–346. *Retrograde cystourethrogram, right oblique view.* **Inflammatory stricture of urethra.** Although main portion of stricture is in bulbomembranous segment, entire urethra seems to be considerably narrowed, as is typical of these cases. (Courtesy of Dr. J. J. Alvarez-Ierena.)

Figure 11–347. *Retrograde urethrogram.* **Long-standing stricture involving primarily bulbous urethra.** Stricture is long and diffuse, and there is also some reduction in caliber of anterior urethra. Ejaculatory ducts and some prostatic ducts are outlined with contrast medium.

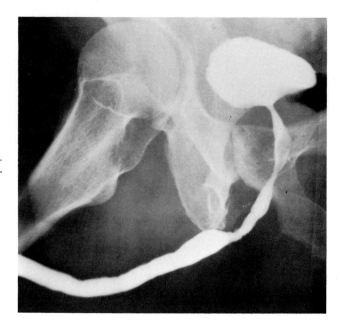

Figure 11–348. *Retrograde urethrogram.* Old Neisserian stricture of bulbous urethra. Note minimal narrowing of entire urethra.

main stricture appears to be confined to one relatively short segment, the entire urethra is narrowed (Figs. 11–346 through 11–349). The urethrogram can illustrate false passages made by sounds during dilation of strictures. Often communication of these false passages with the venous circulation may be seen, providing a graphic explanation of the frequency of chills and fever following urethral instrumentation (Figs. 11–350 through 11–357). Perineal fistula resulting from Neisserian stricture (so-called watering-pot perineum) is infrequent (Fig. 11–358; see also Chapter 15).

Text continued on page 1157

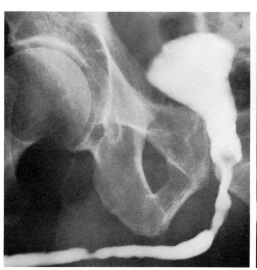

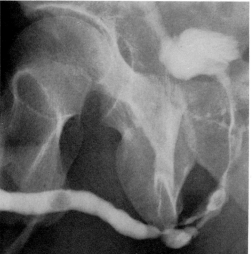

Fig. 11–349   Fig. 11–350

Figure 11–349. *Retrograde urethrogram.* Inflammatory stricture primarily of penoscrotal juncture but, to lesser degree, involving both pendulous and bulbous portions of urethra.

Figure 11–350. *Retrograde urethrogram.* Stricture of bulbomembranous urethra with false passage from recent dilation.

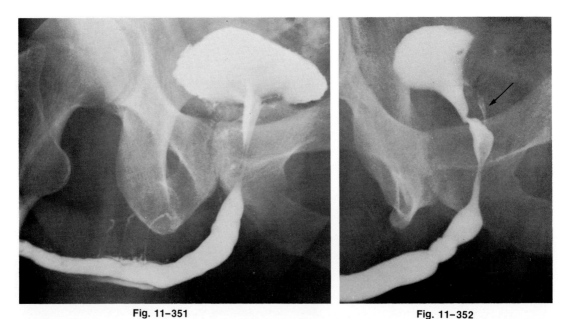

Fig. 11–351   **Fig. 11–352**

Figure 11–351. *Retrograde urethrogram.* **Recently dilated stricture in region of penoscrotal juncture.** Note some extravasation of contrast medium filling veins which apparently communicate with dorsal vein of penis.

Figure 11–352. *Retrograde urethrogram.* **Stricture of bulbomembranous urethra recently dilated.** Note false passage *(arrow)* between floor of prostatic urethra and trigone of bladder (under posterior vesical lip).

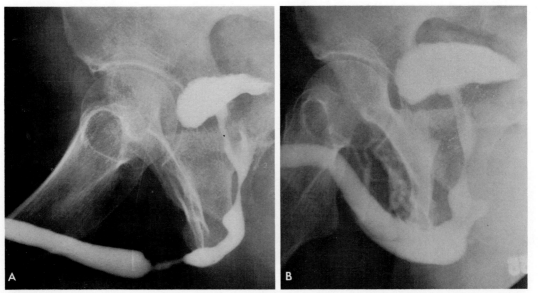

Figure 11–353. Stricture of perineal urethra just proximal to penoscrotal juncture. *Retrograde urethrograms.* **A,** *Before dilation.* **B,** *Immediately after dilation.* "False passage" and extravasation of contrast medium. Note contrast medium filling periurethral veins anteriorly.

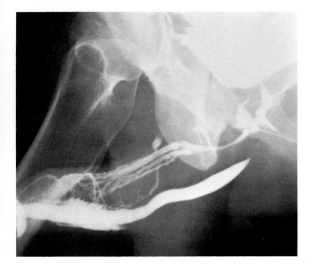

Figure 11–354. *Retrograde urethrogram.* Large-caliber stricture at penoscrotal juncture in man, 30 years of age. Periurethral extravasation of medium fills dorsal vein of penis and communicating veins. Urethrogram made prior to dilation of stricture.

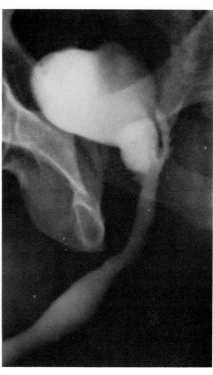

Figure 11–355. *Cystourethrogram.* **Fistula between bladder and bulbous urethra after dilation of urethral stricture** with sounds, during which false passage was made. Patient was incontinent as result of this fistula.

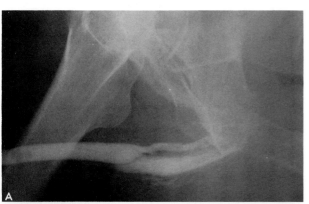

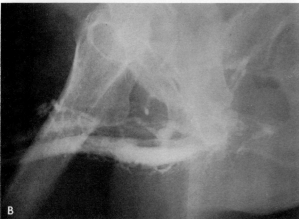

Figure 11–356. Stricture of bulbous urethra with false passage made on attempted dilation. *Retrograde urethrograms.* **A,** *Initial film.* False passage is evident. **B,** *Second film,* after injection of more contrast medium. Extravasation of contrast medium which outlines dorsal vein of penis.

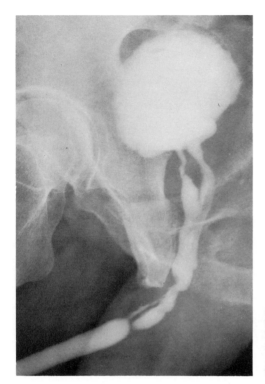

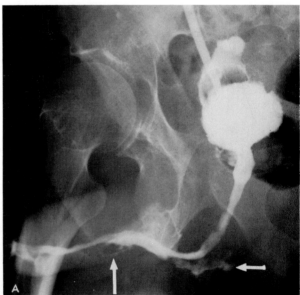

Figure 11–357. *Retrograde urethrogram.* Stricture of bulbous urethra with false passage extending into bladder.

Figure 11–358. Multiple small-caliber strictures of pendulous portion of urethra with urethrocutaneous fistula at penoscrotal juncture and false passage in perineal portion of urethra. **A**, *Voiding cystourethrogram* (contrast medium introduced through suprapubic cystostomy tube). Fistula at penoscrotal juncture (*vertical arrow*) and false passage proximally (*horizontal arrow*). **B**, *Retrograde urethrogram*, made after internal urethrotomy and drainage with indwelling catheter (suprapubic tube had been removed). Small amount of medium is escaping from fistula (*arrow*). Well-filled false passage appears to begin in region of penoscrotal juncture and to extend into bulbous urethra.

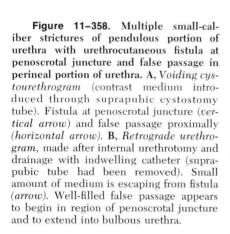

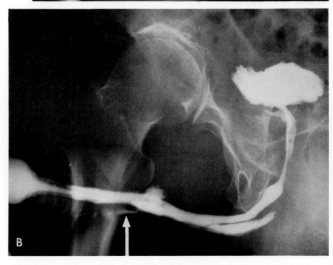

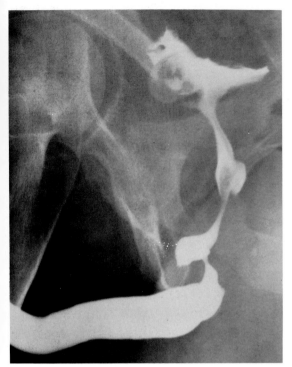

Figure 11–359. *Retrograde urethrogram.* Traumatic stricture of perineal portion of urethra from previous fracture of pelvis. Urethra had been repaired through perineum, resulting in deformity and re-forming of stricture.

TRAUMATIC AND IATROGENIC STRICTURE

Traumatic strictures result from either accidents (fracture of pelvis, straddle injuries, and others) or urethral instrumentation. Because of the large numbers of transurethral prostatic resections and transurethral resections of bladder tumors being done, iatrogenic instrumental strictures (caused by the resectoscope) are now encountered much more commonly. They are caused by the use of instruments of a caliber too large for the urethra.

Traumatic strictures differ from inflammatory strictures in that they usually are shorter and more localized, and the caliber of the remainder of the urethra may be normal or relatively normal. In the case of fracture of the pelvis, the urethra is usually sheared off at the apex of the prostate, and the stricture occurs at that point (in the membranous urethra). Straddle injuries, blows, and other injuries may cause stricture in the perineal segment (Fig. 11–359). Stricture at the site of vesicourethral anastomosis after radical prostatectomy is occasionally encountered (Fig. 11–360).

Iatrogenic (instrumental) strictures are most commonly located in the anterior urethra at its two normally narrow locations: (1) the penoscrotal juncture and (2) the urethral meatus and fossa navicularis. Like traumatic strictures, they may remain localized and short, with the remainder of the urethra of more or less normal caliber (Figs. 11–361 through 11–364). On the other hand, the entire anterior urethra may have been damaged so that it may be completely strictured (Figs. 11–365 through 11–368). Also, strictures of the bulbomem-

Text continued on page 1161

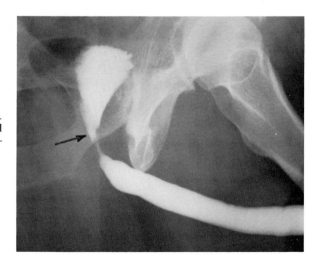

Figure 11–360. *Retrograde urethrogram.* Postoperative stricture at site of vesicourethral anastomosis *(arrow)* which followed radical perineal prostatectomy.

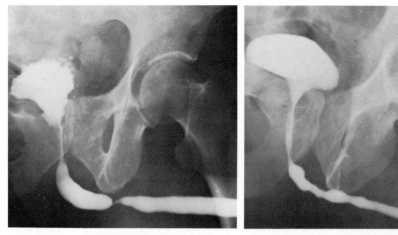

Fig. 11–361   Fig. 11–362

Figure 11–361. *Retrograde urethrogram.* Iatrogenic stricture at penoscrotal juncture from previous transurethral resection.

Figure 11–362. *Retrograde urethrogram.* Iatrogenic (instrumental) stricture of entire urethra.

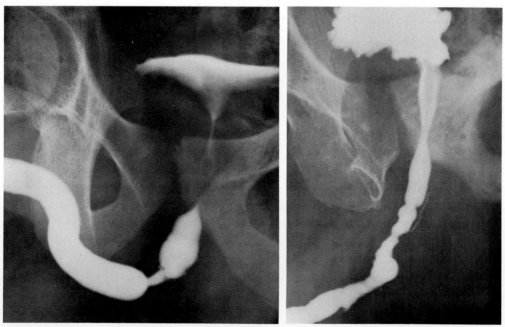

Fig. 11–363   Fig. 11–364

Figure 11–363. *Retrograde urethrogram.* Iatrogenic stricture of bulbous urethra in boy, 17 years of age, caused by prolonged use of indwelling catheter after automobile accident. (Patient had severe brain injury.)

Figure 11–364. *Retrograde urethrogram.* Iatrogenic stricture of urethra in region of penoscrotal juncture and extending proximally. Stricture had persisted in spite of Johannsen's operation. Note contrast medium outlining vein parallel to bulbous urethra.

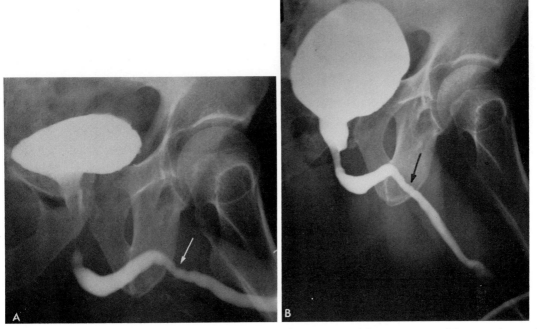

Figure 11–365. Iatrogenic (post-transurethral resection) stricture mainly at penoscrotal juncture *(arrows)*, but also involving pendulous portion of urethra. **A,** *Retrograde urethrogram.* **B,** *Voiding cystourethrogram.*

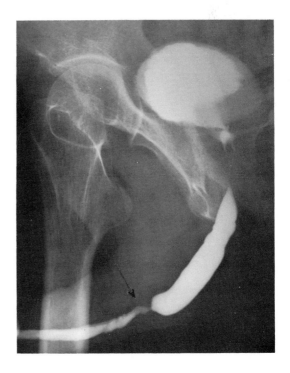

Figure 11–366. *Retrograde urethrogram.* Iatrogenic (post-transurethral resection) stricture at penoscrotal juncture *(arrow)* and pendulous urethra. Postoperative contracture of vesical neck also is present.

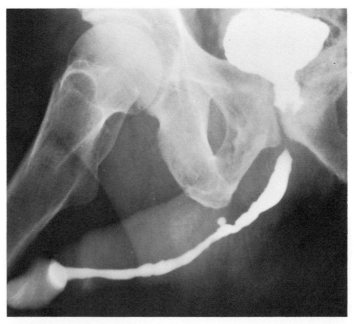

Figure 11–367. Iatrogenic (post-transurethral resection) stricture involving penoscrotal juncture, entire pendulous portion of urethra, and distal half of bulbous portion.

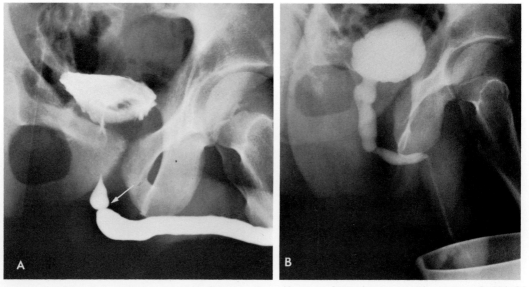

Figure 11–368. Iatrogenic stricture of bulbous urethra of boy, aged 18, after transurethral removal of bladder polyps. **A,** *Retrograde urethrogram.* Stricture *(arrow)* is short. **B,** *Voiding cystourethrogram.* Note dilatation of urethra proximal to stricture.

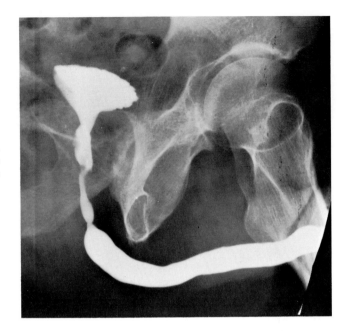

Figure 11-369. *Retrograde urethrogram.* **Iatrogenic (post-transurethral resection) stricture of bulbous portion of urethra.** Remainder of urethra is normal.

branous urethra may be secondary to the use of the electroresectoscope (Fig. 11–369). In contrast, lesions of the penoscrotal juncture are more common after use of the punch instrument.

Instrumental strictures may be prevented by preliminary careful calibration of the urethra with Otis diagnostic bougies. If the anterior urethra does not admit a size 30-F bougie easily, three procedures are available: (1) use of a size 24-F resectoscope, (2) introduction of the resectoscope through a perineal urethrostomy, or (3) enlargement of the urethra by means of internal urethrotomy (Emmett, Kirchheim, and Greene).

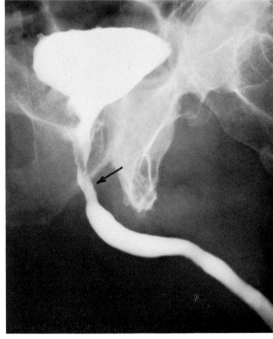

Figure 11-370. *Retrograde urethrogram.* **Post-transurethral-resection incontinence.** Note lack of tonicity of external urethral sphincter *(arrow).*

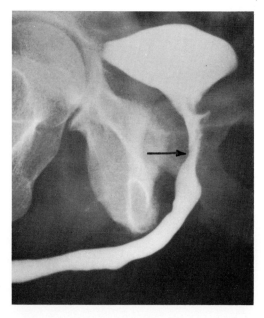

Figure 11–371. *Retrograde urethrogram.* **Post-transurethral-resection incontinence.** Note relaxation (lack of tonicity) of external urethral sphincter *(arrow)*. Also, some residual adenomatous prostatic tissue remains near apex of prostatic urethra.

POSTOPERATIVE INCONTINENCE IN THE MALE

Urinary incontinence occurring after various types of prostatectomy usually results from damage to the external urethral sphincter or the vesical neck. In some cases, this can be demonstrated by a retrograde urethrogram, which will show reduction or absence of the normal tonicity of the external sphincter (Figs. 11–370 and 11–371). See discussion of the external urethral sphincter under the heading of Neurogenic Bladder.

REFERENCES

Abeshouse, B. S.: Diverticula of the Anterior Urethra in the Male: A Report of Four Cases and a Review of the Literature. Urol. Cutan. Rev. 55:690–707, 1951.

Allen, T. D.: Congenital Ureteral Strictures. J. Urol. 104:196–204 (July) 1970.

Amar, A. D.: Vesicoureteral Reflux Associated With Congenital Bladder Diverticulum in Boys and Young Men. J. Urol. 107:966–968 (June) 1972.

Amar, A. D., and Chabra, K.: Reflux in Duplicated Ureters: Treatment in Children. J. Pediat. Surg. 5:419–430 (Aug.) 1970.

Amar, A. D., Singer, B., Lewis, R., and Nocks, B.: Vesicoureteral Reflux in Adults: A Twelve-year Study of 122 Patients. Urology 3:184–189 (Feb.) 1974.

Ambrose, S. S.: Reflux Pyelonephritis in Adults Secondary to Congenital Lesions of the Ureteral Orifice. J. Urol. 102:302–304 (Sept.) 1969.

Ambrose, S. S., and Nicolson, W. P., III: Vesicoureteral Reflux Secondary to Anomalies of the Ureterovesical Junction: Management and Results. J. Urol. 87:695–700 (May) 1962.

Ansell, J. S., and Paterson, J. R. S.: Intermittent Hydronephrosis. N. Engl. J. Med. 267:447–448 (30 Aug.) 1962.

Bailey, R. R.: The Relationship of Vesico-ureteric Reflux to Urinary Tract Infection and Chronic Pyelonephritis—Reflux Nephropathy. Clin. Nephrol. 1:132–141 (May–June) 1973.

Bartrina, J.: Some Considerations on Insufficiency of the Vesicoureteral Valve. Urol. Cutan. Rev. 39:167–172 (Jan.) 1935.

Baum, S., and Gillenwater, J. Y.: Renal Artery Impressions on the Renal Pelvis. J. Urol. 95:139–145 (Feb.) 1966.

Berquist, T. H., Hattery, R. R., Hartman, G. W., Kelalis, P. P., and DeWeerd, J. H.: Vesicoureteral Reflux in Adults. Am. J. Roentgenol. 125:314–321 (Oct.) 1975.

Bialestock, D.: Renal Malformations and Pyelonephritis: The Role of Vesico-ureteral Reflux. Aust. NZ J. Surg. 33:114–127 (Aug.) 1963.

Bischoff, P.: Operative Treatment of Megaureter. J. Urol. 85:268–274 (Mar.) 1961.

Blight, E. M., Jr., and O'Shaughnessy, E. J.: Vesicoureteral Reflux in Children: A Prospective Study. J. Urol. 102:44–46 (July) 1969.

Blumel, J., Evans, E. B., and Eggers, G. W. N.: Partial and Complete Agenesis or Malformation of the Sacrum With Associated Anomalies: Etiologic and

Clinical Study With Special Reference to Heredity; a Preliminary Report. J. Bone and Joint Surg. *41A*:497–518 (Apr.) 1959.

Bors, E.: Neurogenic Bladder. *In* Piersol, G. M.: The Cyclopedia of Medicine, Surgery Specialties. Philadelphia, F. A. Davis Company, Ed. 3, vol. 9, 1951, pp. 603–614.

Bors, E.: Neurogenic Bladder. Urol. Survey 7:177–250 (June) 1957.

Bourne, R. B.: Intermittent Hydronephrosis as a Cause of Abdominal Pain. J.A.M.A. *198*:1218–1219 (12 Dec.) 1966.

Bumpus, H. C., Jr.: Urinary Reflux. J. Urol. *12*:341–346 (Oct.) 1924.

Burger, R. H.: Familial and Hereditary Vesicoureteral Reflux (Letter to the Editor). J.A.M.A. *216*:680–681 (26 Apr.) 1971.

Burke, E. C., Shin, M. H., and Kelalis, P. P.: Prune-belly Syndrome: Clinical Findings and Survival. Am J. Dis. Child. *117*:668–671 (June) 1969.

Campbell, J. B.: Neurosurgical Treatment of Bladder and Bowel Dysfunction Resulting From Anomalous Development of the Sacral Neural Axis. Clin. Neurosurg. 8:133–156 (Oct.) 1960.

Campbell, M. F.: Clinical Pediatric Urology, Philadelphia, W. B. Saunders Company, 1951, 1,113 pp.

Cass, A. S., and Lenaghan, D.: The Influence of Posture on the Occurrence of Vesicoureteral Reflux. Invest. Urol. 2:523–529 (May) 1965.

Chang, C.-Y.: Anterior Urethral Valves: A Case Report. J. Urol. *100*:29–31 (July) 1968.

Cobb, B. G., Wolf, J. A., Jr., and Ansell, J. S.: Congenital Stricture of the Proximal Urethral Bulb. J. Urol. 99:629–631 (May) 1968.

Colabawalla, B. N.: Anterior Urethral Valve: A Case Report. J. Urol. 94:58–59 (July) 1965.

Conway, J. J., Belman, A. B., King, L. R., and Filmer, R. B.: Direct and Indirect Radionuclide Cystography. J. Urol. *113*:689–693 (May) 1975.

Cooper, D. G. W.: Bladder Studies in Children With Neurogenic Incontinence: With Comments on the Place of Pelvic Floor Stimulation. Br. J. Urol. *40*:157–174, 1968.

Culp, O. S.: Treatment of Ureteropelvic Obstruction. Am. Urol. A., North Central Sect., Postgrad. Seminar 278–288, 1955.

Culp, O. S.: Experiences With 200 Hypospadiacs: Evolution of a Therapeutic Plan. Surg. Clin. North Am. 39:1007–1029 (Aug.) 1959.

Culp, O. S.: Choice of Operations for Ureteropelvic Obstruction: Review of 385 Cases. Can. J. Surg. 4:157–165 (Jan.) 1961.

Culp, O. S.: Management of Ureteropelvic Obstruction. Bull. N.Y. Acad. Med. *43*:355–377 (May) 1967.

Culp, O. S., and DeWeerd, J. H.: A Pelvic Flap Operation for Certain Types of Ureteropelvic Obstruction: Observations After Two Years' Experience. J. Urol. 71:523–529 (May) 1954.

Damanski, M.: Cystourethrography in Paraplegia as a Guide to Catheter-Free Life: 17 Years' Experience of a Paraplegic Center. J. Urol. 93:466–471 (Apr.) 1965.

Damanski, M., and Kerr, A. S.: The Value of Cystourethrography in Paraplegia. Br. J. Urol. 44:398–407, 1956–1957.

Daniel, J., Stewart, A. M., and Blair, D. W.: Congenital Anterior Urethral Valve — Diagnosis and Treatment. Br. J. Urol. *40*:589–591 (Oct.) 1968.

Devereux, M. H., and Williams, D. I.: The Treatment of Urethral Stricture in Boys. J. Urol. *108*:489–493 (Sept.) 1972.

Dockray, K. T.: The Perirenal P Sign: A New Roentgenogram Index to the Cause and Treatment of Urinary Ascites in Babies. Am. J. Dis. Child. *119*:179–181 (Feb.) 1970.

Doppman, J. L., and Fraley, E. E.: Arteriography in the Syndrome of Superior Infundibular Obstruction: A Simplified Technic for Identifying the Obstructing Vessel. Radiology 99:1039–1041 (Nov.) 1968.

Duffy, P.: Primary Vesico-ureteric Reflux in Adults. Med. J. Aust. 2:1056–1060 (4 Nov.) 1972.

Dwoskin, J. Y., and Perlmutter, A. D.: Vesicoureteral Reflux in Children: A Computerized Review. J. Urol. *109*:888–890 (May) 1973.

Ellis, D. G., Fonkalsrud, E. W., and Smith, J. P.: Congenital Posterior Urethral Valves. J. Urol. 95:549–554 (Apr.) 1966.

Emmett, J. L.: Further Observations in the Management of Cord Bladder by Transurethral Resection. J. Urol. 57:29–41 (Jan.) 1947.

Emmett, J. L.: Neuromuscular Disease of the Urinary Tract. 1. Physiology of the Normal Bladder: Neurophysiology of Micturition. 2. Neurogenic Vesical Dysfunction (Cord Bladder) and Neuromuscular Ureteral Dysfunction. *In* Campbell, M. F.: Urology, Philadelphia, W. B. Saunders Company, vol. 2, 1954, pp. 1255–1383.

Emmett, J. L., and Simon, H. B.: Transurethral Resection in Infants and Children for Congenital Obstruction of the Vesical Neck and Myelodysplasia. J. Urol. 76:595–608 (Nov.) 1956.

Emmett, J. L., Daut, R. V., and Dunn, J. H.: Role of the External Urethral Sphincter in the Normal Bladder and Cord Bladder. J. Urol. 59:439–454 (Mar.) 1948.

Emmett, J. L., Kirchheim, D., and Greene, L. F.: Prevention of Postoperative Stricture From Transurethral Resection by Preliminary Internal Urethrotomy: Report of Experience With 447 Cases. J. Renol. 78:456–465 (Oct.) 1957.

Emmett, J. L., Simon, H. B., and Mills, S. D.: Neuromuscular Disease of the Urinary Tract in Infants and Children. Pediat. Clin. North Am. 803–818 (Aug.) 1955.

Engle, W. J., and Schlumberger, F. C.: Urinary Extravasation in New Born Infant Associated With Congenital Stenosis of Urethra: Report of Case. Cleveland Clin. Quart. 5:278–283, 1938.

Ericsson, N. O.: Personal communication.

Ericsson, N. O., Hellström, B., Negårdh, A., and Rudhe, U.: Micturition Urethrocystography in Children With Myelomeningocele: A Radiologic and Clinical Investigation. Acta Radiol. [Diagn.] (Stockh.) *11*:321–336, 1971.

Estes, R. C., and Brooks, R. T.: Vesicoureteral Reflux in Adults. J. Urol. *103*:603–605 (May) 1970.

Falk, D.: Intermittent Obstruction at the Ureteropelvic Juncture. J. Urol. 79:16–20 (Jan.) 1958.

Fehrenbaker, L. G., Kelalis, P. P., and Stickler, G. B.: Vesicoureteral Reflux and Ureteral Duplication in Children. J. Urol. *107*:862–864 (May) 1972.

Filly, R. A., Friedland, G. W., Fair, R. W., and Govan,

D. E.: Late Ureteric Obstruction Following Ureteral Implantation for Reflux: A Warning. Urology 4:540–543 (Nov.) 1974.

Fisher, O. D., and Forsythe, W. I.: Micturating Cystourethrography in the Investigation of Enuresis. Arch. Dis. Child. 29:460–471 (Oct.) 1954.

Fraley, E. E.: Dismembered Infundibuloplasty: Improved Technique for Correcting Vascular Obstruction of the Superior Infundibulum. J. Urol. 101:144–148 (Feb.) 1969.

Garrett, R. A., and Schlueter, D. P.: Complications of Antireflux Operations: Causes and Management. J. Urol. 109:1002–1004 (June) 1973.

Geist, R. W., and Antolak, S. J., Jr.: The Clinical Problems of Children With Sterile Ureteral Reflux. J. Urol. 108:343–346 (Aug.) 1972.

Giertz, G., and Lindblom, K.: Urethrocystographic Studies of Nervous Disturbances of the Urinary Bladder and the Urethra: A Preliminary Report. Acta Radiol. 36:205–216 (Sept.) 1951.

Glenn, J. F., and Anderson, E. E.: Distal Tunnel Ureteral Reimplantation. J. Urol. 97:623–626 (Apr.) 1967.

Gonzales, E. T., Glenn, J. F., and Anderson, E. E.: Results of Distal Tunnel Ureteral Reimplantation. J. Urol. 107:572–575 (Apr.) 1972.

Gould, H. R., and Peterson, C. G., Jr.: Voiding Cystourethrography in Children. Am. J. Roentgenol. 98:192–199 (Sept.) 1966.

Govan, D. E., and Palmer, J. M.: Urinary Tract Infection in Children: The Influence of Successful Antireflux Operations in Morbidity From Infection. Pediatrics 44:677–684 (Nov.) 1969.

Graham, J. B., King, L. R., Kropp, K. A., and Uehling, D. T.: The Significance of Distal Urethral Narrowing in Young Girls. J. Urol. 97:1045–1049 (June) 1967.

Graves, R. C., and Davidoff, L. M.: Studies on the Ureter and Bladder With Especial Reference to Regurgitation of the Vesical Contents. J. Urol. 10:185–231 (Sept.) 1923.

Graves, R. C., and Davidoff, L. M.: II. Studies on the Ureter and Bladder With Especial Reference to Regurgitation of the Vesical Contents. J. Urol. 12:93–103 (Aug.) 1924.

Greene, L. F., and Robinson, H. P.: Postoperative Contracture of the Vesical Neck. V. Clinical Findings, Symptoms, and Diagnosis. J. Urol. 94:141–147 (Aug.) 1965.

Greene, L. F., and Robinson, H. P.: Postoperative Contracture of the Vesical ·Neck. VI. Prophylaxis and Treatment. J. Urol. 95:520–525 (Apr.) 1966.

Greene, L. F., Priestley, J. T., Simon, H. B., and Hempstead, R. H.: Obstruction of the Lower Third of the Ureter by Anomalous Blood Vessels. J. Urol. 71:544–548 (May) 1954.

Greene, L. F., Robinson, H. P., and Campbell, J. C.: Postoperative Contracture of the Neck of the Bladder. Abstr. Am. Acad. Gen. Pract. 431–432, 1961.

Grégoir, W., and Van Regemorter, G.: Le reflux vésico-urétéral congénital. Urol. Internat. 18:122–136, 1964.

Griesbach, W. A., Waterhouse, R. K., and Mellins, H. Z.: Voiding Cysto-urethrography in the Diagnosis of Congenital Posterior Urethral Valves. Am. J. Roentgenol. 82:521–529 (Sept.) 1959.

Gross, K. E., and Sanderson, S. S.: Cineurethrography and Voiding Cinecystography, With Special Attention to Vesico-ureteral Reflux. Radiology 77:573–585 (Oct.) 1961.

Gruber, C. M.: I. A Comparative Study of the Intravesical Ureters (Uretero-vesical Valves) in Man and in Experimental Animals. J. Urol. 21:567–581 (May) 1929a.

Gruber, C. M.: II. The Uretero-vesical Valve. J. Urol. 22:275–292 (Sept.) 1929b.

Halverstadt, D. B., and Leadbetter, G. W., Jr.: Internal Urethrotomy and Recurrent Urinary Tract Infection in Female Children. I. Results in the Management of Infection. J. Urol. 100:297–302 (Sept.) 1968.

Hamm, F. C., and Waterhouse, K.: Changing Concepts in Lower Urinary-Tract Obstruction in Children. J.A.M.A. 175:854–857 (11 Mar.) 1961.

Hanley, H. G.: The Pelvi-ureteric Junction: A Cinepyelographic Study. Br. J. Urol. 31:377–384, 1959.

Hanley, H. G.: Hydronephrosis. Lancet 2:664–667 (24 Sept.) 1960.

Helmholz, H. F.: Experimental Studies in Urinary Infection of the Bacillary Type. J. Urol. 31:173–191 (Feb.) 1934.

Hendren, W. H.: Ureteral Reimplantation in Children. J. Pediat. Surg. 3:649–664 (Dec.) 1968.

Hendren, W. H.: Operative Repair of Megaureter in Children. J. Urol. 101:491–507 (Apr.) 1969.

Hendren, W. H.: Posterior Urethral Valves in Boys: A Broad Clinical Spectrum. J. Urol. 106:298–307 (Aug.) 1971.

Heptinstall, R. H.: The Enigma of Chronic Pyelonephritis. J. Infect. Dis. 120:104–107 (July) 1969.

Hinman, F.: The Principles and Practice of Urology, Philadelphia, W.B. Saunders Company, 1935, 1,111 pp.

Hodson, C. J.: The Radiological Contribution Toward the Diagnosis of Chronic Pyelonephritis. Radiology 88:857–871 (May) 1967.

Hodson, C. J., and Craven, J. D.: The Radiology of Obstructive Atrophy of the Kidney. Clin. Radiol. 17:305–320 (Oct.) 1966.

Hodson, C. J., and Edwards, D.: Chronic Pyelonephritis and Vesico-ureteric Reflux. Clin. Radiol. 11:219–231 (Oct.) 1960.

Hodson, C. J., and Wilson, S.: Natural History of Chronic Pyelonephritis Scarring. Br. Med. J. 2:191–194 (24 July) 1965.

Hodson, C. J., McManamon, P. J., and Lewis, M.: A New Concept of the Pathogenesis of Atrophic Pyelonephritis. Abstract 598. In Abstracts of the Fifth International Congress of Nephrology, Mexico City, 1972.

Holm, H.: On Pyelogenic Renal Cysts. Acta Radiol. 29:87–94, 1948.

Hutch, J. A.: Vesico-ureteral Reflux in the Paraplegic: Cause and Correction. J. Urol. 68:457–467 (Aug.) 1952.

Hutch, J. A.: The Ureterovesical Junction. Berkeley and Los Angeles, University of California Press, 1958, 178 pp.

Hutch, J. A.: A New Theory of the Anatomy of the Internal Urinary Sphincter and the Physiology of Micturition. Invest. Urol. 3:36–58 (July) 1965.

Hutch, J. A., and Smith, D. R.: Sterile Reflux: Report of 24 Cases. Urol. Internat. 24:460–465, 1969.

Hutch, J. A., Hinman, F., Jr., and Miller, E. R.: Reflux as a Cause of Hydronephrosis and Chronic Pyelonephritis. J. Urol. 88:169–175 (Aug.) 1962.

Iannaccone, G., and Panzironi, P. E.: Ureteral Reflux in Normal Infants. Acta Radiol. 44:451–456 (Dec.) 1955.

Immergut, M. A., and Wahman, G. E.: The Urethral Caliber of Female Children With Recurrent Urinary Tract Infections. J. Urol. 99:189–190 (Feb.) 1968.

Johnston, J. H.: Vesico-ureteric Reflux in the Child. Clin. Pediat. 2:72–80 (Feb.) 1963.

Johnston, J. H.: Reconstructive Surgery of Megaureter in Childhood. Br. J. Urol. 39:17–21, 1967.

Johnston, J. H., and Kulatilake, A. E.: The Sequelae of Posterior Urethral Valves. Br. J. Urol. 43:743–748, 1971.

Jones, B. W., and Headstream, J. W.: Vesicoureteral Reflux in Children. J. Urol. 80:114–115 (Aug.) 1958.

Jorup, S., and Kjellberg, S. R.: Congenital Valvular Formations in the Urethra. Acta Radiol. 30:197–208, 1948.

Karlin, I. W.: Incidence of Spina Bifida Occulta in Children With and Without Enuresis. Am. J. Dis. Child. 49:125–134 (Jan.) 1935.

Keeton, J. E.: Urethral Stenosis in Female Children With Urinary Tract Infection: An Overview. South. Med. J. 67:1313–1316 (Nov.) 1974.

Kelalis, P. P.: Proper Perspective on Vesicoureteral Reflux. Mayo Clin. Proc. 46:807–818 (Dec.) 1971.

Kelalis, P. P.: The Present Status of Surgery for Vesicoureteral Reflux. Urol. Clin. North Am. 1:457–469 (Oct.) 1974.

Kelalis, P. P., Culp, O. S., Stickler, G. B., and Burke, E. C.: Ureteropelvic Obstruction in Children: Experiences With 109 Cases. J. Urol. 106:418–422 (Sept.) 1971.

Kelalis, P. P., Malek, R. S., and Segura, J. W.: Observations on Renal Ectopia and Fusion in Children. J. Urol. 110:588–592 (Nov.) 1973.

Kendall, A. R., and Karafin, L.: Intermittent Hydronephrosis: Hydration Pyelography. J. Urol. 98:653–656 (Dec.) 1967.

King, L. R., Kazmi, S. O., and Belman, A. B.: Natural History of Vesicoureteral Reflux: Outcome of a Trial of Nonoperative Therapy. Urol. Clin. North Am. 1:441–445 (Oct.) 1974.

King, L. R., Kazmi, S. O., Campbell, J. A., and Belman, A. B.: The Case for Nonsurgical Management in Vesicoureteral Reflux. In Scott, R., Jr., Gordon, H. L., Scott, F. B., Carlton, C. E., and Beach, P. D.: Current Controversies in Urologic Management. Philadelphia, W. B. Saunders Company, 1972, pp. 200–215.

Kjellberg, S. R., Ericsson, N. D., and Rudhe, U.: The Lower Urinary Tract in Childhood: Some Correlated Clinical and Roentgenologic Observations. (Tr. by Erica Odelberg) Almqvist, Year Book Publishers, Inc., 1957, 298 pp.

Koontz, W. W., Jr., and Prout, G. R., Jr.: Agenesis of the Sacrum and the Neurogenic Bladder. J.A.M.A. 203:481–486 (12 Feb.) 1968.

Kreel, L., and Pyle, R.: Arterial Impressions on the Renal Pelvis. Br. J. Radiol. 35:609–613 (Sept.) 1962.

Landes, H. E., and Rall, R.: Congenital Valvular Obstruction of the Posterior Urethra. J. Urol. 34:254–267 (Sept.) 1935.

Langworthy, O. R., and Kolb, L. C.: Histological Changes in the Vesical Muscle Following Injury of the Peripheral Innervation. Anat. Rec. 71:249–263 (July) 1938.

Lapides, J., Anderson, E. C., and Petrone, A. F.: Urinary-Tract Infection in Children. J.A.M.A. 195:248–253 (24 Jan.) 1966.

Lapides, J., and Stone, T. E.: Usefulness of Retrograde Urethrography in Diagnosing Strictures of the Anterior Urethea. J. Urol. 100:747–750 (Dec.) 1968.

Larson, J. W., Swenson, W. M., Utz, D. C., and Steinhilber, R. M.: Psychogenic Urinary Retention. J.A.M.A. 184:697–700 (June) 1963.

Lattimer, J. K., Apperson, J. W., Gleason, D. M., Baker, D., and Fleming S. S.: The Pressure at Which Reflux Occurs: An Important Indicator of Prognosis and Treatment. J. Urol. 89:395–404 (Mar.) 1963.

Lattimer, J. K., Dean, A. L., Jr., Dougherty, L. J., Iu, D., Ryder, C., and Uson, A.: Functional Closure of the Bladder in Children With Exstrophy: A Report of Twenty-eight Cases. J. Urol. 83:647–655 (May) 1960.

Leadbetter, G. W., Jr., and Leadbetter, W. F.: Urethral Strictures in Male Children. J. Urol. 87:409–415 (Mar.) 1962.

Leadbetter, G. W., Jr., Duxbury, J. H., and Dreyfuss, J. R.: Absence of Vesicoureteral Reflux in Normal Adult Males. J. Urol. 84:69–70 (July) 1960.

Lenaghan, D., and Cussen, L. J.: Vesicoureteral Reflux in Pups. Invest. Urol. 5:449–461 (Mar.) 1968.

LeVine, M., Allen, A., Stein, J. L., and Schwartz, S.: The Crescent Sign. Radiology 81:971–973 (Dec.) 1963.

Levitt, S. B., and Sandler, H. J.: The Absence of Vesicoureteral Reflux in the Neonate With Myelodysplasia. J. Urol. 114:118–121 (July) 1975.

Lewin, L., and Goldschmidt, H.: Versuche über die Beziehungen zwischen Blase, Harnleiter und Nierenbecken. Virchows Arch. Path. Anat. 134:33–70, 1893.

Lich, R., Jr., Howerton, L. W., and Davis, L. A.: Vesicourethrography. Tr. Am. A. Genito-Urin. Surgeons 52:43–44, 1960.

Lich, R., Jr., Howerton, L. W., and Davis, L. A.: Vesicourethrography. J. Urol. 85:396–397 (Mar.) 1961a.

Lich, R., Jr., Howerton, L. W., and Davis, L. A.: Recurrent Urosepsis in Children. J. Urol. 86:554–558 (Nov.) 1961b.

Lowsley, O. S., and Kerwin, T. J.: Clinical Urology, Ed. 3, Baltimore, Williams & Wilkins Company, 1956, Vol. 1.

Lyon, R. P., and Smith, D. R.: Distal Urethral Stenosis. J. Urol. 89:414–421 (Mar.) 1963.

Lyon, R. P., and Tanagho, E. A.: Distal Urethral Stenosis in Little Girls. J. Urol. 93:379–388 (Mar.) 1965.

Lyon, R. P., Marshall, S., and Tanagho, E. A.: The Ureteral Orifice: Its Configuration and Competency. J. Urol. 102:504–509 (Oct.) 1969.

MacCarty, C. S.: The Treatment of Spastic Paraplegia by Selective Spinal Cordectomy. J. Neurosurg. 11:539–545 (Nov.) 1954.

Mackie, G. G., Awang, H., and Stephens F. D.: The

Ureteric Orifice: The Embryologic Key to Radiologic Status of Duplex Kidneys. J. Pediatr. Surg. 10:473–481 (Aug.) 1975.

Magnus, R. V.: Vesicoureteral Reflux in Babies With Myelomeningocele. J. Urol. 114:122–125 (July) 1975.

Malek, R. S., and Greene, L. F.: Corticosteroid Therapy of Postoperative Contractures of the Vesical Neck. J. Urol. 110:297–298 (Sept.) 1973.

Malek, R. S., Kelalis, P. P., Burke, E. C., and Stickler, G. B.: Simple and Ectopic Ureterocele in Infancy and Childhood. Surg. Gynec. Obstet. 134:611–616 (Apr.) 1972.

Mandler, J. I., and Pool, T. L.: Primary Diverticulum of the Male Urethra. J. Urol. 96:336–338 (Sept.) 1966.

Markland, C., and Kelly, W. D.: Experiences With the Severely Damaged Urinary Tract. J. Urol. 99:327–336 (Mar.) 1968.

McLellan, F. C.: The Neurogenic Bladder. Springfield, Illinois, Charles C Thomas, 1939, 206 pp.

McRae, C. U., Shannon, F. T., and Utley, W. L. F.: Effect on Renal Growth of Reimplantation of Refluxing Ureters. Lancet 1:1310–1312 (29 June) 1974.

Meadows, J. A., Jr., and Quattlebaum, R. B.: Polyps of the Posterior Urethra in Children. J. Urol. 100:317–320 (Sept.) 1968.

Melick, W. F., Brodeur, A. E., and Karellos, D. N.: A Suggested Classification of Ureteral Reflux and Suggested Treatment Based on Cineradiographic Findings and Simultaneous Pressure Recordngs by Means of the Strain Gauge. J. Urol. 88:35–37 (July) 1962.

Michel, J. R., and Barsamian, J.: Les empreintes vasculaires sur les calices et le bassinet. Ann. Radiol. (Paris) 14:15–26 (Jan.–Feb.) 1971.

Mitchell, G. F., Makhuli, Z., and Frittelli, G.: Congenital Urethral Valve in a Female. Radiology 89:690–693 (Oct.) 1967.

Moore, T.: Hydrocalicosis. Br. J. Urol. 22:304–317, 1950.

Motzkin, D.: The Clinical Significance of Visually Determined Vesicoureteral Reflux. J. Urol. 95:711–712 (May) 1966.

Mulcahy, J. J., Kelalis, P. P., Stickler, G. B., and Burke, E. C.: Familial Vesicoureteral Reflux. J. Urol. 104:762–764 (Nov.) 1970.

Murnaghan, G. F.: Experimental Aspects of Hydronephrosis. Br. J. Urol. 31:370–376, 1959.

Nesbit, R. M.: Diagnosis of Intermittent Hydronephrosis: Importance of Pyelography During Episodes of Pain. J. Urol. 75:767–771 (May) 1956.

Nesbit, R. M., McDonald, H. P., Jr., and Busby, S.: Obstructing Valves in the Female Urethra. J. Urol. 91:79–83 (Jan.) 1964.

Ney, C., and Duff, J.: Cysto-urethrography: Its Role in Diagnosis of Neurogenic Bladder. J. Urol. 63:640–652 (Apr.) 1950.

Notley, R. G.: Electron Microscopy of the Upper Ureter and the Pelvi-ureteric Junction. Br. J. Urol. 40:37–52, 1968.

Palken, M.: Surgical Correction of Vesicoureteral Reflux in Children: Results With the Use of a Single Standard Technique. J. Urol. 104:765–768 (Nov.) 1970.

Pellman, C.: The Neurogenic Bladder in Children With Congenital Malformations of the Spine: A Study of 61 Patients. J. Urol. 93:472–475 (Apr.) 1965.

Penn, I. A., and Breidahl, P. D.: Ureteric Reflux and Renal Damage. Aust. NZ J. Surg. 37:163–168 (Nov.) 1967.

Perkash, I.: Modified Approach to Sphincterotomy in Spinal Cord Injury Patients: Indications, Technique and Results in 32 Patients. Paraplegia 13:247–260 (Feb.) 1976.

Politano, V. A., and Leadbetter, W. F.: An Operative Technique for the Correction of Vesicoureteral Reflux. J. Urol. 79:932–941 (June) 1958.

Prather, G. C.: Calyceal Diverticulum. J. Urol. 45:55–64 (Jan.) 1941.

Raper, F. P.: The Recognition and Treatment of Congenital Urethral Valves. Br. J. Urol. 25:136–141, 1953.

Rolleston, G. L., Maling, T. M. J., and Hodson, C. J.: Intrarenal Reflux and the Scarred Kidney. Arch. Dis. Child. 49:531–539 (July–Dec.) 1974.

Rolleston, G. L., Shannon, F. T., and Utley, W. L. F.: Relationship of Infantile Vesicoureteric Reflux to Renal Damage. Br. Med. J. 1:460–463 (21 Feb.) 1970a.

Rolleston, G. L., Shannon, F. T., and Utley, W. L. F.: The Significance and Management of VUR in Infancy. In Kincaid-Smith, P., and Fairley, K. F.: Renal Infection and Renal Scarring. Melbourne, Mercedes Publishing Services, 1970b, p. 241.

Roper, B. A., and Smith, J. C.: Vesico-ureteric Reflux Following Operations on the Ureteric Orifice. Br. J. Urol. 37:531–535, 1965.

Ross, J. C., and Damanski, M.: Pudendal Neurectomy in the Treatment of the Bladder in Spinal Injury. Br. J. Urol. 25:45–50, 1953.

Ross, J. C., Damanski, M., and Gibbon, N.: Resection of the External Ureteral Sphincter in the Paraplegic—Preliminary Report. J. Urol. 79:742–746 (Apr.) 1958.

Salvatierra, O., Kountz, S. L., and Balzer, F. O.: Primary Vesicoureteral Reflux and End-stage Renal Disease. J.A.M.A. 226:1454–1456 (17 Dec.) 1973.

Sampson, J. A.: Ascending Renal Infection: With Special Reference to the Reflux of Urine From the Bladder Into the Ureters as an Etiological Factor in Its Causation and Maintenance. Bull. Johns Hopkins Hosp. 14:334–350 (Dec.) 1903.

Schlegel, J. U., and Bakule, P. T.: A Diagnostic Approach in Detecting Renal and Urinary Tract Disease. J. Urol. 104:2–10 (July) 1970.

Scott, J. E. S.: A Critical Appraisal of the Management of Ureteric Reflux. In Johnston, J. H., and Scholtmeijer, R. J.: Problems in Paediatric Urology. Amsterdam, Excerpta Medica, 1972, pp. 271–298.

Scott, J. E. S., and De Luca, F. G.: Further Studies on the Ureterovesical Junction of the Dog. Br. J. Urol. 32:320–323, 1960.

Scott, J. E. S., and Stansfeld, J. M.: Treatment of Vesico-ureteric Reflux in Children. Arch. Dis. Child. 43:323–328 (June) 1968a.

Scott, J. E. S., and Stansfeld, J. M.: Ureteric Reflux and Kidney Scarring in Children. Arch. Dis. Child. 43:468–470 (Aug.) 1968b.

Segura, J. W., Kelalis, P. P., Stickler, G. B., and Burke, E. C.: Urinary Tract Infection in Children: A Retrospective Study. J. Urol. 105:591–594 (Apr.) 1971.

Servadio, C., and Shachner, A.: Observations on Vesicoureteral Reflux and Chronic Pyelonephritis in Adults. J. Úrol. *103*:722–726 (June) 1970.

Shelden, C. H., and Bors, E.: Subarachnoid Alcohol Block in Paraplegia: Its Beneficial Effect on Mass Reflexes and Bladder Dysfunction. J. Neurosurg. *5*:385–391 (July) 1948.

Shopfner, C. E.: Nonobstructive Hydronephrosis and Hydroureter. Am. J. Roentgenol. *98*:172–180 (Sept.) 1966b.

Shopfner, C. E.: Roentgen Evaluation of Distal Urethral Obstruction. Radiology *88*:222–231 (Feb.) 1967a.

Shopfner, C. E.: Analysis of Hydronephrosis. Postgrad. Seminar, unit 6 pp. 1–6 (Mar.) 1967b.

Shopfner, C. E.: Roentgenological Evaluation of Bladder Neck Obstruction. Am. J. Roentgenol. *100*:162–176 (May) 1967c.

Shopfner, C. E., and Hutch, J. A.: The Trigonal Canal. Radiology *88*:209–221 (Feb.) 1967.

Siegelman, S. S., and Bosniak, M. A.: Renal Arteriography in Hydronephrosis. Radiology *85*:609–616 (Oct.) 1965.

Silber, I., and McAlister, W. H.: Longitudinal Folds as an Indirect Sign of Vesicoureteral Reflux. J. Urol. *103*:89–91 (Jan.) 1970.

Smellie, J., Edwards, D., Hunter, N., Normand, I. C. S., and Prescod, N.: Vesico-ureteric Reflux and Renal Scarring. Kidney Internat. *8*:S-65-S-72, 1975.

Smith, D. R.: Critique on the Concept of Vesical Neck Obstruction in Children. J.A.M.A. *207*:1686–1692 (3 Mar.) 1969.

Stark, G.: The Pathophysiology of the Bladder in Myelomeningocele and Its Correlation With the Neurological Picture, Dev. Med. Child. Neurol. [Suppl.] *16*:76–86, 1968.

Stephens, F. D.: Preliminary Follow-up study of 101 Children With Reflux Treated Conservatively. *In* Kincaid-Smith, P., and Fairley, K. F.: Renal Infection and Renal Scarring. Melbourne, Mercedes Publishing Services, 1970, pp. 283–285.

Stephens, F. D., and Lenaghan, D.: The Anatomical Basis and Dynamics of Vesicoureteral Reflux. J. Urol. *87*:669–680 (May) 1962.

Stephens, F. D., Joske, R. A., and Simmons, R. T.: Megaureter With Vesico-ureteric Reflux in Twins. Aust. NZ J. Surg. *24*:192–194 (Feb.) 1955.

Stevens, W. E.: Congenital Obstructions of the Female Urethra. J.A.M.A. *106*:89–92 (11 Jan.) 1936.

Stewart, C. M.: Delayed Cystography and Voiding Cystourethrography. J. Urol. *74*:749–759 (Dec.) 1955.

Stickler, G. B., Kelalis, P. P., Burke, E. C., and Segar, W. E.: Primary Interstitial Nephritis With Reflux: A Cause of Hypertension. Am. J. Dis. Child. *122*:144–148 (Aug.) 1971.

Tanagho, E. A., and Pugh, R. C. B.: The Anatomy and Function of the Ureterovesical Junction. Br. J. Urol. *35*:151–165, 1963.

Tanagho, E. A., Guthrie, T. H., and Lyon, R. P.: The Intravesical Ureter in Primary Reflux. J. Urol. *101*:824–832 (June) 1969.

Tanagho, E. A., Hutch, J. A., Meyers, F. H., and Rambo, O. N., Jr.: Primary Vesicoureteral Reflux: Experimental Studies of Its Etiology. J. Urol. *93*:165–176 (Feb.) 1965.

Tanagho, E. A., Meyers, F. H., and Smith, D. R.: The Trigone: Anatomical and Physiological Considerations. 1. In Relation to the Ureterovesical Junction. J. Urol. *100*:623–632 (Nov.) 1968.

Thornbury, J. R., and Immergut, M. A.: Polyview Voiding Cystourethrography in Children. Am. J. Roentgenol. *95*:475–478 (Oct.) 1965.

Tobenkin, M. I.: Hereditary Vesicoureteral Reflux. South Med. J. *57*:139–147 (Feb.) 1964.

Uehling, D. T.: Effect of Vesicoureteral Reflux on Concentrating Ability. J. Urol. *106*:947–950 (Dec.) 1971.

Vermooten, V.: Congenital Cystic Dilatation of the Renal Collecting Tubules. Yale J. Biol. Med. *23*:450–453 (June) 1951.

Vermooten, V., and Schweinsberg, M.: Radiographic Estimation of the Size of the Prostate. Radiology *182*:1010–1015 (June) 1964.

Vlahakis, E., Hartman, G. W., and Kelalis, P. P.: Comparison of Voiding Cystourethrography and Expression Cystourethrography. J. Urol. *106*:414–415 (Sept.) 1971.

Walker, D., Richard, G., Dobson, D., and Finlayson, B.: Maximum Urine Concentration: Early Means of Identifying Patients With Reflux Who May Require Surgery. Urology *1*:343–346 (Apr.) 1973.

Warren, J. W., Jr.: Congenital Diverticulum of the Urethra. Am. Surg. *21*:385–387, 1955.

Warren, M. M., Kelalis, P. P., and Stickler, G. B.: Unilateral Ureteroneocystostomy: The Fate of the Contralateral Ureter. J. Urol. *107*:466–468 (Mar.) 1972.

Waterhouse, K.: Voiding Cystourethrography: A Simple Technique. J. Urol. *85*:103–104 (Jan.) 1961.

Watkins, K. H.: Cysts of the Kidney Due to Hydrocalycosis. Br. J. Urol. *11*:207–215, 1939.

Weiss, R. M., and Lytton, B.: Vesicoureteral Reflux and Distal Ureteral Obstruction. J. Urol. *111*:245–249 (Feb.) 1974.

Weiss, R. M., Schiff, M., Jr., and Lytton, B.: Late Obstruction After Ureteroneocystostomy. J. Urol. *106*:144–148 (July) 1971.

Whitaker, R. H.: The Ureter in Posterior Urethral Valves. Br. J. Urol. *45*:395–403, 1973.

Widén, T.: Renal Angiography During and After Unilateral Ureteric Occlusion: A Long-Term Experimental Study in Dogs. Acta. Radiol. (Suppl.) *162*:1–103, 1958.

Williams, D. I.: Urology in Childhood. *In* Encyclopedia of Urology. XV. Berlin, Springer-Verlag, 1958, pp. 127–137.

Williams, D. I., and Abbassian, A.: Solitary Pedunculated Polyp of the Posterior Urethra in Children. J. Urol. *96*:483–486 (Oct.) 1966.

Williams, D. I., and Burkholder, G. V.: The Prune Belly Syndrome. J. Urol. *98*:244–251 (Aug.) 1967.

Williams, D. I., and Mininberg, D. T.: Hydrocalycosis: Report of Three Cases in Children. Br. J. Urol. *40*:541–545 (Oct.) 1968.

Williams, D. I., and Nixon, H. H.: Agenesis of the Sacrum. Surg. Gynec. Obstet. *105*:84–88 (July) 1957.

Williams, D. I., and Sturdy, D. E.: Recurrent Urinary Infection in Girls. Arch. Dis. Child. *36*:130–136 (Apr.) 1961.

Williams, D. I., Scott, J., and Turner-Warwick, R. T.: Reflux and Recurrent Infection. Br. J. Urol. *33*:435–441 (Dec.) 1961.

Williams, D. I., Whitaker, R. H., Barratt, T. M., and

Keeton, J. E.: Urethral Valves. Br. J. Urol. *45*:200–210, 1973.

Willscher, M. K., Bauer, S. B., Zammuto, P. J., and Retik, A. B.: Renal Growth and Urinary Infection Following Antireflux Surgery in Infants and Children. J. Urol. *115*:722–725 (June) 1976.

Winberg, J., Larson, H. and Bergström, T.: Comparison of the Natural History of Urinary Infection in Children With and Without Vesicoureteric Reflux. *In* Kincaid–Smith, P., and Fairley, K. F.: Renal Infection and Renal Scarring. Melbourne, Mercedes Publishing Services, 1970, pp. 293–302.

Witherington, R.: Experimental Study on Role of Intravesical Ureter in Vesicoureteral Regurgitation. J. Urol. *89*:176–179 (Feb.) 1963.

Woodard, J. R., and Keats, G.: Ureteral Reimplantation: Paquin's Procedure After 12 Years. J. Urol. *109*:891–894 (May) 1973.

Woodburne, R. T.: Anatomy of the Ureterovesical Junction. J. Urol. *92*:431–435 (Nov.) 1964.

Young, H. H., Frontz, W. A., and Baldwin, J. C.: Congenital Obstruction of the Posterior Urethra. J.Urol. *3*:289–354, 1919.

Zel, G., and Retik, A. B.: Familial Vesicoureteral Reflux. Urology *2*:249–251 (Sept.) 1973.

Zinner, N. R., and Paquin, A. J., Jr.: Experimental Vesicoureteral Reflux. IV. Role of Neuromuscular Activity. J. Urol. *104*:262–266 (Aug.) 1970.

ADDITIONAL BIBLIOGRAPHY

Alvarez Colodrena, J. W., and di Lella, P.: Estrechez blenorrágica rebelde de la uretra en la infancia: consideraciones a propósito de tres casos. Rev. Especialid. *4*:429–431 (June) 1929.

Bapna B. C., Singh, S. M., Chally, R., Thomas, K., and Chargavo, S.: Bladder Neck Obstruction in Children. Indian J. Pediatr. *37*:11–14 (Jan.) 1970.

Berman, L. B., Crotty, J. J., and Tina, L. U.: The Pediatric Implications of Bladder Neck Obstructions. Pediatrics *28*:816–821 (Nov.) 1961.

Bodian, M.: Some Observations on the Pathology of Congenital "Idiopathic Bladder-neck Obstruction" (Marion's Disease). Br. J. Urol. *29*:393–398, 1957.

Boissonnat, P., and Bouteau, P.: Valvule de l'urèthre antérieur, canal accessoire diverticulaire et maladie du col vésical, chez un garçon de dix ans. J. Urol. Nephrol. (Paris) *60*:949–954 (Dec.) 1954.

Brandesky, G.: Conservatively Treated Urethral Valves. J. Pediatr. Surg. *8*:945–947 (Dec.) 1973.

Cass, A. S., and Stephens, F. D.: Posterior Urethral Valves: Diagnosis and Management. J. Urol. *112*:519–525 (Oct.) 1974.

Cendron, J., DeBurge, J. P., and Karlaftis, C.: Valvules de l'urèthre postérieur. J. Urol. Nephrol. (Paris) *75*:15–38, 1969.

Cibert, J., Gilloz, A., Salaheddine, N., and Sato, T.: Polype de l'urèthre postérieur chez le garçon. J. Urol. Nephrol. (Paris) *72*:83–86, 1966.

Cox, C. E.: The Urethra and Its Relationship to Urinary Tract Infection: The Flora of the Normal Female Urethra. South. Med. J. *59*:621–626 (May) 1966.

Cox, C. E., Lacy, S. S., and Hinman, F. Jr.: The Urethra and Its Relationship to Urinary Tract Infection. II. The Urethral Flora of the Female With

Recurrent Urinary Infection. J. Urol. *99*:632–638 (May) 1968.

Devine, P. C., Sakati, I. A., Poutasse, E. F., and Devine, C. J., Jr.: One Stage Urethroplasty: Repair of Urethral Strictures With a Free Full Thickness Patch of Skin. J. Urol. *99*:191–193 (Feb.) 1968.

DeWolf, W. C., and Fraley, E. E.: Congenital Urethral Polyp in the Infant: Case Report and Review of the Literature. J. Urol. *109*:515–516 (Mar.) 1973.

Downs, R. A.: Congenital Polyps of the Prostatic Urethra: A Review of the Literature and Report of Two Cases. Br. J. Urol. *42*:76–85, 1970.

Draper, J. W., Braasch, W. F.: The Function of the Ureterovesical Valve: An Experimental Study of the Feasibility of the Ureteral Meatotomy in Human Beings. J.A.M.A. *60*:20–24 (4 Jan.) 1913.

Duckett, J. W., Jr.: Current Management of Posterior Urethral Valves. Urol. Clin. North Am. *1*:471–483 (Oct.) 1974.

Emmett, J. L., and Helmholz, H. F.: Transurethral Resection of the Vesical Neck in Infants and Children. J. Urol. *60*:463–478 (Sept.) 1948.

Everett, H. S., and Brack, C. B.: Unusual Lesions of the Female Urethra. Obstet. Gynecol. *1*:571–578 (May) 1953.

Field, P. L., and Stephens, F. D.: Congenital Urethral Membranes Causing Urethral Obstruction. J. Urol. *111*:250–255 (Feb.) 1974.

Filly, R., Friedland, G., Govan, D. E., and Fair, W. R.: Development and Progression of Clubbing and Scarring in Children With Recurrent Urinary Tract Infections. Radiology *113*:145–153 (Oct.) 1974.

Firlit, C. F., and King, L. R.: Anterior Urethral Valves in Children. J. Urol. *108*:972–975 (Dec.) 1972.

Forsythe, W. I., and McFadden, G. D. F.: Congenital Posterior Urethral Valves: A Study of Thirty-five Cases. Br. J. Urol. *31*:63–70, 1959.

Friedland, G. W., Axman, M. M., and Love, T.: Neonatal "Urinothorax" Associated With Posterior Urethral Valves. Br. J. Radiol. *44*:471–474 (June) 1971.

Gleason, D. M., Bottaccini, M. R., and Lattimer, J. K.: What Does the Bougie à Boule Calibrate? J. Urol. *101*:114–116 (Jan.) 1969.

Gute, D. B., Chute, R., and Baron, J. A., Jr.: Bladder Neck Revision for Obstruction in Men: A Clinical Study Reporting Normal Ejaculation Postoperatively. J. Urol. *99*:744–749 (June) 1968.

Harrow, B. R.: The Rarity of Bladder-neck Obstruction in Children. J. Pediatr. *69*:853–854 (Nov.) 1966.

Hendren, W. H.: A New Approach to Infants With Severe Obstructive Uropathy: Early Complete Reconstruction. J. Pediatr. Surg. *5*:184–199 (Apr.) 1970.

Hodson, C. J.: The Mechanism of Scar Formation in Chronic Pyelonephritis. *In* Kincaid-Smith, P., and Fairley, W. F.: Renal Infection and Renal Scarring, Melbourne, Mercedes Publishing Services, 1970, pp. 327–329.

Kaplan, G. W., and King, L. R.: An Evaluation of Y-V Vesicourethroplasty in Children. Surg. Gynecol. Obstet. *130*:1059–1066, 1970.

Kaplan, G. W., and King, L. R.: Cystitis Cystica in Childhood. J. Urol. *103*:657–659 (June) 1970.

Kaplan, G. W., Sammons, T. A., and King, L. R.: A

Blind Comparison of Dilatation, Urethrotomy, and Medication Alone in the Treatment of Urinary Tract Infection in Girls. J. Urol. *109*:917–919 (May) 1973.

Keer, W. S., Jr.: Results of Internal Urethrotomy in Female Patients for Urethral Stenosis. J. Urol. *102*:449–450 (Oct.) 1969.

Keitzer, W. A., and Benavent, C.: Bladder Neck Obstruction in Children. J. Urol. 89:384–388 (Mar.) 1963.

Kelalis, P. P.: Hydronephrosis in Infants and Children. Am. Fam. Physician 7:90–99 (May) 1973.

Kelalis, P. P., Burke, E. C., and Stickler, G. B.: The Riddle of Vesicoureteral Reflux. Clin. Pediatr. *11*:495–496 (Sept.) 1972.

King, L. R., and Idriss, F. S.: The Effect of Vesicoureteral Reflux on Renal Function in Dogs. Invest. Urol. *4*:419–427 (Mar.) 1967.

Knutrud, O., and Hendren, W. H.: Diversion Vs. Immediate Reconstruction for Megaureter. Presented at the 42nd Annual Meeting of the American Academy of Pediatrics, Section on Surgery, Chicago, October 20, 1973.

Krøigaard, N.: The Lower Urinary Tract in Infancy and Childhood: Micturition Cinematography With Simultaneous Pressure-flow Measurement. Acta Radiol. [Suppl.] *300*:1–174, 1970.

Kuppusami, K., and Moors, D. E.: Fibrous Polyp of the Verumontanum. Can. J. Surg. *11*:388–390, (July) 1968.

Lattimer, J. K., and Hubbard, M.: Relative Incidence of Pediatric Urological Conditions. J. Urol. *71*:759–764 (June) 1954.

Lead Article. V.U.R. + I. R. R. = C. P. N.? Lancet 2:1120–1121, 1974.

Leadbetter, G. W., Jr.: A Simplified Urethroplasty for Strictures of the Bulbous Urethra. J. Urol. 83:54–59 (Jan.) 1960.

Lewy, P. R., and Belman, A. B.: Familial Occurrence of Nonobstructive Noninfectious Vesicoureteral Reflux With Renal Scarring. J. Pediatr. 86:851–856 (June) 1975.

Lich, R., Jr., Howerton, L. W., Davis, L. A.: Vesicourethrography. J. Urol. 85:396–397 (Mar.) 1961.

Lich, R., Jr., Howerton, L. W., and Davis, L. A.: Recurrent Urosepsis in Children. J. Urol. 86:554–558 (Nov.) 1961.

Lyon, R. P., and Marshall, S.: Urinary Tract Infections and Difficult Urination in Girls: Long-term Followup. J. Urol. *105*:314–317 (Feb.) 1971.

Mahony, D. T.: Studies of Enuresis. I. Incidence of Obstructive Lesions and Pathophysiology of Enuresis. J. Urol. *106*:951–958 (Dec.) 1971.

Malek, R. S., Kelalis, P. P., Stickler, G. B., and Burke, E. C.: Observations on Ureteral Ectopy in Children. J. Urol. *107*:308–313 (Feb.) 1972.

Marion, G.: Surgery of the Neck of the Bladder. Br. J. Urol. 5:351–356, 1933.

McGovern, J. H., and Marshall, V. F.: Reflux and Pyelonephritis in 35 Adults. J. Urol. *101*:668–672 (May) 1969.

Mogg, R. A.: Congenital Anomalies of the Urethra. Br. J. Urol. *40*:638–648, 1968.

Nesbit, R. M., and Labardini, M. M.: Urethral Valves in the Male Child. J. Urol. 96:218–228 (Aug.) 1966.

Nunn, I. N.: Bladder Neck Obstruction in Children. J. Urol. 93:693–699 (June) 1965.

O'Donnell, B., Vella, L., and Maloney, M.: The Measurement of Lower Urinary Tract Obstruction in Infants and Children. J. Pediatr. Surg. 2:518–522 (Dec.) 1967.

Presman, D., Ross, L. S., and Nicosia, S. V.: Fibromuscular Hyperplasia of the Posterior Urethra: A Cause for Lower Urinary Tract Obstruction in Male Children. J. Urol. *107*:149–153 (Jan.) 1972.

Randall, A.: Congenital Valves of the Posterior Urethra. Ann. Surg. *73*:477–480 (Apr.) 1921.

Reisman, D. D.: Bladder Neck Obstructions in Children. J.A.M.A. *188*:1057–1061 (22 June) 1964.

Retief, P. J. M.: Urethral Valve Obstruction. S. Afr. Med. J. *44*:181–189 (14 Feb.) 1970.

Rickham, P. P.: Advanced Lower Urinary Obstruction in Childhood. Arch. Dis. Child. *37*:122–131 (Apr.) 1962.

Robertson, W. B., and Hayes, J. A.: Congenital Diaphragmatic Obstruction of the Male Posterior Urethra. Br. J. Urol. *41*:592–598, 1969.

Rudhe, U., and Ericsson, N. O.: Roentgen Evaluation of Primary Bladder Neck Obstruction in Children. Acta Radiol. [Diagn.] (Stockh.) 3:237–248 (May) 1965.

Scott, F. B., and Caffarena, E.: Diagnosis of Anterior Urethral Valves. J. Urol. *110*:261–263 (Aug.) 1973.

Scott, W. F., Collins, T. A., and Singer, P. L.: Papilloma of Urethra in Infant. J. Med. Assoc. State Ala. 7:370–371 (Apr.) 1938.

Smellie, J. M., Hodson, C. J., Edwards, D., and Normand, I. C. S.: Clinical and Radiological Features of Urinary Infection in Childhood. Br. Med. J. 2:1222–1226 (Nov. 14) 1964.

Smith, D. R.: Critique on the Concept of Vesical Neck Obstruction in Children. J.A.M.A. *207*:1686–1692 (3 Mar.) 1969.

Stadaas, J. O.: Pedunculated Polyp of Posterior Urethra in Children Causing Reflux and Hydronephrosis. J. Pediatr. Surg. 8:517–521 (Aug.) 1973.

Stephens, F. D.: Urethral Obstruction in Childhood: The Use of Urethrography in Diagnosis. Aust. NZ J. Surg. 25:89–109 (Nov.) 1955.

Stephens, F. D.: Congenital Malformations of the Rectum, Anus and Genito-urinary Tracts. Edinburgh, E. and S. Livingstone, 1963, 370 pp.

Stewart, C. M.: Congenital Bladder Neck Obstruction: Diagnosis by Delayed and Voiding Cystography and Surgical Removal by Use of a New Cold, Crush-Cutting Punch. J. Urol. 83:679–681 (May) 1960.

Stueber, P. J., and Persky, L.: Solid Tumors of the Urethra and Bladder Neck. J. Urol. *102*:205–209 (Aug.) 1969.

Walker, D, and Richard, G. A.: A Critical Evaluation of Urethral Obstruction in Female Children. Pediatrics *51*:272–277 (3 Mar.) 1973.

Waterhouse, K., and Hamm, F. C.: The Importance of Urethral Valves as a Cause of Vesical Neck Obstruction in Children. J. Urol. 87:404–408 (Mar.) 1962.

Waterhouse, K., and Scordamaglia, L. J.: Anterior Urethral Valve: A Rare Cause of Bilateral Hydronephrosis. J. Urol. 87:556–559 (Apr.) 1962.

Whitaker, J., and Johnston, G. S.: Estimation of Urinary Outflow Resistance in Children: Simultaneous Measurement of Bladder Pressure, Flow Rate, and Exit Pressure. Invest. Urol. 3:379–389 (Jan.) 1966.

Whitaker, J., and Johnston, G. S.: Correlation of Urethral Resistance and Shape in Girls. Radiology *91*:757–761 (Oct.) 1968.

Williams, D. I., and Eckstein, H. B.: Obstructive Valves in the Posterior Urethra. J. Urol. *93*:236–246 (Feb.) 1965.

Williams, D. I., and Retik, A. B.: Congenital Valves and Diverticula of the Anterior Urethra. Br. J. Urol. *41*:228–234, 1969.

Young, B. W.: Lower Urinary Tract Obstruction in Childhood. Philadelphia, Lea and Febiger, 1972, 203 pp.

Chapter 12

CALCULOUS DISEASE OF THE GENITOURINARY TRACT

by Reza S. Malek

GENERAL CONSIDERATIONS

Rate of Incidence

Urinary calculi have plagued man since history began. One of the most outstanding features of urolithiasis is its widely varying geographic incidence. In the United States urolithiasis is very common: at the Mayo Clinic, 1,500 cases of renal stone are seen annually (i.e., in approximately 1 of every 150 patients) (Wilson and associates), and it is estimated that annual patient cost for urolithiasis in the United States is at least $47.3 million (Finlayson). In general, with an annual stone incidence of 1 or more cases per 1,000 of population, the United States ranks higher than other major human urinary "stone quarries" in the world such as the British Isles, Scandinavia, and Mediterranean countries, where annual frequencies average about 0.2 to 0.5 per 1,000 of population. In some villages in Thailand, however, the annual frequency is as high as 8 per 1,000 (Finlayson).

In the United States the highest incidence of calculous disease has been reported from the southeastern states, with the second highest rate of incidence occurring in New England (Boyce, Garvey, and Strawcutter). A survey of these so-called stone areas yields no common denominator on which to base the etiology of stone formation.

The frequent occurrence of stones of the upper urinary tract, which is reportedly becoming more prevalent, strongly correlates with the more sedentary life in technologically developed countries (Andersen; Lonsdale; Mates; Sutor). Several groups of people are apparently protected to various degrees from stone disease. They include Central and South American Indians, Bantu Africans, and the blacks in the United States (Boyce, Garvey, and Strawcutter; Butt; Modlin). Men are affected four times as frequently by uninfected stone disease as are women; however, if all forms of stone disease are considered, its frequency is almost the same in both sexes (Clark and Nordin; Sutor).

Upper tract stones occur primarily in middle age; the peak incidence is in people 20 to 40 years old (Blacklock; Fetter and associates; Inada and associates). Estimates of the recurrence rate of upper urinary tract calculi range from 9 to 73 per cent, with a recurrence interval of approximately 9 years. Tragically, about one third of patients having one or more episodes of upper tract calculi will eventually lose a kidney (Finlayson).

Composition, Architecture, and Formation of Urinary Calculi

Calcium oxalate, calcium phosphate, diammonium calcium phosphate, magnesium ammonium phosphate (struvite), magnesium phosphate, uric acid, cystine, various urates (sodium, ammonium, calcium, magnesium, alone or in combination), and rarely, xanthine, indigo, sulfonamide (Fig. 12–1), steatin, phenazopyridine, and other crystals, have all been identified as components of human urinary calculi (Finlayson). For all practical purposes, approximately 95 per cent of all upper urinary tract calculi are composed of calcium oxalate, calcium phosphate, and magnesium ammonium phosphate (struvite). Uric acid and urates account for about 4 per cent and cystine for about 1 per cent.

Urinary calculogenesis is not a singular, simple, or direct process but the result of multiple, complex, and interrelated processes. All human urinary concretions, despite their varied appearance and irrespective of their origin in the urinary tract, manifest a remarkably characteristic internal architecture. The basic morphologic features may be described in terms of various combinations of spherules, concentric laminations, and radial striations with or without frond formation. No natural concretion is ever formed as a sedimentary mass of crystals; both crystals and matrix are invariably fundamental components of each stone and, morphologically, are intimately associated (Boyce, 1968; Malek and Boyce, 1977).

Matrix is a mucoprotein that exists in fibrous (laminar) and quasi-amorphous (interlaminar, gel-like) forms. With respect to its composition, 85 per cent of its mass is formed by matrix substance A, which, as

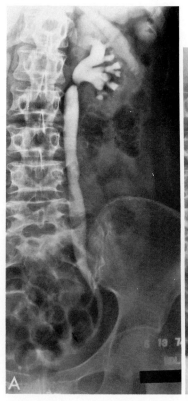
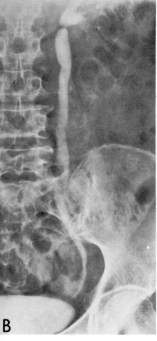

Figure 12–1. Sulfonamide stone in patient receiving sulfapyridine for dermatitis herpetiformis. **A**, *Excretory urogram.* Nonopaque calculus near left ureterovesical juncture *(arrow).* Note left ureteropyelectasis. **B**, *Excretory urogram.* Note normal left lower ureter after partial dissolution and spontaneous passage of calculus as a result of hydration, urinary alkalinization, and discontinuation of sulfapyridine.

immunologic techniques have demonstrated, is of renal origin. The same substance is present in large quantities in the urine of active stone-formers and in smaller concentrations in the urine of occasional stone-formers; it is absent from normal urine (Malek and Boyce, 1973). Currently, it is thought that uromucoid (also of renal origin), which is present in all human urine, is converted to mineralizable matrix substance by sialidase (N-acetyl neuraminidase) in the renal tubular epithelium (Malek and Boyce, 1973). Rarely, radiolucent calculi that consist almost completely of matrix are found in infected, poorly functioning kidneys (see Figures 12–9 and 12–73).

Crystals of both organic and inorganic composition, on a weight-to-weight basis, form the major portion of urinary calculi. The fibrous matrix of even the purest calculi of any crystalline composition is covered by crystals that are presumed to be calcium phosphate in the form of apatite. Calcium oxalate (monohydrate and dihydrate) appears in greatest concentrations on the apatite-covered fibrils but fills the interlaminar gel-like matrix to varying extents, depending on the extent of mineralization of the particular stone. Uric acid, cystine, and struvite crystals, in contrast, have a predilection for the interlaminar gel-like areas (Boyce, 1968; Malek and Boyce, 1977).

Intranephronic calculosis is miniaturized calculogenesis within the tubular epithelium and is consistently demonstrable in the kidneys of all formers of calcium oxalate stones. These microcalculi may indeed migrate to subepithelial or intralymphatic positions to represent Randall's plaques or Carr's bodies, respectively. Their calculogenic potential is emphasized by the direct relationship between their abundance and the activity of the stone disease (Malek and Boyce, 1973).

Several factors, including urinary pH, solute load, and the activity of urinary inhibitors, influence crystal formation. The urinary pH directly affects the cystine, uric acid, and struvite crystal systems. The relative solute load per unit volume of urine is important in any crystal system—though perhaps not as important as was formerly thought—but in all types of stone disease there are patients with the disorder who, despite increased solute loads, fail to form stones. Known inhibitors include magnesium, citrate, pyrophosphate, and other polyphosphates, all of which account for 30 to 40 per cent of the total inhibition of calcium crystal systems; their amounts do not vary between stone-formers and normal persons. The remaining 60 to 70 per cent of inhibition is attributable to unidentified inhibitors whose action or actions are similar to those of polyphosphates (Smith, 1972b).

Secondary factors, including obstruction with stasis and infection with urea-splitting bacteria, appear to be important, primarily in the patient with an underlying metabolic disorder associated with stone formation (Smith, 1974). An understanding of these factors in calculogenesis is essential because their imbalance permits stone formation, and all therapy is aimed at correcting these imbalances.

CLASSIFICATION

There are two main types of urolithiasis. **Primary calculi** (in the Western Hemisphere) are predominantly of renal origin. They form as a result of various well-recognized or hitherto unknown urinary abnormalities. Their spontaneous migration down the urinary conduits may give rise to ureteral, vesical, or urethral calculi. Primary bladder stones, once common in Europe, are now endemic in the developing countries.

Secondary calculi almost invariably develop from the encrustation of crystal-matrix complexes on foreign bodies in the urinary passages or in *association* with obstructed or chronically infected urinary tracts, or both. Urologic lesions (usually obstructive), urosepsis, or both are commonly found in stone-formers (35 per cent in adults and 65 per cent in children) (Boyce,

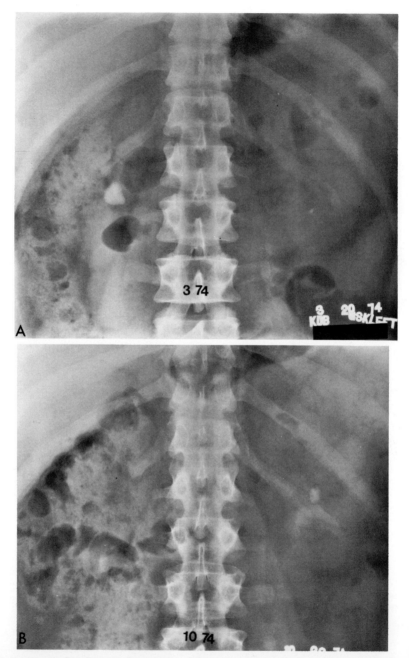

Figure 12–2. Surgical and metabolic activity of stone disease in 41-year-old man with idiopathic hypercalciuria. **A,** *Plain film.* Large symptomatic calcium oxalate stone at right ureteropelvic juncture (surgical activity) and small stone in lower pole of left kidney. **B,** *Plain film.* Left renal stone has enlarged (metabolic activity). Note absence of new or residual calculous material on right side after right pelviolithotomy.

Legend continued on opposite page

1967; Malek and Kelalis, 1975b). However, in only a few (5 per cent) cases can true primary obstruction or urinary tract anomalies be demonstrated. The obstructive process in the remaining patients is·usually related to previous passage of calculi or surgical procedures for their removal

(Boyce, 1967). Furthermore, the incidence of stone disease among patients with infected, obstructed, or anomalous urinary tracts is extremely low (0 to 5 per cent) (Boyce, 1967; Malek and Kelalis, 1975b). These observations tend to establish urinary infection and obstruction not as *initiat-*

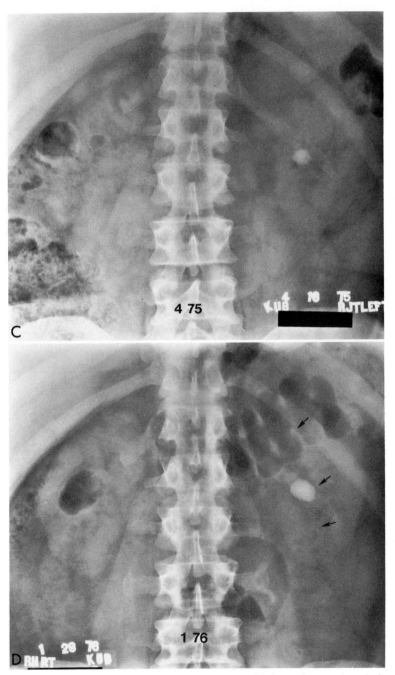

Figure 12–2 *Continued.* **C**, *Plain film.* Further enlargement of left renal stone (metabolic activity) despite thiazide therapy. **D**, *Plain film.* Further enlargement of left renal calculus *(middle arrow)* and appearance of two additional stones *(upper and lower arrows)* in left kidney (metabolic activity).

Illustration continued on following page

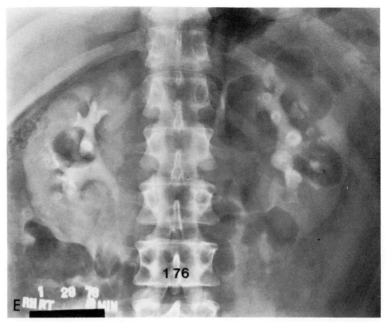

Figure 12–2 *Continued.* E, *Excretory urogram.* Symptomatic left ureteropelvic obstruction by stone (surgical activity). Note normal appearance of right kidney after pelviolithotomy.

ing factors (contrary to common belief) but rather as *promoting* factors for calculogenesis, which indeed follows a pathologic deviation of normal biologic mineralization in the renal tubular cells or in the abnormal pelviocalyceal urine (Malek and Boyce, 1973).

As urolithiasis—whatever the cause—may be sporadic, the determination of the activity or rate of stone formation in each patient becomes an invaluable guide to therapy. An arbitrary classification of the activity of stone disease, as used at the Mayo Clinic, is as follows:

1. Metabolically active—one or more of the following has occurred: (a) New stone formation in the past year. (b) Growth of existing stones in the past year. (c) Documented passage of gravel in the past year.

2. Metabolically inactive: none of the above has occurred; in other words, there has been no change in stone formation within the past year.

3. Indeterminate activity: available data are inadequate for classification.

4. Surgical activity: a stone-bearing kidney becomes obstructed, infected, painful, or hematuric, so that surgical intervention is necessary.

Surgical activity in no way implies metabolic activity; the symptomatic calculus may have been formed several years previously and may have remained unchanged during this period. Obviously, surgical and metabolic activities may occur together; however, surgical activity does not in itself mean that the patient is actively forming stones (Fig. 12–2).

Urolithiasis may be regarded as a solitary complication or as one of several manifestations of a large number of underlying disorders. A practical classification of such diseases is provided in Table 12–1.

RENAL CALCULI

Clinical Features of Renal Calculi

Accurate evaluation of the patient's past history, his family history, and his past and present geographic residence is of the utmost importance. Special attention must be paid to growth and development, dietary habits, vitamin intake, periods of pro-

Table 12–1. **Classification of Urolithiasis**

RENAL TUBULAR SYNDROMES
Renal tubular acidosis
Distal defect, type I
Carbonic anhydrase inhibition
Cystinuria
Glycinuria

ENZYME DISORDERS
Primary hyperoxaluria
Type I, glycolic aciduria
Type II, L-glyceric aciduria
Xanthinuria

HYPERCALCEMIC STATES
Primary hyperparathyroidism
Sarcoidosis
Hypervitaminosis D
Milk-alkali syndrome
Neoplasms
Cushing's syndrome
Hyperthyroidism
Idiopathic infantile hypercalcemia
Immobilization

URIC ACID LITHIASIS
Idiopathic uric acid lithiasis
Gout
Increased purine metabolism
Low urine-output states
Idiopathic renal lithiasis
Hyperparathyroidism

UROLITHIASIS ASSOCIATED WITH INTESTINAL
DISEASE
Acquired hyperoxaluria
Uric acid lithiasis

IDIOPATHIC RENAL LITHIASIS

INFECTED UROLITHIASIS AND URINARY STASIS

NEPHROCALCINOSIS

ENDEMIC CALCULI (See Vesical Calculi.)

longed illness with immobilization or dehydration, endocrinopathies, and exposure to any forms of medical treatment and surgical procedures both on and outside the genitourinary tract.

Gross hematuria, urosepsis (with or without fever), abdominal or flank pain, and renal colic are the commonest presenting symptoms. These seem to occur with approximately equal frequency in either sex. Spontaneous passage of a calculus along the urethra frequently may be the first and only symptom; the stone may be discovered protruding from the urethral meatus. Enuresis, polydipsia, and sudden anuria due to calculous obstruction of both kidneys, of a solitary kidney, or of the urethra are less common. Single or multiple asymptomatic and unsuspected calculi are discovered in some patients through interpretation of abnormal findings on urinalysis, during evaluation of an anomalous urinary tract, or during unrelated radiologic examination of the chest or abdomen.

The physical examination may reveal characteristic signs of metabolic disorders such as the typical "elfin" facies of idiopathic infantile hypercalcemia (Williams and Eckstein), overt signs of hyperadrenocorticism or flaccid paralysis, and cardiac arrhythmias associated with hypokalemia of renal tubular acidosis. Obviously, varying degrees of azotemia may complicate any form of stone disease and may indeed dominate the clinical picture. A mass in the flank may lead to the diagnosis of hydronephrosis. Rarely, in thin patients or in children, stones may be palpated along the ureter, in the bladder, or in the urethra.

Although individuals with vesicoureteral reflux seldom have renal calculi, investigation and correction of reflux in a stone-forming patient with urosepsis are prerequisites for successful management of the stone disease (Fig. 12–3). Furthermore, urosepsis—especially with a urea-splitting organism—or obstruction (or both) precludes assessment of metabolic activity until the infection or obstruction has been eliminated or corrected.

Gross or microscopic hematuria, pyuria, and urosepsis should not be dismissed as simply being sequelae of stone disease. The possibilities of concurrent renal tuberculosis, glomerulonephritis, and, more commonly, lower urinary tract malignancy should be borne in mind. The status of the entire urinary tract must be determined, and initial excretory urograms may thus be followed by cystoscopic, cineradiographic, and retrograde studies as indications arise.

LABORATORY INVESTIGATIONS OF RENAL CALCULI

A number of screening studies should be carried out routinely (Table 12–2), and

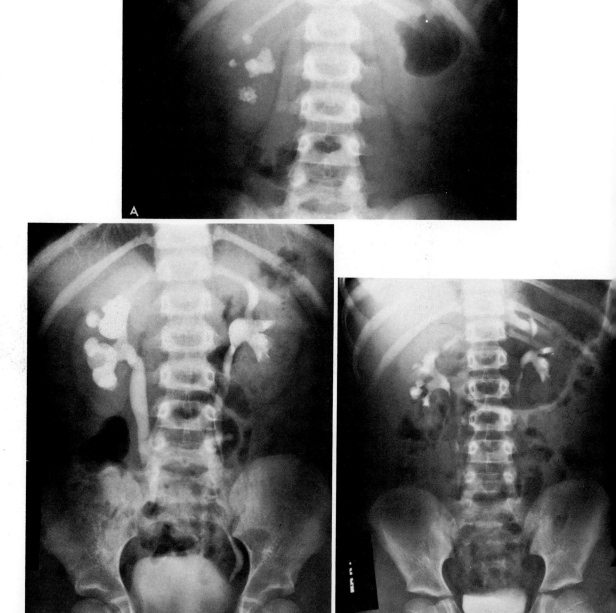

Figure 12–3. Importance of correcting reflux in stone-forming patient with urosepsis. Patient was a 5-year-old girl with primary hyperoxaluria, type I, who presented with enuresis. **A,** *Plain film.* Multiple densely opaque calcium oxalate calculi in right kidney. **B,** *Excretory urogram.* Bilateral ureteropyelocaliectasis, more advanced with scarring on right, from bilateral vesicoureteral reflux and recurrent urosepsis. **C,** *Excretory urogram.* Much-improved appearance of stone-free upper urinary tract four years after removal of right renal stones, bilateral ureteroneocystostomy, and control of metabolic stone disease and infection (From Malek, R. S., 1976.)

Table 12–2. Routine Diagnostic Tests in Urolithiasis

SERUM STUDIES
  Calcium (3 times)
  Phosphorus (3 times)
  Protein electrophoresis
  Uric acid
  Blood acid-base balance
  Potassium
  Creatinine

URINE STUDIES
  Urinalysis
  Fasting urine pH
  Urine culture and antibiotic sensitivities
  24-Hour collections
    Creatinine clearance
    Calcium
    Phosphorus
    Cystine
    Oxalate
    Uric acid

STONE ANALYSIS (when stones are available)

ROENTGENOGRAPHIC STUDIES
  Preliminary plain film (KUB) and tomography
  Excretory urography
  Retrograde ureteropyelography (when indicated)

none should be overlooked, since in rare instances two or more metabolic abnormalities coexist (see sections on primary hyperparathyroidism and uric acid lithiasis, and Figure 12–101). Other more specific diagnostic tests are referred to in the section on medical management.

The urinary sediment should be exam-ined for crystals; their nature may afford a clue as to the type of stone (Fig. 12–4). Cystine and uric acid crystals may be precipitated by adding a few drops of glacial acetic acid (which lowers the pH to about 4.0) to a test tube containing urine, which is then refrigerated. Other types of crystals may be recognized in the fresh urinary sediment.

Roentgen Studies of Renal Calculi

The urographic diagnostic problems associated with urinary calculi can be classified in four categories: (1) identification of calcific shadows that appear in the plain film; (2) localization of those calcific shadows that prove to be stones in the urinary tract; (3) the demonstration of nonopaque urinary calculi that are not apparent on the plain film; and (4) appraisal of pathologic and physiologic changes in the urinary tract produced by calculi.

Importance of Preliminary Plain Film (KUB)

In Chapter 1 and Chapter 7 the importance of making a preliminary plain film before urograms are made is discussed at length. As is stated in those chapters, no-

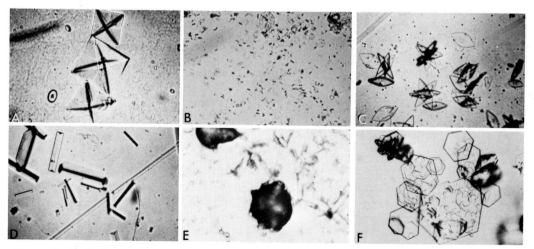

Figure 12–4. Light microscopic appearance of common urinary crystals. **A,** Calcium oxalate. **B,** Calcium carbonate. **C,** Uric acid. **D,** Triple phosphate (struvite). **E,** Ammonium urate (calcium phosphate in background). **F,** Cystine. (From Malek, R. S., 1976.)

where is a plain film more important than in the diagnosis of urinary calculi. The reason for this is apparent. Urographic medium may completely obscure calculi so that they would not be suspected if no preliminary plain film were available. Likewise, localized collections of urographic medium in a ureter bent back on itself or in a calyx projected in the anteroposterior plane might suggest a calculus when none was present. It is axiomatic that one should never attempt the interpretation of urograms if no preliminary plain film is available.

RADIOGRAPHIC CHARACTERISTICS OF URINARY CALCULI

Most urinary calculi are sufficiently opaque to roentgen rays to cast a shadow in the plain film. Stones vary greatly in radiopacity (density). All stones have some opacity to roentgen rays, but when the opacity

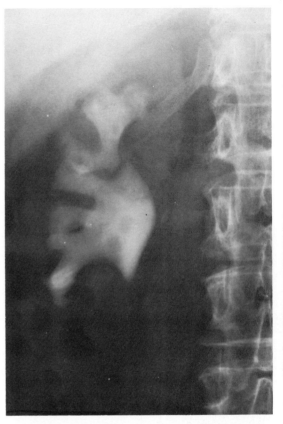

Figure 12–6. *Plain film.* Branched calculus composed of magnesium ammonium phosphate (struvite). Note relative radiolucency as compared with calcium phosphate stone (Fig. 12–5).

of the stones is no greater than that of the surrounding soft tissues, they will not cast shadows on the film.

The roentgenographic density of a stone varies according to the atomic weight of the salt of which it is composed (Arcelin). The greater the atomic weight, the greater the opacity of the stone. Stones that are regarded as opaque to roentgen rays are (in decreasing order of opacity) calcium oxalate, calcium carbonate, and the phosphates (Lagergren and Öhrling; Winsbury-White). Cystine stones vary considerably in opacity. Stones that are considered to be of poor opacity (or nonopaque) are composed of uric acid and the urates (ammonium, sodium, magnesium, and potassium), xanthine (Prien and Frondel), and "matrix" concretions. "Pure" stones, those containing only one chemical substance, are rare. Most stones are mixtures of the various

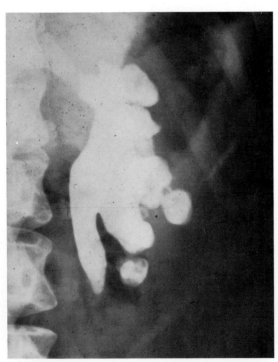

Figure 12–5. *Plain film.* Branched calculus composed of calcium phosphate. Note uniform dense radiopacity. (From Boyce, W. H., 1965)

chemical substances, so all degrees of opacity are encountered.

The roentgen appearance of calculi may suggest their composition. For instance, calcium phosphate calculi usually have smooth contours and are of uniform maximum opacity (Fig. 12–5). Calcium oxalate calculi are also very radiopaque and are difficult to distinguish from calcium phosphate (see Figures 12–102 through 12–106; also see Figure 12–3). On the other hand, magnesium ammonium phosphate hexahydrate calculi are of considerably less opacity (Fig. 12–6); calculi of this type are often seen in patients with persistent urinary infection. Laminated calculi result from the deposition of alternate layers of densely radiopaque material (such as calcium phosphate or calcium oxalate) and material of relatively low radiopacity such as magnesium ammonium phosphate hexahydrate or urates (Fig. 12–7). Calcium oxalate is present in more than half of all urinary calculi, but a "pure" calcium oxalate calculus is rarely encountered.

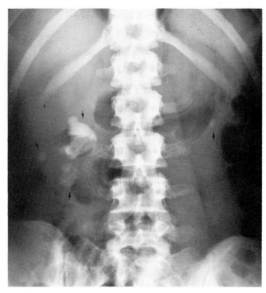

Figure 12–8. *Plain film.* **Bilateral cystine calculi** *(arrows).* Typical "ground-glass" appearance with uniform radiopacity and absence of lamination. Note "satellite" stones *(outer arrows)* in peripheral calyces of staghorn-stone–containing right kidney. This is rather characteristic for cystine stone disease.

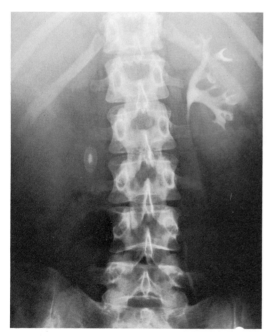

Figure 12–7. *Excretory urogram, 45-minute film.* **Laminated stone with very dense center (probably calcium oxalate).** Stone situated at right ureteropelvic juncture. No function seen. Left kidney normal.

Cystine calculi have been erroneously thought of as essentially nonopaque, but in reality they are moderately opaque and present a "frosted" or "ground-glass" appearance (Fig. 12–8).

The only almost completely radiolucent calculi are pure uric acid or urates (ammonium, sodium, magnesium, or potassium), xanthine, and matrix concretions, although impurities may frequently make them faintly opaque.

Matrix concretions are composed largely of a mucoprotein matrix laminated with sparsely distributed crystals of magnesium ammonium phosphate and basic calcium phosphate as hydroxyapatite (Boyce, 1965). The calcific material is in such low concentration, however, that it usually casts no shadow in the plain film (Fig. 12–9; see also Figure 12–73). The gross specimen has a "waxy" surface and is yellow (Fig. 12–9D).

A peculiar, poorly understood type of small calculus occurs in such conditions as nephrocalcinosis, sponge kidney, and calyceal diverticula or cysts filled with "milk of

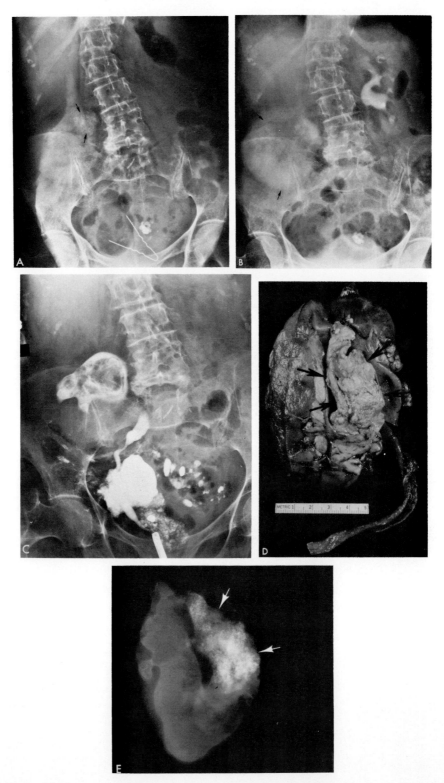

Figure 12–9. Matrix stone in 83-year-old woman with *Proteus mirabilis* urosepsis. **A,** *Plain film.* Punctate calcification above right sacro-iliac joint *(arrows).* **B,** *Excretory urogram (delayed film).* Functionless right pelvic kidney *(arrows).* **C,** *Retrograde ureteropyelogram.* Radiolucent filling defect in dilated right renal pelvis and calyces. Note ureteropelvic obstruction and residual barium in large bowel. **D,** *Surgical specimen.* Right kidney containing yellowish "waxy" matrix calculus *(arrows).* **E,** *Specimen radiograph* shows collection of spherules forming stone *(arrows).*

calcium" stone. Boyce (1965) has grouped these under the heading *seed calculi*. He describes them as perfect spherules, usually composed of calcium phosphate as hydroxyapatite in an organic matrix, varying in size from microscopic to 1 mm in diameter. They may be formed in the renal tubular cells and peritubular interstitium. If they enter larger drainage ducts, they frequently acquire additional layers of calcium oxalate and become larger, as may be the case in nephrocalcinosis (both with and without associated sponge kidney). If excreted into a relatively closed calyceal "diverticulum" or calyceal "cyst," they may remain small and discrete and are spoken of as "milk of calcium" stones (see discussion on pages 1234 to 1236).

During investigation for calculi, it is useful to remember that calculogenesis resulting from metabolic disorders is usually bilateral and that branched (partial or complete staghorn) calculi are usually composed of struvite, cystine, or uric acid.

Confusing Extraurinary Calcific Shadows

The problem of extraurinary shadows is discussed in detail in Chapter 7. For emphasis, a few of the commonly confusing extraurinary shadows are mentioned here. Calcified costal cartilages, blood vessels, and, occasionally, calcified pulmonary granulomas are common sources of confusion, since they may appear in such fragmentary outline as to suggest renal stone (Figs. 12–10 through 12–13). Calcified mesenteric lymph nodes must always be kept in mind. Their more or less characteristic appearance, plus the fact that they change position in relation to each other as well as to the bony pelvis, makes their recognition quite easy (Fig. 12–14). Increased density of the tips of the transverse processes of the lumbar vertebrae may suggest ureteral stone if not closely scrutinized (Fig. 12–15). Fragmentary calcification of the iliac vessels just below the sacroiliac joints is

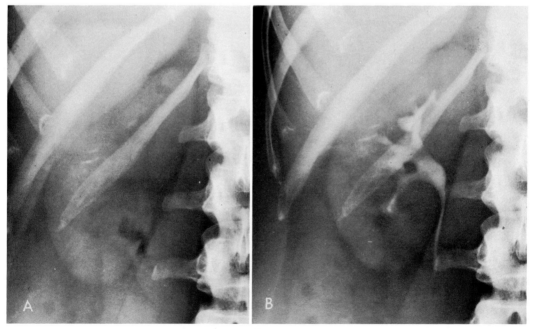

Figure 12–10. A, *Plain film.* Shadows over renal area caused by **calcified costal cartilages. Could be mistaken for renal calculi. B,** *Excretory urogram.* Calcific shadows excluded.

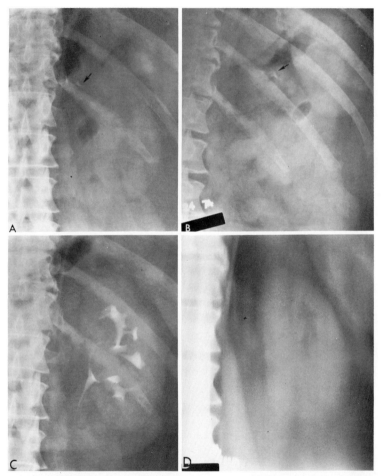

Figure 12–11. A, *Plain film.* Shadow over left renal area *(arrow)* caused by **calcified costal cartilage.** **B,** *Plain film, oblique view.* Shadow appears as branched calculus *(arrow).* **C,** *Excretory urogram.* Shadow hidden by rib **could be mistaken for branched calculus.** Note left parapelvic cyst. **D,** *Plain film (tomogram).* Excludes shadow from left renal area.

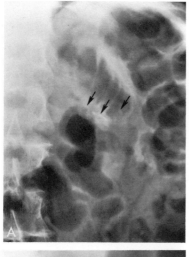
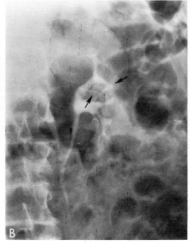
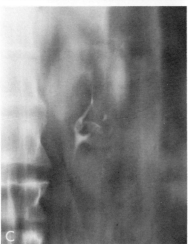

Figure 12–12. A, *Plain film.* Shadows over renal area caused by **calcified renal artery** *(inner two arrows)* and **small renal calculus** *(outer arrow).* **Former could be mistaken for branched calculus. B,** *Excretory urogram.* Excludes renal arterial calcification seen in midportion of kidney outside collecting system *(inner arrow).* Small renal calculus is included in a middle calyx *(outer arrow).* **C,** *Excretory urogram (tomogram).* Renal arterial calcification is well visualized and excluded from collecting system.

commonly mistaken for ureteral calculi. Although the physician experienced in urographic interpretation often is able to identify these shadows in the plain film, urographic methods frequently must be used for their identification (Fig. 12–16). Phleboliths are not difficult to recognize in most cases, because they have a smooth outline, a dense periphery, and less-dense centers. However, the fact that they are nearly always located in the areas of the lower portions of the ureters may make identification with a lead catheter or a urogram necessary (Fig. 12–17). Laminated and faceted shadows over the right renal area should always make one suspect gallstones (Fig. 12–18), although laminated renal stones do occur.

Because they tend to produce urinary stasis of some degree, urinary calculi furnish an ideal situation for the use of excretory urography. The stasis prevents too-rapid excretion of medium, so delineation of the urinary tract may be better than in normal patients who have no obstruction. In some cases, however, it is necessary to resort to retrograde pyelography for adequate diagnosis.

Small calculi may be exceedingly difficult to visualize, either in the kidneys or in the ureters. It has been the not uncommon experience of every urologist to have a patient spontaneously pass a small stone after a most exhaustive urologic examination had failed to disclose its presence. This diagnostic difficulty is caused not only

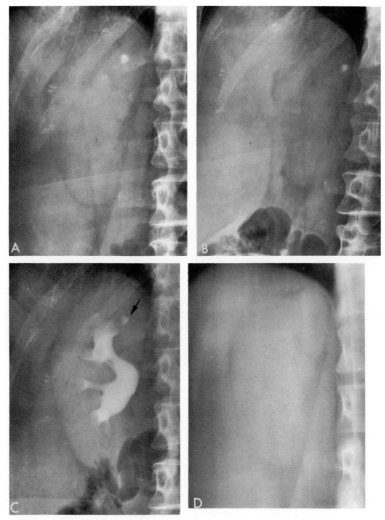

Figure 12–13. **A,** *Plain film.* Shadow over upper right renal area caused by **calcified lung granuloma. Could be mistaken for renal stone. B,** *Plain film.* Oblique view does not completely exclude shadow. **C,** *Excretory urogram.* Calcified shadow *(arrow)* could represent stone in a calyceal diverticulum, but for practical purposes it is excluded from collecting system. **D,** *Plain film (tomogram).* Excludes shadow from right renal area.

by the small size of the stone but also by other factors such as the degree of opacity, overlying fluid or gas in the intestine, or adjacent bony structures. Renal tomography with and without excretory urography is now widely used. Structures of urologic interest are in different planes. These planes, and by the same token small calculi not readily seen on plain film, may be brought into focus by tomography (Fig. 12–19; see also Figures 12–106, 12–112, 12–116, 12–125, 12–131, and 12–133). Renal tomography has thus become routine

in investigation of the stone-forming patients at the Mayo Clinic. This technique can also exclude such confusing extraurinary calcific shadows as costal cartilages (see foregoing discussion and Figures 12–11 through 12–13).

Opaque Calcific Shadows

Methods of Identification and Localization. One suspects a urinary calculus on the plain film when a calcific shadow overlies the areas where the kidneys, ureters,

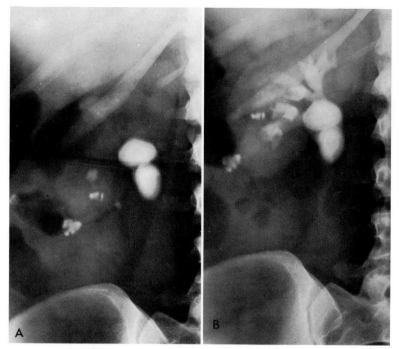

Figure 12–14. Calcified mesenteric lymph nodes and renal calculi. **A,** *Plain film.* Multiple shadows over right renal area suggest calcified mesenteric lymph nodes and renal calculi. Identification with urogram will be necessary. **B,** *Excretory urogram.* Large shadows are two stones in right renal pelvis. Remainder of shadows are calcified mesenteric lymph nodes. Note how shadows of calcified lymph nodes change position in relation to each other, as well as to renal calculi.

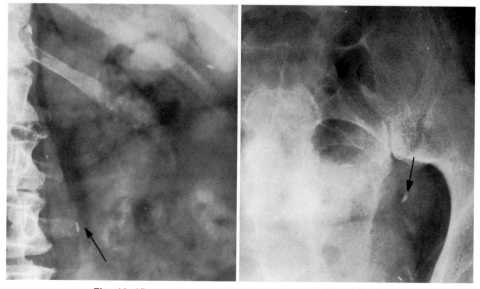

Fig. 12–15   **Fig. 12–16**

Figure 12–15. *Plain film.* Increased density of left transverse process of third lumbar vertebra that could be mistaken for ureteral calculus.

Figure 12–16. *Plain film.* Fragmentary calcification of iliac vessel below left sacro-iliac joint that is commonly confused with ureteral calculus.

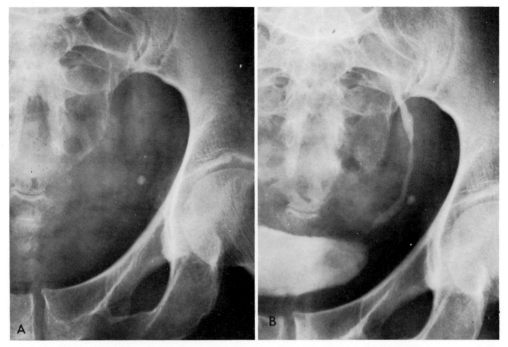

Figure 12–17. **A,** *Plain film.* **Phlebolith could be confused with ureteral stone.** Shadow opposite left ischial spine, circular in outline, with dense periphery and less dense center, suggests phlebolith. **B,** *Excretory urogram.* Left ureter is outlined, and shadow is excluded and demonstrated to be phlebolith.

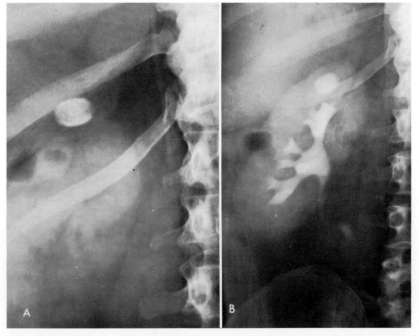

Figure 12–18. **Gallstone that could be mistaken for renal calculus. A,** *Plain film.* Laminated shadow overlying upper border of right kidney. **B,** *Excretory urogram.* Shadow excluded; it is definitely produced by gallstone.

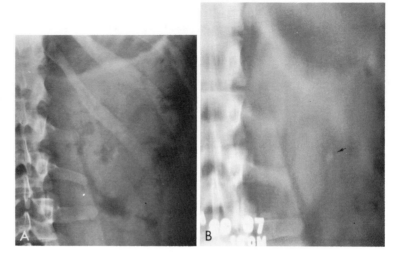

Figure 12–19. A, *Plain film.* **Stone of poor radiopacity (cystine)** barely visible near lower pole of left kidney. **B,** *Plain film (tomogram).* Stone distinctly demonstrable *(arrow)* once brought into "focus" by tomography.

bladder, and prostate gland are normally situated. Shadows in other areas, however, cannot be entirely identified in this manner because of possible mobility of the kidneys and ureters, not to mention other factors such as the possibility of anomalous renal position, large hydronephrosis, and distended urinary bladder or diverticula. Factors other than position, therefore, should

be relied on for identification of urinary calculi. Data obtained by use of the lead catheter and by means of urography and tomography also may be necessary.

Shape or Contour of Shadow. The shape or contour of a shadow is of great diagnostic importance. Often a calculus assumes the shape of a calyx or may even form a cast of the pelvis and calyces. In the

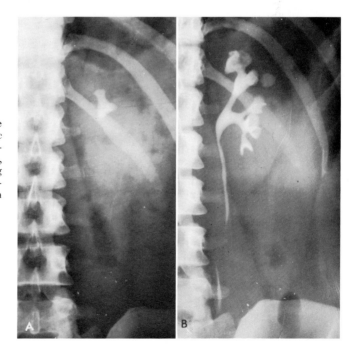

Figure 12–20. A, *Plain film.* **Stone forming cast of upper calyx.** Calcific shadow overlying upper pole of left kidney, assuming contour of renal calyx. **B,** *Excretory urogram.* Stone is seen forming cast of portion of upper calyx, with resulting caliectasis. Small calyceal diverticulum adjacent to lateral branch of upper calyx.

Fig. 12–21

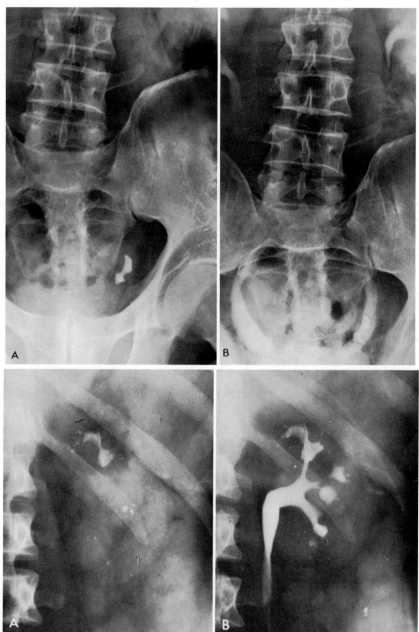

Fig. 12–22

Figure 12–21. A, *Plain film.* Shadow of stone forming cast of composite calyx of left kidney, which has dropped into lower segment of ureter. B, *Excretory urogram.* Both ureters dilated. Shadow is demonstrated to be included in lower portion of left ureter.

Figure 12–22. A, *Plain film.* Multiple calcific shadows overlying left renal area. Largest shadow appears to be cast of composite calyx. B, *Left retrograde pyelogram.* Largest shadow is seen to be stone forming cast of composite upper calyx. Other shadows are smaller stones in various calyces.

latter case it is spoken of as a branched or staghorn calculus (Figs. 12–20, 12–21, and 12–22).

Use of Opaque Ureteral Catheter and Additional Plain Films. Although identification of shadows in the plain film when an opaque catheter is in place may be feasible, it is not so accurate a procedure as urography. However, if one can introduce an opaque catheter so that in the plain film the catheter or its tip is adjacent to the shadow and maintains its position in oblique and lateral views, one can assume with reasonable assurance that the shadow in question is a urinary calculus. Parenthetically, it should be stated that opaque catheters are of more value in the identification of ureteral than renal calculi (Figs. 12–23 and 12–24).

The Urogram. Urography is by far the most useful method for identification and localization of urinary calculi. Both the excretory and retrograde methods are useful, one complementing the other. The problem of which to use is discussed in detail in Chapter 1. An excretory urogram is the procedure to employ first in nearly all cases. If visualization is sufficient for identification, one obviates the danger of introducing contrast medium above an obstructing stone by retrograde means, which always carries some risk of febrile reaction and pain.

The object of the urogram, of course, is to show that the shadow in question is within some portion of the pelviocalyceal system. Often it is possible to do this simply by making an anteroposterior urogram. If the shadow and the opaque medium coincide and the stone produces an increase or decrease in density of the contrast medium or a "negative" shadow, or if its shape coincides with the contour of some part of the pelviocalyceal system, one may be reasonably sure of its identification. If, however, the positions of the contrast medium and of the stone coincide, but the medium is so dense that it obscures the shadow completely, or if the shape of the stone is not of diagnostic value, or both,

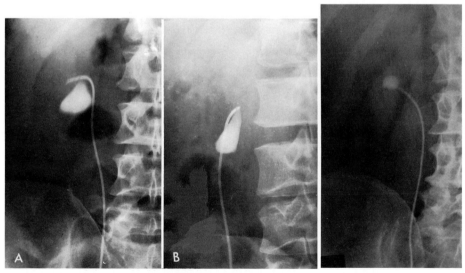

Fig. 12–23   Fig. 12–24

Figure 12–23. A, *Plain film.* **Identification of renal calculus with opaque catheter.** In anteroposterior view, catheter surrounds and is adjacent to shadow. **B,** *In oblique view,* catheter is still adjacent to shadow, a fact which would seem to indicate that it is definitely renal stone.

Figure 12–24. *Plain film.* **Identification of renal calculus with opaque catheter.** Lead catheter in right ureter. Shadow overlying middle portion of right kidney. Tip of catheter adjacent to shadow, suggesting that it is definitely renal calculus. Oblique view would be necessary to be certain of this diagnosis, as it is possible that shadow in question could be in plane anterior or posterior to that of kidney.

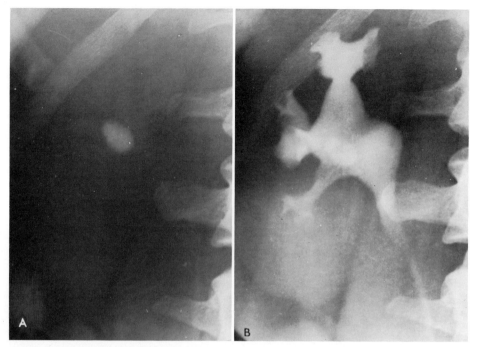

Figure 12–25.   Identification of renal calculus by means of urogram. **A,** *Plain film.* Calcific shadow overlying right midrenal area. **B,** *Right retrograde pyelogram.* Shadow is seen to be stone in renal pelvis; it is of greater density than urographic medium and can be seen through it.

one could assume that the shadow in question could be outside the kidney but lying in such a position that it coincides with the pelviocalyceal system in the anteroposterior view. In such a case oblique or lateral views and tomograms are necessary for diagnosis. Films made with the patient erect may help "throw out" shadows that lie over the kidney or ureter in the routine film made with the patient supine. If the shadow cannot be "thrown out" in these urograms, it is usually reasonably safe to assume that the shadow is a renal calculus (Figs. 12–25 through 12–36). If still in doubt, one may resort either to pyelograms made with medium of less density or to air pyelograms (Figs. 12–37, 12–38, and 12–39).

Text continued on page 1201

Figure 12–26.   Multiple renal calculi of greater density than contrast medium. **A,** *Plain film.* Multiple calcific shadows over lower pole of right kidney. **B,** *Excretory urogram.* Shadows are seen to be stones in renal pelvis and in lower calyces of right kidney.

Figure 12–27.   **A,** *Plain film.* **Stone in lower calyx of left kidney; calcified splenic vessel.** Irregular calcific shadow overlying lower pole of left kidney. Shadow suggesting calcified splenic vessel overlying upper pole. **B,** *Left retrograde pyelogram.* Lower shadow definitely included in calyx, as is demonstrated by contour of lower calyx, which matches that of stone. Oblique view would not be necessary for accurate identification.

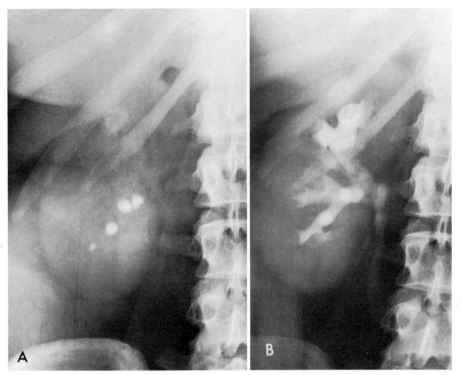

Figure 12–26. *See opposite page for legend.*

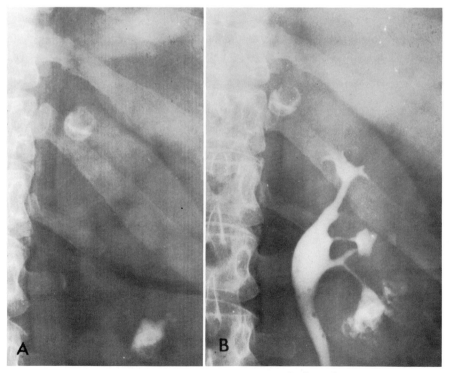

Figure 12–27. *See opposite page for legend.*

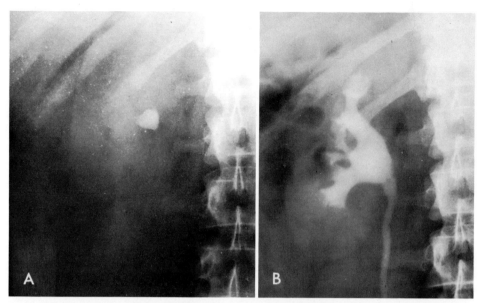

Figure 12-28. *See opposite page for legend.*

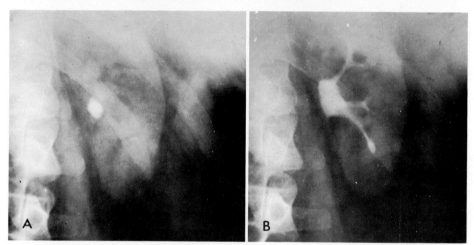

Figure 12-29. *See opposite page for legend.*

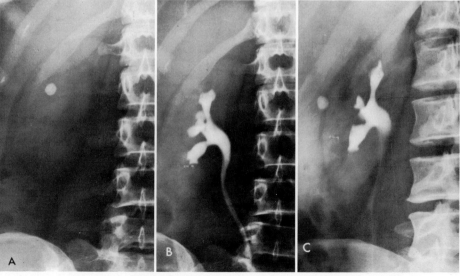

Figure 12-30. *See opposite page for legend.*

Figure 12–28. Stone in renal pelvis of almost same density as contrast medium. **A,** *Plain film.* Calcific shadow overlying right renal area. **B,** *Excretory urogram.* Shadow obscured by pelviocalyceal system. One would need oblique view to be absolutely sure that shadow is renal stone.

Figure 12–29. Stone in left renal pelvis. Essentially same diagnostic situation as in Figure 12–28. **A,** *Plain film.* Calcific shadow overlying left renal area. **B,** *Left retrograde pyelogram.*

Figure 12–30. Extraurinary shadow suggests renal stone. Was excluded only with oblique urogram. **A,** *Plain film.* Calcific shadow overlying right renal area. **B,** *Right retrograde pyelogram. Anteroposterior view* shows shadow obscured by pelviocalyceal system. Suggests that shadow is renal stone. **C,** *Oblique view.* Shadow definitely excluded from kidney. This case illustrates how easily errors can be made in diagnosis if oblique views are not made when indicated.

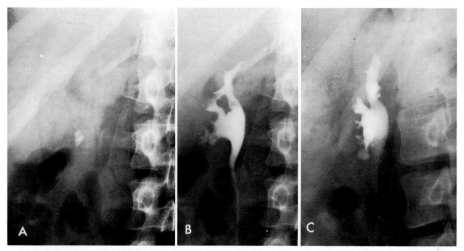

Figure 12–31. Right renal calculus. Identification required oblique urogram. **A,** *Plain film.* Calcific shadow overlying lower pole of right kidney. **B,** *Right retrograde pyelogram, anteroposterior view.* Shadow obscured by pelviocalyceal system, suggesting that it is included in pelvis or lower calyces. **C,** *Oblique view.* Shadow is not excluded, corroborating diagnosis of right renal stone.

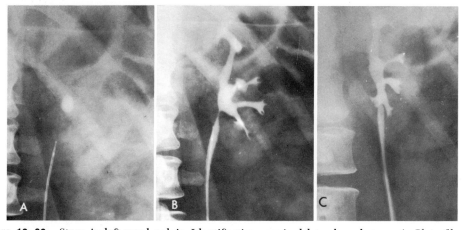

Figure 12–32. Stone in left renal pelvis. Identification required lateral pyelogram. **A,** *Plain film.* Calcific shadow overlying left kidney. **B,** *Left retrograde pyelogram, anteroposterior view.* Shadow obscured by renal pelvis, suggesting that shadow is included in pelvis. **C,** *Lateral view.* Shadow is not excluded, corroborating diagnosis of left renal stone.

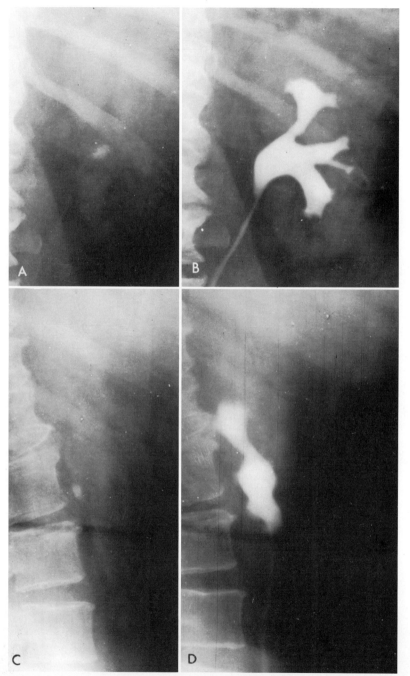

Figure 12–33. Stone in left renal pelvis. Identification required lateral pyelogram. **A,** *Plain film.* Calcific shadow overlying left midrenal area. **B,** *Left retrograde pyelogram, anteroposterior view.* Shadow of stone is obscured by contrast medium filling pelvis but is not accurately identified. **C,** *Lateral plain film.* Shadow lying just anterior to bony structure of third lumbar vertebra. **D,** *Left lateral retrograde pyelogram.* Stone definitely included in pelvis.

Fig. 12–34

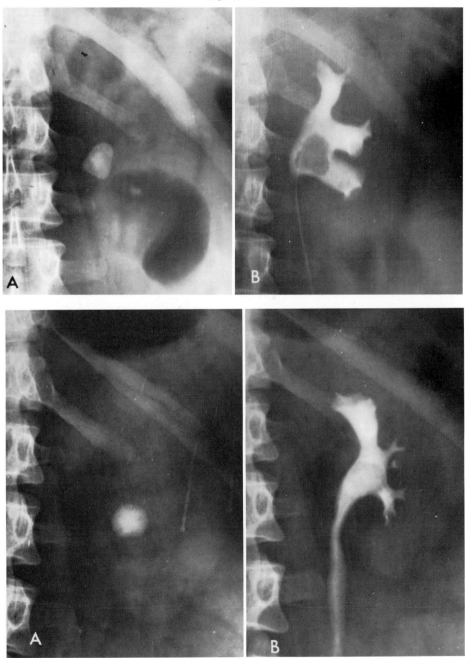

Fig. 12–35

Figure 12–34. Laminated stones in left renal pelvis and lower calyx, producing "negative" filling defects in pyelogram. **A,** *Plain film.* Two calcific shadows of good density. **B,** *Left retrograde pyelogram.* Stones displace contrast medium and cast "negative" shadow in renal pelvis and tip of lower calyx. Oblique views would not be necessary for accurate diagnosis.

Figure 12–35. Laminated stone in left renal pelvis producing partial "negative" filling defect in pyelogram. **A,** *Plain film.* Calcific shadow of good density overlying midrenal area. **B,** *Left retrograde pyelogram.* Stone displaces contrast medium and produces partial negative shadow in pelvis, making accurate diagnosis possible without use of oblique views.

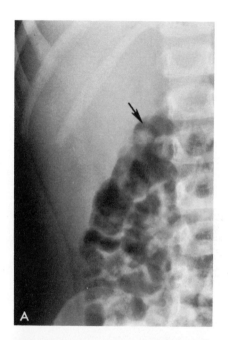

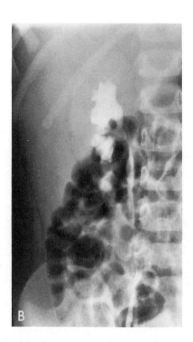

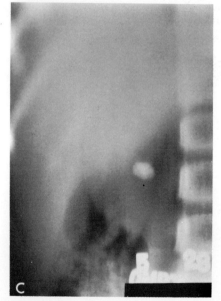

Figure 12–36. Large stone in right renal pelvis not well seen on plain film and obscured by contrast medium during excretory urography but dramatically demonstrated by plain tomogram. **A,** *Plain film.* Shadow of poor radiopacity *(arrow)* in right renal area. Could be mistaken for bowel gas. **B,** *Excretory urogram.* Mild right caliectasis. Contrast medium in normal intrarenal pelvis obscures stone. **C,** *Plain film (tomogram)* dramatically shows stone.

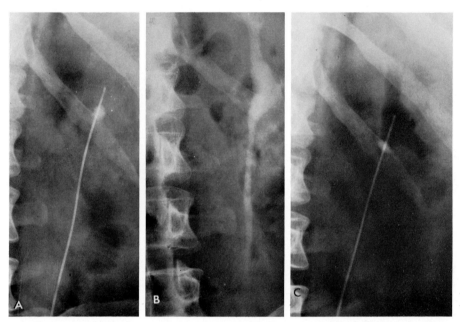

Figure 12–37. Stone at left ureteropelvic juncture identified with an air pyelogram. **A,** *Plain film.* Lead catheter in left ureter. Calcific shadow over left midrenal area suggests stone in renal pelvis. **B,** *Left retrograde pyelogram using contrast medium.* Shadow obscured by pelviocalyceal system, but identity of shadow cannot be accurately determined from this pyelogram, because shadow and contrast medium are apparently of equal density. **C,** *Left retrograde air pyelogram.* Shadow is seen to be stone localized at ureteropelvic juncture.

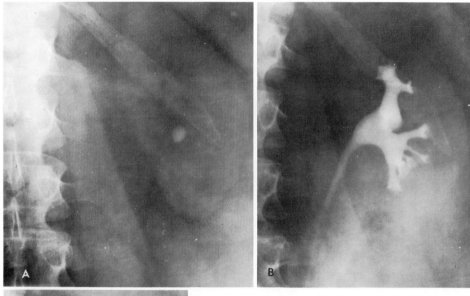

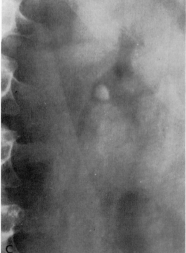

Figure 12–38.   Stone in left renal pelvis identified with an air pyelogram. **A,** *Plain film.* Calcific shadow over left midrenal area suggests renal stone. **B,** *Left retrograde pyelogram, using contrast medium.* Shadow obscured by pelviocalyceal system, but shadow cannot be accurately identified because shadow and contrast medium are apparently of equal density. **C,** *Left retrograde air pyelogram.* Shadow is seen to be stone in renal pelvis.

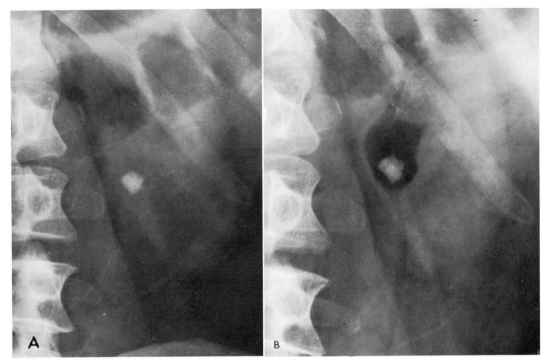

Figure 12–39. Stone in left renal pelvis identified with an air pyelogram. **A,** *Plain film.* Calcific shadow over left midrenal area. **B,** *Left retrograde air pyelogram.* Shadow demonstrated to be stone in pelvis of left kidney.

Nonopaque Calculi and Calculi of Poor Density

Stones of poor density and completely nonopaque stones are easily overlooked in both plain films and urograms. Stones of poor density may cast shadows so dim that they are easily obscured by gas in the intestine. They can be seen only if carefully looked for. Soft stones composed of putty-like material, uric acid, cystine, xanthine, and organic substance, so-called matrix calculi, may fall into this category. Urographic medium may help interpretation by casting a negative shadow of the stone. Just as often, however, it will obscure the stone, which will not be recognized unless the plain film is closely scrutinized. Under these circumstances renal tomograms, both plain and with excretory urography, may be extremely helpful (see Figures 12–19 through 12–54).

Various combinations, such as dense center and less dense periphery, or vice versa, yield roentgenograms of unusual appearance (Figs. 12–40 through 12–48). Completely nonopaque stones are the bugaboo of urologists. If small, they may be almost impossible to demonstrate. When of sufficient size and volume, they cast a negative shadow or filling defect, which furnishes excellent visualization (Figs. 12–49 through 12–53). Negative shadows and filling defects, however, must be differentiated from a host of lesions, including tumors, blood clots, ectopic renal papillae, renal artery aneurysms or other vascular malformations and impressions, inclusion cysts, and cholesteatomas (Malek, Aguilo and Hattery) (Fig. 12–54). When the diagnosis is in doubt, subsequent roentgenograms made several days or weeks later, especially if a chemolytic program is undertaken, will show a change in contour or absence of the negative shadow (Fig. 12–55; see sections on cystinuria and uric acid lithiasis, and also Chapter 14).

Text continued on page 1213

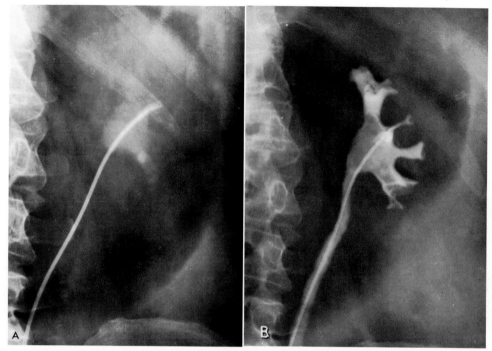

Figure 12–40. Branched stone of poor density yields "negative" shadow in pyelogram. **A,** *Plain film.* Shadow of soft stone of poor density outlining pelvis and lower calyces of left kidney. **B,** *Left retrograde pyelogram.* Contrast medium is displaced by stone, forming partially negative shadow. Stone forms cast of pelvis and lower calyx.

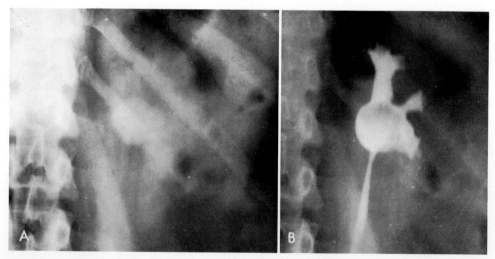

Figure 12–41. Renal calculus of poor density identified as "negative" shadow in pyelogram. **A,** *Plain film.* Indefinite shadow suggesting soft stone of poor density overlying left midrenal area. **B,** *Left retrograde pyelogram.* Medium displaced by stone. Partial filling defect of left renal pelvis, indicating that stone is in pelvis and portion of lower calyx.

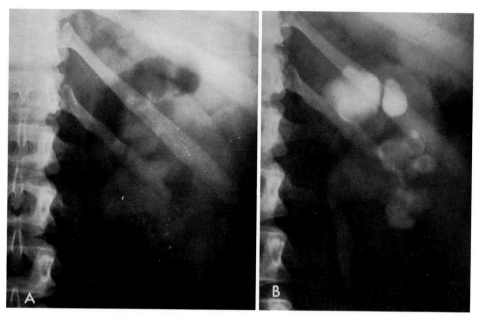

Figure 12–42. Branched stone of poor density. **A**, *Plain film.* Branched stone of poor density filling pelvis and calyces of left kidney. **B**, *Excretory urogram.* Moderate caliectasis beyond projections of stone. Pelvis does not fill with medium because it is completely filled with stone.

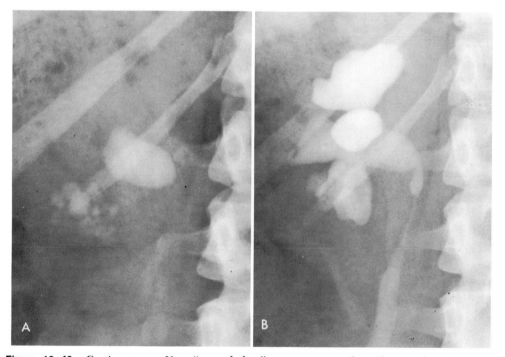

Figure 12–43. Cystine stones. Note "ground-glass" appearance in plain film. **A**, *Plain film.* **B**, *Excretory urogram.* Cystine stones in pelvis and lower calyx of right kidney. Density of stone is less than that of contrast medium.

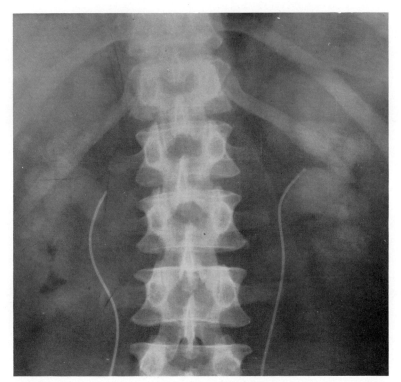

Figure 12–44.   Bilateral uric acid stones with some calcium impurities. **Poor density.** *Plain film* with opaque ureteral catheters in place. Branched calculi of poor density filling pelvis and calyces of both kidneys.

Fig. 12–45

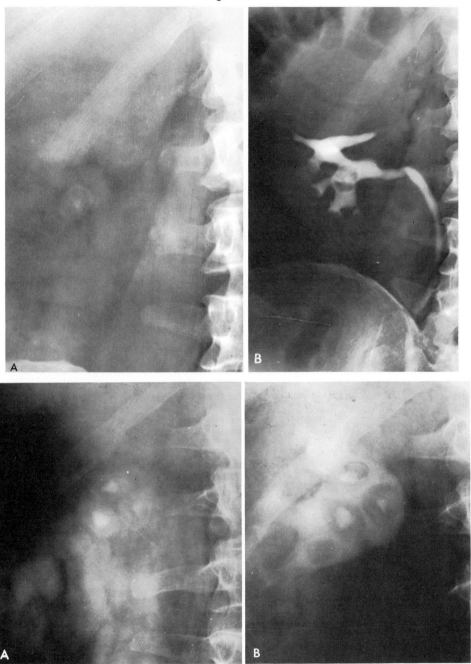

Fig. 12–46

Figure 12–45. Laminated renal stone with dense center and less dense periphery. **A,** *Plain film.* Shadow over right renal area, with dense center but remainder of poor density. **B,** *Right retrograde pyelogram.* Shadow is seen to be stone with dense center and periphery, situated in pelvis. Because of its poor density, **stone casts negative shadow. Simple cyst in upper pole of kidney.**

Figure 12–46. Laminated calculi with dense centers but peripheries of poor density which could be easily **overlooked in plain film.** Well-demonstrated as "negative" shadows in pyelogram. **A,** *Plain film.* Three triangular calcific shadows over right renal area. **B,** *Right retrograde pyelogram.* Four filling defects in dilated renal pelvis. Filling defects are larger than shadows seen in plain film. They are caused by four stones, one of which is completely nonopaque and three of which have nonopaque peripheries.

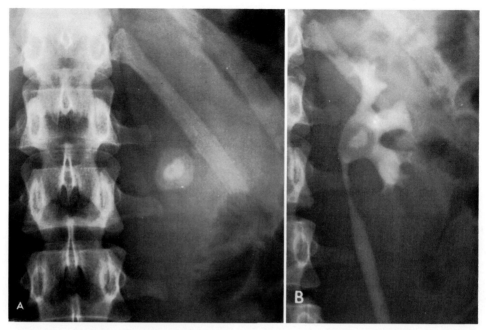

Figure 12–47. A, *Plain film.* **Stone** with dense center and less dense periphery. **B,** *Left retrograde pyelogram.* Negative shadow cast by **laminated stone** as it displaces contrast medium. Note that dense center of stone is easily visualized.

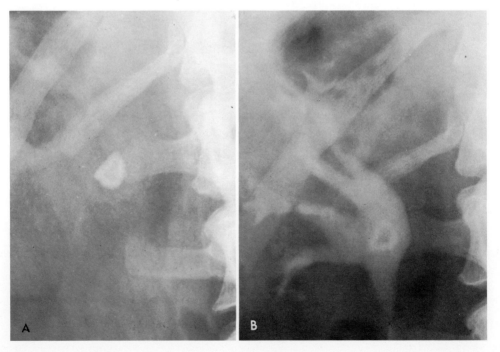

Figure 12–48. Laminated stone; periphery is more dense then center. **A,** *Plain film.* **B,** *Excretory urogram.* Stone is in renal pelvis; "negative" shadow of center of stone is most prominent.

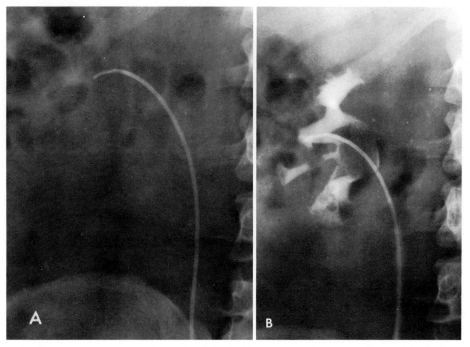

Figure 12–49. Nonopaque stone in renal pelvis. **A,** *Plain film.* Catheter in right ureter. Otherwise negative. **B,** *Right retrograde pyelogram.* Nonopaque stone. **Negative shadow occupying most of renal pelvis is due to nonopaque stone.**

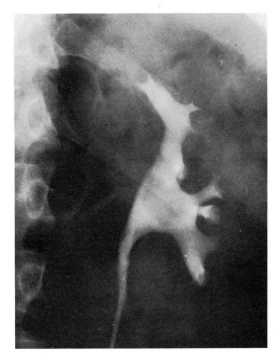

Figure 12–50. Nonopaque stone in renal pelvis. *Left retrograde pyelogram.* Indistinct "negative" shadow occupying left renal pelvis and proximal portion of infundibulum of upper calyx, caused by nonopaque stone. Plain film was negative (not shown).

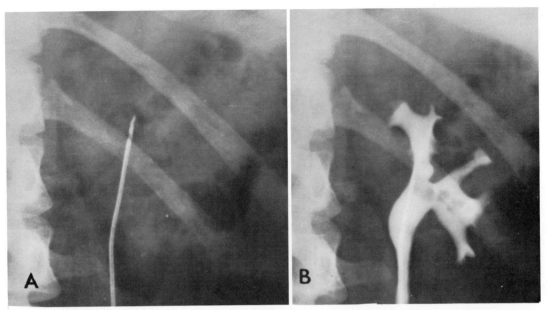

Figure 12–51. Nonopaque calculi in pelvis and lower calyces. **A,** *Plain film.* Negative. **B,** *Left retrograde pyelogram.* Multiple negative shadows caused by nonopaque stones in pelvis and lower calyx of left kidney.

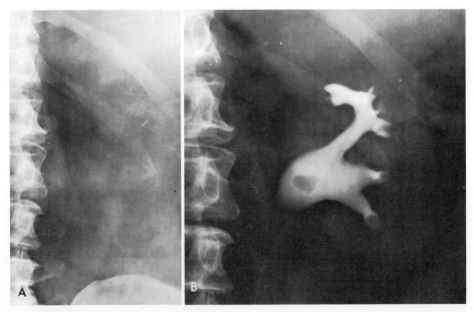

Figure 12–52. Nonopaque renal calculi. **A,** *Plain film.* Negative. **B,** *Left retrograde pyelogram.* Two discrete negative shadows in pelvis of left kidney, indicating nonopaque stones.

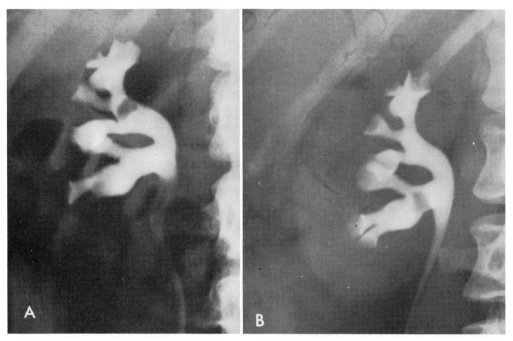

Figure 12–53. "Migratory" nonopaque stone. **A,** *Right retrograde pyelogram.* Filling defect in upper major calyx, caused by nonopaque stone. Plain film was negative (not shown). **B,** *Right retrograde pyelogram,* made 2 days later. Stone is now in lower major calyx, indicating migratory stone.

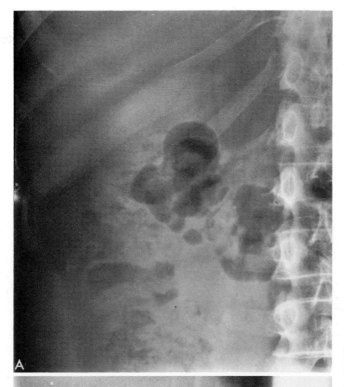

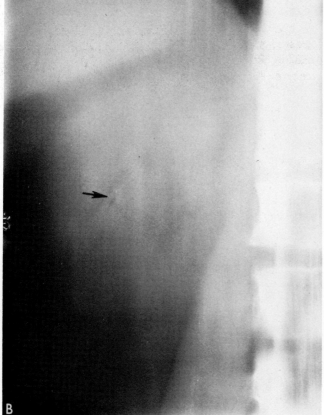

Figure 12–54. Poor-density stone (uric acid) and vascular impression of lower pole infundibulum mimicking nonopaque stone or other lesion. **A,** *Plain film.* Poor-density stone barely visible near superior border of last rib. **B,** *Plain film (tomogram)* shows poorly calcified uric stone *(arrow).*

Legend continued on opposite page

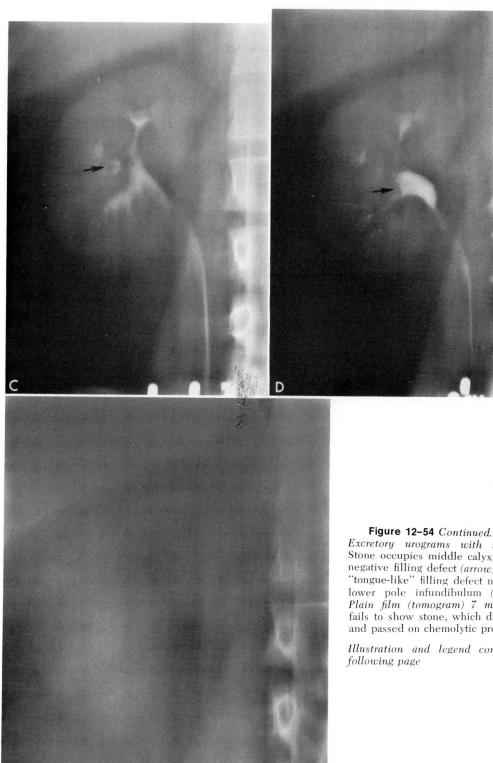

Figure 12–54 *Continued.* **C** and **D**, *Excretory urograms with tomograms.* Stone occupies middle calyx, producing negative filling defect *(arrow)*. Note also "tongue-like" filling defect near base of lower pole infundibulum *(arrow).* **E**, *Plain film (tomogram) 7 months later* fails to show stone, which disintegrated and passed on chemolytic program.

Illustration and legend continued on following page

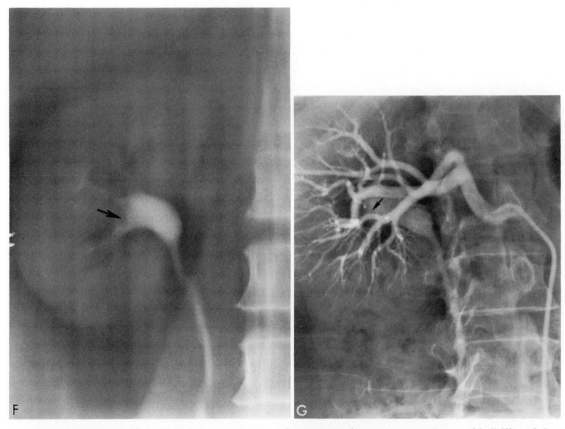

Figure 12–54 *Continued.*   **F,** *Excretory urogram with tomogram* shows persistent "tongue-like" filling defect *(arrow)* unchanged in size or position. **G,** *Selective renal arteriogram* shows area of vascular impression producing "tongue-like" filling defect *(arrow).*

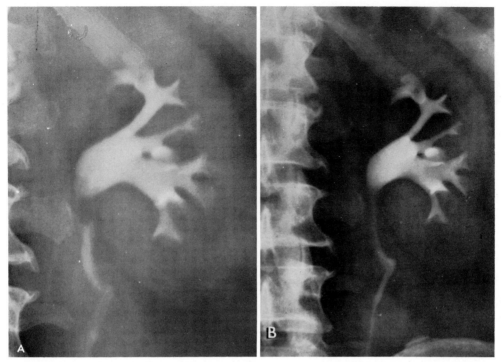

Figure 12–55. Air bubble simulating nonopaque stone. **A,** *Left retrograde pyelogram.* Oval negative shadow at or just below ureteropelvic juncture suggests nonopaque stone. **B,** *Left retrograde pyelogram* made 2 days later. Filling defect has disappeared. It was apparently result of air bubble.

PATHOLOGIC RENAL CHANGES RESULTING FROM CALCULI

As might be expected, the most common pathologic condition produced by stone is obstruction, with dilatation of the renal pelvis, the calyces, or both. The location and degree of dilatation depend on the position of the stone and the degree of obstruction produced. A stone lodged in the infundibulum of a calyx may produce localized caliectasis or hydrocalyx. Stones in calyces may produce dilatation simply because of their presence and associated infection. Stones in dilated calyces usually are recognized quite easily, especially if the stone assumes somewhat the shape of the calyx (Figs. 12–56, 12–57, and 12–58). A stone in the renal pelvis may produce pyelectasis or caliectasis or both (Figs. 12–59, 12–60, and 12–61).

The presence of a stone in the renal pelvis may cause spasm and contraction of the pelvis rather than dilatation. In such cases the pelvis is seen tightly contracted around the stone, with an associated spasticity and contracture of the ureteropelvic juncture, apparently a result of irritation (Figs. 12–62, 12–63, and 12–64).

Secondary Calculi

Calculi may develop in association with urinary stasis (see section on classification). One example of this is the calculi of recumbency, which occur in patients who are bedridden for a long time, usually after accidents that have caused multiple fractures (Fig. 12–65) (see section on immobilization; also see sections on infected urolithiasis and urinary stasis). Another example is the patient with obstruction of the ureteropelvic juncture and associated pyelectasis (Figs. 12–66 through 12–71). A majority of these patients have underlying metabolic abnormalities, and their stone-forming tendency is merely *promoted* by stasis.

Text continued on page 1222

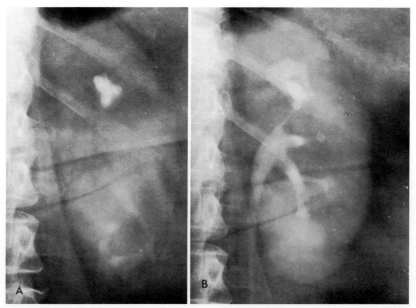

Figure 12–56. Stone obstructing upper calyx. **A,** *Plain film.* Calcific shadow overlying upper pole of left kidney, suggesting stone forming cast of portion of upper calyx. **B,** *Excretory urogram.* Dilatation of upper calyx caused by stone, which obstructs minor calyx and infundibulum. Remainder of kidney normal.

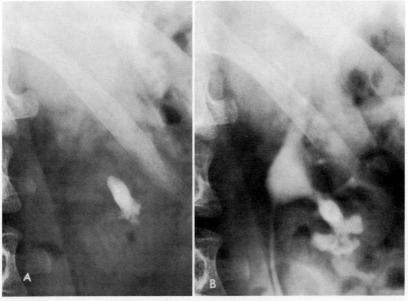

Figure 12–57. Stone obstructing lower calyx. **A,** *Plain film.* Irregular calcific shadow overlying lower pole of left kidney. **B,** *Excretory urogram.* Shadow is stone impacted in infundibulum of lower calyx, producing localized dilatation of lower minor calyx.

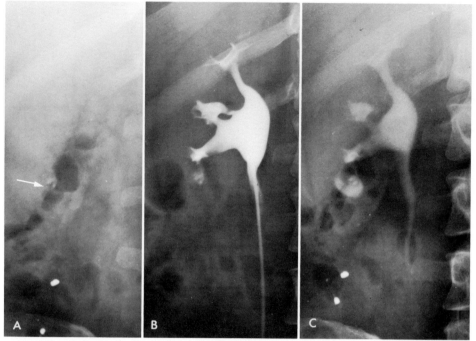

Figure 12–58. **Stone obstructing lower calyx.** Caliectasis proximal to stone demonstrated by excretory urogram. **A,** *Plain film.* Irregular calcific shadow overlying lower pole of right kidney *(arrow).* **B,** *Right retrograde pyelogram.* Shadow is included in branch of lower calyx, which does not appear to be greatly dilated. **C,** *Excretory urogram.* Marked dilatation of lower calyx proximal to stone. This would have been missed if excretory urogram had not been made.

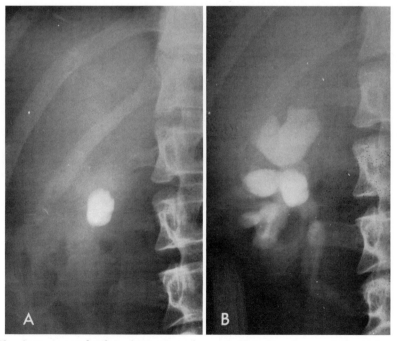

Figure 12–59. **Stone in renal pelvis obstructing calyces. A,** *Plain film.* Large calcific shadow overlying right renal pelvis. **B,** *Excretory urogram.* Shadow is stone in pelvis of kidney, causing moderate caliectasis and adjacent ureterectasis.

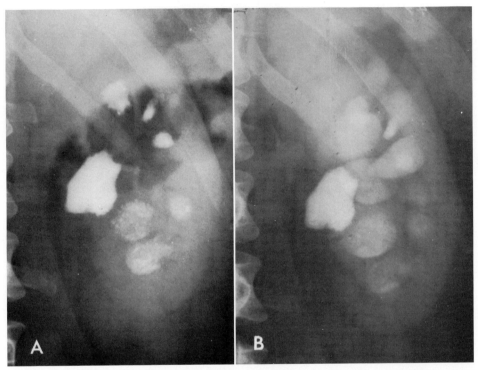

Figure 12–60.   Stone in renal pelvis with secondary (?) calculi in dilated (obstructed) calyces. A, *Plain film.* Calcific shadows outlining pelvis and calyces of left kidney. B, *Excretory urogram.* Larger shadow is stone filling pelvis and producing marked caliectasis. There are secondary calculi in all calyces as a result of obstructive dilatation.

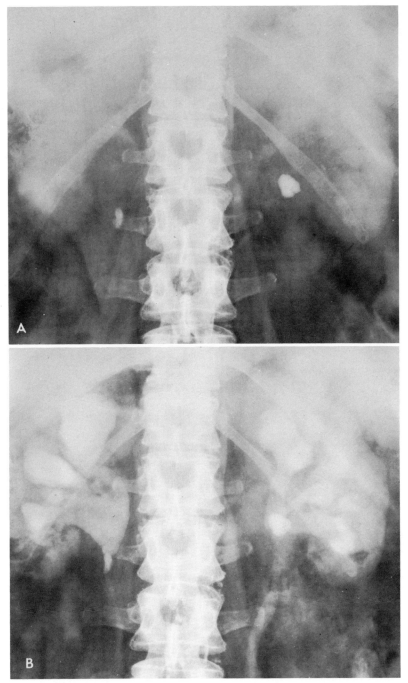

Figure 12–61. A, *Plain film.* B, *Excretory urogram.* Stone is blocking each ureteropelvic juncture and producing caliectasis, especially marked on right.

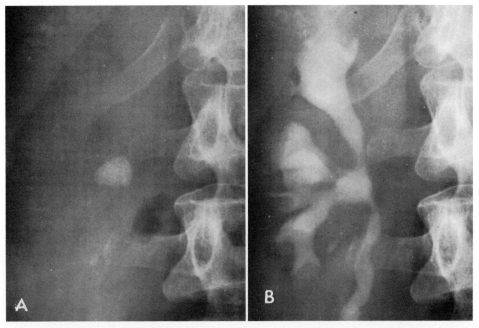

Figure 12–62.   Stone in renal pelvis, which is tightly contracted around it. **A,** *Plain film.* Calcific shadow overlying right renal area. **B,** *Right retrograde pyelogram.* Some evidence of caliectasis.

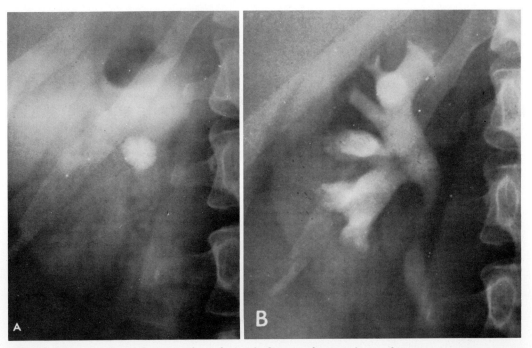

Figure 12–63.   **A,** *Plain film.* Irregular calcific shadow overlying right renal area. **B,** *Excretory urogram.* **Right renal pelvis and adjacent portion of ureter spastic and contracted around pelvic stone,** with some evidence of caliectasis. Very little obstruction is present.

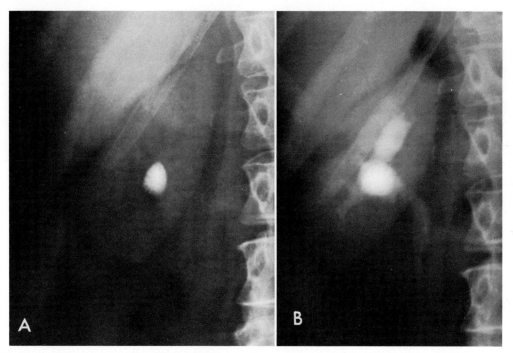

Figure 12–64. A, *Plain film.* Calcific shadow overlying right renal area. **B,** *Excretory urogram.* Right renal pelvis contracted around stone, causing moderate caliectasis.

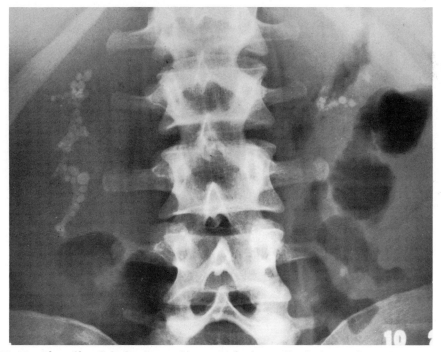

Figure 12–65. *Plain film.* **Calculi of recumbency.** Multiple small calculi in calyces. (Patient immobilized with fracture of pelvis.) Might be confused with nephrocalcinosis.

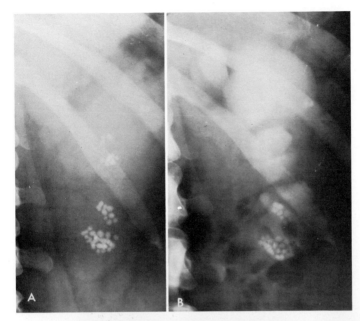

Figure 12-66. Secondary calculi in hydronephrosis. **A,** *Plain film.* Multiple small calculi scattered throughout left renal area. **B,** *Excretory urogram.* Incomplete filling of left renal pelvis. Marked caliectasis. Stones are grouped in large dilated calyces.

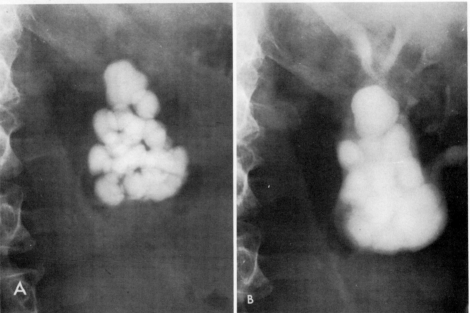

Figure 12-67. Secondary calculi in hydronephrosis. **A,** *Plain film.* Large number of calculi overlying left renal area. **B,** *Excretory urogram.* Marked pyelectasis with minimal caliectasis. Large pelvis is filled with calculi. Obstruction at ureteropelvic juncture. Left nephrectomy.

Figure 12-70. *Excretory urogram.* **Bilateral obstruction of ureteropelvic junctures, with secondary nonopaque calculi.** On right, three large oval calculi produce negative shadows. On left, pelvis and calyces are filled with numerous small nonopaque calculi which give a mottled appearance. Both kidneys explored; calculi removed, and plastic operation performed on ureteropelvic juncture.

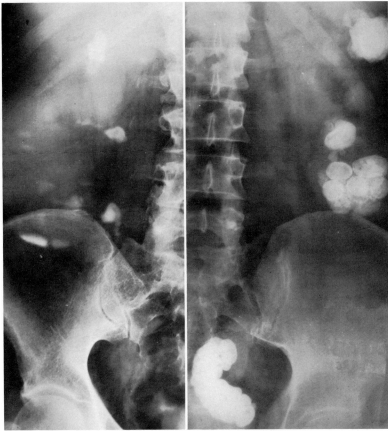

Fig. 12–68   Fig. 12–69

Figure 12–68.   Secondary calculi in hydronephrosis. *Plain film.* Multiple calcific shadows overlying entire right side of abdomen. Excretory urogram (not shown here) showed no function on right. Left kidney normal. Exploration showed extreme hydronephrosis with secondary calculi. Right nephrectomy. Hydronephrosis and stones.

Figure 12–69.   Secondary calculi in hydronephrosis and hydroureter. *Excretory urogram.* Nonfunctioning left kidney, which is site of extreme hydronephrosis and ureterectasis. Large secondary calculi situated in kidney and lower portion of ureter. Right kidney was normal.

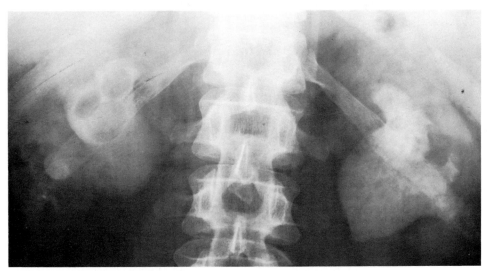

Figure 12–70.   *See opposite page for legend.*

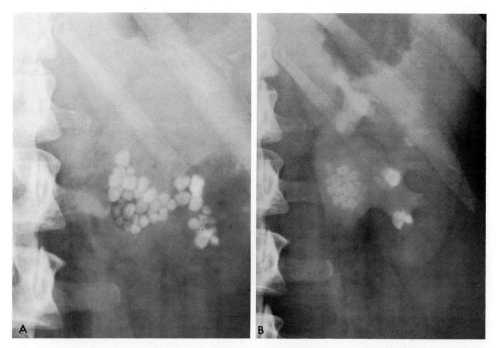

Figure 12–71. Obstruction of ureteropelvic juncture, with pyelectasis and multiple secondary calculi. **A,** *Plain film.* **B,** *Excretory urogram.*

At times it may be difficult to know whether there is sufficient functioning renal tissue to permit a conservative operation (removal of calculi) or whether a nephrectomy will be required. The excretory urogram is not an accurate indication of the actual absence or diminution of function (Wilkiemeyer and associates). When the function of the kidney with secondary calculi is in question, the demonstration of good blood supply by means of renal angiography and [^{99m}Tc] DTPA renal blood flow studies may be distinctly helpful (Figs. 12–72 and 12–73).

Caliectasis With Calculi Simulating Tuberculosis With Calcification

At times, stones may be of such contour and density and may produce such caliectasis that they suggest renal tuberculosis with calcification. This type of stone usually is irregular, with many fragments lying close together in an irregularly dilated calyx that simulates the cortical destruction characteristic of tuberculosis

(Figs. 12–74 and 12–75) (see also Chapter 10, Renal Tuberculosis).

Miscellaneous Types and Locations of Calculi

Laminated calculi are occasionally seen (see Figure 12–7). "Burr-like" stones, more common in the bladder, are also seen in the renal pelvis (Figs. 12–76 through 12–79).

Branched (Staghorn) Calculi

Branched calculi produce the most dramatic-appearing roentgenograms in urography. They practically always consist of magnesium ammonium phosphate (struvite), uric acid (with or without impurities), or cystine. Forming a cast of part or all of the pelviocalyceal system, they may reach enormous proportions, especially in patients in whom pyelectasis becomes severe. There is usually no problem in identifying or localizing such calculi, but it may be extremely difficult to estimate renal

Text continued on page 1230

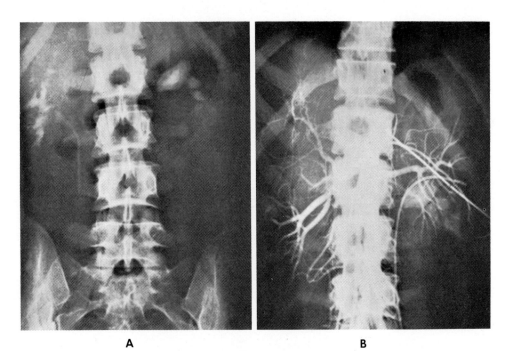

A   B

Figure 12–72. Evaluation of "recovery potential" of damaged kidney by arteriography. **A,** *Excretory urogram.* **Multiple stones in nonfunctioning left kidney.** Normal right kidney. **B,** *Aortogram* shows excellent arterial supply to both right and left kidneys. *Comment:* In this case excretory urogram suggested presence of partially destroyed, nonfunctioning left kidney. Aortogram, by virtue of demonstrating equally good arterial supply bilaterally, suggested that conservative operation, with preservation of kidney, was indicated. Excretory urogram made 5 months after removal of stone showed excellent function of left kidney. (Courtesy of Dr. A. K. Doss.)

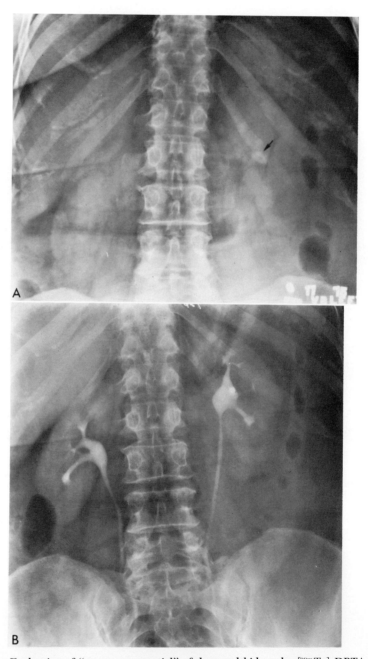

Figure 12-73.   Evaluation of "recovery potential" of damaged kidney by [^{99m}Tc] DPTA blood flow studies and selective renal arteriography. **A,** *Plain film.* Stone in region of left renal pelvis *(arrow).* **B,** *Excretory urogram* is normal. Generous left renal pelvis. No evidence of obstruction. Patient's asymptomatic urinary infection was treated. She elected to undergo pelviolithotomy later.

Legend continued on opposite page.

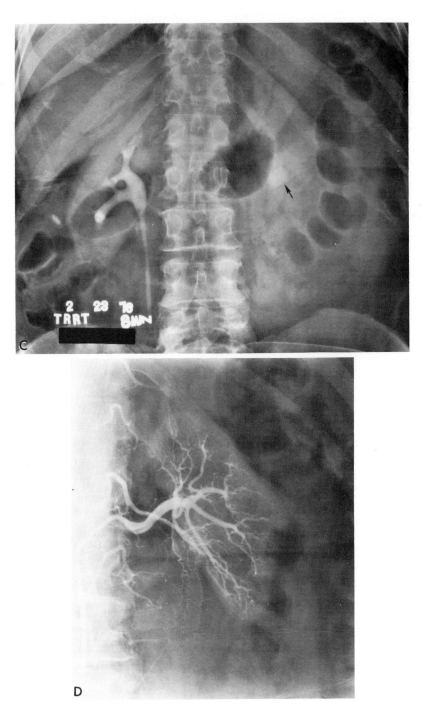

Figure 12–73. *Continued.*   C, *Excretory urogram made 8 months later* shows some increase in size of left renal stone *(arrow)* and no function in left kidney. Patient was uninfected and asymptomatic. **D,** *Selective renal arteriography.* Main renal artery and its divisions are normal. Corticomedullary vessels are rather attenuated, and renal cortex appears thin.

Illustration and legend continued on following page

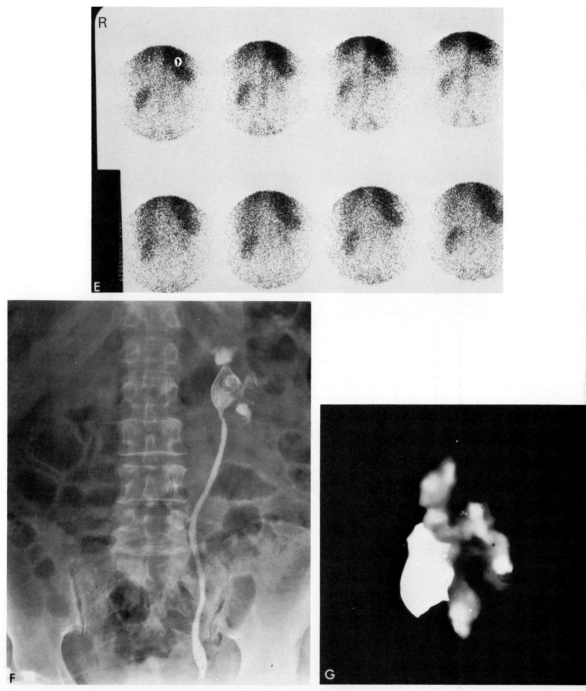

Figure 12–73. *Continued.* **E,** [^{99m}Tc] *DPTA blood flow study* shows practically no blood flow on left side despite relatively good blood flow suggested by arteriography. **F,** *Retrograde ureteropyelogram.* Left renal pelvis and calyces filled with calculus and surrounding matrix, producing "negative" filling defect. Calyces appear "moth-eaten." **G,** *Specimen radiograph* shows calculus (very dense) and surrounding matrix (less dense) found in calyces after nephrectomy. Entire left kidney was practically destroyed by pyelonephritis and papillary necrosis. *Comment:* Arteriographic findings in this case were misleading.

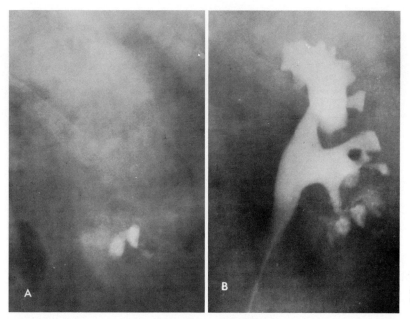

Figure 12–74. Renal calculi simulating tuberculosis with calcification. **A,** *Plain film.* Irregular areas of calcification over lower pole of left kidney. **B,** *Left retrograde pyelogram.* Marked irregularity of lower calyx, which could suggest cortical destruction with calcification from tuberculosis. This, however, was stone in dilated, infected lower calyx. Inoculated guinea pigs were negative for tuberculosis.

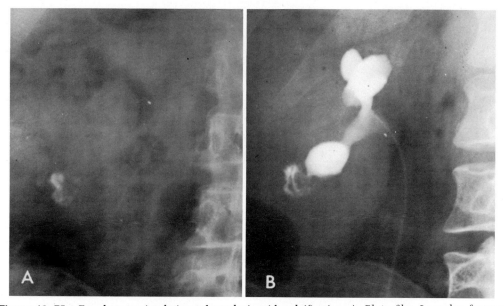

Figure 12–75. Renal stone simulating tuberculosis with calcification. **A,** *Plain film.* Irregular, fragmentary type of calcification in lower pole of right kidney. **B,** *Right retrograde pyelogram.* Unusual caliectasis, with apparent absence of middle calyx. Calcification seems to communicate with, and is adjacent to and below, dilated lower calyx. Could easily be mistaken for tuberculous calcification.

Fig. 12–76   Fig. 12–77

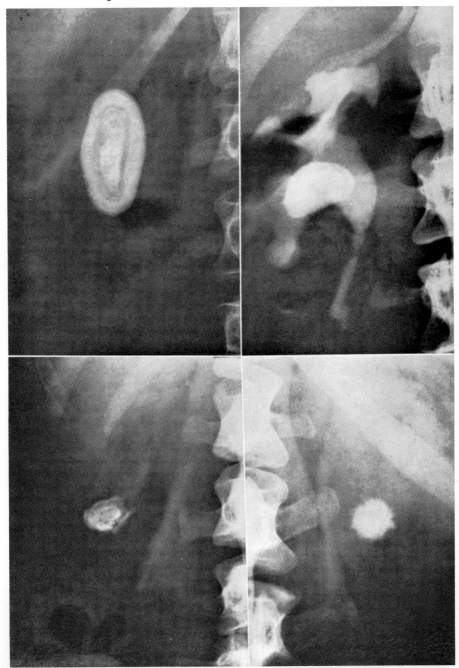

Fig. 12–78   Fig. 12–79

Figure 12–76. *Plain film.* Large laminated stone in right kidney, associated with marked pyelectasis.
Figure 12–77. Laminated stone in renal area. *Right retrograde pyelogram.* Stone free in renal pelvis.
Figure 12–78. *Plain film.* Unusual type of laminated stone in lower calyx of right kidney.
Figure 12–79. *Plain film.* "Burr-like" type of renal stone situated in left renal pelvis.

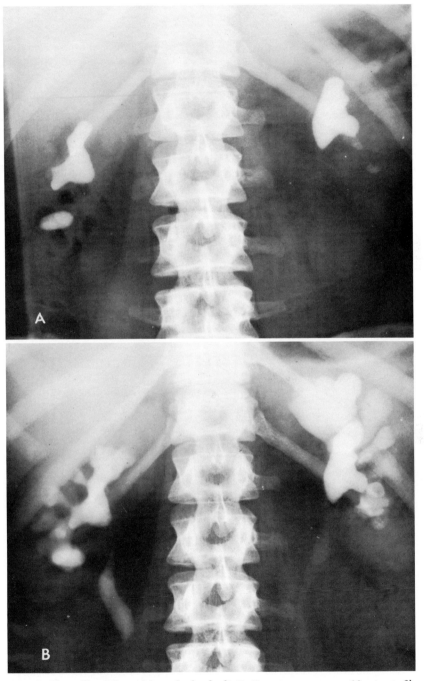

Figure 12–80. A, *Plain film.* **Bilateral branched calculi.** B, *Excretory urogram, 20-minute film.* Moderately good function bilaterally. Considerable caliectasis on left due to obstruction from stone.

function by means of excretory urography. The reason for this is that often the stone completely fills the pelvis and calyces so that no medium can collect around its periphery. If contrast medium cannot be demonstrated in the ureter, some other test of renal function must be used (see previous section on secondary calculi). In some cases the calyces are dilated beyond the tips of the branched calculi so that varying degrees of caliectasis may be demonstrated (Figs. 12–80 through 12–83).

Recurring Calculi

Calculi that recur following surgical removal may assume bizarre shapes because of postoperative deformity of the pelvis and calyces, including calyceal deformity caused by nephrostomy tubes (Figs. 12–84 and 12–85). Calculi that have been spilled in the wound during operation may present some problem in identification (Fig. 12–86).

Calculi in Anomalies

Calculi in anomalous conditions of the kidneys and ureters are discussed in Chapter 9.

"Cortical" Stones; Stones in Calyceal Diverticula or Pyelogenic Cysts

"Cortical" stones may present difficult problems in diagnosis. In most cases they are situated near the calyces, so that the problem nearly always is one of determining whether the stone is in the tip of a calyx, in a walled-off portion of the calyx, in a pyelogenic cyst, diverticulum,* or hydrocalyx, or in the adjacent cortex, not communicating with the pelviocalyceal system. Differential diagnosis here requires use of an excretory urogram to determine whether

---

*See discussion of calyceal diverticulum and pyelogenic cyst, Chapter 11, Urinary Stasis.

Text continued on page 1234

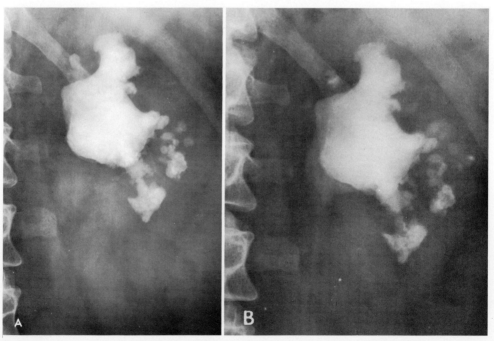

Figure 12–81. A, *Plain film.* Large branched stone forming cast of pelvis and calyces. B, *Excretory urogram, 20-minute film.* Moderately good function, as seen by areas of medium in pelvis and upper ureter just medial to margin of stone.

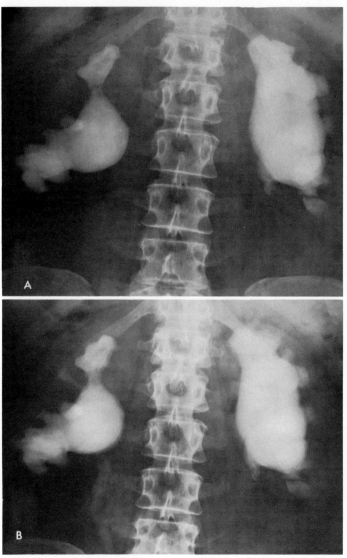

Figure 12–82. A, *Plain film.* **Huge bilateral branched calculi filling pelvis and calyces of both kidneys. B,** *Excretory urogram, 20-minute film.* Evidence of function on right, as shown by contrast medium in lateral branch of upper calyx and ureter. Function also retained in left kidney, as shown by collection of contrast medium around periphery of stone.

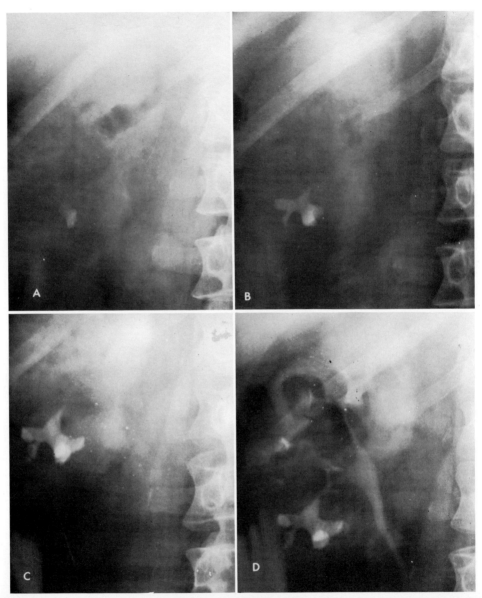

Figure 12–83. Progression in growth of branched calculus from single calculus in tip of minor calyx to one filling entire lower group of calyces, including infundibulum of major calyx. **A,** *Plain film.* Small stone in tip of lower calyx of right kidney. **B,** *Plain film,* 6 months later than **A.** Stone has grown and now fills two branches of lower calyces. **C,** *Plain film,* 19 months later than **B.** Stone has increased in size and now fills larger group of calyces, part of major calyx, and infundibulum. **D,** *Excretory urogram,* same date as **C.** Pelvis and middle and upper calyces normal. Lower group of calyces completely filled by branched calculus.

Fig. 12–84

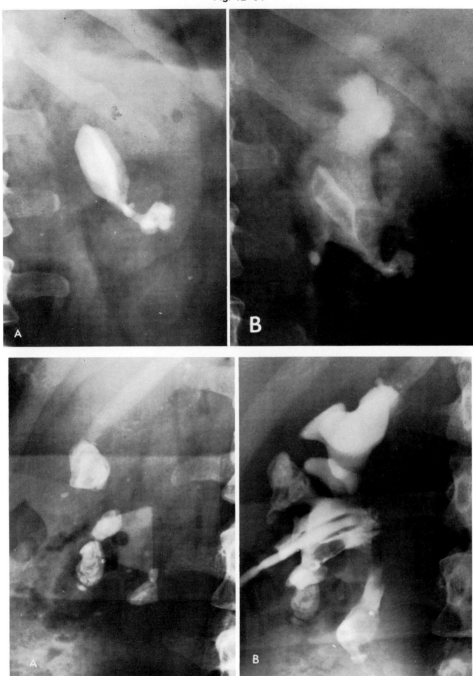

Fig. 12–85

Figure 12–84. Recurring calculi in postoperatively deformed kidney. **A,** *Plain film.* Laminated calculus of unusual shape in left renal area. **B,** *Excretory urogram.* Stone is seen lying in pelvis and postoperatively deformed lower calyx. Moderate pyelectasis.

Figure 12–85. Recurring calculi in postoperatively deformed right kidney and upper part of ureter. **A,** *Plain film.* Multiple calculi of varying sizes, some of which are laminated, overlying right kidney. Adhesive tape, which is securing nephrostomy tube, is also visible. The tube is nonopaque, so it can be seen only with difficulty. **B,** *Right retrograde pyelogram.* Medium injected through nephrostomy tube, which is now visible. Marked deformity, cicatrization, and dilatation of calyces. Stones located in upper and lower calyces and in pelvis. Lowermost large stone is included in deformed, dilated upper part of ureter, just below ureteropelvic juncture.

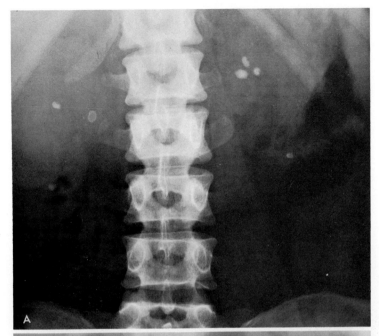

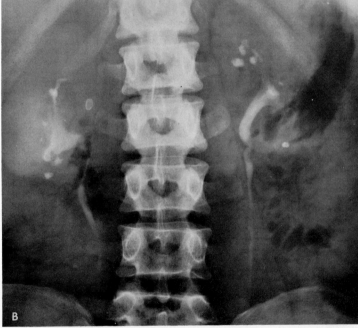

Figure 12–86. Multiple renal calculi, spilled in wound at time of operation. **A,** *Plain film.* Multiple calculi overlying and in vicinity of both kidneys. **B,** *Excretory urogram.* Postoperative deformity of pelves and calyces. Stones are seen to lie outside pelviocalyceal system.

medium surrounds the stone, showing that it communicates with the calyx, or whether there is no communication. Urograms must be made in various oblique positions as well as in the lateral position. In many cases it is not possible to make the distinction accurately until the involved kidney has been explored surgically (Figs. 12–87 through 12–91).

"Milk of Calcium" Renal Stone

Several cases of "milk of calcium" renal stone have been reported in the literature (Benendo and Litwak; Berg and associates; Henken; Howell; Maurer and Wildin; Pullman and King; Rosenberg; Walker and associates). The term "milk of calcium" has been borrowed from a some-

Fig. 12–87

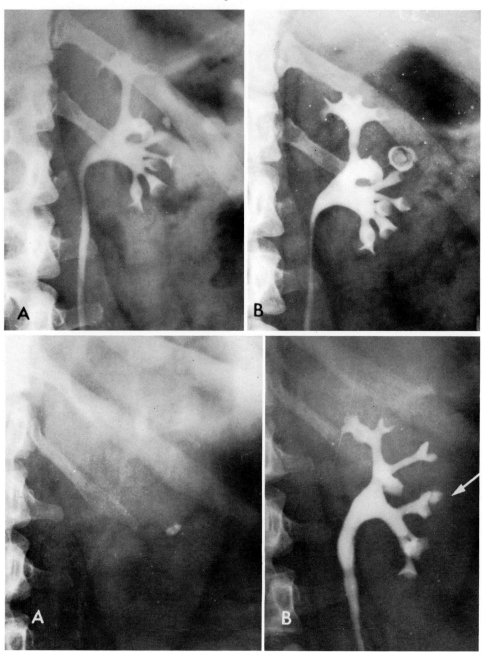

Fig. 12–88

Figure 12–87. Renal cortical or encysted stone. **A,** *Left retrograde pyelogram.* Stone adjacent to, but well removed from, tips of middle and upper calyces. **B,** *Left retrograde pyelogram* made 4 years later. Marked increase in size of cortical stone, which still occupies same position and apparently does not communicate with pelviocalyceal system.

Figure 12–88. Renal cortical or encysted stone. **A,** *Plain film* (made following retrograde pyelography—a little contrast medium remains in upper calyx and ureter). Calcific shadow overlying left renal area. **B,** *Left retrograde pyelogram.* Shadow adjacent to and beyond middle calyx *(arrow);* impossible to tell from these films whether contrast medium surrounds stone.

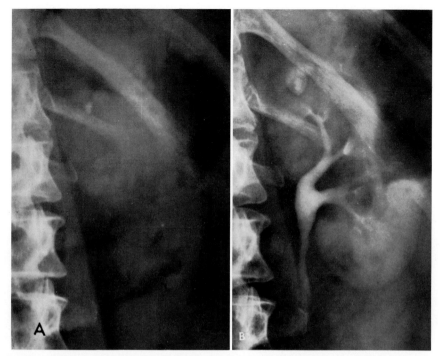

Figure 12–89. A, *Plain film.* **Stone in calyceal diverticulum.** Renal cortical or encysted stone over upper pole of left kidney? **B,** *Excretory urogram.* Shadow seems to be at least 1 cm beyond tip of upper calyx. However, contrast medium surrounds stone, suggesting stone in calyceal diverticulum.

what similar condition encountered in the gallbladder. The "milky" fluid is a suspension of a fine calcific sediment, which has been alleged to be calcium carbonate.

In all reported cases, the "milk of calcium" fluid has been contained, at least initially, either in a calyceal diverticulum with restricted drainage into the calyx or in a pyelogenic cyst (calyceal cyst*) in which no communication with the calyx could be found.

In most cases the condition was asymptomatic and was found only accidentally. In the plain film taken with the patient supine, the appearance suggests an ordinary round or oval solid calculus. With the patient upright or sitting, however, the calcific material gravitates to the bottom of the cyst, resulting in the characteristic "half-moon" contour (Figs. 12–92 and 12–93).

———
*See discussion of calyceal diverticulum and pyelogenic cyst, Chapter 11, Urinary Stasis.

In all of the case reports it has been stated that the material consists of calcium carbonate, as is the case in the gallbladder. However, in only one of the seven reported cases (autopsy case of Walker and associates) was the material actually analyzed, the authors stating that it was calcium carbonate. Boyce (1965) reports that the material consists of small spherules of calcium phosphate (see discussion of "seed calculi," page 1183). Some of the patients have been operated on. In Howell's case (the first reported), the true diagnosis was not suspected before operation, as no film had been made with the patient upright. The condition was considered to be a solid stone, which could not be found at operation. Postoperative films in the upright and lateral positions disclosed the true nature of the lesion. In another case, associated with an infected staghorn calculus, squamous cell carcinoma of the renal pelvis was also found (Berg and associates).

Text continued on page 1241

Fig. 12–90

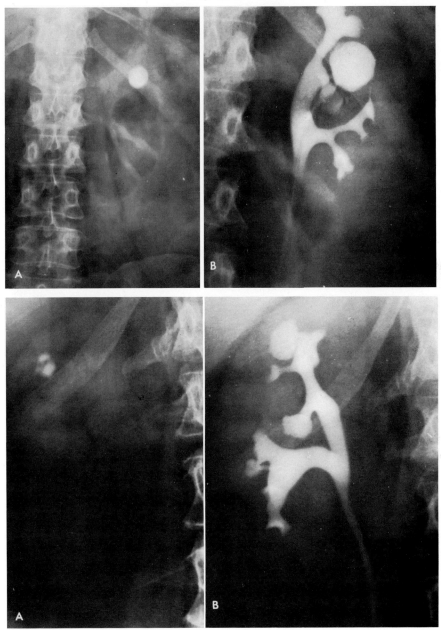

Fig. 12–91

Figure 12–90.   Stone in calyceal diverticulum. **A,** *Plain film.* Calcific shadow over upper pole of left kidney. **B,** *Left retrograde pyelogram.* Medium fills diverticulum and surrounds stone; there apparently is communication with branch of upper calyx.

Figure 12–91.   Stone in calyceal diverticulum. **A,** *Plain film.* Irregular calcific shadow over upper pole of right kidney. **B,** *Right retrograde pyelogram.* Contrast medium fills circular pocket which surrounds stone and apparently communicates with upper calyx.

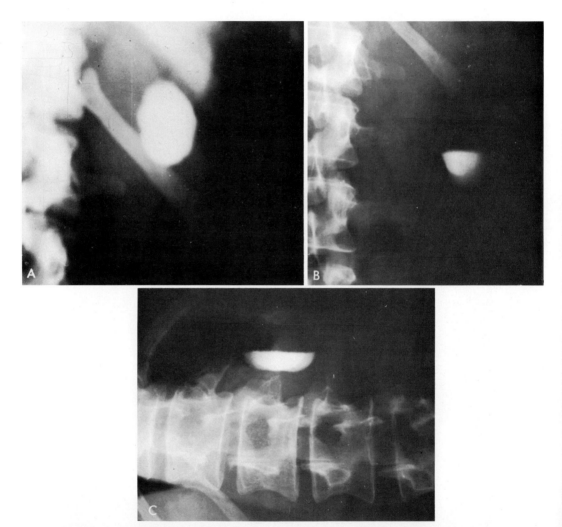

Figure 12–92. "Milk of calcium" stone. A, *Plain film,* supine position. Shadow appears to be oval solid calculus over upper pole of kidney. B, *Upright film.* Calcium material has "layered out," resulting in typical "half-moon" shape. C, *Horizontal right lateral position.* "Half-moon" appearance with convex border projected against spine. (From Boyce, W. H., 1965.)

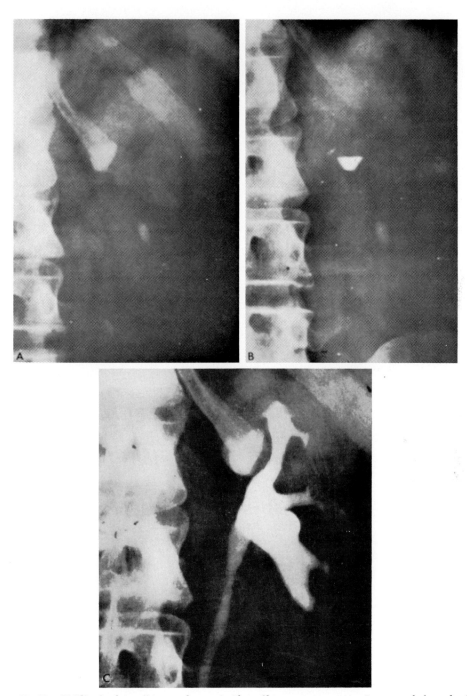

Figure 12–93. "Milk of calcium" in renal cyst. **A,** *Plain film,* supine position. Large oval-shaped calculus in upper pole of left kidney. Smaller stone of less density over lower pole. **B,** *Plain film* in erect position. Upper shadow has "layered out," causing shadow to assume typical "half-moon" contour. Lower shadow unchanged. **C,** *Retrograde pyelogram,* supine position. Upper shadow now assumes original shape. It is "milk of calcium" material in cyst adjacent to upper calyx. No apparent communication with calyx or pelvis. Lower stone is in lower calyx and is obscured by contrast medium. (From Benendo, B., and Litwak, A.)

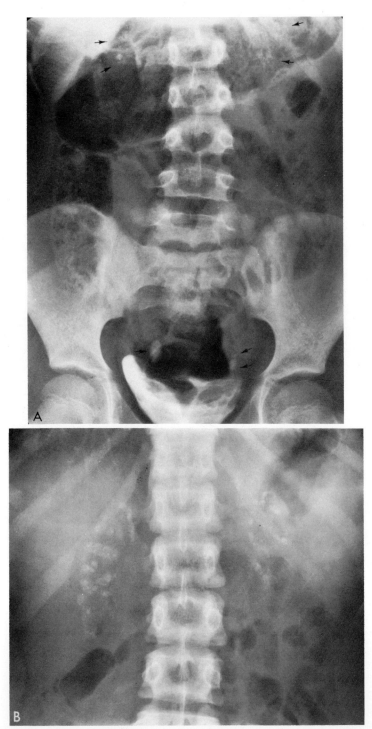

Figure 12–94. Nephrocalcinosis (medullary type), nephrolithiasis, and bilateral ureterolithiasis in 8-year-old girl with type I renal tubular acidosis who presented with hematuria. **A,** *Excretory urogram.* Bilateral renal calculi and ureteral calculi *(arrows).* **B,** *Plain film made 6 years later* shows nephrocalcinosis. **C,** *Excretory urogram (tomogram),* shows thin parenchyma, pyelocaliectasis, and nephrocalcinosis, bilaterally. *Comment:* Patient underwent bilateral ureterolithotomies (calcium oxalate and phosphate calculi) initially and again 4 years later while stone disease remained metabolically inactive on alkali and orthophosphate therapy. (Figures **B** and **C** from Malek, R. S., 1976.)

Illustration continued on opposite page.

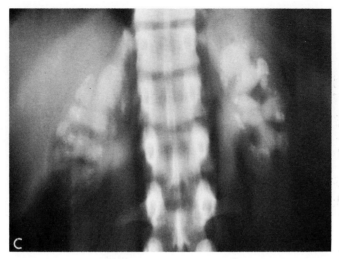

Figure 12–94. *Continued.*

Pathogenesis and Medical Management

The derangements in the internal environment that lead to stone formation are caused by a diversity of metabolic disorders (see Table 12–1). An account of the mechanisms underlying these disorders and of the acceptable methods for their correction is presented in this chapter.

RENAL TUBULAR SYNDROMES

Renal Tubular Acidosis

Renal tubular acidosis (RTA) represents a group of syndromes characterized by defects of hydrogen ion (H^+) excretion (type I) or bicarbonate conservation (type II) by the kidney (Seldin and Wilson).

Type I, the classic type of RTA (because it has been studied longest), results from a defect in the distal tubule, which is unable to generate or maintain the normally steep pH gradient between blood and tubular urine. The most plausible explanation of the defect is an excessive back-diffusion of secreted hydrogen ion from tubular urine to blood, probably because of increased permeability of the distal tubular cells to hydrogen ion; bicarbonate reabsorption is usually normal.

The condition is characterized by a constellation of biochemical disorders, including hyperchloremic acidosis and excessive urinary loss of sodium, potassium, calcium, and phosphate. Its complications are those of systemic acidosis, urolithiasis, nephrocalcinosis, muscular weakness or paralysis, cardiac arrhythmias, osteomalacia, and polyuria; renal failure may supervene.

Calculogenesis is considered to result from hypercalciuria and associated low urinary citrate excretion (the result of systemic acidosis). Not infrequently, however, patients with type I continue to form stones despite correction of metabolic abnormalities when normal quantities of calcium and citrate are being excreted.

Type I RTA may occur in a pure primary form as a transient disease. In this form it usually affects infant boys, who rarely develop radiologic evidence of nephrocalcinosis and who usually recover fully without sequelae after adequate therapy. Alternatively, type I RTA may occur as a persistent disease. This form is found predominantly in girls aged 2 years or older and in adults of both sexes. In 73 per cent of patients with the persistent form, there is associated nephrocalcinosis or lithiasis (Figs. 12–94 through 12–97). The persistent variety occasionally may be

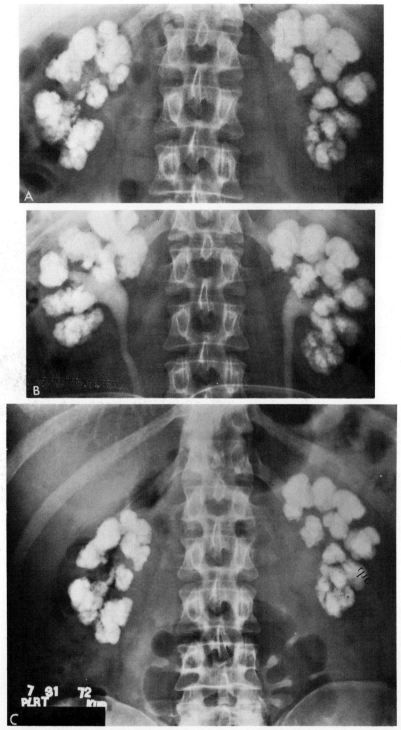

Figure 12–95. Severe nephrocalcinosis (medullary type) in 33-year-old man with type I renal tubular acidosis and recurrent passage of calculi for 11 years (brother also has renal stones). **A,** *Plain film.* Severe bilateral nephrocalcinosis and papillary-tip calcification. **B,** *Excretory urogram* shows medullary calcification, caliectasis, and parenchymal thinning **C,** *Plain film made 4 years later* shows some increase in nephrocalcinosis. *Comment:* During 4 years of alkali therapy, stone disease had remained metabolically and surgically active. Orthophosphate therapy was initiated and stone disease stabilized. (Fig. C from Smith, L H., 1974.)

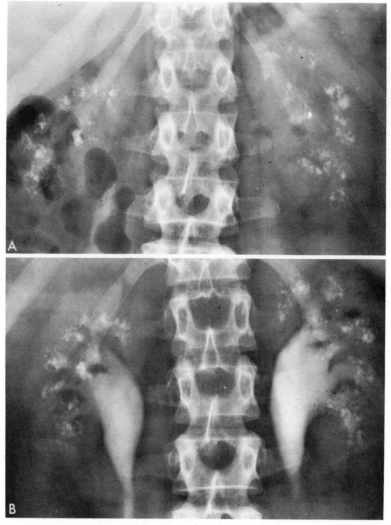

Figure 12–96. Nephrocalcinosis (medullary type) in 38-year-old woman with type I renal tubular acidosis, recurrent passage of calculi (calcium phosphate), and four surgical procedures for removal of calculi, over 11 years. **A,** *Plain film.* Bilateral nephrocalcinosis and papillary-tip calcifications. **B,** *Excretory urogram.* Bilateral cortical scarring and pyelectasis. Calcifications are in medulla and papillary tips. *Comment:* Stone disease remained stable on alkali therapy alone (Courtesy of Dr. C. J. Van Den Berg.)

incomplete, in which case nephrocalcinosis occurs in the absence of hypercalciuria and hyperchloremic acidosis. The transient variety is rarely familial, but dominant transmission with variable expression has been described for the persistent variety. Secondary causes of the type I disorder include various states of hypercalcemia, hyperglobulinemia, and poisoning (amphotericin B) (Seldin and Wilson).

Type II RTA results from defective bicarbonate reabsorption in the proximal tubule. It occurs in a primary form, either as an isolated defect or as part of Fanconi's syndrome, and as a secondary phenomenon in disorders such as heavy metal poisoning, dysproteinemia, rejection reaction to a renal transplant, and hereditary fructose intolerance. The common factor in these diverse disorders is lysozymuria, which results from either systemic overproduction or renal injury. Proximal tubular binding of

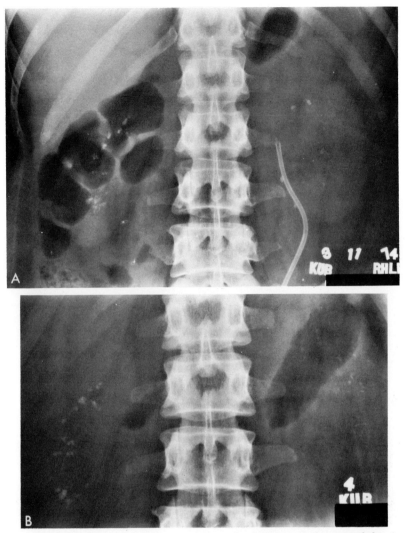

Figure 12–97. Nephrocalcinosis (medullary type), nephrolithiasis, and ureterolithiasis in 39-year-old woman with type I renal tubular acidosis, recurrent colic, and previous left pelviolithotomy. **A,** *Plain film.* Bilateral nephrocalcinosis and lithiasis. Note upper left ureteral calculi and opaque left ureteral catheter. **B,** *Plain film.* Diminution in stone material bilaterally. *Comment:* Several stones passed spontaneously and new stones have not formed (metabolically inactive) during one year of treatment with alkali.

lysozyme could be responsible for impaired bicarbonate reabsorption (Seldin and Wilson).

Only type I RTA has been associated with nephrocalcinosis and lithiasis. The diagnosis depends on demonstration of the inability of the patient to form an acid urine (pH <5.5) in the presence of systemic acidosis (i.e., a plasma bicarbonate concentration of 20 mEq per liter) with normal bicarbonate conservation by the kidney. In health, the kidney can usually acidify the urine (pH <5.5) after a twelve-hour fast, whereas in type I disease the kidney cannot lower the urine pH below 6.0; these facts are used as the basis for a screening test. The diagnosis may be confirmed by an ammonium chloride challenge (100 mg per kg of body weight daily in four divided doses): the diagnosis is confirmed if, when the plasma bicarbonate concentration has reached 20 mEq per liter (without bicarbonate wasting by the kidney), the pH of urine has not diminished to less than 5.5.

The test must be carried out when the urine is sterile because urinary pH is altered by bacterial metabolism.

Correction of the metabolic derangements with replacement of bicarbonate, sodium, and potassium is the first line of treatment. It is convenient to use a solution (Polycitra*) that consists of sodium citrate, potassium citrate, and citric acid to provide 1 to 3 mEq of bicarbonate per kilogram of body weight in 24 hours; it is given in four divided doses. Administration of sodium bicarbonate with a potassium supplement is another form of replacement therapy. Additional therapy with orally administered phosphate (to provide 1.5 to 2.0 g daily of inorganic phosphorus) has been effective in patients who continue to form stones despite achieving metabolic balance (see Figures 12–94 through 12–97).

Carbonic Anhydrase Inhibition

Carbonic anhydrase inhibitors (e.g., acetazolamide) can induce metabolic derangements that are similar to type I RTA. Calculogenesis usually stops after the drug has been discontinued. The oral administration of phosphate also may be beneficial (Smith, 1974).

Cystinuria

Cystinuria is an inborn error of amino acid transport in the kidney and intestine. Excessive amounts of cystine, ornithine, arginine, and lysine are excreted in the urine. The only recognized complication of this disorder is stone formation, which results from the limited solubility of cystine in urine (Thier and Segal). Cystinuria must not be confused with cystinosis (a manifestation of the Fanconi-Lignac syndrome), which is complicated by the deposition of cystine in the reticuloendothelial system and elsewhere *without* stone formation.

Cystinuria is inherited in an autosomal recessive manner. It is the homozygote, in

*Willen Drug Company, Baltimore, MD 21202.

whom the daily excretion of cystine and the other three amino acids usually amounts to more than 500 mg, who is the stone-former. The completely recessive heterozygote (type I) is normal, but the incompletely recessive heterozygote (types II and III) manifests cystinuria (150 to 300 mg per 24 hours) and lysinuria without stone formation (Smith, 1974).

A screening test with the cyanide-nitroprusside reaction is positive when cystinuria is in excess of 75 mg per gram of urine creatinine. But because the screening test may be positive in heterozygotes as well as in homozygotes, quantitative analysis of urinary amino acids is also necessary (Thier and Segal).

Therapy is designed to decrease the concentration of urinary cystine (by increasing urine volume) and concomitantly to increase its solubility (by raising urinary pH). Diuresis exceeding 2.5 liters every 24 hours is achieved by having the patient take drinks hourly during the waking hours and at least once nightly (at 0200). The urine is made alkaline by means of a solution of sodium and potassium citrate and citric acid (Polycitra). A dose of 15 ml is taken after each meal and again at 0200.

At maximal urine alkalinity (pH 7.5 to 7.8), the amount of cystine that can be held in solution is doubled. Adherence to nocturnal treatments is most critical in patients with cystinuria, for it is during the night that urine volume and pH both decrease. Methionine is a primary source of cystine, and therefore rigid dietary restriction of protein can diminish urinary cystine levels, but protein restriction is poorly tolerated, not recommended in children, and seldom used.

For chemolysis of existing cystine stones and control in occasional stone formers who do not respond to conservative measures, D-penicillamine (with supplemental vitamin B_6) may be added to the regimen (Figs. 12–98 and 12–99). D-Penicillamine combines with cysteine, the precursor of cystine, to form a disulfide complex ten times as soluble in urine as is cystine; as a result, the urinary cystine

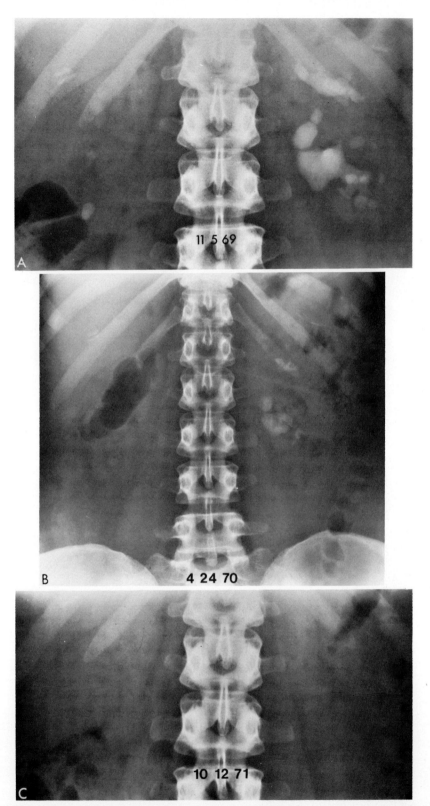

Figure 12–98. **Effect of chemolysis on cystine stones** in 32-year-old cystinuric woman with a twelve-year history of recurrent passage of calculi and multiple bilateral renal and ureteral operations. (Sister and maternal aunt and uncle are also stone formers.) **A,** *Plain film.* Bilateral homogeneous opaque cystine calculi. (From Smith, L. H., 1974.) **B,** *Plain film.* Diminution of stone materal bilaterally on therapy. **C,** *Plain film.* Complete dissolution of calculi. *Comment:* Treatment consisted of hydration, urinary alkalinization, and *d*-penicillamine with vitamin B_6 supplement.

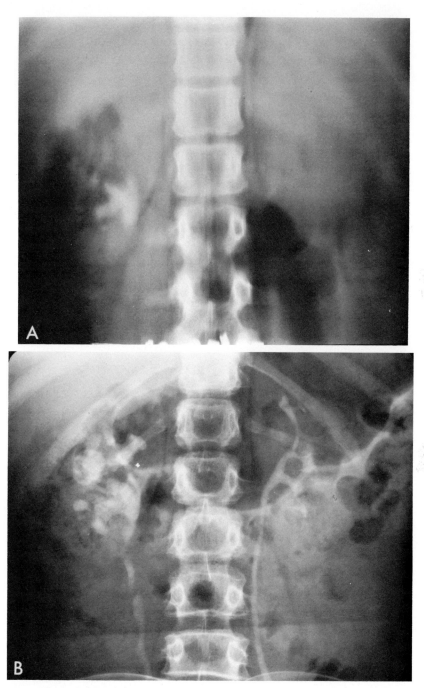

Figure 12–99.   Effect of chemolysis on cystine stones in 14-year-old cystinuric boy with a ten-year history of hematuria, recurrent stone formation, and multiple surgical procedures for removal of calculi. **A,** *Plain film (tomogram).* Homogeneous branched stone and smaller "satellite" cystine stones on right side. **B,** *Excretory urogram.* Postoperative deformities of right calyces and upper ureter. Note that there is no significant obstruction.

Illustration and legend continued on following page

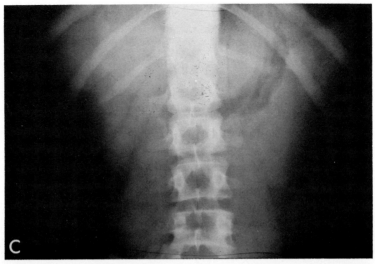

Figure 12–99. *Continued.* **C,** *Plain film.* Complete dissolution of right renal calculi. *Comment:* Treatment consisted of hydration, urinary alkalinization, and *d*-penicillamine with vitamin B$_6$ supplement. (Figures **A** and **C,** from Malek, R. S., 1976.)

concentration is diminished. For the dissolution of preexisting stones, 1.0 to 2.0 g is administered daily in four divided doses (30 minutes before meals and at bedtime) to reduce the urinary cystine concentration to less than 200 mg every 24 hours. For patients who require D-penicillamine in addition to conservative measures, the dosage should be the minimum amount sufficient to arrest the stone disease. The drug has serious side effects, including acute hypersensitivity, agranulocytosis, proteinuria, the nephrotic syndrome, and vitamin B$_6$ deficiency; it is not therefore a substitute for an otherwise adequate conservative program. Surgical activity or calcification of the stone during therapy which prevents its dissolution may make it necessary to remove the calculus before subsequent maintenance on conservative therapy (Figs. 12–100 and 12–101).

Glycinuria

Glycinuria is a rare genetically transmitted tubular defect that is clinically manifested by oxalate urolithiasis (de Vries and associates). No effective treatment exists except hydration and alkalinization.

ENZYME DISORDERS

Primary Hyperoxaluria

Primary hyperoxaluria is a rare genetic disorder of glyoxylic acid metabolism that results in the increased synthesis and excretion of oxalate. The mode of transmission is autosomal recessive (Williams and Smith).

Two enzyme defects are recognized; they both result in the accumulation of glyoxylic acid and its conversion to the end-product, oxalic acid. Type I hyperoxaluria (glycolic aciduria) is characterized by an increase in the urinary excretion of oxalic acid, glyoxylic acid, and glycolic acid; it is due to deficiency of 2-oxo-glutarate: glyoxylate *carboligase;* this is the most common form of the inherited disorder. In type II hyperoxaluria (L-glyceric aciduria), there is a great increase in the excretion of L-glyceric acid; glycolic acid excretion is normal. This condition is due to a deficiency in D-glyceric *dehydrogenase.*

Clinical manifestations of the disease usually relate to nephrocalcinosis and lithiasis (Figs. 12–102, 12–103, and 12–104; also see Figure 12–3). The onset of symp-

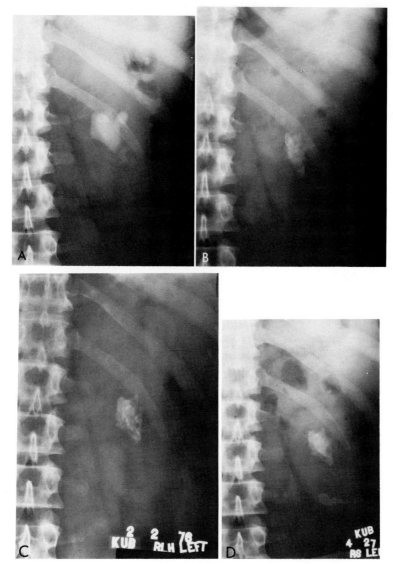

Figure 12–100. Failure of chemolytic program owing to subsequent calcifications of partially lysed cystine stone in 41-year-old cystinuric man with solitary left kidney (right nephrectomy elsewhere for stone disease). **A,** *Plain film.* Typical cystine stone on left side. **B,** *Plain film.* Some decrease in size of stone on chemolytic program for 1 year. **C,** *Plain film 1 year later* shows stone is unchanged in size, but increase in density suggests calcification of matrix. **D,** *Plain film 6 years later* shows stone is still unchanged. *Comment:* Patient is asymptomatic and faithfully follows usual program.

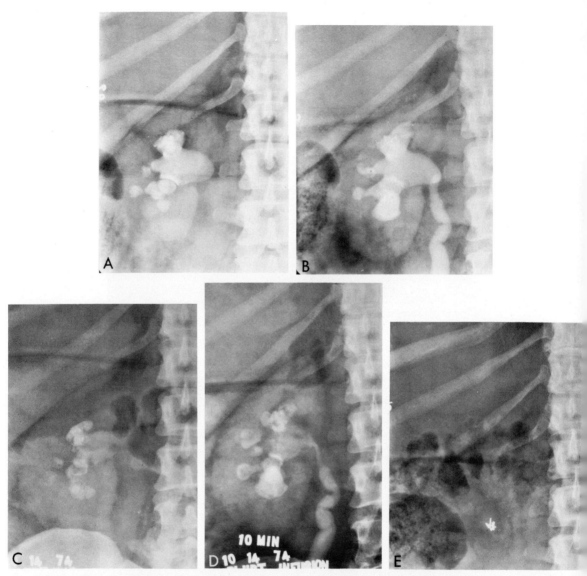

Figure 12–101.   Failure of chemolytic program owing to urinary infection in 49-year-old cystinuric man who also has primary hyperparathyroidism. **A,** *Plain film.* Staghorn calculus in right kidney. Urine is infected. **B,** *Excretory urogram.* Good excretion of contrast medium by stone-bearing right kidney. Right ureter is dilated. **C,** *Plain film.* Some diminution of stone material, but not impressive after 1½ years of treatment. **D,** *Excretory urogram.* Right kidney remains unobstructed, but patient has symptomatic urosepsis. **E,** *Plain film 4 months after right pelviolithotomy.* Right kidney is free of stone and infection. Note surgical metallic clips in right renal area. *Comment:* Parathyroidectomy was performed before chemolytic program of hydration, urinary alkalinization, and *d*-penicillamine with vitamin B$_6$ supplement was begun. Antibiotics were also used, but infection persisted. Stone composition was cystine, calcium oxalate, calcium phosphate, and calcium carbonate. Patient is now maintained on hydration and urinary alkalinization only.

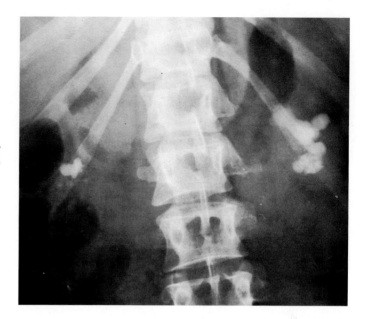

Figure 12–102. *Plain film.* **Primary hyperoxaluria** in 35-year-old woman with dense, bilateral stones.

toms usually occurs before the age of 5 years; both sexes are equally affected. Some patients present with uremia and growth retardation; rarely, acute arthritis and cardiac symptoms ensue, owing to widespread deposition of oxalate in tissues (oxalosis). The majority of undiagnosed and untreated patients die of renal failure before they reach the age of 20 (Williams and Smith).

Hyperoxaluria may be acquired in several ways, including the ingestion of ethylene glycol, excessive amounts of rhubarb, or doses of ascorbic acid (vitamin C) in excess of 2.0 grams within 24 hours. Pyridoxine (vitamin B_6) is a coenzyme in the conversion of glyoxylic acid to glycine, and hyperoxaluria has been reported in states of pyridoxine deficiency. Increased oxalate excretion can also occur in association with

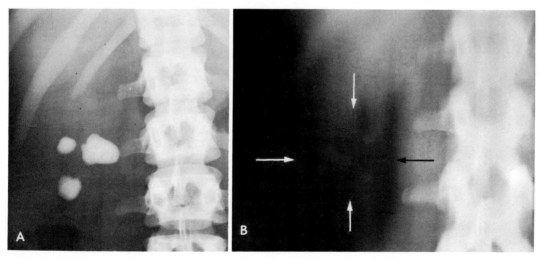

Figure 12–103. **Primary hyperoxaluria. A,** *Plain film.* Original stones present in right kidney in 1959 were dense and homogeneous. **B,** *Plain film.* Patient developed *Proteus* bacteriuria postoperatively and formed five stones. These contained small amounts of calcium oxalate, but the major crystal component was struvite (magnesium ammonium phosphate). The stones were much less dense on roentgenogram (*arrows*).

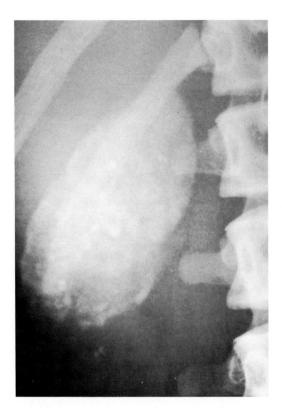

Figure 12–104. *Plain film.* **Primary hyperoxaluria.** **Diffuse nephrocalcinosis** in solitary right kidney of 26-year-old woman with renal insufficiency due to primary hyperoxaluria. She also had oxalate crystals in her bone marrow.

cirrhosis, renal tubular acidosis, and sarcoidosis; the mechanism is obscure (Smith, Fromm, and Hofmann). (The syndrome of hyperoxaluria, nephrolithiasis, and intestinal disease is discussed separately on page 1269).

The diagnosis of primary hyperoxaluria is based on the finding of an increased excretion of urinary oxalate (the normal urinary oxalate excretion is less than 40 mg per 24 hours). Yet the absolute quantity of oxalate excreted within a 24-hour period varies greatly among individual patients with this condition, and the amount in the urine cannot always be used to predict the severity and progression of the disease (Smith, Jones, and Keating).

Experience with the treatment of primary hyperoxaluria is very limited, but stone formation may be controlled by the oral administration of pyridoxine, 50 mg three times daily, and phosphate (as inorganic phosphorus), 1.5 to 2.0 g daily in four divided doses (Figs. 12–105 and 12–106) (Smith, Jones, and Keating).

Xanthinuria

Xanthinuria is an exceedingly rare genetic disorder of purine metabolism in which a deficiency of xanthine oxidase results in an increased secretion of xanthine, decreased amounts of uric acid in the serum and urine, and xanthine stone formation (Fig. 12–107). In modern medical practice, the use of allopurinol, a xanthine oxidase inhibitor, is by far the commonest cause of xanthinuria; indeed, xanthine stones have occasionally occurred in patients taking allopurinol (Wyngaarden). To prevent xanthine stone formation, a high fluid intake and, if necessary, alkalinization of the urine are helpful.

HYPERCALCEMIC STATES

Acute hypercalcemia initially damages the collecting ducts, resulting in ADH-resistant polyuria with hypotonic urine. Clinical uremia may follow days or weeks

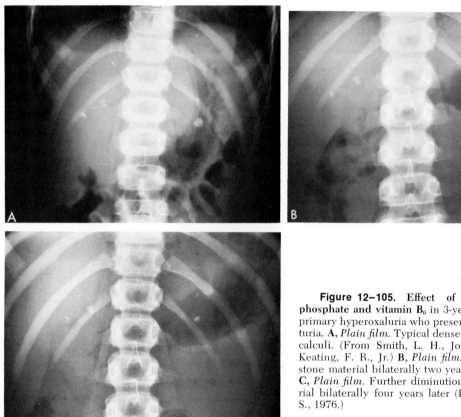

Figure 12–105. Effect of therapy with phosphate and vitamin B_6 in 3-year-old girl with primary hyperoxaluria who presented with hematuria. **A,** *Plain film.* Typical dense calcium oxalate calculi. (From Smith, L. H., Jones, J. D., and Keating, F. R., Jr.) **B,** *Plain film.* Diminution of stone material bilaterally two years after therapy. **C,** *Plain film.* Further diminution of stone material bilaterally four years later (From Malek, R. S., 1976.)

of sustained elevation of the serum calcium concentration to 15 mg/dl or higher.

Chronic hypercalcemia causes renal calcification—initially in the collecting tubules and next in Henle's loop, convoluted tubules, glomeruli, and blood vessels. Radiographically, the calcification is usually seen in the medulla, but it may spread to the cortex. Renal tubular blockage with dilatation and interstitial and periglomerular fibrosis initially results in polydipsia and polyuria that are disproportionate to the depression in the glomerular filtration rate. Later, chronic renal failure, hypertension, and metastatic calcification follow.

The usual causes of hypercalcemia that may be associated with stone disease are listed in Table 12–1. Correction of the primary disorder prevents further stone formation.

Primary Hyperparathyroidism

Primary hyperparathyroidism is the hypercalcemic disorder that is most commonly associated with stones. An estimated 2 to 10 per cent of stone-formers have been found to have hyperparathyroidism (Pyrah and associates). Renal lithiasis (in 46 per cent of cases), nephrocalcinosis (in 5 per

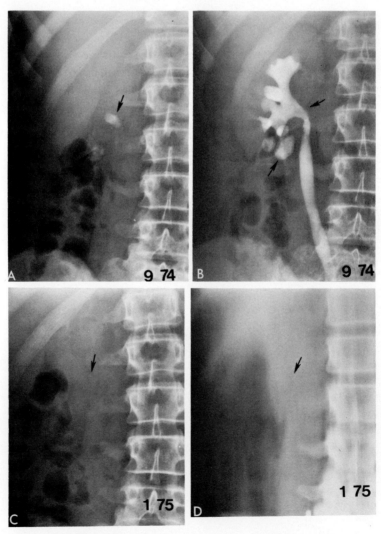

Figure 12–106. *See opposite page for legend.*

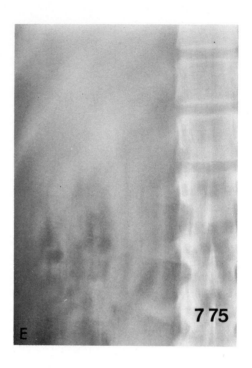

Figure 12–106. Effect of therapy with phosphate and vitamin B_6 in 12-year-old boy with primary hyperoxaluria who presented with colic and passage of gravel. **A,** *Plain film.* Calcium oxalate stone impacted at right ureteropelvic juncture *(upper arrow).* Collection of calcium phosphate, carbonate, and oxalate calculi in region of right lower pole. **B,** *Excretory urogram.* Impacted stone at right ureteropelvic juncture with resultant caliectasis and edema of upper right ureter *(upper arrow).* Lower-pole calculi are in diseased dilated lower-pole calyx *(lower arrow).* **C,** *Plain film.* Tiny recurrent right renal stone *(arrow)* barely visible 4½ months after pelviolithotomy and excision of diseased stone-bearing lower-pole calyx. **D,** *Plain film (tomogram).* Stone is definitely identified. **E,** *Plain film (tomogram).* No evidence of stone formation 6 months after more intensive phosphate therapy. *Comment:* Importance of using tomography to detect tiny recurrent calculi early, thereby identifying metabolic activity and allowing institution of more effective therapy, is well demonstrated in this case.

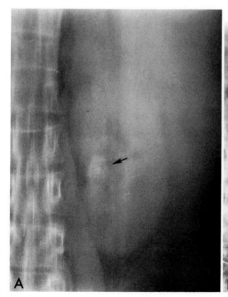
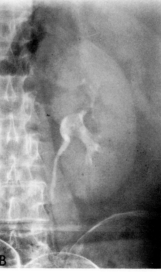

Figure 12–107. Xanthinuria with stone formation in 38-year-old man with severe liver disease (sclerosing cholangitis and secondary biliary cirrhosis) and related deficiency of xanthine oxidase. **A,** *Plain film (tomogram).* Stone of poor radiopacity in left renal pelvis *(arrow).* **B,** *Excretory urogram.* Negative filling defect produced by faintly opaque branched stone.

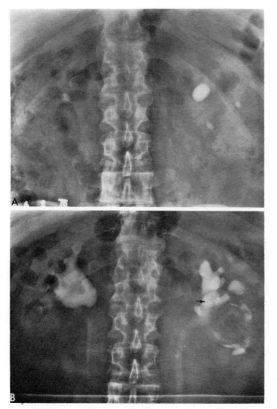

Figure 12–108. Bilateral renal calculi in patient with primary hyperparathyroidism. **A,** *Plain film.* Bilateral renal calculi. **B,** *Excretory urogram.* **Congenital diverticulum of right stone-containing renal pelvis.** Large left renal stone causes partial obstruction to upper-pole infundibulum *(arrow).* Other smaller left renal calculi are in lower-pole calyces deformed by large renal cyst.

cent), and significant impairment of renal function (in 8 per cent) are the most common complications (Figs. 12–108 and 12–109). Yet only in 10.5 per cent of the stone-forming patients is the stone disease metabolically active (Malek, 1974). No significant differences in urinary excretion of calcium and magnesium have been observed among those with metabolically active stone disease, those with inactive stone disease, and those without stones; thus, other factors such as hydroxyprolinuria must also contribute (Malek 1974; Malek and Kelalis, June 1976). The exact nature of and reasons for the earliest, reversible changes in renal function, manifested by tubular inability to concentrate (polyuria, nocturia) and acidify urine, are poorly understood. More advanced functional impairment accompanied by histologic evidence of renal parenchymal damage, reflected in diminished renal plasma flow and glomerular filtration rate, has been reported in a significant proportion of patients. The most severe and irreversible changes have occurred in patients with advanced bone disease or nephrocalcinosis (Pyrah and Hodgkinson). Relief of calculous obstruction, treatment of urinary infection, and parathyroidectomy obviously would help to normalize renal function (Malek, 1974).

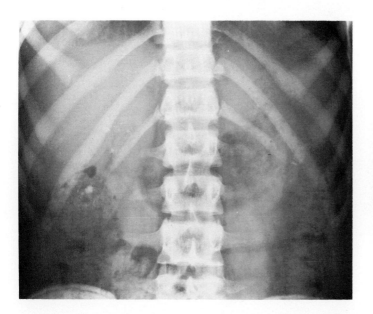

Figure 12–109. Nephrocalcinosis (medullary type) and nephrolithiasis in 15-year-old girl with primary hyperparathyroidism who presented with painful hematuria. *Plain film.* Bilateral nephrocalcinosis, more severe on right, and stone in right lower-pole calyx (From Malek, R. S , 1976.)

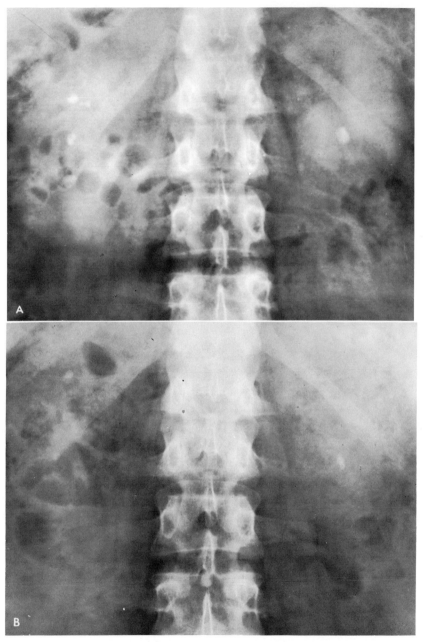

Figure 12–110 Partial dissolution of calculi following removal of parathyroid adenoma. Bilateral renal calculi in woman, 27 years of age, with hyperparathyroidism (serum calcium, 15.0 mg; serum phosphate, 1.9 mg per 100 ml). **A,** *Plain film* made before excision of right superior parathyroid gland because of parathyroid adenoma, chief cell type. **B,** *Plain film* made 6 months after operation. Note substantial reduction in size of all calculi

At this time, the key to the diagnosis of primary hyperparathyroidism still is accurate determination of the serum calcium in a clinical setting compatible with the diagnosis. Recently, determination of the serum immunoreactive parathyroid hormone (iPTH) has proved to be an invaluable diagnostic adjunct (see below). Almost all stone-formers with primary hyperparathyroidism remain well, with inactive stone disease, after parathyroid adenectomy, which should be carried out before appropriate treatment of calculous disease is undertaken; the reverse order is fraught with dangers of postoperative hypercalcemic crisis and rapid recurrence of calculi (Malek, 1974) (Figs. 12–110 and 12–111).

Stone disease may continue to be active even after parathyroidectomy. This represents the coexistence of hyperparathyroidism and idiopathic stone disease and requires phosphate therapy (also see sec-

tion on uric acid lithiasis) (Fig. 12–112). Complicated situations such as the coexistence of tumors producing parathormone-like substances with primary hyperparathyroidism tax the judgment of most clinicians. An increase in the serum immunoreactive parathyroid hormone (iPTH) that shows a positive correlation with the degree of hypercalcemia appears to be produced specifically by the hyperfunctioning parathyroid gland. In our experience, this correlation serves as a useful aid in differentiating this entity from the hypercalcemia of malignancy (Malek, 1974). Exceptionally, a substance produced by renal cell carcinomas seems to have immunoreactive characteristics identical with those of true parathyroid hormone. The actual cause of hypercalcemia occurring under such circumstances may be determined only in a step-by-step fashion by elimination and careful reevaluation (Fig. 12–113).

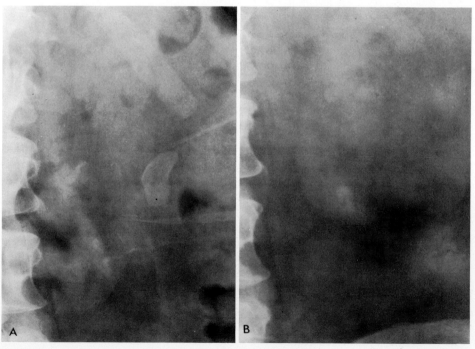

Figure 12–111.   Partial dissolution of calculi following removal of parathyroid adenoma. Left renal calculus and hyperparathyroidism in man, 48 years of age. **A,** *Plain film* shows **large calculus in lower pole of left kidney. B,** *Plain film* made 4 months after surgical removal of parathyroid adenoma. Great reduction in size of stone.

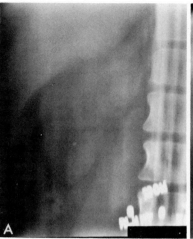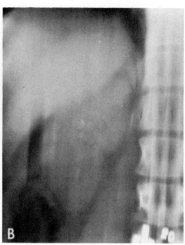

Figure 12–112. Example of stone disease remaining active after successful parathyroidectomy. **A,** *Plain film (tomogram).* Small stone in lower pole of right kidney in patient with hyperparathyroidism. **B** *Plain film (tomogram) made 6 months after parathyroidectomy and normalization of serum calcium* shows additional new stone formation near upper pole of right kidney. Lower-pole stone is also present but is out of focus.

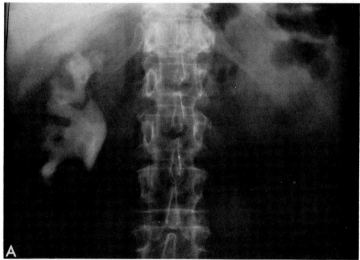

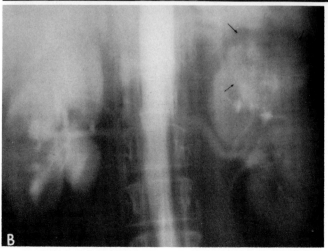

Figure 12–113. Example of primary hyperparathyroidism, nephrolithiasis, and renal cell carcinoma discovered simultaneously in 62-year-old woman with ten-year history of recurrent renal calculi **A,** *Plain film.* Staghorn calculus (struvite) right kidney. **B,** *Nephrotomogram.* Hypernephroma of upper pole left kidney (*arrows*).

Illustration and legend continued on following page

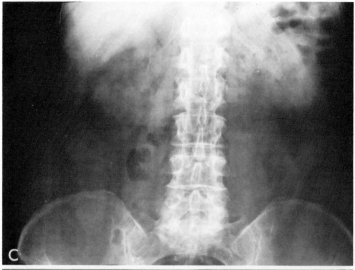

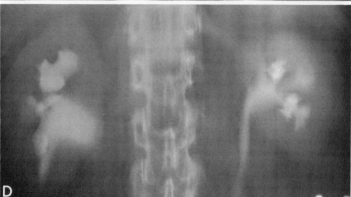

Figure 12–113. *Continued.* **C,** *Plain film.* No residual or recurrent calculi 2 years later. **D,** *Excretory urogram.* Normal right kidney after nephrolithotomy. Small left kidney after partial (upper pole) nephrectomy for removal of renal cell carcinoma. *Comment:* Patient underwent left partial nephrectomy followed by right nephrolithotomy 6 months later. Parathyroidectomy was carried out almost 2 years later because serum calcium remained elevated and serum iPTH was also elevated.

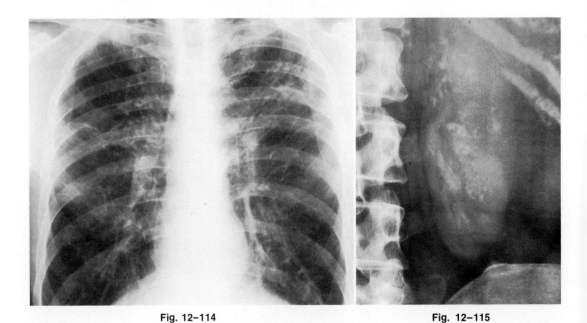

Fig. 12–114   Fig. 12–115

Figure 12–114. Sarcoidosis. Pulmonary involvement.
Figure 12–115. *Plain film.* **Nephrocalcinosis** in woman, 64 years of age, with sarcoidosis of many years' standing.

Sarcoidosis

Nephrocalcinosis, lithiasis, metastatic calcification, and renal insufficiency all may complicate sarcoidosis (Figs. 12–114 and 12–115). Sarcoidosis affects women more frequently than men (ratio 3 to 2), but life-threatening complications are more likely to occur in men. An estimated 5 to 30 per cent of patients have hypercalcemia (Scholz and Keating, 1956). Calcific deposits occur within the tubular lumina, in the interstitium, and in the cortex. Hypercalciuria (600 to 1,000 mg per 24 hours) may occur, with or without hypercalcemia; it seems to be caused by the increased intestinal absorption of dietary calcium resulting from hypersensitivity to vitamin D (Smith, 1972a). Additionally, hyperuricosuria and hyperoxaluria may occur (Fig. 12–116).

The administration of corticosteroids to patients with sarcoidosis is followed by a decrease in urinary calcium excretion and an increase in fecal calcium content. The mode of action of steroids in this respect is

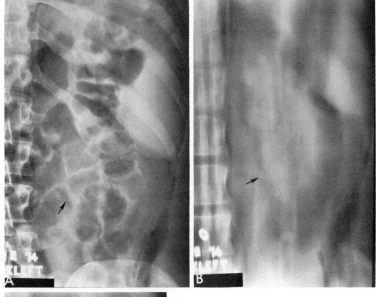

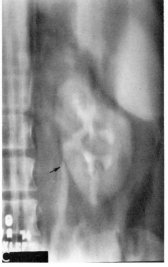

Figure 12–116. Sarcoidosis, hypercalcemia, hyperuricemia, hypercalciuria, and hyperuricosuria in 35-year-old man with four-year history of recurrent passage of calculi. **A,** *Plain film.* Stone of poor radiopacity in region of left kidney *(arrow).* **B,** *Plain film (tomogram).* Better delineation of calculus *(arrow).* **C,** *Excretory urogram.* Calculus is at ureteropelvic juncture *(arrow).* Also note additional stone causing negative filling defect in lower-pole calyx. *Comment:* Pelviolithotomy was carried out. Calculi consisted of calcium oxalate and phosphate. Patient was treated with steroids.

not understood, but temporary or permanent healing of sarcoid granulomas may follow.

Hypervitaminosis D

Excessive intake of vitamin D may cause hypercalcemia with subsequent stone formation and nephrocalcinosis. Other conditions may also result from excessive intake of this vitamin or an abnormal sensitivity to it (Smith, 1974) (see section on idiopathic infantile hypercalcemia).

Milk-Alkali Syndrome

The features of the milk-alkali syndrome, which results from prolonged intake of excessive amounts of milk, milk products (especially cheese), and absorbable alkali (any or all of these), include hypercalcemia without hypercalciuria, normal concentrations of serum alkaline phosphatase and phosphorus, alkalosis, renal insufficiency, and metastatic calcification.

The calculogenic potential of this syndrome is clearly corroborated by our findings of intranephronic calculosis in a group of patients treated by a dietary regimen

unusually high in milk; a substantial number of these patients form stones (Malek and Boyce, 1973).

Neoplasms

Neoplasms of the thyroid, prostate, breast, kidney, and lung often metastasize to bones. Hypercalcemia reportedly develops at some stage in approximately 9 per cent of patients who have such neoplasms (Myers) and in 70 per cent of patients with multiple myeloma, although nephrocalcinosis has rarely been demonstrated radiographically in multiple myeloma (Gutman and Yü (Fig. 12–117). Hypercalcemia may also occur in leukemia and lymphoma.

Certain tumors such as carcinoma of the lung, kidney, ovary, testis, penis, or bladder can cause hypercalcemia in the absence of bony metastases. These families of tumors have been shown to elaborate parathormone-like substances (see section on primary hyperparathyroidism). Oncolytic therapy is the treatment of choice.

In patients with metastatic rhabdomyosarcoma, the use of strontium-87 has made it possible to detect renal parenchymal calcification that is not visible roentgenogra-

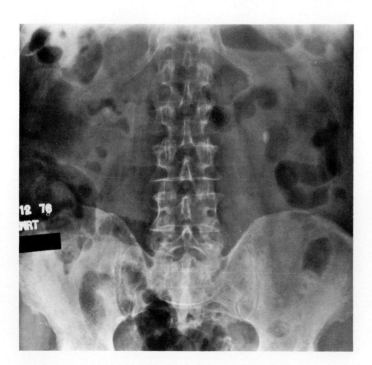

Figure 12–117. *Plain film.* **Left renal calculus.** Patient was a 75-year-old man who presented with widespread multiple myeloma (involving skull, bony pelvis, and ribs) and resultant hypercalcemia.

phically. In ⁸⁷ᵐSr whole-body scans done on such patients, uptake of ⁸⁷ᵐSr is intense and localized to the renal outline; radiographically visible but stable nephrocalcinosis, on the other hand, shows little if any radiostrontium uptake (Samuels and Smith). This technique has obvious potentialities, among which determination of metabolic activity of stone disease may prove useful.

Cushing's Syndrome

In Cushing's syndrome and in prolonged corticoid therapy, abnormal breakdown of protein results in loss of bone matrix. This, in turn, is followed by resorption of calcium, hypercalciuria, and associated urolithiasis in as many as 30 per cent of patients with Cushing's syndrome (Hurxthal and O'Sullivan).

Nephrocalcinosis (Fig. 12–118) and urolithiasis (Figs. 12–119 and 12–120) may be associated with endogenous or exogenous hypercorticism. The latter may result when steroids are used in the treatment of patients with myopathies, the nephrotic syndrome, aplastic anemia, or other conditions requiring prolonged use of large amounts of steroids (Malek and Kelalis, 1975a).

Hyperthyroidism

Hyperthyroidism is often associated with osteoporosis, increased calcium excretion, and accelerated turnover of calcium stores. Hypercalcemia secondary to hyperthyroidism is uncommon; it may result in urolithiasis, nephrocalcinosis, and renal insufficiency that may be reversible with effective treatment of thyrotoxicosis (Epstein and associates) (Fig. 12–121).

Idiopathic Infantile Hypercalcemia

Idiopathic infantile hypercalcemia, which begins in the first year of life, may be classified as an inborn error of metabolism of vitamin D or related substances, whose serum activity in these children may be 20 to 30 times that found in normal infants (Fellers and Schwartz). An identical picture may be produced by hypervitaminosis D. Hypercalcemia, hypercalciuria, and nephrocalcinosis are the usual manifestations; azotemia and hypertension may follow. Elfin facies, dwarfism, mental retardation, and osteosclerosis may be features of severe forms of the condition.

The **blue-diaper syndrome** results from a defect in the intestinal transport of tryptophan. Bacterial degradation of the tryp-

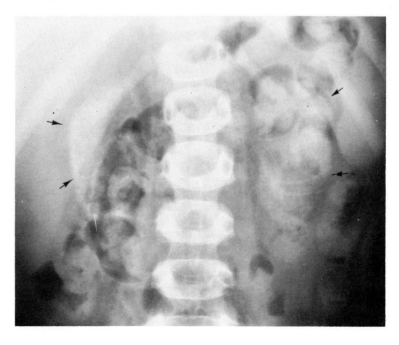

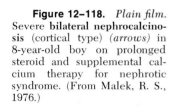

Figure 12–118. *Plain film.* Severe **bilateral nephrocalcinosis** (cortical type) *(arrows)* in 8-year-old boy on prolonged steroid and supplemental calcium therapy for nephrotic syndrome. (From Malek, R. S., 1976.)

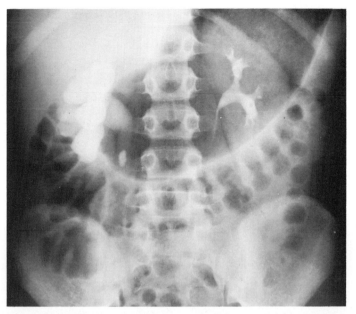

Figure 12–119. *Excretory urogram.* Hydronephrotic right kidney with **large calcium oxalate stone** in upper ureter. Patient was an 8-year-old boy on prolonged steroid therapy for nephritis. (From Malek, R. S., 1976.)

tophan, followed by excessive production of indole, leads to indicanuria; oxidation causes the urine to become indigo blue, producing the blue coloration of the diaper. This condition is also associated with hypercalcemia and nephrocalcinosis (Drummond and associates).

Treatment of these conditions consists of avoidance of vitamin D, reduction of die-

tary intake of calcium, and administration of cortisone for a few weeks.

Immobilization

Immobilization is accompanied by bone resorption, which causes severe hypercalcemia, hypercalciuria, and stone formation. Children and young adults are

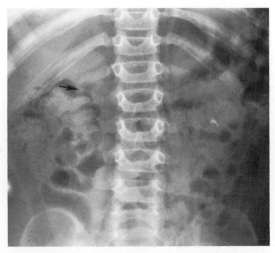

Figure 12–120. *Plain film.* Tiny stone in right kidney *(arrow)* and larger linear calculus in left kidney of young girl on prolonged steroid therapy for myopathy.

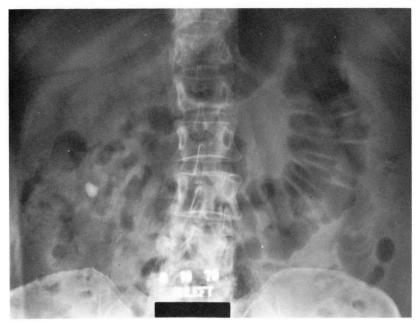

Figure 12–121. *Plain film.* **Stone in right kidney** of 60-year-old woman with long-standing, incompletely treated thyrotoxicosis.

particularly susceptible (Bennett and Colodny; Smith, 1974) (also see the section on infected urolithiasis) (Fig. 12–122; also see Figure 12–65).

URIC ACID LITHIASIS

The incidence of uric acid lithiasis among the stone-forming population varies from 5 to 39 per cent (Atsmon and associates). Conditions associated with this type of calculogenesis are listed in Table 12–1 (Gutman and Yü). The most common variety of uric acid lithiasis is the idiopathic. This condition occurs in families with a history of gout. These stone-formers have normal levels of serum and urinary uric acid but tend to excrete abnormally acidic urine.

Approximately 25 per cent of people with gout form uric acid stones; conversely, gout is present in 25 per cent of patients who form uric acid stones. In persons with untreated gout, calculogenesis does not correlate well with the degree of uricosuria. On the other hand, among those patients treated with uricosuric agents but

without urinary alkalinization, the incidence of uric acid stone disease is definitely increased.

In myeloproliferative disorders and some other states of increased purine turnover, excessive uric acid production may rapidly lead to stone formation; indeed, this may be the presenting abnormality of the underlying disorder (Fig. 12–123). Uric acid lithiasis may pose a serious problem during the treatment of these conditions if purine breakdown is significantly increased. Occasionally, the entire upper collecting system may be filled with uric acid crystals; consequent azotemia with oliguria or anuria can usually be relieved by insertion of ureteral catheters and appropriate medical treatment (see below) (Fig. 12–124).

Uric acid lithiasis may also occur in conditions associated with low urine output secondary to obstructive processes such as bladder neck obstruction. In patients with ileostomies, loss of water and bicarbonate results in urine of low volume and unusually high acidity—an ideal situation for uric acid stone formation (see Figure 12–130). Occasionally, patients with

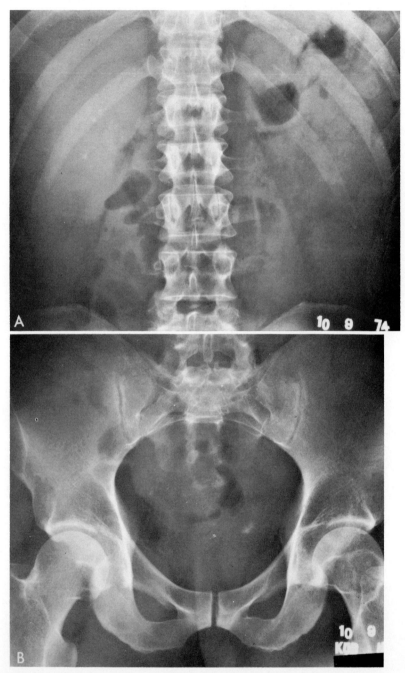

Figure 12–122   Calculi of recumbency. **A,** *Plain film.* Multiple right renal calculi of poor radiopacity. **B,** *Plain film.* Left lower ureteral calculus. **C,** *Plain film 1 year after left ureterolithotomy.* Most of right renal calculi have spontaneously and painlessly passed. *Comment:* Patient was a 36-year-old man immobilized for 3 months as a result of multiple injuries.

Illustration continued on opposite page.

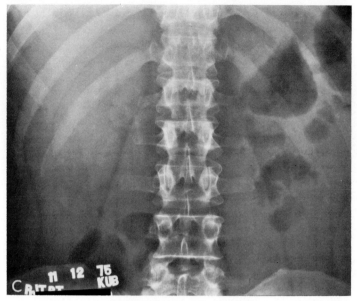

Figure 12–122. *Continued*

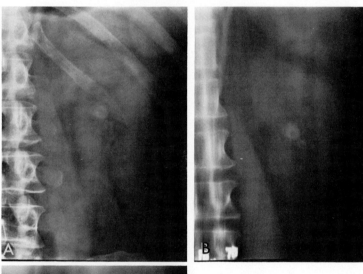

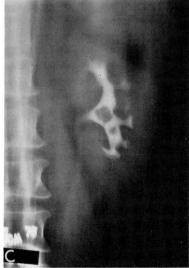

Figure 12–123. Uric acid lithiasis in 57-year-old man with gammopathy. **A,** *Plain film.* Uric acid calculi of poor radiopacity in left kidney. **B,** *Plain film (tomogram).* Left renal calculi better visualized; they seem to contain calcium impurities. **C,** *Tomogram.* Filling defect in left renal pelvis and lower-pole infundibulum produced by calculi. *Comment:* Chemolytic program of hydration, urinary alkalinization, and allopurinol administration failed to dissolve these calculi because of much calcium impurity.

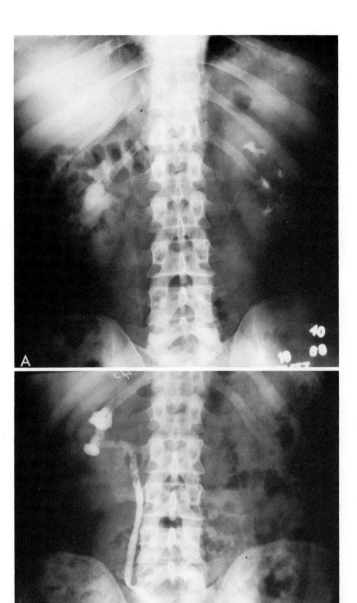

Figure 12–124. Uric acid "sludge" obstructing right renal pelvis and ureter in hyperuricemic patient. **A,** *Excretory urogram.* Right pyelocaliectasis. Ureter not seen in vicinity of ureteropelvic juncture. **B,** *Retrograde ureteropyelogram.* Uric acid sludge in ureteropelvic juncture and upper ureter producing negative filling defects. **C,** *Excretory urogram.* Normal upper urinary tract 1 month after treatment. *Comment:* Some uric acid crystals were washed out endoscopically and others were dissolved by hydration, urinary alkalinization, and allopurinol administration.

Illustration continued on opposite page.

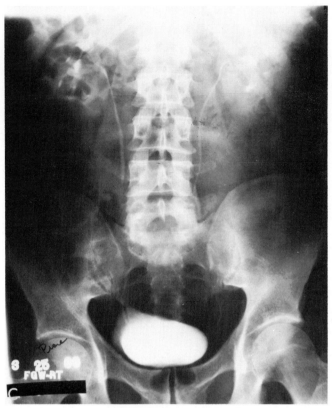

Figure 12–124. *Continued.*

primary hyperparathyroidism or idiopathic renal lithiasis form pure or mixed uric acid calculi. The mechanism for this is not clear, but complete evaluation of calcium metabolism in patients with uric acid lithiasis is strongly indicated.

The results of treatment of uric acid lithiasis have been gratifying. In alkaline urine (pH ≥6.5), uric acid ionizes as very soluble urate. Thus a high fluid intake (to produce a urine volume in excess of 2.5 liters per 24 hours) and the addition of alkali (to maintain a urine pH of >6.5) usually suffice in most patients. Allopurinol, by inhibiting xanthine oxidase, diminishes the concentration of uric acid in the urine and is particularly useful in the chemolysis of uric acid calculi, unless the collecting system is infected or totally obstructed or both (Figs. 12–125, 12–126, and 12–127). This drug is also beneficial in states of increased purine metabolism; in such cases it is often used prophylactically to decrease the production of uric acid.

Successful chemolysis of uric acid stones can be achieved in almost every instance if the affected kidney is making urine, if the stone is not of a mixed type, and if calcification of the stone does not occur during therapy (see Figure 12–123). A substantial decrease in the size of the stone is usually observed within one month of starting treatment. In the patient who becomes stone-free, allopurinol administration can be discontinued unless the patient has gout or a myeloproliferative disorder. High fluid intake and, at times, urinary alkalinization should, however, be continued.

UROLITHIASIS ASSOCIATED WITH INTESTINAL DISEASE

The incidence of nephrolithiasis in patients with inflammatory diseases of the intestine is 7.2 per cent, which is much higher than that in hospitalized patients in

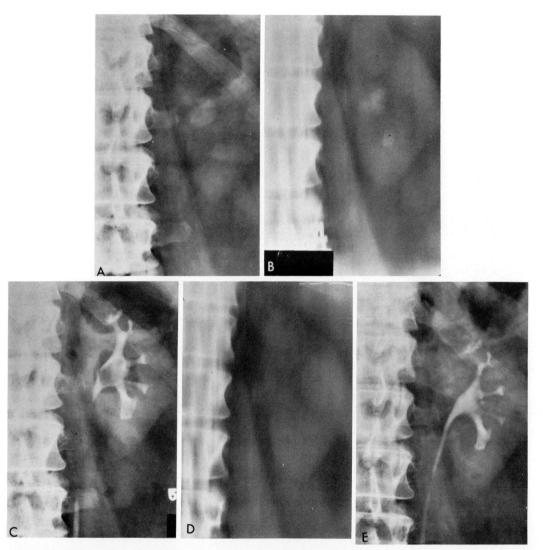

Figure 12–125. **Effect of chemolysis on large uric acid stones** in 54-year-old man with long-standing gout who presented with hematuria. **A,** *Plain film.* Calculi of poor radiopacity in left kidney. **B,** *Plain film (tomogram).* Left renal calculi better visualized. **C,** *Excretory urogram.* Large calculus in left renal pelvis and smaller one in lower-pole calyx, producing negative filling defect. **D,** *Plain film (tomogram).* No calculi are demonstrable 4 months after chemolytic program (hydration, urinary alkalinization and allopurinol) was started. **E,** *Excretory urogram.* Normal. No evidence of negative filling defects.

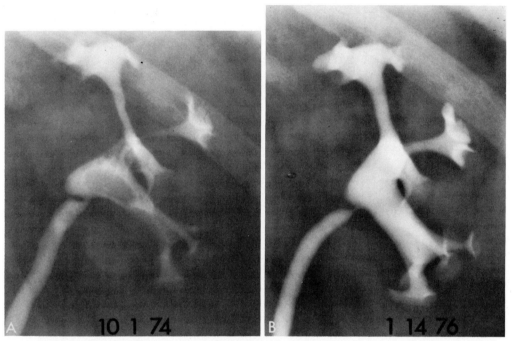

Figure 12–126. Effect of chemolysis on large uric acid stone in 49-year-old patient with idiopathic uric acid lithiasis. **A,** *Excretory urogram.* Negative filling defect in renal pelvis produced by radiolucent uric acid stone. Also note clinically insignificant ureteropelvic stenosis. **B,** *Excretory urogram.* No evidence of filling defect after chemolysis of calculus with hydration, urinary alkalinization, and administration of allopurinol.

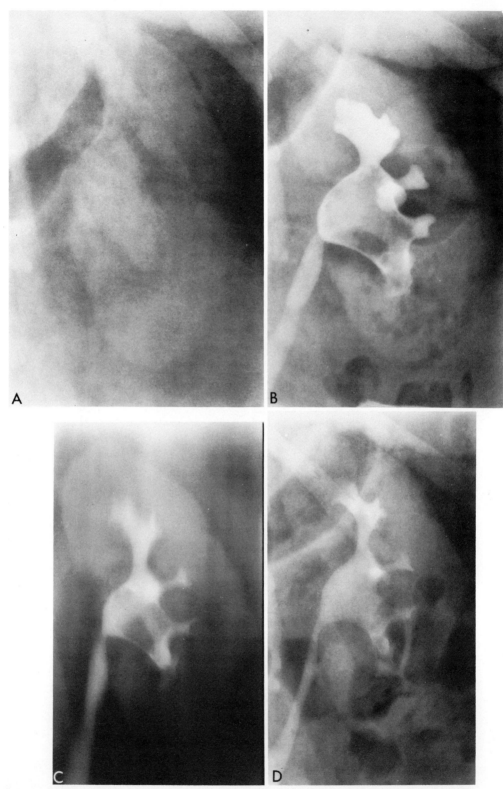

Figure 12–127. **Effect of chemolysis on branched uric acid stone** in 56-year-old hyperuricemic man who presented with abdominal pain. **A,** *Plain film* Large stone of poor radiopacity in left kidney. **B,** *Excretory urogram.* Branched uric acid stone producing negative filling defect in left renal pelvis and lower calyces. **C,** *Excretory urogram.* Renal stone diminished in size 2 months after chemolytic program (hydration, urinary alkalinization and allopurinol) was started. **D,** *Excretory urogram.* Complete dissolution of calculus 3 months later.

general (1 per 1,000). The majority (72 per cent) of these calculi are radiopaque; presumably they contain calcium (Gelzayd and associates).

Two metabolic abnormalities appear to dominate the picture. The more common abnormality is the development of hyperoxaluria (Smith, Fromm, and Hofmann) (Fig. 12–128). Its causation, though not clearly understood, seems to be related to disturbances of bile acid metabolism, malabsorption of bile acids, and bacterial deconjugation. Recent experiments at the Mayo Clinic with radioactive cholylglycine have shown an association among increased bile acid glycine turnover, excessive intestinal absorption of oxalate, and hyperoxaluria, but they have shed no light on the pathogenesis of hyperoxaluria in patients with intestinal disease (Hofmann and associates). Treatment with cholestyramine or taurine in a limited number of adults has been effective in decreasing the urinary oxalate concentration to a normal value (Fig. 12–129).

The less common abnormality is the formation of uric acid stones, especially in association with the excessive loss of fluid and alkali that occurs under these circumstances (Fig. 12–130). Treatment with allopurinol, as described in the foregoing section on uric acid lithiasis, is often necessary because adequate replacement of the fluid and alkali is often difficult in these settings.

IDIOPATHIC RENAL LITHIASIS

In approximately 70 to 80 per cent of the adult stone-formers in the United States, renal lithiasis is idiopathic. In the reported series, 50 to 80 per cent of the patients have had hypercalciuria; the remaining 20 to 50 per cent have been normocalciuric. In a large series of patients with idiopathic renal lithiasis, only 19 per cent had had evidence of urinary infection at any time in their history, and only 4 per cent had active infection at the time of their evaluation (Smith, 1974). The syndrome of idiopathic renal lithiasis is much more common in men, with an approximate sex ratio of 5 to 1, and it is only diagnosed by exclusion, after all other known causes of calculogenesis have been carefully elim-

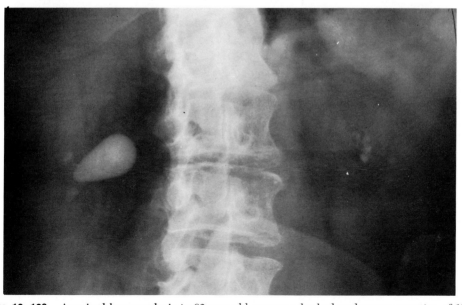

Figure 12–128. **Acquired hyperoxaluria** in 62-year-old woman who had undergone resection of 15 feet of small intestine for mesenteric thrombosis. *Plain film.* Both large and small radiopaque stones but no staghorn formation.

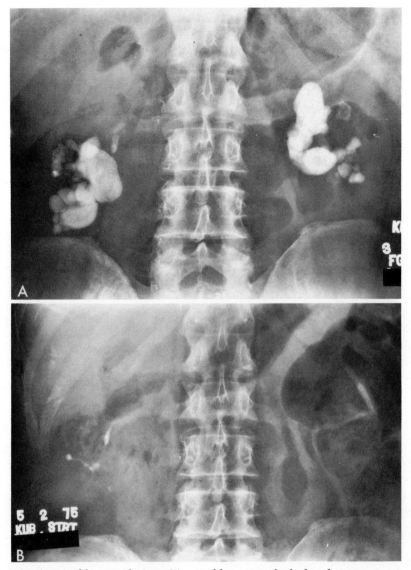

Figure 12–129.   Acquired hyperoxaluria in 65-year-old woman who had undergone resection of 135 cm. of small and portion of large bowel for regional enteritis. She had rapidly recurrent nephrolithiasis. **A,** *Plain film.* Bilateral branched calcium oxalate calculi **B,** *Plain film.* Postoperative calcification of right kidney and no calculi in left kidney 3 years later. *Comment:* Calculi were removed surgically, and patient's active stone disease was stabilized by administration of cholestyramine (4 g three times a day). (Courtesy of Dr. L H. Smith.)

inated. There are several categories of the idiopathic variety:

　　1. Persistent hypercalciuria (primary renal calcium leak).

　　2. Stress hypercalciuria (primary intestinal hyperabsorption of calcium).

　　3. Normocalciuria (primary inhibitor defects).

Additionally, mild hyperoxaluria, increased urine alkalinity, abnormalities of uric acid metabolism, and "normocalcemic" hyperparathyroidism have been described (Smith, 1974).

　　In our experience, idiopathic renal lithiasis, with or without hypercalciuria, is also the most common form of metabolic stone disease during childhood (Malek and Kelalis, 1975b). Calculogenesis in idio-

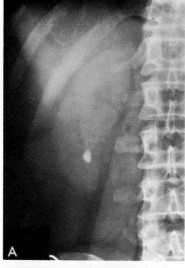

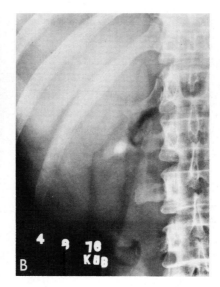

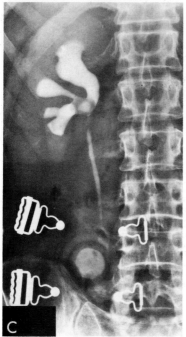

Figure 12–130. Uric acid stone formation in patient with previous calcium oxalate stone who had undergone total colectomy with creation of permanent ileostomy. **A,** *Plain film.* Calcium oxalate stone in lower pole of right kidney. **B,** *Plain film.* Stone has moved to renal pelvis and has enlarged (less opaque periphery). **C,** *Excretory urogram.* Caliectasis due to stone impacted at ureteropelvic juncture. Note dense center (calcium oxalate) and radiolucent periphery (uric acid) causing negative filling defect. *Comment:* Treatment consisted of pelviolithotomy and maintenance on allopurinol.

pathic renal lithiasis is commonly intermittent; thus, in order to determine the need for specific medical therapy, the definition of metabolic activity becomes important (see section on classification).

Only those patients with metabolically active stone disease require specific therapy. A high fluid intake should be maintained in all patients, and in patients with hypercalciuria (i.e., more than 275 mg per 24 hours in men and 250 mg per 24 hours in women on general diet containing 600 to 700 mg of calcium), the dietary calcium intake should be restricted. Specific medication includes the use of thiazides, magnesium oxide with or without pyridoxine, and phosphate. Methylene blue, a crystal poison, has not proved of great value.

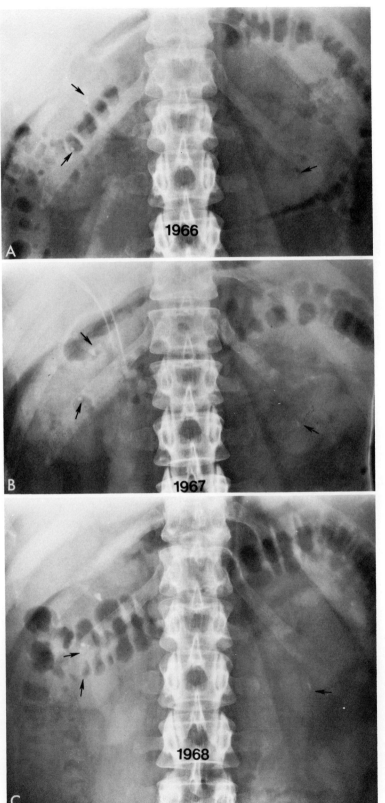

Figure 12–131. Effectiveness of phosphate therapy in idiopathic renal lithiasis with hypercalciuria in 41-year-old man with long history of recurrent renal calculi. **A,** *Plain film.* Bilateral small renal calculi *(arrows).* Patient managed conservatively with hydration and dietary calcium restriction. **B,** *Plain film.* Increase in stone material bilaterally 1 year later *(arrows).* Patient had also passed calculi in interim (metabolically active). Phosphate therapy was started. **C,** *Plain film.* Increase in stone material on right side *(arrows).* Left side stable *(arrow).* Patient had not adhered to therapeutic program. **D,** *Plain film (tomogram) (same time as C)* shows increase in right renal stone material more distinctly. **E,** *Plain film (tomogram).* Diminution of stone material on right side. Left side stable. Patient has not passed any stones in intervening 4 years while on adequate phosphate therapy.

Illustration continued on opposite page

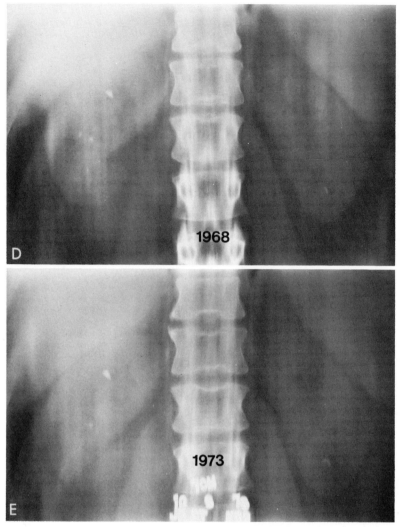

Figure 12–131. *Continued.*

Hydrochlorothiazide causes a decrease of 50 per cent or more in the urinary calcium concentration and a concomitant slight increase in urinary magnesium (Yendt and associates). Reabsorption of sodium and calcium in the ascending limb of Henle's loop and of sodium in the distal tubule is inhibited. A considerable loss of sodium and water (and a small amount of calcium) thus diminishes the extracellular fluid volume. This is followed by a compensatory increase in proximal tubular reabsorption of the glomerular filtrate, with which large amounts of calcium are also reabsorbed, so that much less calcium appears in the urine (Suki and associates).

The use of hydrochlorothiazide may be associated with hypokalemia, hyperglycemia, hyperuricemia, and hypercalcemia. It has been effective in about 70 per cent of patients with hypercalciuria and ineffective in those whose urinary calcium concentration is normal (Smith, 1974) (see Figure 12–132).

Magnesium oxide, with or without pyridoxine, is reportedly effective in some patients (Melnick and associates; Mukai and Howard). The usefulness of this regimen is limited by intestinal intolerance to magnesium oxide—hence the difficulty in achieving adequate urinary concentrations.

Phosphate, given orally as neutral sodium potassium phosphate (Neutra-Phos*) or as neutral potassium phosphate (K-Phos Neutral tablets†) to provide 1.5 to 2 grams of inorganic phosphorus daily in three or four divided doses, is one of the most effective therapeutic agents (it has been 92 per cent effective in Mayo Clinic experience) (Figs. 12–131 and 12–132). Occasionally, a patient who is an extremely active stone-former may require more than 2 grams of phosphorus daily (Smith, 1974).

The exact mode of action of phosphate

_____

*Willen Drug Company, Baltimore, MD 21202.
†Beach Pharmaceuticals, Tampa, FL 33611.

is unknown; it appears to increase the ability of urine to hold calcium salts in solution. In some patients there is a decrease in urinary calcium excretion, but this does not seem to be the basis of the therapeutic response. Pyrophosphate excretion is increased with this therapy but usually not sufficiently to explain the action of the phosphorus. Furthermore, differential renal function studies in hypercalciuric patients indicate that the actively stone-forming kidney may actually excrete normal amounts of calcium (Malek, Wilkiemeyer, and Boyce).

Some patients may experience diarrhea during the first few weeks of therapy.

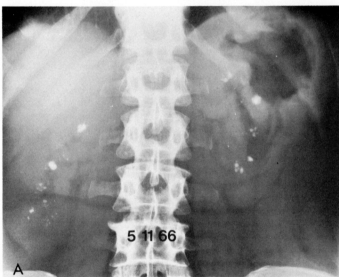
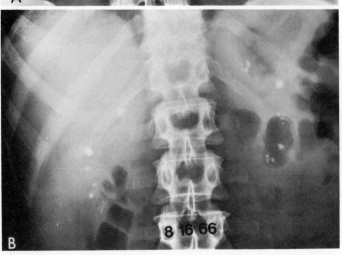

Figure 12–132. Effectiveness of phosphate therapy in idiopathic renal lithiasis with normocalciuria in 49-year-old woman with fifteen-year history of stone disease **A,** *Plain film.* Bilateral nephrolithiasis and papillary-tip calcification. Patient treated with thiazide. **B,** *Plain film.* Increase in stone material. Thiazide discontinued and phosphate therapy started. **C,** *Plain film.* Diminution of stone material bilaterally 8 months later **D,** *Plain film.* Marked diminution of stone material bilaterally 8 years later on phosphate therapy.

Illustration continued on opposite page.

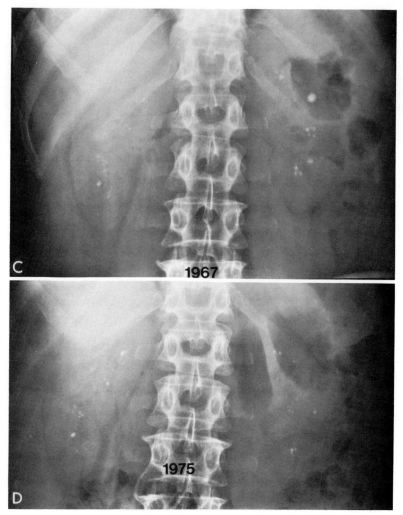

Figure 12–132. *Continued.*

This usually subsides; otherwise, antidiarrheal medication can be used in conjunction with phosphate therapy. The neutral phosphate salts seem to be tolerated better. Patients with stones may pass some of the calculi while under treatment and should be warned accordingly at the beginning of treatment. Infection with urea-splitting bacteria and struvite stone formation are contraindications to phosphate therapy. The phosphate is ineffective under these circumstances and may actually cause stone growth.

INFECTED UROLITHIASIS AND URINARY STASIS

All forms of urinary calculous disease may be complicated by urosepsis. It has long been maintained by many that obstruction or infection (or both) is primarily calculogenic. Our studies of stone-formers with and without obstruction or infection tend to support the belief that the initiation of stone formation is a pathologic deviation of normal biologic mineralization in the renal tubular cells (Malek and

Boyce, 1973). Cumulative data obtained from a large number of centers do not establish urinary obstruction or infections as a primary *initiating* factor but rather as a sequel to renal calculus formation (Boyce, 1967; Malek and Kelalis, 1975b). Urinary obstruction may contribute to infection and to the retention of preformed intra-nephronic stone nidi; these consist of microspherules of hydroxyapatite-matrix complexes that rarely form "pure" matrix calculi but more frequently harbor calcium oxalate, calcium phosphate, uric acid, cystine, struvite, or a combination of these crystals, as the case may be (Malek and Boyce, 1973).

Subsequently, the urinary tract may be invaded by urea-splitting bacteria. These include all *Proteus* species and some strains of staphylococci; rarely, organisms of the *Aerobacter-Klebsiella* group, *Pseudomonas* species, *Escherichia coli,* and enterococci may also produce alkaline urine (Smith, 1967). The crystalline nature of the stone then becomes struvite (Fig. 12–133), consisting of magnesium ammonium phosphate in addition to calcium and carbonate (i.e., a triple-phosphate stone). Stone growth under these circumstances may be extremely rapid; surprisingly, a

small calculus may grow to form a staghorn stone within a few weeks.

Urologic lesions (commonly obstructive), or urosepsis, or both are found in association with stone disease in 35 per cent of stone-forming adults and 65 per cent of children. The majority of these stoneformers have bacilluria attributable to *Proteus mirabilis,* with alkaline urine. Conversely, the incidence of stone disease among patients with infected, obstructed, or anomalous urinary tracts is very low (0 to 5 per cent) (Boyce, 1967; Malek and Kelalis, 1975b).

Immobilization for even as short a time as three weeks may be followed by stone formation (Bennett and Colodny; Smith, 1967). Hypercalciuria from bone demineralization in association with *functional* obstruction from prolonged recumbency is the predisposing factor. Uropathogens may also gain entry through indwelling catheters (including nephrostomy tubes, and so forth) or in the course of diagnostic studies (Fig. 12–134). An insidious onset with complicating urinary infection is more likely than an acute episode. High fluid intake, urinary acidification, and frequent changes of position are good prophylactic measures. Once stones have formed, conservative

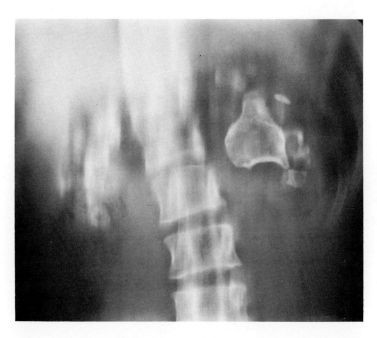

Figure 12–133. *Plain film (tomogram).* **Bilateral staghorn uric acid calculi** (lucent center) **covered by radiopaque shell of struvite** from *Proteus mirabilis* urosepsis. Right side not in focus. (From Malek, R. S., 1976.)

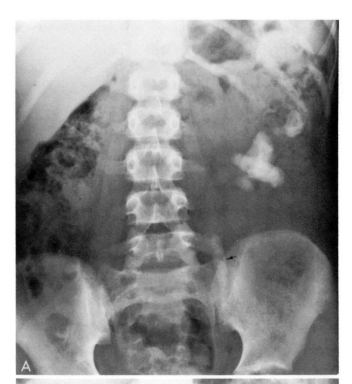

Figure 12–134. Infected renal lithiasis in 13-year-old boy with solitary
nephrostomy-tube-bearing left kidney.
Previous right nephrectomy. Left
nephrostomy tube has been in place for 5
years. **A**. *Plain film.* Typical appearance
of struvite calculi in left kidney and
ureter *(arrow)*. **B**, *Excretory urogram.*
Enlarged left kidney with caliectasis and
marked cortical loss.

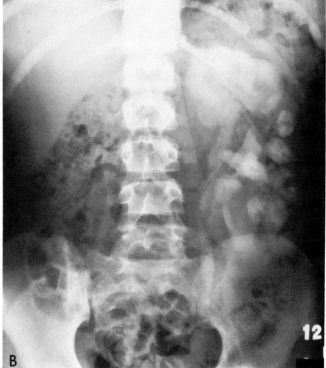

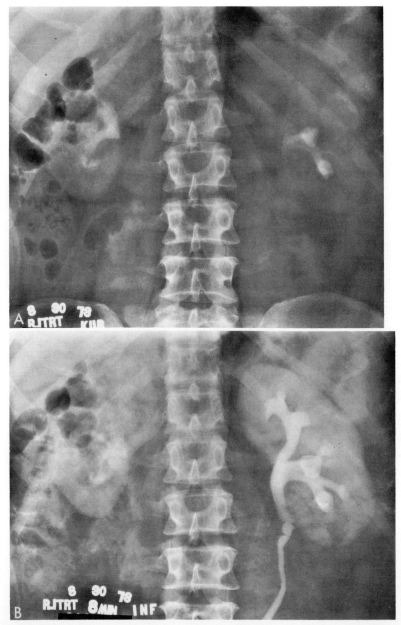

Figure 12–135. Recurrent infected renal lithiasis in 45-year-old man with unrecognized primary hyperparathyroidism. Previous left renal stone surgery **A,** *Plain film.* Typical branched struvite calculi **B,** *Excretory urogram.* Functionless right kidney. Postoperative deformity of left upper ureter from previous surgical procedure. *Comment:* This case typifies how failure to recognize underlying metabolic etiology can produce a renal invalid.

measures deserve a trial in these patients because of the possibility of breakup and spontaneous passage of the fragments.

Treatment of Infected Renal Lithiasis

Successful treatment of infected renal lithiasis requires an aggressive approach. Specific metabolic abnormalities may be defined in more than 60 per cent of patients with struvite stones (Smith, 1974); if these abnormalities are not sought, both surgical and antimicrobial measures will fail (Fig. 12–135). Renal function and its degree of impairment will also have bearing on the possible therapeutic approaches and must be carefully assessed. The importance of high fluid intake (in excess of 2,500 ml) throughout the 24-hour period must be stressed.

The infection should be treated initially with bactericidal antibiotics according to in vitro sensitivities of the isolated uropathogens. If an operation is scheduled, treatment should be started 48 to 72 hours beforehand and continued for 8 to 12 days afterward. If urine culture obtained at renal operation is still positive, the chemotherapeutic regimen may have to be altered according to the newly determined bacterial sensitivities. The urine is then cultured again in 48 hours to determine the effectiveness of the new program. Surgical correction of the obstructive element or stasis and removal of the calculous material in its entirety is the ideal form of treatment; the presence of residual stone material is almost always followed by recurrent infection and growth of any remaining fragments. At times, the surgical goal is best achieved by removal of diseased, stone-bearing, and poorly functioning kidney, provided the contralateral kidney is relatively normal and free of infection; at other times, bilateral operation at reasonable intervals is necessary.

Long-term suppressive therapy is indicated for most patients who have or have had struvite stones with infection. It is started during the last few days of post-operative antibiotic therapy. A number of regimens have been useful. At the Mayo Clinic, a combination of methenamine mandelate (1 g four times daily) or methenamine hippurate (1 g twice daily) and ammonium chloride (500 to 1,000 mg four times daily) given for 6 to 12 months after surgery has increased the cure rate. The urine pH should be kept at 5.5 or less. Metabolic activity is assessed during the follow-up period when the patient is free of infection. Although rare, vesicoureteral reflux in infected stone-forming patients must be sought and corrected. Urosepsis perpetuated by reflux or obstruction precludes assessment of metabolic activity until the infection and its perpetuating factors have been eliminated or corrected (see Figure 12–3).

The urine should be cultured monthly during the first three months and every three months thereafter if the patient remains uninfected. Relapse or reinfection should be treated with appropriate antibiotics in the meantime. Plain films (KUB) and tomograms should be obtained every three months during the first year after operation. If the patient remains stone-free, the follow-up interval may be increased to six months, but continued follow-up is imperative.

Renacidin* and other buffered solutions may be used for calculus chemolysis. The presence of an unobstructed and preferably sterile urinary tract with a nephrostomy or other similar tubes is essential; otherwise, severe renal damage as well as systemic toxicity may result.

Surgical Management of Renal Calculi

A description of the various surgical techniques for the management of renal calculi is beyond the scope of this book, but the following points deserve emphasis.

1. Control of metabolic derangements and urinary infection is the preoperative,

---

*Guardian Chemical Corp., Hauppauge, Long Island, NY 11787.

intraoperative, and postoperative requisite of successful surgery for urinary calculi. All stones, regardless of their size and position, are potentially harmful. Some stones are spontaneously passable, others may be too small to be recovered surgically, and renal papillary calcifications masquerading as calyceal stones cannot readily be removed.

2. The proper operative approach to the stone-bearing urinary conduit and the timing of surgical intervention must be individually and carefully considered. Aside from emergent situations such as complete urinary obstruction, sepsis, intractable pain or hemorrhage, and unremitting ileus, surgery for stone may be elective.

3. Kidneys that are anatomically or functionally solitary demand special consideration. Under these and other circumstances requiring prolonged clamping of the renal pedicle, localized renal hypothermia is an important adjunct.

4. Duplex collecting systems, ureteropelvic obstruction, and anomalies of the position, shape, or rotation of the kidney all are indices of supernumerary vascular pedicles.

5. When peripelvic and periureteral adhesions from previous operations or infection are suspected, a ureteral catheter inserted cystoscopically serves as a useful guide for easier dissection.

6. Patency of the ureter must be ascertained before and during operation lest urinary extravasation from disrupted suture lines and fistulization occur.

7. In general, surgically active or infected calculi should be removed. Renal lithiasis that is metabolically inactive, indeterminate, or active but rendered inactive by medical management may be carefully followed. The subsequent development of urosepsis, stone growth, or surgical activity may necessitate surgical intervention. In any event, the need for preservation of the nephron, restoration of effective internal drainage, removal of all calculous material, accurate and preferably watertight closure with fine absorbable sutures, return of the urinary structures into their fat-padded sur-

roundings for normal peristalsis, and, finally, continued control of urinary infection if present is axiomatic. Recurrence of stone disease, usually owing to inability to eradicate infection, occurs in at least 15 per cent of the patients with infected renal lithiasis (Boyce and Elkins). Thus, the need for careful and regular follow-up of all stone-formers cannot be overemphasized.

Renal Calculi in Childhood

Calculous disease of the urinary tract during childhood is relatively uncommon in the Western Hemisphere. In comparison with the 1 to 3 new cases seen annually at urologic centers in North America, 10 or 12 new ones are encountered in the British centers (Malek and Kelalis, 1975b). In sharp contrast stands the common occurrence of so-called endemic calculi in Asia (see discussion in section on vesical calculi), where this is one of the most frequent pediatric urologic problems; 1,250 such cases were recorded in Thailand within seven years (Passmore).

Our 20-year experience with 101 stone-bearing children encountered among 145,000 new pediatric admissions at the Mayo Clinic (Malek and Kelalis, 1975b) indicates that the majority are in the older age group (mean 9.8 years) and that boys outnumber girls by a ratio of 2 to 1. In two thirds of the children, stone disease is likely to have identifiable metabolic causes: idiopathic renal lithiasis, 31 per cent (Fig. 12–136); renal tubular acidosis (distal type), 8 per cent; cystinuria, 6 per cent; primary hyperoxaluria, 6 per cent; primary hyperparathyroidism, 6 per cent; hypercortisonism, 5 per cent; uric acid lithiasis, 3 per cent; milk-alkali syndrome, 1 per cent; and idiopathic infantile hypercalcemia, 1 per cent (see Figures 12–3, 12–19, 12–36, 12–94, 12–99, 12–105, 12–106, 12–109, 12–118, 12–119, 12–120, 12–133, and 12–134). The remaining third have the infected type of renal lithiasis. In this last group, the patients are likely to have had multiple uro-

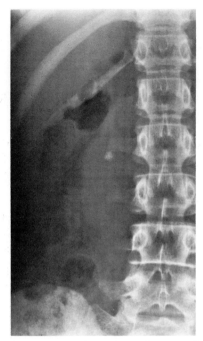

Figure 12-136. *Plain film.* **Calcium oxalate and phosphate calculus** in right kidney of 14-year-old girl with idiopathic renal lithiasis and hypercalciuria.

logic procedures, urinary infection, and stasis, with diversionary and indwelling drainage devices (see Figure 12-134).

With appropriate therapy (see section on pathogenesis and medical management), stone disease may become inactive in 70 per cent of affected children. Those unfortunate children with uncontrollable disease are likely to die from renal failure and should be considered for renal allograft. Stone-formers, irrespective of their age, must never be dismissed. They are cursed with basic metabolic problems that rival cancer, and unless their internal derangements are controlled by various prophylactic regimens, these patients are doomed. With proper and timely attention, up to 90 per cent of the victims of these vicious syndromes can be promised a reasonably normal future.

NEPHROCALCINOSIS

Nephrocalcinosis represents a pathologic deposition of calcium in the renal parenchyma (Malek and Kelalis, 1975a; Mortensen and Emmett). It is a manifestation of a variety of disorders, most of which are referred to in this chapter. In our experience, primary hyperparathyroidism, renal tubular acidosis, and primary hyperoxaluria are the usual underlying causes (Malek, 1974; Malek and Kelalis, 1975a; Mortensen and Emmett). Other causes include chronic nephritides (Arons and associates; Geraci and associates; Randall and associates), hypervitaminosis D, the milk-alkali syndrome (Burnett and associates; Scholz and Keating, 1955), an excess of endogenous or exogenous steroids (Hurxthal and O'Sullivan; Malek and Kelalis, 1975a), sarcoidosis (Richtsmeier; Wilson and Brown), idiopathic infantile hypercalcemia (Lightwood and Payne; Snyder) sulfonamide intoxication (Engel), medullary sponge kidney (Vermooten), thyrotoxicosis (Epstein and associates), neoplastic disease (with or without metastatic bony deposits) (Plimpton and Gellhorn; Thomas and associates), and skeletal atrophy due to disuse (Thomas and associates). Tuberculous, fungal, and nonspecific infections (Mortensen and Emmett) as

Table 12-3. Conditions Associated With Nephrocalcinosis

RENAL TUBULAR SYNDROMES
  Renal tubular acidosis (type 1)

ENZYME DISORDERS
  Primary hyperoxaluria

HYPERCALCEMIC STATES
  Primary hyperparathyroidism
  Sarcoidosis
  Hypervitaminosis D
  Milk-alkali syndrome
  Malignancy (with or without secondary)
  Cushing's syndrome (endogenous or exogenous)
  Hyperthyroidism
  Idiopathic infantile hypercalcemia

PARENCHYMAL RENAL DISEASE
  Nonspecific infections and inflammations (chronic
    glomerulonephritis)
  Tuberculosis
  Mycoses
  Tumors
  Cystic disease (including medullary sponge kidney)

VASCULAR PHENOMENA
  Tubular necrosis (including drug-induced)
  Infarction (acute cortical necrosis)

IDIOPATHIC NEPHROCALCINOSIS

Fig. 12-137

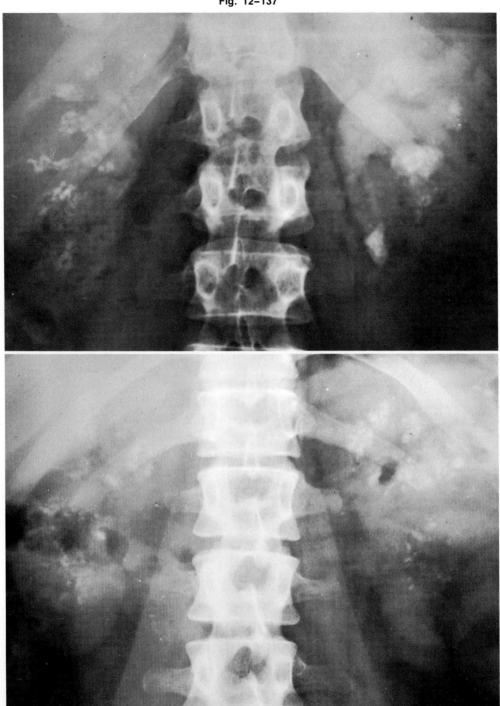

Fig. 12-138

Figure 12-137.   Medullary type of nephrocalcinosis and nephrolithiasis. *Excretory urogram.* Stone impacted just below left ureteropelvic juncture. Pelviolithotomy.

Figure 12-138.   *Plain film.* Nephrocalcinosis. Feathery type of calcification.

well as renal infarcts, cysts, and tumors may cause parenchymal calcification; rarely, the condition is idiopathic (Table 12–3).

Contrary to earlier views and in our experience, a significant number (55 of 100) of patients with renal tubular ectasia ranging in degree from papillary blush to medullary sponge kidney have radiologic evidence of renal calcification, practically all of which is located in the medullary cystic areas. Among 73 such patients with serum calcium and 33 with 24 hour urinary calcium measurements, 13 had disorders of calcium metabolism such as primary hyperparathyroidism, milk-alkali syndrome, or idiopathic renal lithiasis with or without hypercalciuria. However, of the 55 patients adequately followed, only 11 per cent have had metabolically active stone disease (Aguilo and associates). The treatment, after exclusion of all other metabolic causes and treatment of infection, is the same as for patients with idiopathic renal lithiasis (Thomas).

Nephrocalcinosis usually affects both kidneys but occasionally is confined to one kidney. It may be associated with other forms of urolithiasis (Malek, 1974; Malek

and Kelalis, 1975a). The medullary type accounts for 95 per cent of cases (Huth) in which calcification involves the distal tubules and the loop of Henle; the renal pyramids show fine feathery or coarse granular deposits (Figs. 12–137 through 12–142). This form should be carefully distinguished from papillary-tip calcifications (see Figure 12–132).

The rare cortical variety appears as a diffuse stippled calcification that produces a faint "calcium shadow" outlining the entire kidney. Chronic glomerulonephritis (Esposito; Geraci and associates; Pyrah and Hodgkinson) and acute renal cortical necrosis (Riesz and Wagner; Walls and associates) are the underlying causes (Figs. 12–143 through 12–147).

Microcalculi may be shed from areas of parenchymal involvement into the urinary passage. Smaller deposits may pass spontaneously, with or without colic, and larger ones may be retained. Unless the condition is complicated by surgically active and retained calculi, no operative intervention is indicated. The treatment of choice is adequate hydration and control of the underlying disease.

Text continued on page 1294

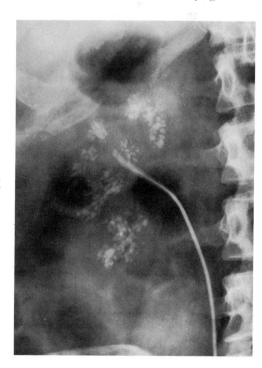

Figure 12–139. *Plain film.* With opaque catheter in right ureter. **Nephrocalcinosis (medullary type). Feathery type of calcification.**

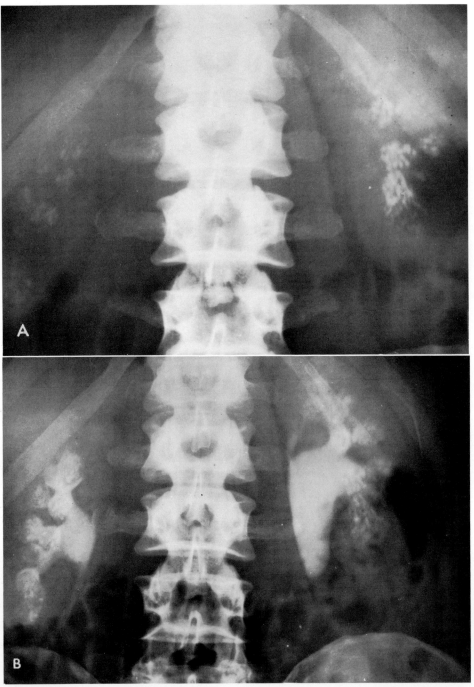

Figure 12–140. A, *Plain film.* Medullary type of nephrocalcinosis. Granular type of calcification. B, *Excretory urogram.* Typical relationship of calcific shadows to wide, cup-shaped calyces, showing calcification in tips of pyramids as they project into calyces.

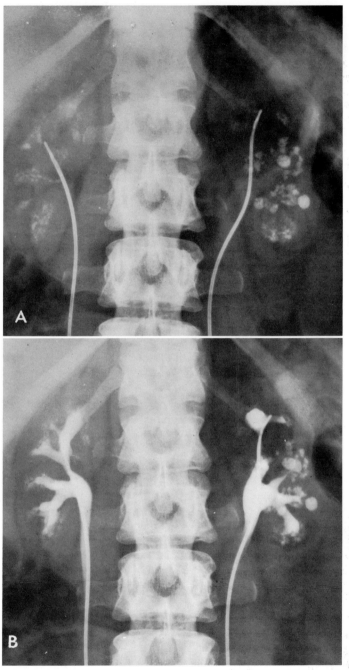

Figure 12–141.   A, *Plain film.* Nephrocalcinosis (medullary type). Coarse granular type of calcification. B, *Bilateral retrograde pyelogram.* Typical involvement of renal pyramids.

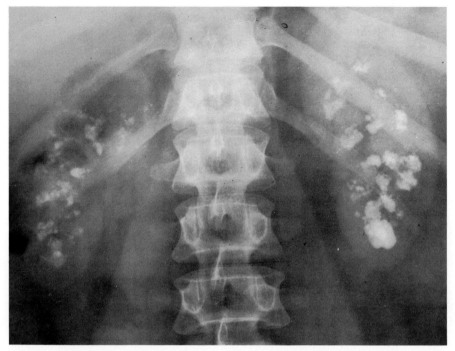

Figure 12–142. *Plain film.* Advanced nephrocalcinosis (medullary type). Coarse granular type of calcification.

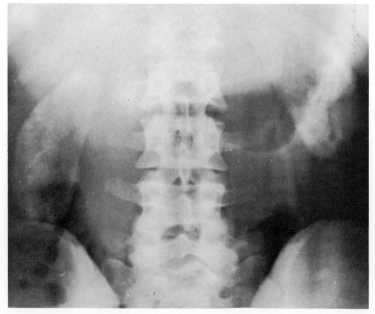

Figure 12–143. *Plain film.* **Nephrocalcinosis of chronic glomerulonephritis.** Increase in renal density caused by diffuse granular calcifications in parenchyma. Note small regular renal outlines. (From Esposito, W. J.)

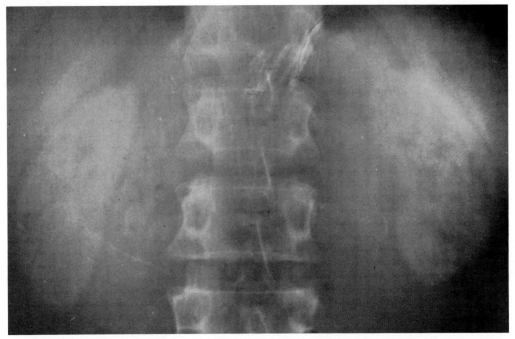

Figure 12–144. *Plain film.* **Nephrocalcinosis of glomerulonephritis.** Note innumerable fine granular calcifications that are primarily cortical in location. (From Esposito, W. J.)

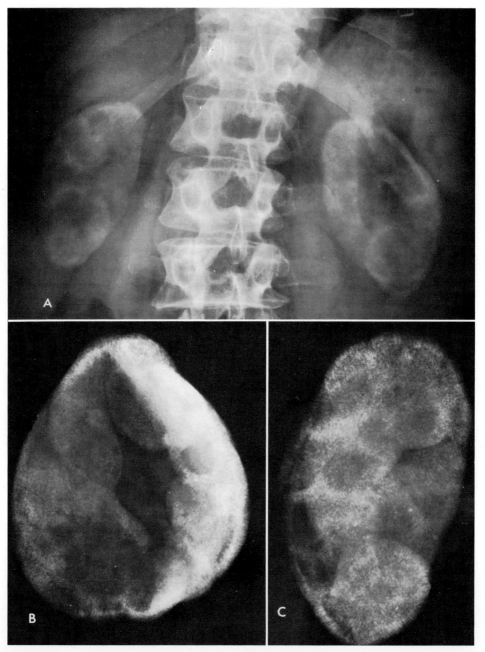

Figure 12–145. A, *Plain film.* Cortical type of nephrocalcinosis. Diffuse involvement of entire kidneys. **B** and **C,** *Roentgenograms made of kidneys removed at necropsy.* (Courtesy of Dr. Richard Lyons.)

Fig. 12-146

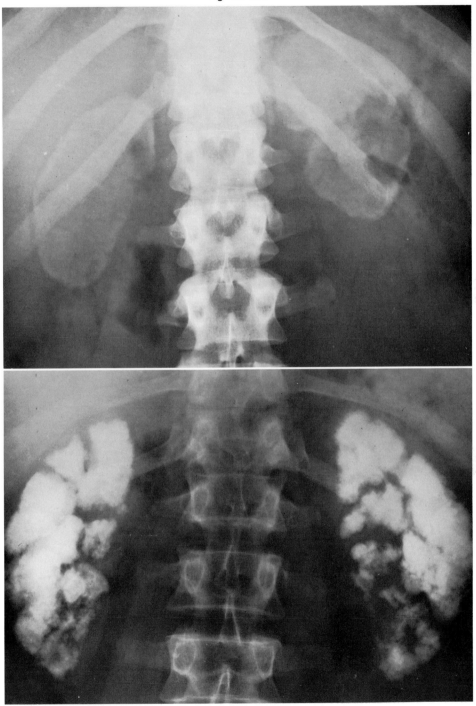

Fig. 12-147

Figure 12-146. *Plain film.* **Nephrocalcinosis from chronic glomerulonephritis.** Fine granular stippling diffusely distributed throughout entire kidney of man, 23 years of age, with renal insufficiency. Apparently end result of glomerulonephritis.

Figure 12-147. *Plain film.* **Advanced nephrocalcinosis.**

URETERAL CALCULI

Clinical Features of Ureteral Calculi

Clinical features of ureteral calculi and their significance are similar to those of renal calculi and will not be further discussed.

Roentgen Studies of Ureteral Calculi

REASONS FOR DIFFICULTIES IN DEMONSTRATING URETERAL CALCULI IN PLAIN FILMS

Difficulties in diagnosis of ureteral stones arise when they are of small size or poor density, or when they are obscured by gas in the intestine or by bony structures that they overlie. The last cause is one of the commonest sources of diagnostic error. The bony structures that most often give trouble are the transverse processes of the lumbar vertebrae and the sacrum. Careful inspection is required to avoid overlooking stones in these areas (Figs. 12–148 through 12–154). Another cause of difficulty is a roentgenogram that is technically poor because of overexposure or underexposure or because of movement of the patient. It is not unusual to see a poorly made roentgenogram in which no shadow is present. However, a good roentgenogram taken immediately afterward may show the stone clearly (Fig. 12–155).

Phleboliths have been discussed previously (see Chapter 7). In most cases they may be recognized by their location, their characteristic circular shape, and the difference in degree of density between the center and the periphery. In some cases, however, ureteral stones may simulate phleboliths, and their differentiation by means of a urogram or plain film with an opaque catheter in place becomes necessary (Figs. 12–156, 12–157, and 12–158).

Text continued on page 1301

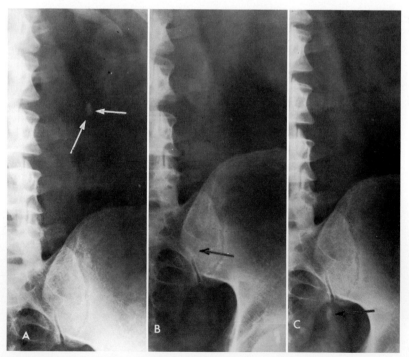

Figure 12–148. Difficulty visualizing stones that overlie bone. **A,** *Plain film.* Shadow of stone in upper third of left ureter, well visualized. **B,** *Plain film,* 1 month later. Could easily be read as normal, since stone is overlying left wing of sacrum *(arrow).* Indefinite shadow could be mistaken for minimal changes in bone. **C,** *Plain film,* 1 week later than **B.** Stone has now descended below left sacroiliac joint and is easily visualized.

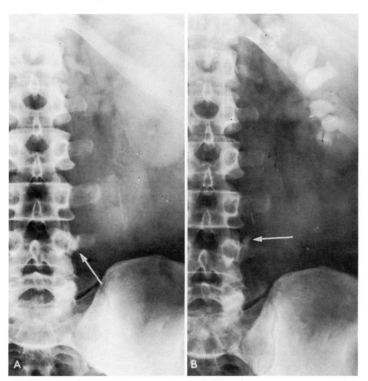

Figure 12–149. Difficulty in visualizing stones that overlie bone. A, *Plain film.* Ureteral stone overlying fourth left lumbar transverse process; could easily be overlooked, as it appears to be part of bony structure *(arrow).* **B,** *Excretory urogram.* In this urogram, position of x-ray tube shifted enough to throw shadow above transverse process, where it can easily be seen. Pyeloureterectasis above.

Fig. 12–150

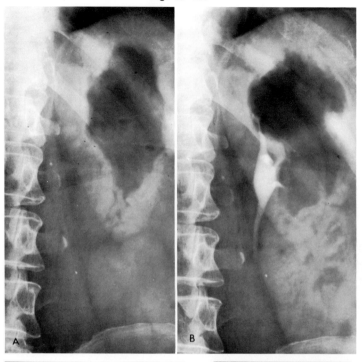

Figure 12–150. Tip of transverse process simulates ureteral stone. **A,** *Plain film.* Increased density of tip of left transverse process of third lumbar vertebra. Might easily be mistaken for ureteral stone. **B,** *Excretory urogram.* Ureter is outlined and is 1 cm lateral to shadow, excluding it from ureter.

Figure 12–151. Difficulty of visualizing stones that overlie tip of transverse process. **A,** *Plain film.* Shadow overlying tip of right transverse process of third lumbar vertebra. Impossible to say whether shadow represents ureteral stone or increased density of tip of transverse process. **B,** *Excretory urogram.* Shadow is ureteral stone included in outline of ureter.

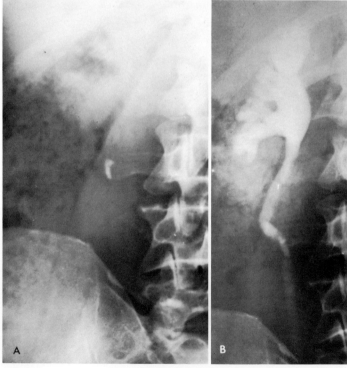

Fig. 12–151

Fig. 12–152

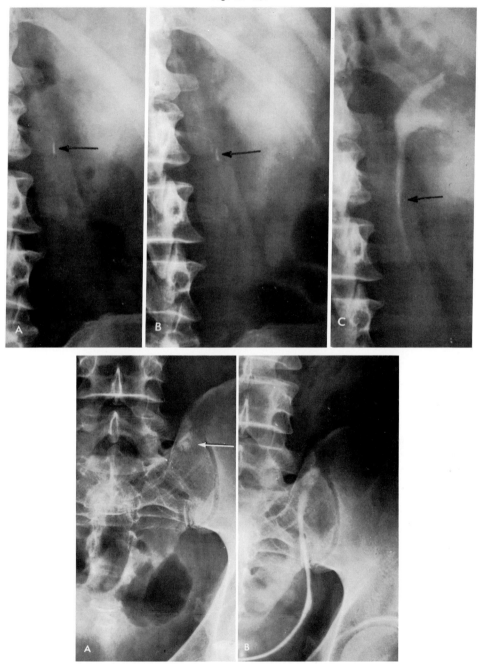

Fig. 12–153

Figure 12–152. Difficulty in visualizing stones that overlie tip of transverse process. **A,** *Plain film.* Shadow overlying tip of left transverse process of second lumbar vertebra; appears to be increased density of tip of transverse process. **B,** *Plain film.* Position of patient in relation to x-ray tube has been changed. Shadow slightly lateral to tip of transverse process, suggesting that it is ureteral stone. **C,** *Excretory urogram.* Shadow shown to be stone included in upper third of left ureter.

Figure 12–153. Difficulty in visualizing stones that overlie bone. **A,** *Plain film.* Indefinite, irregular shadow over left upper margin of sacrum appears to be part of bony structure. **B,** *Left retrograde pyeloureterogram.* Shadow is large irregular stone that completely obstructs left ureter.

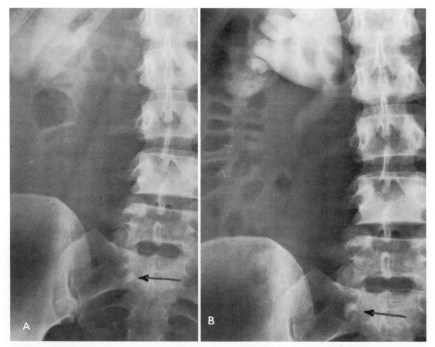

Figure 12–154.   Difficulty in visualizing stones that overlie bone. A, *Plain film.* Indefinite shadow over right wing of sacrum. Might easily be regarded as part of bony structure. **B,** *Excretory urogram.* Shadow is now more definite and is seen to represent large ureteral stone producing pyeloureterectasis above obstruction.

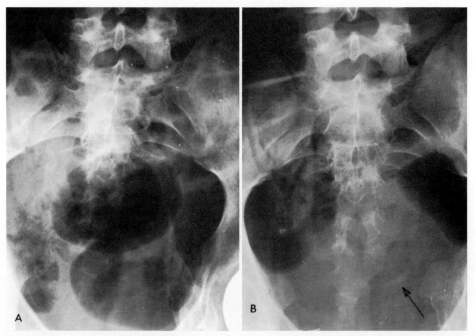

Figure 12–155.   Illustration of manner in which calculi are missed because of poor roentgenograms or gas in bowel. A, *Plain film.* Gas obscures both lower ureteral areas. No definite shadow of ureteral stone apparent. **B,** *Roentgenogram* made 1 day later, with better preparation. Shadow of ureteral calculus now visible in lower third of left ureter opposite left ischial spine *(arrow).*

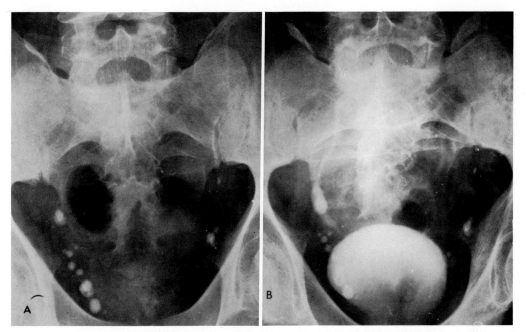

Figure 12–156. Difficulty of distinguishing phleboliths and ureteral calculi. **A,** *Plain film.* Multiple shadows on both sides of bony pelvis which appear to be phleboliths, and fragmentary calcification of iliac vessels. **B,** *Excretory urogram.* Right ureter is visualized and shows uppermost shadow on right to be **large calculus included in ureter.** Remainder of shadows are phleboliths.

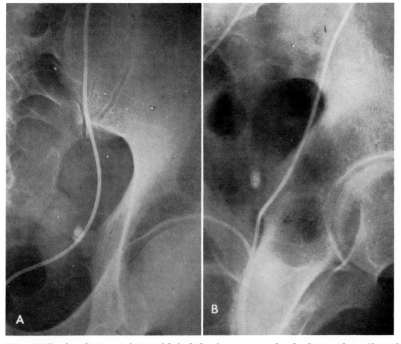

Figure 12–157. Difficulty distinguishing phleboliths from ureteral calculi. **A,** *Plain film.* Shadow opposite left ischial spine, with typical oval shape and center of poor density. Suggests phlebolith but is adjacent to lead catheter in left ureter. **B,** *Lateral view.* Shadow displaced away from ureteral catheter, **indicating that it is phlebolith.**

Fig. 12–158

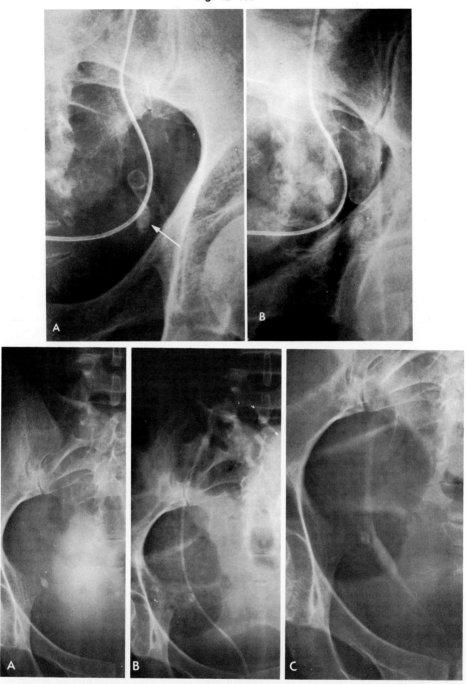

Fig 12–159

Figure 12–158. Phleboliths versus ureteral calculi. **A,** *Plain film.* Large calcific shadow opposite left ischial spine, adjacent to calcified pelvis vessel and ureteral catheter. Identity cannot be accurately determined from this view. **B,** *Oblique view.* Shadow now appears well removed from ureteral catheter, **indicating that it is large phlebolith.**

Figure 12–159. Extraureteral shadow simulating stone. Opaque catheter inadequate for diagnosis. **A,** *Plain film.* Calcific shadow opposite right ischial spine. Could be either ureteral stone or phlebolith. **B,** *Plain film* with opaque catheter in right ureter. Shadow is adjacent to catheter and might erroneously be considered ureteral stone. Oblique roentgenogram or urogram would be necessary for accurate diagnosis. **C,** *Right retrograde ureterogram.* Ureter is outlined and is adjacent to shadow, but contrast medium is definitely removed from shadow and does not include it, **indicating that shadow is extraureteral.**

OPAQUE STONES

Methods of Identification and Localization

Use of Opaque Catheter and Additional Plain Films. When only an opaque catheter is employed for identification of shadows over the ureteral areas, errors in interpretation are likely to occur unless the physician keeps in mind the limitations of this particular examination. The fact that a shadow is in line with a ureteral catheter in the anteroposterior view is not sufficient evidence to make a diagnosis of stone. Oblique and even lateral views should be used to try to "throw out" or exclude the shadow. If, after these procedures, the shadow is still adjacent to or seemingly well removed from the catheter, a possibility of error remains. A phlebolith or other extraureteral shadow may lie so close to the wall of the ureter that only the thickness of the ureteral wall separates it from the lead catheter. In such a case it might be erroneously interpreted as being a ureteral stone. On the other hand, a stone in a dilated ureter or ureteral diverticulum might be so far removed from the opaque catheter as to be considered excluded from the ureter. There is no question that a ureterogram is the more accurate procedure (Figs. 12–159 through 12–162). When the diagnosis is in doubt, stereoscopic roentgenograms may be helpful. Occasionally, a lead catheter may completely obscure a small ureteral stone (Fig. 12–163).

Urograms. As already mentioned, urograms provide the most reliable means of identifying ureteral calculi. In some cases, when there is moderate obstruction but good function, the dilated ureter is well visualized by excretory urography down to and including the stone, so that a definite diagnosis may be made with an anteroposterior view only (Figs. 12–164 through 12–168). On the other hand, the excretory urogram may yield too fractional a visual-

Text continued on page 1307

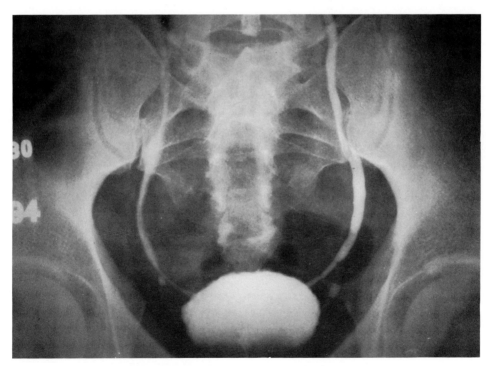

Figure 12–160. Extraureteral shadows identified with ureterogram. *Bilateral retrograde pyelogram.* Calcific shadows in region of lower portions of both ureters, excluded by retrograde pyelography. Although shadow on right is very close to ureter, it can be seen that urographic medium does not include it. Oblique view not necessary in this case.

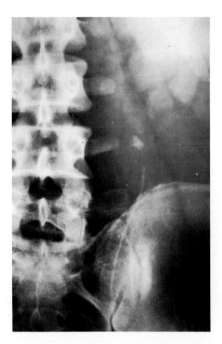

Figure 12–161.   Ureteral stone obstructing midureter. Identification with opaque catheter. *Plain film.* Large irregular shadow in upper part of left ureter, opposite transverse process of fourth lumbar vertebra. **No function is evident from excretory urogram.** Catheter met obstruction in region of stone. Typical appearance of tip of catheter 1 to 2 cm below shadow of stone. This type of picture is commonly seen in cases of ureteral stone completely obstructing ureter.

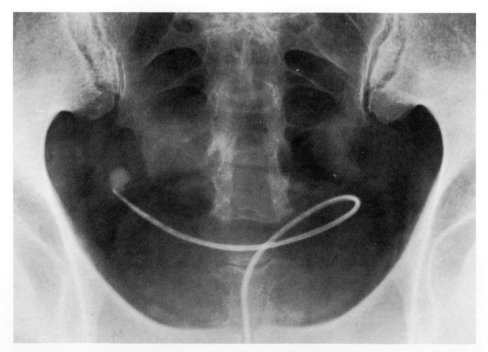

Figure 12–162.   *Plain film.* **Large stone in intramural portion of right ureter.** Tip of catheter adjacent to stone. Oblique view or stereoscopic view would be necessary for accurate urographic diagnosis. However, on *cystoscopic examination,* **grating was felt and catheter would not pass by stone.** With these additional clinical data, no further roentgenograms were necessary.

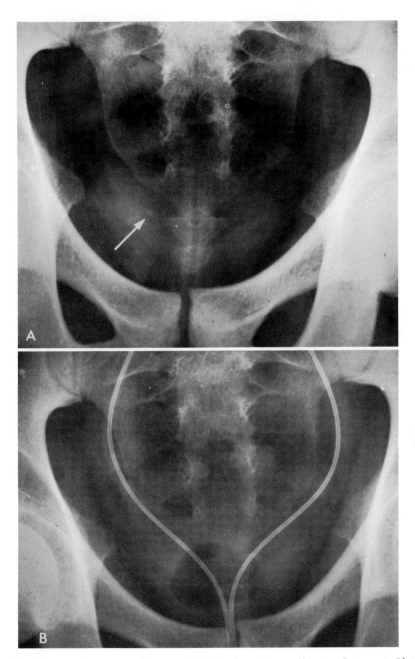

Figure 12–163. Danger of opaque catheter completely obscuring small ureteral stone. A, *Plain film*. Minute indistinct shadow overlying lower right ureteral area *(arrow)*. B, *Plain film* with opaque catheter in each ureter. Catheter in right ureter completely obscures small stone in lower part of right ureter.

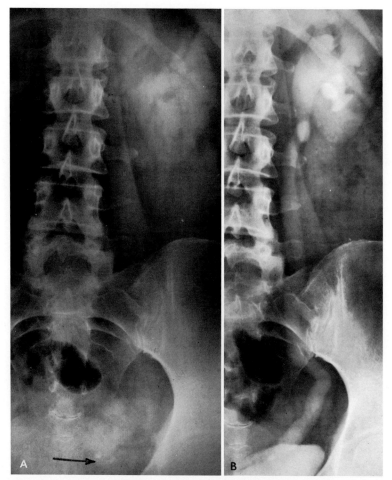

Figure 12–164.   Ureteral stone identified with anteroposterior urogram only. **A,** *Plain film.* Calcific shadow over left lower ureteral area, not identified *(arrow)*. **B,** *Excretory urogram.* Marked dilatation of ureter above shadow. Outline of dilated ureter ends abruptly above shadow, which is sufficient evidence that shadow represents stone in terminal portion of left ureter. Further urographic studies would be unnecessary.

Fig. 12–165

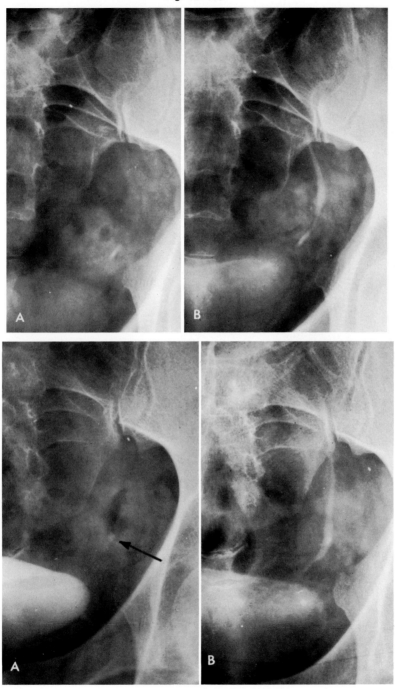

Fig. 12–166

Figure 12–165. Ureteral stone identified with anteroposterior urogram only. **A,** *Plain film.* Linear calcific shadow opposite left ischial spine, not identified. **B,** *Excretory urogram.* Ureter outlined; it is not dilated but is in line with shadow, and medium has collected around shadow, increasing its density and indicating that it is stone in ureter. Necessity of further roentgenograms for diagnosis would seem questionable.

Figure 12–166. Ureteral stone identified with anteroposterior urogram only. **A,** *Excretory urogram.* Shadow over left lower ureteral area was also present in plain film. Not identified. **B,** *Excretory urogram* (later film). Left ureter outlined and in line with shadow. However absence of dilatation or other findings would still leave diagnosis in doubt. Oblique views would be necessary for accurate interpretation. This was proved to be stone.

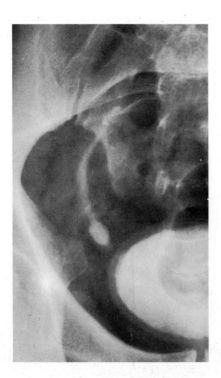

Figure 12–167. Ureteral stone not completely identified with anteroposterior urogram. *Excretory urogram.* Large calcific shadow overlying lower right ureteral area. It is in line with ureter and suggests that shadow may be stone in ureter. However, in absence of deformity, dilatation, or other pathologic changes in region of stone, other diagnostic procedures would be necessary for accurate interpretation. **Shadow was proved to be ureteral stone.**

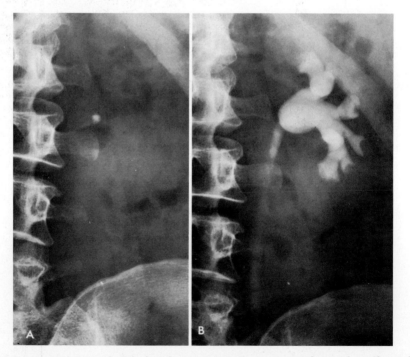

Figure 12–168. Ureteral stone identified with anteroposterior urogram only. **A,** *Plain film.* Calcific shadow above left third lumbar transverse process. **B,** *Excretory urogram.* Shadow identified as stone in upper part of ureter. Pelvis and ureter are dilated above stone, and contrast medium surrounds it.

ization for diagnosis, so that retrograde pyelography is necessary.

THE EXCRETORY UROGRAM THAT DEMONSTRATES TEMPORARY ABSENCE OF FUNCTION

A rather unusual finding peculiar to excretory urography occurs when a kidney fails to excrete urographic medium because of an obstruction from a ureteral stone. Apparently this situation may prevail almost immediately after obstruction occurs. The inability of the kidney to function (as far as excretion of urographic medium is concerned) is a temporary phenomenon, for the excretory ability of the kidney returns in a matter of hours after relief of the obstruction (Figs. 12–169 and 12–170).

THE OBSTRUCTIVE NEPHROGRAM

Opacification of the renal parenchyma from ureteral obstruction (renal colic from stone) was noted in 1932 by Wesson and Fulmer. From this original observation have emerged the diagnostic procedures of renal parenchymal opacification, namely nephrography and nephrotomography. (See discussion of technique and explanation of mechanics of nephrography in Chapter 1.) The consensus has been that although contrast medium in the intrarenal arteries and veins plays some part, most of the parenchymal opacification is from contrast medium in the renal tubules, in the renal tubular cells, and possibly in the interstitial tissues. Absorption of water from the tubules further concentrates the intratubular contrast medium.

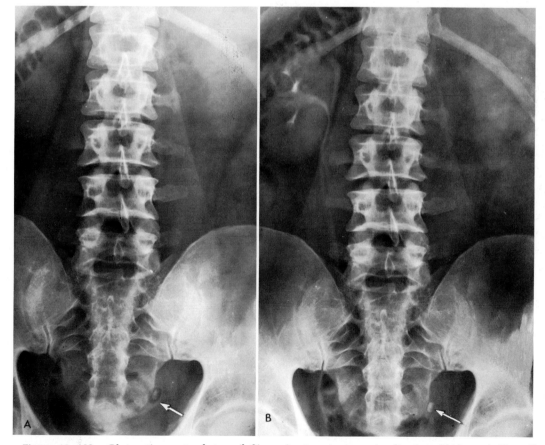

Figure 12–169. Obstructive ureteral stone (left) causing transient nonvisualization of kidney. **A,** *Plain film.* Calcific shadow over left lower ureteral area, not identified. **B,** *Excretory urogram.* Shadow is ureteral stone producing temporary absence of excretion of contrast medium from left kidney. Function returned promptly after removal of stone. Duplication on right, otherwise normal.

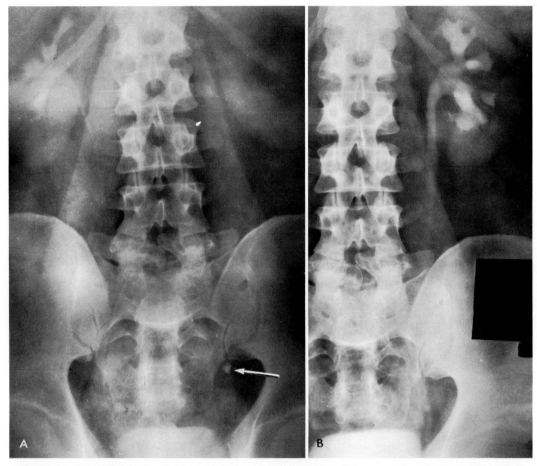

Figure 12–170.   Obstructive (left) ureteral stone causing transient "absence of function" of kidney. **A,** *Excretory urogram.* Stone in lower third of left ureter just below left sacro-iliac joint, which has caused temporary absence of function of left kidney. Right kidney normal. **B,** *Excretory urogram* made 2 weeks later following ureterolithotomy. Function has returned to left kidney. Residual pyeloureterectasis present.

The peculiar phenomenon of renal opacification during acute obstruction (obstructive nephrography) has proved of diagnostic value in acute or subacute obstruction, especially that caused by ureteral calculi. Small ureteral calculi are notoriously difficult to demonstrate radiographically, in which event the presence of parenchymal opacification in the absence of visualization of the collecting system (calyces, pelvis, and ureter) may help confirm the diagnosis (Fig. 12–171). Later films (from one to several hours) may also reveal opacification of the collecting system (Figs. 12–172 and 12–173).

The explanation of the obstructive nephrogram is not entirely clear. Excretion of urine is considered to be a process of ultrafiltration by the glomerulus. The rate of filtration or clearance of the renal plasma depends on the glomerular capillary pressure minus the sum of the osmotic pressure of the plasma and the intratubular (back) pressure.

The prevailing theory suggests that glomerular filtration continues at a decreased rate despite obstruction. The rate of fluid flow in the tubules is decreased and an increased amount of water is reabsorbed from the filtrate, causing an increased concentration of contrast medium in the tubules. The rate of urine formation and flow is markedly reduced, causing delayed opacification of the obstructed col-

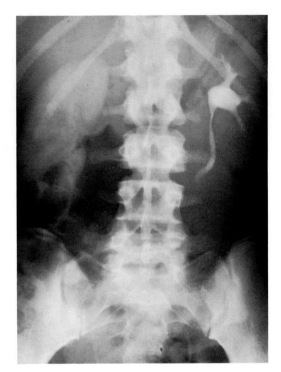

Figure 12–171. *Excretory urogram.* Small, poorly opaque (cystine) **ureteral stone** (right) obscured by gas in bowel. **Renal colic with obstruction causing increased nephrographic effect** but poor filling of pelvis and calyces. Left kidney normal.

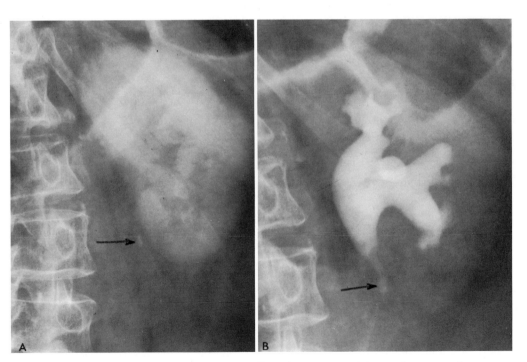

Figure 12–172. **A,** *Excretory urogram, 45-minute film.* **Obstructive nephrogram from ureteral stone** in upper third of ureter. **B,** *Excretory urogram, 6-hour film.* Collecting system now filled with contrast medium. Moderate pyelectasis. Note that intensity of nephrogram has now diminished.

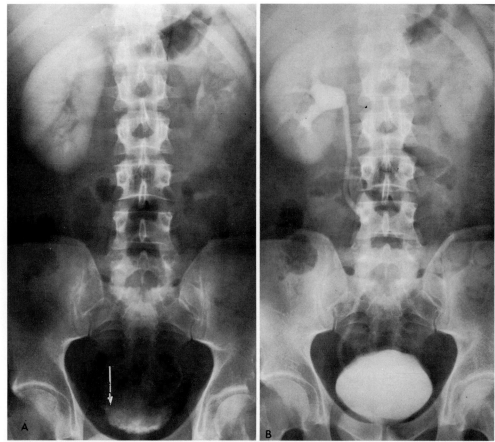

Figure 12–173.   **A,** *Excretory urogram, 2-hour film.* **Obstructive nephrogram** in patient with obstruction by stone in intramural ureter *(arrow).* Only small amount of contrast medium remains in normal left kidney. **B,** *Excretory urogram,* 5¹⁄₂-*hour film.* Collecting system is now filled with contrast medium and nephrogram is of less density.

lecting system. Typically, the intensity of the nephrogram increases slowly for several hours, then gradually diminishes over a period of up to two or more days if obstruction is not released. Jungmann's animal experiments support this view.

OBLIQUE AND LATERAL VIEWS: PYELOURETERECTASIS

Identification of ureteral stones by means of urographic medium presents problems almost identical to those encountered with renal stones. The mere demonstration that the shadow in question and the outline of the ureter coincide in the anteroposterior view may not be sufficient for diagnosis. The use of the oblique and lateral views (as explained previously in con-

nection with diagnosis by means of an opaque catheter) also applies here. Other factors, such as a localized dilatation of the ureter in the region where the stone is lodged (Figs. 12–174 through 12–177) or a collection of medium around the stone, increasing its density, may be most helpful in interpretation (Figs. 12–178, 12–179, and 12–180). Ureteral dilatation just above or below the stone or in both locations may be telltale evidence (Fig. 12–181). In some cases the ureter becomes edematous in the region of the stone, so that urographic medium seems to end abruptly a few millimeters above and below the stone. This phenomenon is observed when the stone is lodged in the intramural portion of the ureter (Figs. 12–182 through 12–186).

Pyeloureterectasis above a shadow is

Text continued on page 1317

Fig. 12–174

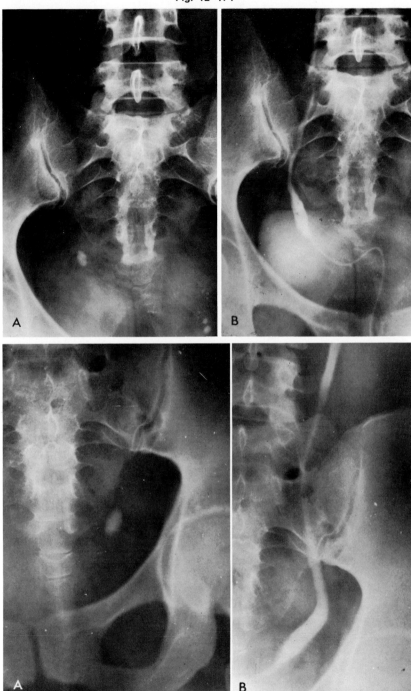

Fig. 12–175

Figure 12–174. Ureteral stone. **A,** *Plain film.* Oval shadow in region of lower portion of right ureter, not identified. **B,** *Right retrograde pyelogram.* Shadow is shown to be in line with ureter, but, in addition, there is **localized dilatation of ureter in region of stone,** which casts negative shadow, thereby offering definite proof that shadow represents stone in lower part of ureter.

Figure 12–175. Ureteral stone. **A,** *Plain film.* Large oval shadow in region of lower portion of left ureter. **B,** *Left retrograde pyelogram.* Shadow is in line with ureter and **ureter is dilated in this area, furnishing reasonably good evidence that shadow represents stone in ureter.**

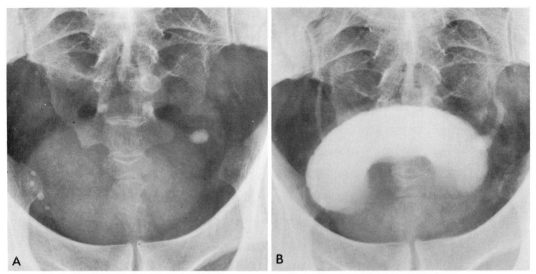

Figure 12–176.   Ureteral stone and enlarged prostate. **A,** *Plain film.* Shadow over lower left ureteral area. **B,** *Excretory urogram.* Hyperplasia of prostate with filling defect in base of bladder and beginning "hook-shape" terminal ureters caused by prostatic enlargement. Shadow is stone in terminal "hook" of ureter.

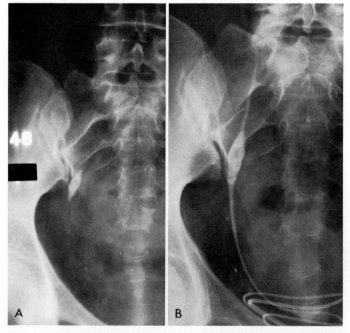

Figure 12–177.   Ureteral stone. **A,** *Plain film.* Elongated calcific shadow overlying lower margin of right sacro-iliac joint. **B,** *Right retrograde ureterogram.* Shadow is identified as representing large ureteral stone, since there is **localized dilatation of ureter and stone casts negative shadow.**

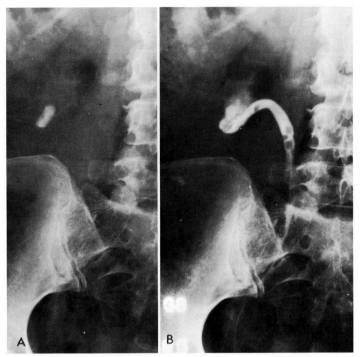

Figure 12–178. Ureteral stone. **A,** *Plain film.* Calcific shadow just above ilium, to right of fourth lumbar vertebra. **B,** *Right retrograde pyelogram.* Shadow is proved to represent stone obstructing ureter just below ureteropelvic juncture. Ureter is angulated at this point and **medium collects around and includes shadow, permitting positive identification of stone** Negative shadows in upper part of ureter from air bubbles.

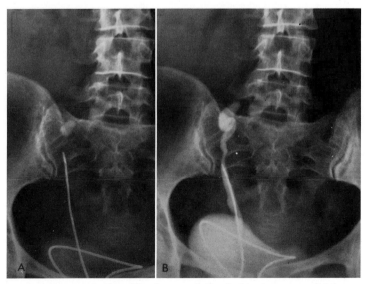

Figure 12–179. Ureteral stone. **A,** *Plain film.* Large calcific shadow in course of right ureter, at upper margin of sacrum. Tip of lead catheter lies just beneath shadow. Shadow not identified. **B,** *Right retrograde ureterogram.* Contrast medium surrounds shadow and ureter is dilated at this point, giving positive evidence that shadow represents stone in ureter.

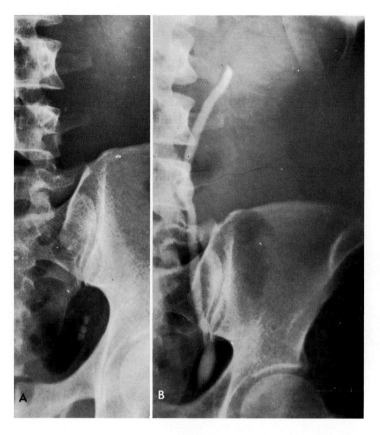

Figure 12–180 Multiple ureteral calculi in stump of ureter (previous nephrectomy). **A** *Plain film.* Multiple calcific shadows in region of lower third of left ureter in patient who had previously undergone left nephrectomy. **B,** *Left retrograde ureterogram.* Entire ureter dilated grade 2, but **ureter in region of shadows is dilated grade 3, indicating that shadows represent ureteral calculi** in terminal portion of ureter. Ureter ends abruptly at level of second transverse process, where it was ligated at previous nephrectomy.

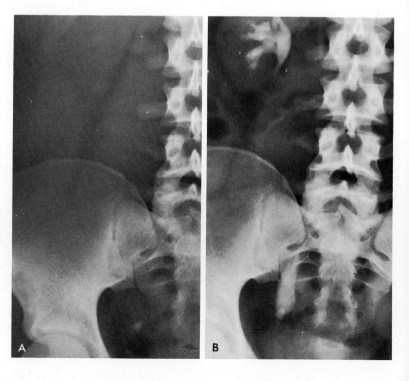

Figure 12–181. Ureteral stone with ureterectasis above. **A,** *Plain film.* Triangular shadow over lower right ureteral area. **B,** *Excretory urogram.* Outline of dilated ureter above shadow demonstrates it to be stone in ureter.

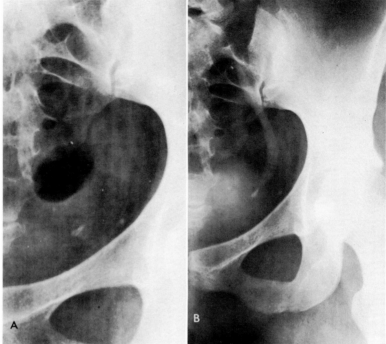

Figure 12–182. Ureteral stone. **A,** *Plain film.* Calcific shadow over left lower ureteral area. **B,** *Excretory urogram.* Dilatation of ureter above shadow with abrupt termination a few millimeters above stone. Typical finding with ureteral stone which is tightly grasped by edematous ureter.

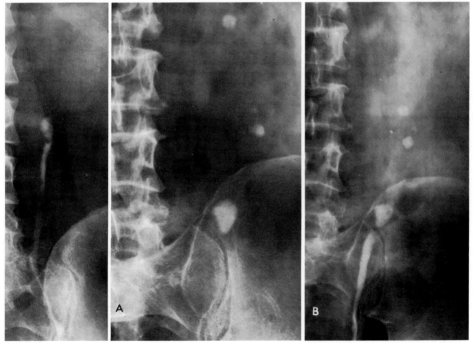

Fig. 12–183   Fig. 12–184

Figure 12–183. Ureteral stone. *Left retrograde pyelogram.* Large oval stone in upper portion of left ureter. Characteristic abrupt termination of contrast medium, which appears to end almost 0.5 cm below stone.

Figure 12–184. Ureteral and renal calculi. **A,** *Plain film.* Large stone in middle portion of left ureter, with multiple stones in left kidney. **B,** *Left retrograde ureterogram.* Stone completely obstructing ureter. No contrast medium above obstruction Characteristic abrupt termination of medium, which ends almost 1 cm below level of stone.

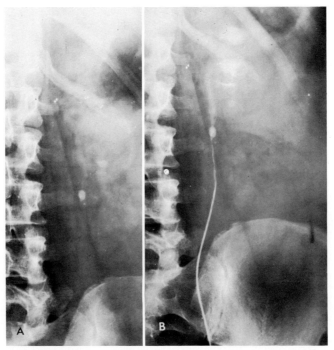

Figure 12–185.   Ureteral stone. **A,** *Plain film.* Stone in upper portion of left ureter and in lower pole of left kidney. **B,** *Left pyeloureterogram.* Stone in line with ureter. **Edema and narrowing of ureter in region of and immediately below, stone.**

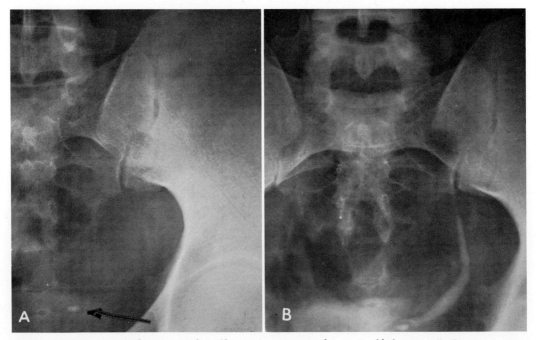

Figure 12–186.   Ureteral stone. **A,** *Plain film.* Stone in terminal portion of left ureter. **B,** *Excretory urogram.* **Characteristic abrupt termination of medium above stone.** with apparently none surrounding it. This form of visualization occurs commonly when stone is located in terminal portion of ureter.

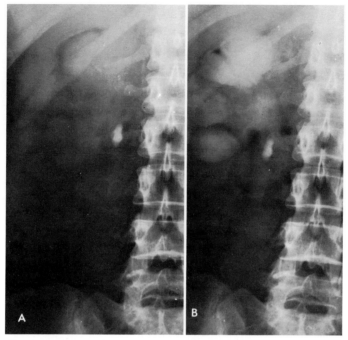

Figure 12–187. Obstructing ureteral stone causing pyeloureterectasis. **A,** *Plain film.* Irregular, elongated calcific shadow overlying tip of right transverse process of second lumbar vertebra. **B,** *Excretory urogram.* Shadow is in line with ureter. In addition, there is **marked pyeloureterectasis above shadow,** furnishing proof that there is stone obstructing upper third of right ureter.

excellent supportive evidence that the shadow represents a calculus. Not uncommonly, however, considerable pyelectasis may be present, yet the ureter above the stone may appear to be only minimally dilated. In some cases the ureter may not be outlined with contrast medium, because contrast medium diffuses very slowly into the stagnant urine in the dilated part above the obstruction (Figs. 12–187 through 12–191). The use of reinjection, infusion technique, or delayed films (1 to 2 hours) may overcome this problem and provide adequate filling and visualization. If these methods are not successful, additional data may be obtained by means of an opaque ureteral catheter. The retrograde introduction of urographic medium above an obstructing ureteral stone should be avoided when possible, as it may result in an acute renal infection.

NONOPAQUE STONES AND STONES OF POOR DENSITY

Stones of poor density and nonopaque stones may be most difficult to recognize. Often the only method available is to elicit "grating" or obstruction on passage of a ureteral catheter. Ureterectasis or ureteral edema may suggest the presence of a stone. Collections of urographic medium around a nonopaque stone in an excretory urogram may point to its presence. The classic finding, of course, is a "negative" shadow or filling defect in the urographic medium (Fig. 12–192). A nonopaque stone may suggest ureteral obstruction from a stricture or a primary ureteral tumor (Fig. 12–193). Various degrees of density of a stone, such as an opaque center and nonopaque periphery, or vice versa, may produce unusual varieties of urograms (Fig. 12–194).

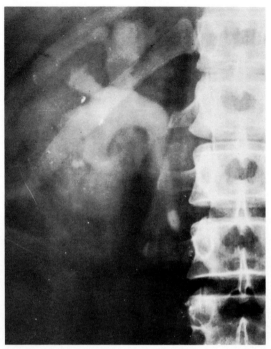

Figure 12–188. Obstructing ureteral stone causing pyeloureterectasis. *Excretory urogram.* Stone in upper third of right ureter, producing pyeloureterectasis above obstruction.

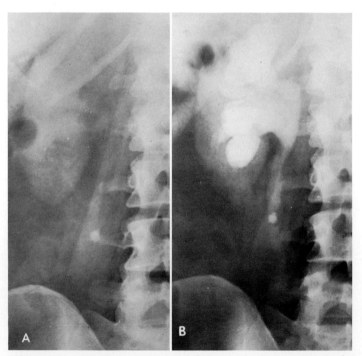

Figure 12–189. Obstructing ureteral stone causing moderate pyeloureterectasis. **A,** *Plain film.* Right ureteral shadow. **B,** *Excretory urogram.* Moderate pyeloureterectasis above stone. **Characteristic abrupt termination of contrast medium just above and below stone.**

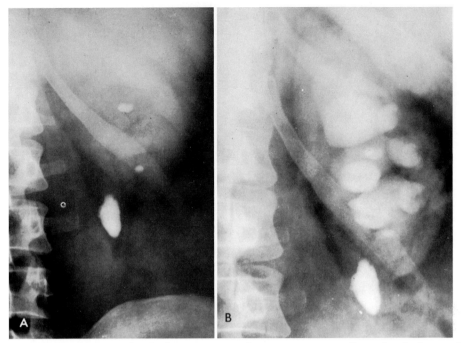

Figure 12–190. Large ureteral calculus causing pyeloureterectasis. Small renal calculi. **A,** *Plain film.* Large calcific shadow opposite transverse process of third lumbar vertebra with two smaller shadows overlying left renal area, suggesting large ureteral calculus and smaller renal calculi. **B,** *Excretory urogram.* Marked caliectasis with two small shadows included in dilated calyces. **Although ureter is not outlined, it might be reasonably safe to surmise that large shadow represents ureteral stone that is cause of obstruction.**

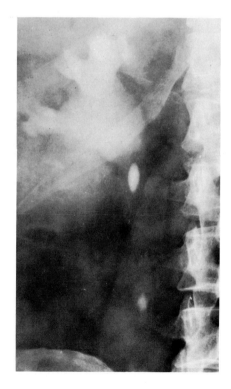

Figure 12–191. Ureteral stones causing pyeloureterectasis. **Ureter not outlined.** *Excretory urogram.* Ureteral stones, one just below ureteropelvic juncture, other in middle portion of ureter. Although ureter is not well outlined, from position of stones and pyelectasis above them, it would seem reasonable to assume that diagnosis of ureteral stones is correct.

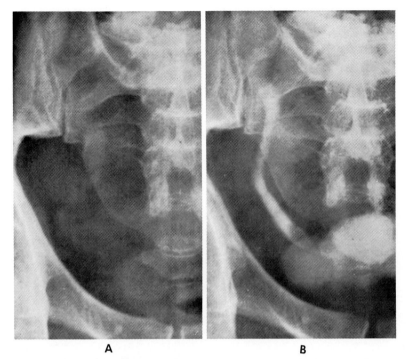

Figure 12–192. Nonopaque ureteral stone. **A,** *Plain film.* No ureteral stones visible. **B,** *Right retrograde.* *ureterogram.* Filling defect in terminal portion of ureter from nonopaque stone.

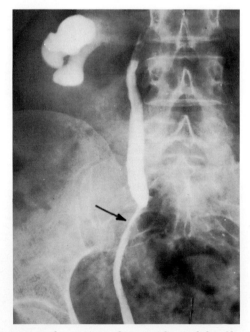

Figure 12–193. Nonopaque ureteral stone simulating either solid infiltrating ureteral tumor or ureteral **stricture.** *Right retrograde pyelogram.* Obstruction in middle portion of ureter over sacral promontory. Pyeloureterectasis above obstruction. Area just below dilatation impossible to fill with contrast medium. Plain film showed no shadow. Diagnosis rested between ureteral tumor, ureteral stricture, and nonopaque stone. Exploration revealed nonopaque ureteral stone.

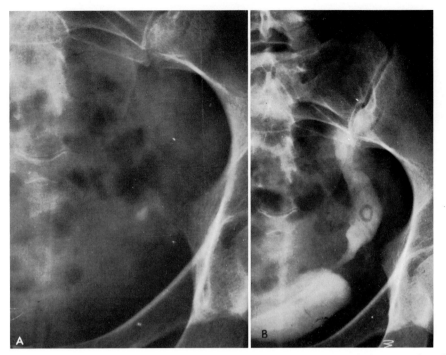

Figure 12–194.   Laminated ureteral stone with dense center and nonopaque periphery. **A,** *Plain film.* Small calcific shadow opposite left ischial spine. **B,** *Excretory urogram.* Moderate dilatation of lower portion of left ureter. Nonopaque periphery of stone forms negative shadow, while center of shadow is of same density as urographic medium.

MISCELLANEOUS TYPES OF URETERAL STONES, LOCATIONS, AND PROBLEMS

Stones in Dilated Ureters; Large Ureteral Stones

In advanced ureterectasis, single or multiple stones may move around freely in the ureter and by so doing change their appearance and location from film to film. The dilatation and tortuosity of the ureters also may be of so great a degree that the shadows observed in the plain film suggest that the stones are extraureteral.* Occasionally, ureteral calculi can assume enormous proportions (Figs. 12–195 through 12–200).

Ureteral Calculi in Anomalies

The problem of ureteral stone in congenital anomalies chiefly concerns ureteral duplication. (This condition is discussed

---

*Stones associated with ureteroceles are described in Chapter 9.

in Chapter 9.) It is not difficult to realize the errors that would be possible in such a situation. If the existence of duplication is not recognized, a stone in one ureter, obstructing one segment of a kidney, may be called an extraurinary shadow if only the other ureter is visualized. Diagnosis may be most difficult in cases of incomplete duplication. In such cases the ureteral catheter usually will pass up only one branch of the ureter because of the anatomic arrangement at the site of bifurcation. It may be impossible to introduce an opaque catheter or contrast medium up the other branch of the ureter, where the stone is lodged. If the renal segment serving this branch of the ureter is temporarily functionless (to excretory urography), diagnosis will be difficult (Fig. 12–201).

Migratory Stones

In most cases a ureteral stone moves only one way in a ureter: down. In the occasional case, however, stones seem to

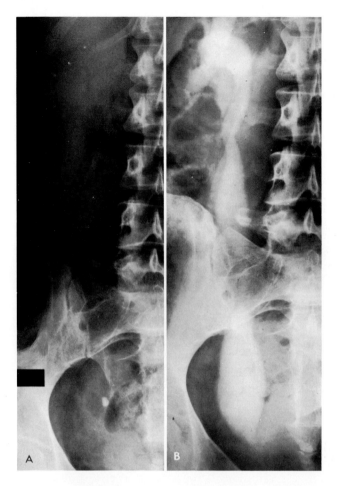

Figure 12–195. Ureteral stone in mega-loureter. **A,** *Plain film.* Triangular ureteral stone in lower third of right ureter. **B,** *Right retrograde pyelogram (10-minute delayed pyelogram).* Congenital (?) megaloureter with greatest amount of dilatation in lower third. Stone is included in ureter and apparently moves around considerably. Patient has recurring colic.

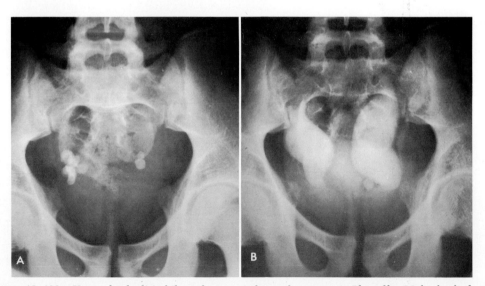

Figure 12–196. Ureteral calculi in bilateral congenital megaloureters. **A,** *Plain film.* Multiple shadows over both ureteral areas. **B,** *Excretory urogram.* Marked congenital (?) dilatation of lower third of each ureter. Shadows of ureteral calculi move around freely in dilated lower portions of ureters. Large shadow on left appears to be excluded from ureter, but in other roentgenograms it was shown to be definitely included. Unusual appearance is evidently result of incomplete filling of ureter.

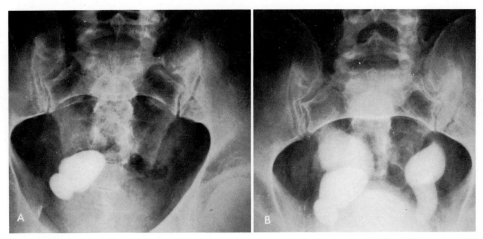

Figure 12-197. Ureteral calculi in dilated ureters suggest vesical calculi. **A,** *Plain film.* Impossible to tell from this roentgenogram whether large calcific shadows are in bladder or in ureter. **B,** *Excretory urogram.* Shadows are demonstrated to be stones in dilated lower portion of right ureter.

change position and move up and down the ureter freely. In one film they may be in the lower part of the ureter, whereas in a later film they may be in the upper part or even in the renal pelvis. Although in most cases this means a dilated ureter, cases are encountered in which there appears to be little or no ureterectasis (Fig. 12–202).

Stones in Intramural Part of Ureter

Mention has already been made (Chapter 8) of the normal urographic relationship between the interureteric ridge and the intramural ureters. Edling demonstrated that in cases of stone, tumor, or other lesions of the intramural ureter, alter-

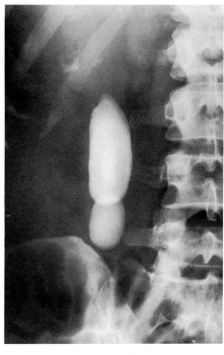

Figure 12-198. *Excretory urogram.* Large ureteral calculi, with poor renal function.

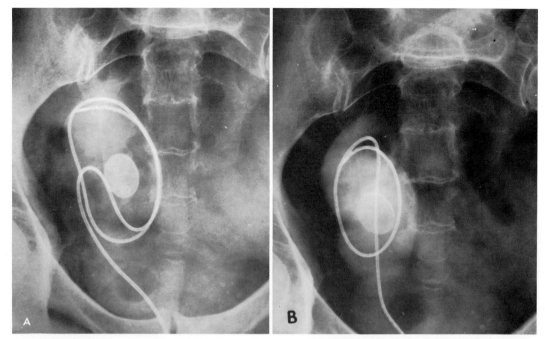

Figure 12–199. Ureteral calculus in dilated ureter suggests vesical calculus. **A,** *Plain film.* Large oval calculus overlying right vesical area. Lead catheter coiled around it. It is impossible to tell from this roentgenogram whether calculus is in vesical diverticulum or in dilated lower portion of ureter. **B,** *Right retrograde ureterogram.* Stone shown definitely to be in hugely dilated lower portion of right ureter.

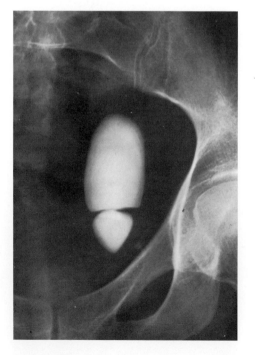

Figure 12–200. *Plain film.* **Huge ureteral stone.** Lower portion of stone still retains shape of minor calyx from which it apparently originated.

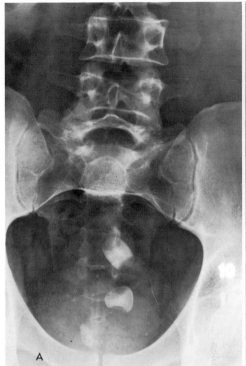
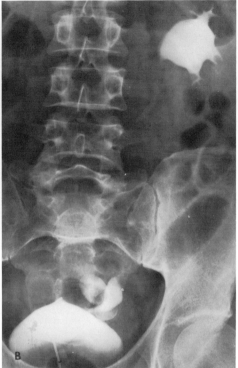
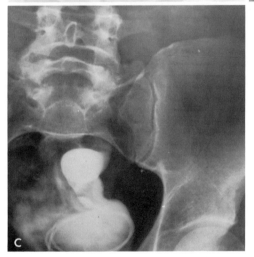

Figure 12–201. Large calculi in ectopic (duplicated) upper-pole ureter of a man. **A,** *Plain film.* Three large calcific shadows over middle and left vesical area. **B,** *Excretory urogram.* Pyelectasis, grade 1+, of lower half of duplicated left kidney. Calyces within normal limits. Ureter normal except lower third, where there is localized ureterectasis that overlies but does not include calcific shadows. **C,** *Left ureterogram.* Catheter introduced into ectopic ureteral orifice situated at 6 o'clock position in vesical neck. This ureter served "functionless" upper segment of left kidney. Dilated terminal portion of ectopic ureter included three calculi seen in **A.**

ation of this normal relationship can be helpful in diagnosis. All urologists are aware of the tremendous amount of edema that may sometimes be present when a stone is impacted in the intramural ureter. Cystoscopically, the lesion appears as a red granular areola often associated with bullous edema, which may reach such proportions that it may be mistaken for an infiltrating carcinoma of the bladder.

Edema of the intramural ureter in-creases the distance between the ureteral lumen and the interureteric ridge. When edema is minimal, the condition may be recognized only by comparing the two sides, which normally are symmetrical. The normal distance between the ureteral lumen and the interureteric ridge is about 2 to 3 millimeters; when mild edema caused by a stone is present, a slight increase in this distance (plus the presence of a small calcific shadow) may indicate the

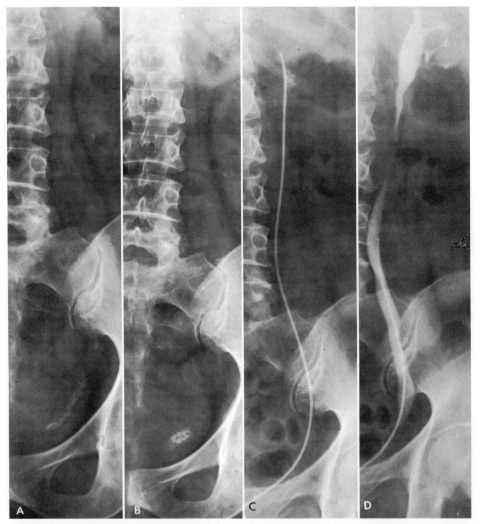

Figure 12–202. Migratory ureteral calculi. **A** and **B,** *Plain films* made on same day show multiple calculi low in left ureter, with different distribution in each film. **C,** *Plain film* with opaque catheter in ureter (made 2 days later). Calculi are now in upper part of ureter and renal pelvis. **D,** *Retrograde pyelogram* shows atrophic kidney with typical vertical pelvis. Calculi are in pelvis.

correct diagnosis of ureteral stone. In a communication on this subject, Camiel emphasized the importance of this urographic observation and pointed out that large radiolucent shadows or filling defects may result from extensive periureteral edema. The edema may involve only the area of the ureteral orifice, or it may include the entire intramural ureter, which will appear as a radiolucent shadow that may be cylindrical, tulip-shaped, oval, or round, or may even appear as a "halo" or "cobra head" effect around the stone or the dilated ureter similar to that seen in cases of ureterocele.

The contour of the interureteric ridge may also be altered by the edema (Figs. 12–203, 12–204, and 12–205).

The edema may be so extensive, diffuse, and poorly defined that the shadow does not appear to be confined strictly to the region of the ureteral orifice and intramural ureter. In some cases irritation around the intramural ureter may cause spastic ipsilateral contraction of the bladder with its typical urographic appearance (Fig. 12–206).

It should be appreciated that all of the findings enumerated may be present for a

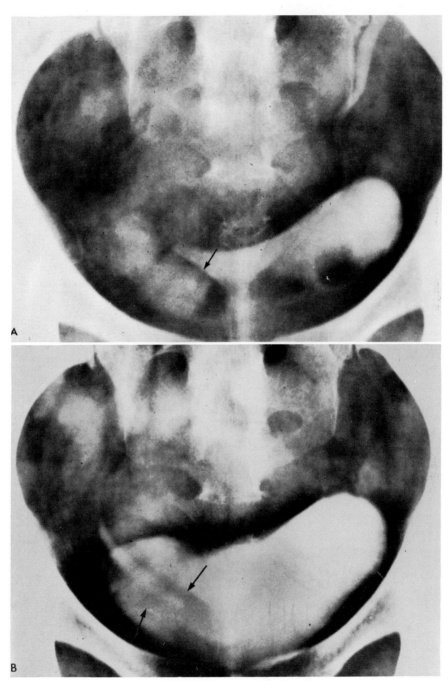

Figure 12–203. Edema of intramural ureter because of stone increases distance between ureteral lumen (and stone) and interureteric ridge. *Excretory urograms.* **A**, *Early film.* Small calculus in terminal right ureter. No medium has yet appeared in right ureter, but cystogram (from contrast medium from left kidney) shows spasm of right half of bladder and increased distance between stone and interureteric ridge (*arrow*). **B**, *Sixty-minute film.* Right ureter now outlined. "Sleeve-like" radiolucent area (*arrows*) surrounds intramural ureter.

Illustration and legend continued on following page

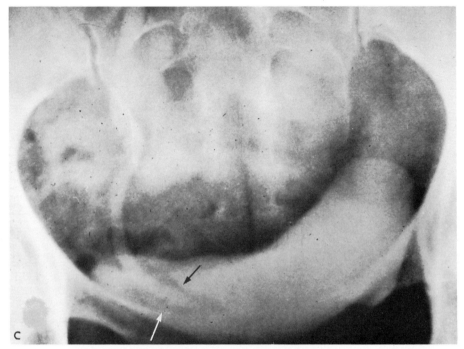

Figure 12–203. *Continued.*   **C,** *Ninety-minute film;* patient erect. Radiolucent area appears V-shaped *(arrows).* (From Camiel, M. R.)

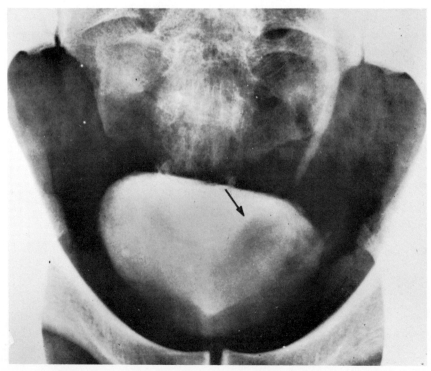

Figure 12–204.   Edema of intramural ureter because of recently passed stone. *Excretory urogram.* Left ureteral stone has recently passed but edema, still present, results in radiolucent filling defect with medial compression of interureteric ridge *(arrow).* (From Camiel, M. R.)

Fig. 12–205

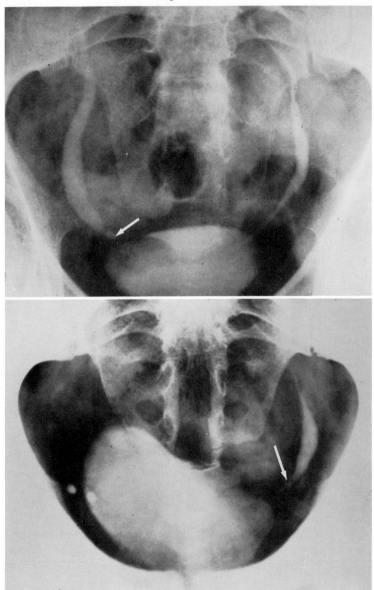

Fig. 12–206

Figure 12–205. Edema of intramural ureter because of stone. *Excretory urogram.* Small stone *(arrow)* in right ureter at point where ureter enters bladder. Tulip-shaped radiolucent filling defect distal to stone with medial compression of interureteric ridge from edema of intramural ureter. (From Camiel, M. R.)

Figure 12–206. *Excretory urogram.* Left ureteral stone just above bladder *(arrow)*, **causing spastic contraction of left wall.** (From Camiel, M. R.)

short time after the stone has passed or may be the result of traumatic edema from manipulation for a ureteral stone (see Figures 12–209 and 12–214). It is important to remember also that even though the kidney on the involved side is not functioning (temporarily), the cystogram produced by contrast medium from the opposite kidney will demonstrate the radiolucent filling defects; it is not necessary for the involved ureter to be outlined with contrast medium before the correct diagnosis is made.

Spontaneous Urinary Extravasation Due to Calculous Ureteral Obstruction

Spontaneous nontraumatic perirenal extravasation of urine is an unusual phenomenon. At one end of the spectrum, its most common form is represented by mild peripelvic extravasation, a form of fornical backflow, which is observed in approximately 2 per cent of the excretory urograms with abdominal compression (Hinman) and which may follow calculous ureteral obstruction (Khan and Malek). At the other end of the spectrum is the uncommon frank rupture of the renal pelvis, which usually occurs in chronically diseased or stone-containing and obstructed kidneys (Joachim and Becker; Shaw).

Patients are usually symptomatic and manifest some combination of colicky or constant flank pain, hematuria, nausea and vomiting, abdominal or flank tenderness, and fever (Khan and Malek).

Excretory urography discloses various degrees of the fornical type of backflow or gross peripelvic extravasation. Ureteral obstruction is the rule in all patients and is most frequently caused by a ureteral calculus (approximately 50 per cent of cases) (Fig. 12–207). When the urinary collecting system is acutely obstructed by a pathologic process or abdominal compression, or both, the resultant increase in intraluminal pressure, augmented by a sudden diuretic load of urographic contrast medium, may lead to rupture at the weakest point. In an otherwise healthy upper urinary tract, this

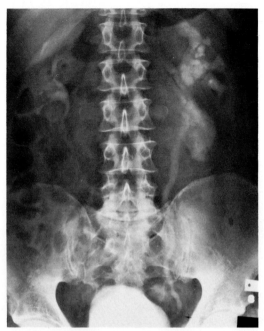

Figure 12–207. Spontaneous nontraumatic urinary extravasation. *Excretory urogram.* Gross peripelvic (fornical) and periureteral extravasation due to small obstructive left lower ureteral calculus *(arrow).* (From Khan, A. U., and Malek, R. S.)

point is usually at the calyceal fornix; the extravasated urine (peripelvic extravasation) dissects in the loose connective tissue of the sinus renalis and is absorbed by the lymphatics. This form of urinary extravasation is transient and relatively innocuous and may represent essentially a physiologic "safety valve." In contrast, extravasation of urine from a tear in a renal collecting system affected by chronic calculous obstruction, infection, and eventual erosion is usually of grave significance and requires early surgical intervention (Khan and Malek).

Excretory urography *without* abdominal compression is the most important diagnostic step when extravasation or predisposing calculous ureteral obstruction is suspected. Retrograde ureteropyelography may be necessary, not only to determine the site and possibly the nature of obstruction but also to provide relief if the obstructive element can be bypassed. In calculous ureteral obstruction, removal of the stone (commonly in the lower ureter) is usually all that is required (Khan and Malek).

Stone-bearing Ureteral Stumps

After nephrectomy and partial ureterectomy for conditions other than urothelial carcinomas, approximately 1 per cent of remaining ureteral stumps produce symptoms (from 3 months to 25 years later). These symptoms are usually nonspecific (lower urinary tract irritation and pain with or without urinary infection) and therefore may completely mislead the urologist. Indeed, even colicky pain emanating from the side where a nephrectomy has previously been performed may be perplexing to the unwary (Fig. 12–208). In the absence of infection, neoplastic change, and fibrosis, the ureteral stump remains as an integral normal part of the urinary tract and retains the physiologic properties of its parent ureter, and thus peristalsis and colic can occur (Malek and associates, 1971). Of the symptomatic stumps, 30 per cent contain calculi, and in our experience only 69 per cent are diagnosed roentgenologically. Excision of the symptomatic stump is the treatment of choice.

Management of Ureteral Calculi

SURGICAL MANAGEMENT OF URETERAL CALCULI

Surgically active ureteral calculi (see classification of renal calculi), as well as those that continue to remain asymptomatically in any part of the ureter despite the usual conservative measures, should be removed.

Transurethral Manipulation of Ureteral Calculi

Ureteral stones less than 1 centimeter in their greatest diameter that initially present in the pelvic ureter or subsequently migrate down into such a position and fail to pass spontaneously are usually amenable to transurethral extraction. The caliber of the ureter through which the stone must pass is as important as the size of the calculus. The presence of fused hips, urethral stricture, hydronephrosis from chronic impaction of the stone, multiple stones, and ureteral deformities (anomalies and so forth) are the usual contraindications to transurethral manipulation. Children, especially young boys, are particularly unsuitable candidates for these maneuvers.

Ideally the feasibility of introducing any type of stone extractor should first be determined by advancing a 5- or 6-F ureteral catheter to a point proximal to that of calculous impaction. The transurethral manipulation of ureteral stones presents urographic problems that are usually not too difficult to evaluate. Occasionally, a stone may be engaged in an Ellik looped catheter or a Councill, Johnson, or Dormia (wire basket) stone extractor and held up in the ureter so that it cannot be withdrawn. In such a case a plain film may reveal the position of the stone in relation to the extractor so that suitable means may be employed to dislodge it (Figs. 12–209 through 12–212). Edema of the ureter and ureteral orifice following traumatic manipulation may cause obstruction and temporary cessation of the ability of the kidney to excrete urographic medium. The edema may be so severe in the region of the ureteral orifice as to cause a filling defect in the cystogram which suggests a vesical tumor (Figs. 12–213 and 12–214).

Ureterolithotomy

Ureteral stones 1 centimeter in diameter or larger as well as smaller ones that fail to pass spontaneously or by transurethral manipulation require open surgical intervention. Other indications for ureterolithotomy include ureteral stones in infants and children, impacted stones of any size above the true bony pelvis, ureteral obstruction below the stone, and disease of the ipsilateral urinary tract requiring concomitant

Text continued on page 1338

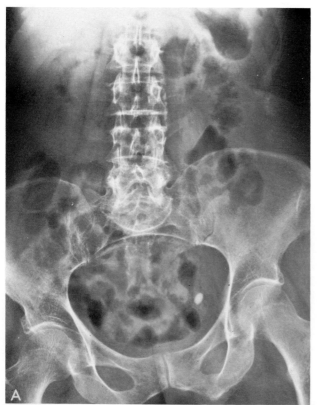

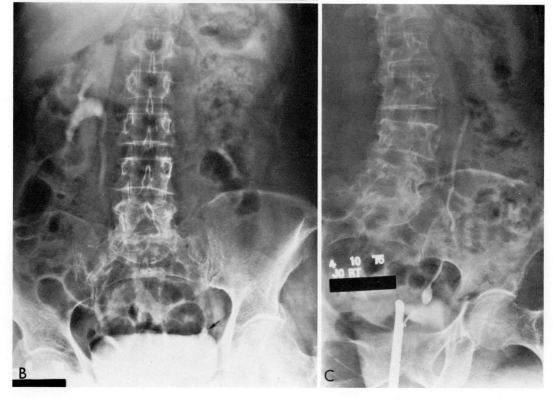

Figure 12–208. Stone-bearing ureteral stump manifesting as colic and urinary infection. Patient was a 75-year-old woman who had undergone left nephrectomy 28 years previously. **A,** *Plain film.* Calcific density in left hemipelvis was thought to be a phlebolith. **B,** *Excretory urogram.* Normal solitary right kidney. Calcific density *(arrow)* almost obscured by contrast medium in bladder. **C,** *Retrograde ureterogram* outlines long left ureteral stump. Dilated terminal portion contains calculus.

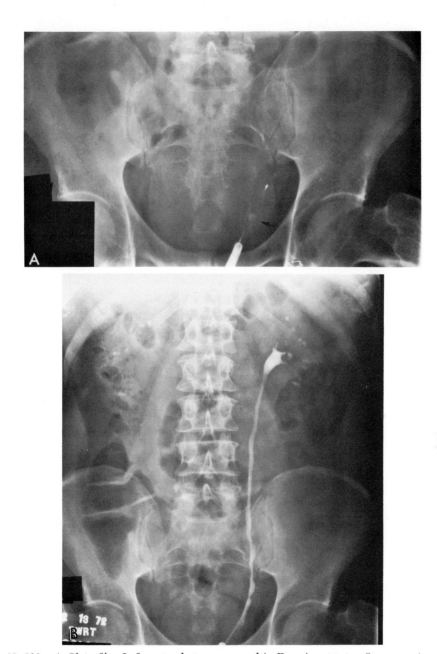

Figure 12–209.   A, *Plain film.* **Left ureteral stone engaged in Dormia extractor.** Stone was immediately extracted. **B,** *Retrograde ureteropyelogram.* Edema of left lower ureter due to trauma of stone extraction. Ureteral catheter was left indwelling for 48 hours.

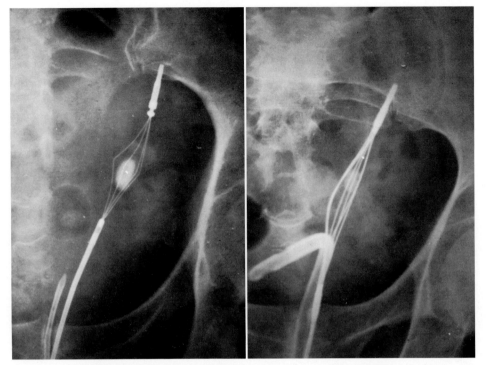

Fig. 12–210   Fig. 12–211

Figure 12–210. *Plain film.* Ureteral stone engaged in Johnson extractor. Twenty-four hours later, stone and extractor were withdrawn.

Figure 12–211. *Plain film.* Ureteral stone engaged in Councill extractor. Since it could not be withdrawn, extractor was left in place with urethral catheter alongside. Extractor with stone withdrawn successfully 48 hours later.

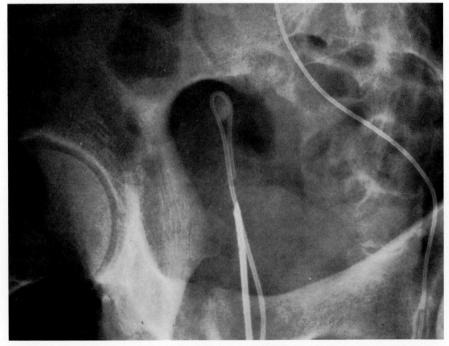

Figure 12–212. *Plain film.* Ureteral stone is engaged in Ellik looped catheter and is held up in lower third of ureter.

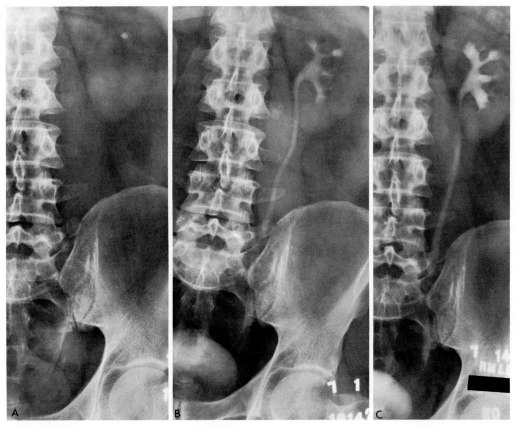

Figure 12–213.   Edema of terminal ureter following transurethral manipulation and removal of stone. **A,** *Plain film.* Shadow of ureteral calculus in lower third of left ureter; also one in left kidney. **B,** *Excretory urogram.* Moderate dilatation of ureter down to and including ureteral stone in lower third of ureter. Shadow in kidney is included in branch of upper calyx. **C,** *Excretory urogram* made several days after transurethral manipulation and removal of ureteral calculus. **Residual edema of lower third of left ureter prevents normal filling of ureter in this region.**

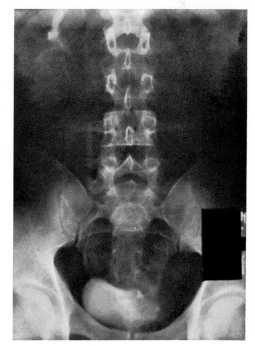

Figure 12–214.   *Excretory urogram.* Temporary absence of function of left kidney, with filling defect in left half of bladder, from edema secondary to unsuccessful transurethral manipulation of ureteral calculus impacted in intramural portion of left ureter. Stone subsequently passed, and renal function returned to normal.

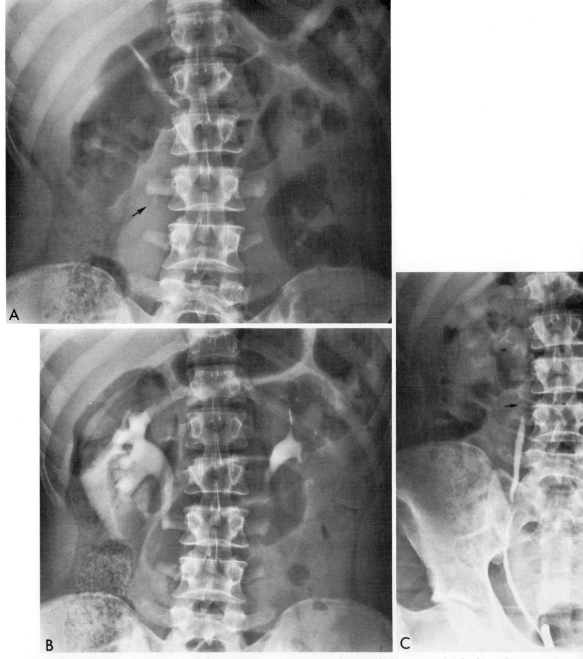

Figure 12–215.   Importance of determination of patency of ureter below area of calculous obstruction. **A,** *Plain film.* Cystine stone of poor radiopacity *(arrow)* just below transverse process of third lumbar vertebra. **B,** *Excretory urogram.* Complete obstruction at level of right ureteral calculus. Similar calculi of poor radiopacity may exist in lower ureter and be missed during surgical removal, with resultant postoperative obstruction and urinary extravasation. **C,** *Retrograde ureterogram.* Normal right ureter up to point of complete obstruction by calculus *(arrow).*

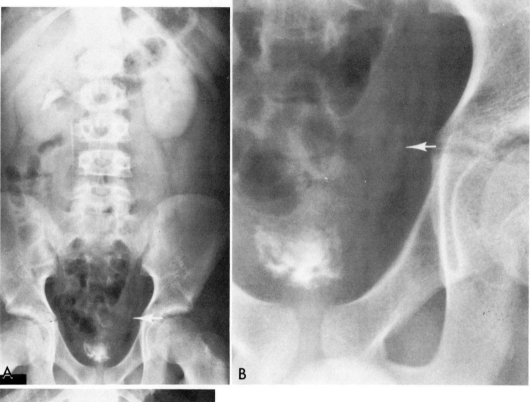

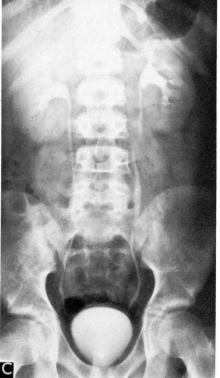

Figure 12–216. Effect of chemolysis on uric acid ureteral calculus in 12-year-old hyperuricemic boy with abdominal pain and hematuria. **A**, *Excretory urogram.* Left ureteral calculus of poor radiopacity *(arrow)* causing partial left ureteral obstruction. Note early obstructive nephrogram. **B**, *Excretory urogram.* Localized view of pelvis shows stone slightly better *(arrow).* **C**, *Excretory urogram.* Normal. Stone has dissolved after 10 days of hydration, urinary alkalinization, and allopurinol administration. (Courtesy of Dr. Ovidio E. Vitas.) (From Malek, R. S., 1976.)

surgical correction. Passage of a ureteral catheter in patients who have previously undergone ureterolithotomies may serve as an invaluable guide for identification of the ureter amid the scar tissue and may also serve as a stent to promote better healing of a ureter that has been previously operated upon. The importance of obtaining a pre-operative plain film (KUB) and of determining the patency of the ureter below the area of calculous obstruction cannot be overemphasized (Fig. 12–215).

CHEMOLYSIS OF URETERAL CALCULI

Dissolution of *pure* uric acid and cystine ureteral calculi can be successfully achieved if the affected kidney is not infected, or totally obstructed, or both (see sections on cystinuria and uric acid lithiasis). A substantial decrease in the size of the stone is usually observed within one month of starting treatment. Passage of small fragments during treatment may induce transient colic, of which the patient must be forewarned (Fig. 12–216).

VESICAL CALCULI

Vesical calculus is predominantly a disease of the male sex in all races and nationalities. Calculi frequently migrate down the ureter from the upper urinary tract and are occasionally retained in the bladder (migrant calculi), but of those that are formed in the bladder, usually in association with obstruction or infection of the lower urinary tract (secondary calculi), the majority (98 per cent), in the United States, occur in older men (Straffon and Higgins). The usual associated lesions include bladder outlet obstruction, urethral stricture, neurogenic bladder, vesical diverticulum, and cystocele.

Phosphatic encrustations (secondary calculi) are formed on a variety of foreign bodies in the urinary tract. These include nonabsorbable sutures; pins or clips swallowed accidentally with subsequent perforation of the bowel and entry into the urin-

ary tract; a variety of objects introduced transurethrally by the patient during the course of genital manipulation; and catheters that are left indwelling for prolonged drainage. Occasionally, the balloon of a Foley catheter may break while indwelling and a portion of it may thus be left behind to act as a stone nidus (Fig. 12–217).

Endemic Calculi

The much-used term *endemic stone disease* is of dubious validity when one considers that this entity is not regularly prevalent in any country or race and that there are historical variations in the rate of incidence within given countries and population groups. However, the term may be retained until the causative factors have been defined more clearly.

This type of stone disease was once common in England but gradually disappeared after World War I; today, it remains widely distributed in Middle and Far Eastern countries. The older reports were concerned exclusively with bladder stones, but more recent studies suggest that upper urinary tract calculi also occur commonly in endemic disease (Fig. 12–218) (Eckstein).

Primary or endemic stones form in the urinary tracts of children in whom obstruction or infection or other usual calculogenic factors are not demonstrable. Recurrence after removal is low, and the stones are usually composed of ammonium hydrogen urate with calcium oxalate and a minimum of calcium phosphate (Valyasevi and Van Reen). The disease is prevalent in children of low socioeconomic class, predominantly in boys under 5 years of age.

Studies in Thailand have shown the following:

1. Bladder stones are almost seven times as prevalent among village children as among city children.

2. In contrast to the common practice of giving village infants supplemental feedings of glutenous rice, only very few city infants would receive such a diet.

3. The 24-hour urine volume and os-

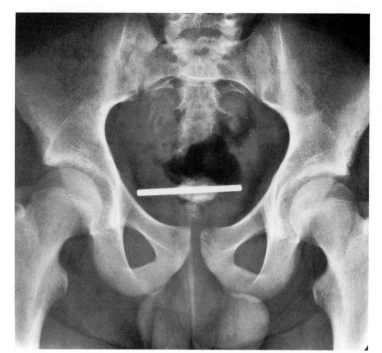

Figure 12–217. Foreign body calculus. *Plain film.* Metal rod (self-introduced, transurethrally) found on routine examination in bladder of 14-year-old boy with pyuria. Note infected calculous material around midportion of rod. (From Malek, R. S., 1976.)

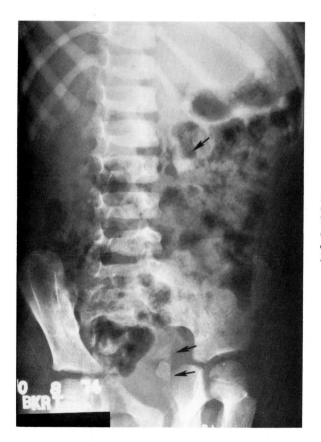

Figure 12–218. Endemic calculi. *Plain film.* Large left renal calculus *(upper arrow)* and two ureteral calculi *(lower arrows)* in 5-year-old Asian boy. Patient had previous renal and bladder calculi (urate) removed at age 1 year. Present stones also consisted of urates with struvite shell caused by *Proteus mirabilis* urosepsis.

molality both are frequently lower in new-born infants and older children in villages than in their counterparts in the city.

4. Urinary phosphate and sulfate excretion is lower in village children, and, conversely, higher concentrations of urinary calcium and significant oxalate crystalluria are observed in village children. (Uric acid crystalluria, on the other hand, is found equally often among village and city children.) It is likely that low urinary phosphate and sulfate concentrations in village infants reflect the deficiency of milk and high-quality protein in their diets (Chutikorn and associates).

Hydroxyproline is thought to have several roles in stone formation. Not only is it a precursor of oxalate but it is also thought to have an effect on oxalate crystal transformation and clumping. Also, hydroxyproline excretion is increased under several abnormal conditions during which calculogenesis is common, including hyperparathyroidism, malnutrition, immobilization, and bone tumors. Recent studies indicate that dietary supplementation with hydroxyproline for infants living in areas of Thailand where bladder stones are endemic results in oxalate crystalluria and clumping of oxalate crystals accompanied by increased excretion of hydroxyproline, oxalate, and calcium in the urine (Dhanamitta and Valyasevi). These elegant studies do not identify the exact cause of vesical calculogenesis but certainly help to shed light on some factors that may be involved in these areas of such high incidence.

Clinical Features and Investigations of Vesical Calculi

The typical symptoms of vesical calculus consist of dull or sharp pain and hematuria, which may be aggravated by exercise and sudden movement. These symptoms may be more pronounced at the end of urination when the bladder is empty, and the discomfort may be relieved when the patient lies supine. Although some vesical calculi are asymptomatic, irritative

lower urinary tract symptoms and interruption of the urinary stream may be observed in 30 to 50 per cent of patients (Straffon and Higgins).

Sudden excruciating pain may be referred to the tip of the penis or to the scrotum in boys, or to the perineum via the third and fourth sacral nerves in boys and girls. Occasionally the pain may be referred to the back, the hip, or the sole of the foot. Additionally, in longstanding cases, hemorrhoids or rectal prolapse due to straining, and, in boys, abnormally frequent erections induced by trigonal irritation may occur. Foreign-body calculi in the bladder are usually associated with foul-smelling infected urine. Longstanding vesical calculous disease with or without infection may lead to contracture of the bladder (transient from edema or permanent from fibrosis), vesicoureteral reflux, and ureterovesical obstruction (Taneja).

Although correction of the associated obstructive lesion(s) and elimination of urinary infection may prevent the recurrence of vesical calculi, other possible underlying etiologic factor(s) must be carefully ruled out. Indeed, a bladder stone may be the only presenting symptom of the stone-forming tendency (Potter and associates), and the affected patient deserves a complete evaluation.

ROENTGEN STUDIES OF VESICAL CALCULI

Poor Radiopacity of Most Vesical Calculi

Of all urinary calculi, those situated in the urinary bladder are the most often overlooked when one is examining the plain film. In many cases this is due to the fact that the physician examining the roentgenograms does not scrutinize the vesical area thoroughly. On the other hand, even if the roentgenograms are most carefully examined, a large number of vesical calculi will be missed. Primarily responsible for this situation is the fact that many vesical calculi are composed of uric acid or urates and either are radiolucent or cast shadows of poor density. Also, these calculi usually lie over bone (sacrum), and this further increases the difficulty of roentgen visualization. Incomplete preparation of the patient's bowel often results in various rounded, indefinite shadows in the bony pelvis produced by fecal material in the rectosigmoid; these shadows may simulate the faint outlines of poorly visualized vesical calculi.

It is estimated that in 50 per cent to 60 per cent of cases vesical calculus cannot be diagnosed roentgenographically. For this reason one should never state that vesical calculi are not present until the bladder has been thoroughly examined with the cystoscope. Some nonopaque calculi can be seen as negative shadows in either an excretory or a retrograde cystogram (Figs. 12–219 through 12–222).

Roentgenographic Characteristics of Vesical Calculi

Vesical calculi vary in quantity from a single calculus to many and in size from

Fig. 12–219　　　　　　　　**Fig. 12–220**

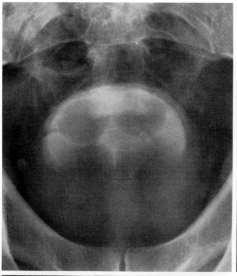 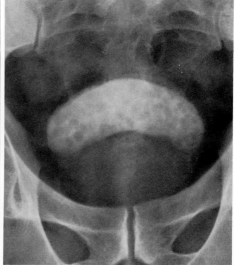

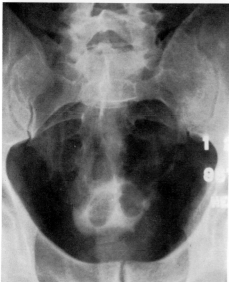

Figure 12–219. *Excretory cystogram.* Non-opaque vesical calculi producing negative shadows. Hypertrophy of prostate, producing negative filling defect in base of bladder. Plain film was negative.

Figure 12–220. *Excretory cystogram.* Multiple negative shadows from many small, round, nonopaque calculi in bladder. Note filling defect in base of bladder from hypertrophy of prostate. Plain film was negative.

Figure 12–221. *Excretory cystogram.* Nonopaque calculi in bladder produce large oval negative shadows. Plain film was negative.

Fig. 12–221

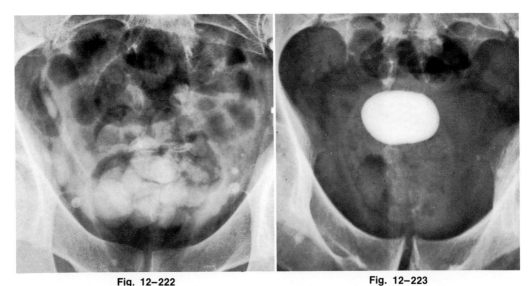

Fig. 12–222   Fig. 12–223

Figure 12–222. *Excretory urogram.* Fecal material in rectum suggests multiple vesical calculi of poor density.

Figure 12–223. *Plain film.* Vesical calculus.

that of a grain of sand to enormous proportions. Usually the calculi are circular or oval in outline, but almost any shape may be encountered (Figs. 12–223 through 12–229). One of the most unusual-appearing types of stone is the hard burr or jackstone variety (Figs. 12–230 and 12–231), which gets its name from the many irregular prongs that project from its surface. This stone usually is composed of calcium oxalate. The commonest position of vesical calculi is in the center of the bony pelvis, well above the

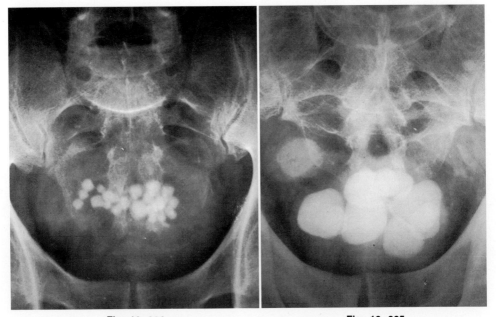

Fig. 12–224   Fig. 12–225

Figures 12–224 and 12–225. *Plain films.* Multiple radiopaque vesical calculi.

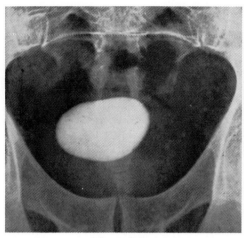 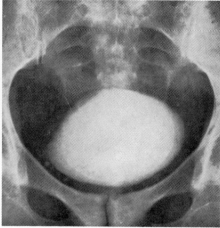

Fig. 12–226   Fig. 12–227

Figure 12–226. *Plain film.* Large vesical calculus.
Figure 12–227. *Plain film.* Huge vesical calculus removed suprapubically. Obstetrical forceps used to deliver stone from bladder. (Courtesy of Dr. W. N. Wishard.)

symphysis pubis. Intravesical protrusion of enlarged prostatic lobes may cause a rather odd configuration of vesical calculi, since they tend to arrange themselves around the intravesical encroachment of the enlarged prostate gland (Figs. 12–232, 12–233, and 12–234).

Stones Situated Partially or Entirely Within Vesical Diverticula

Stones situated either partially or entirely within vesical diverticula may present a rather bizarre appearance as to both location and shape. In such a situation they may be confused with large ureteral stones in a hugely dilated ureter. Dumb-bell-shaped stones, with one end lodged in a diverticulum and the other projecting into the bladder, are not uncommonly seen (Figs. 12–235 and 12–236). Figure 12–237 illustrates a rather unusual case of a dumb-bell-shaped calculus in the bladder of a woman. One part of the stone was fixed in an area where vesicovaginal fistula had been repaired previously. Vesical calculi in

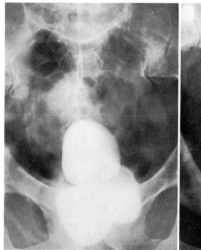 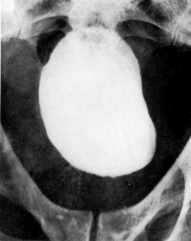

Fig. 12–228   Fig. 12–229

Figure 12–228. *Excretory urogram.* Multiple large vesical calculi.
Figure 12–229. *Plain film.* Large vesical calculus. Multiple small prostatic calculi.

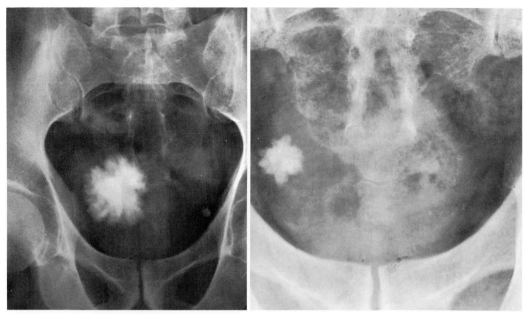

Fig. 12–230   Fig. 12–231

Figure 12–230. *Plain film.* Vesical calculus of burr-like type.
Figure 12–231. *Plain film.* Jackstone variety of stone in bladder of patient with hypertrophy of prostate.

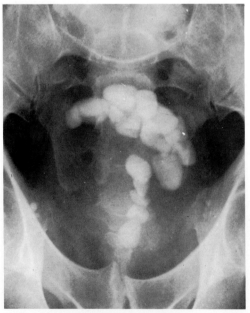

Figure 12–232. *Plain film.* Multiple vesical calculi in male patient with hypertrophy of prostate gland. Calculi are arranged around intravesical projection of enlarged prostate.

Fig. 12–233

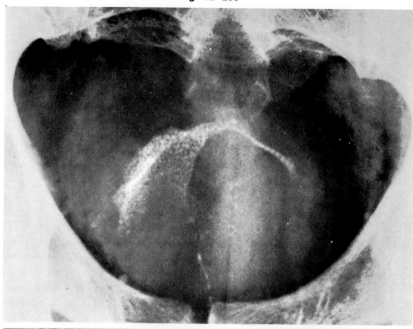

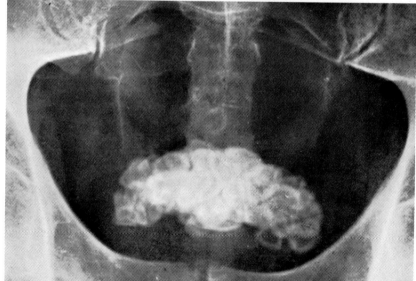

Fig. 12–234

Figure 12–233. *Plain film.* Large number of very small vesical calculi distributed around intravesical projection of enlarged prostatic lobes.

Figure 12–234. *Plain film.* Large number of small calculi in bladder distributed around intravesical projection of prostate.

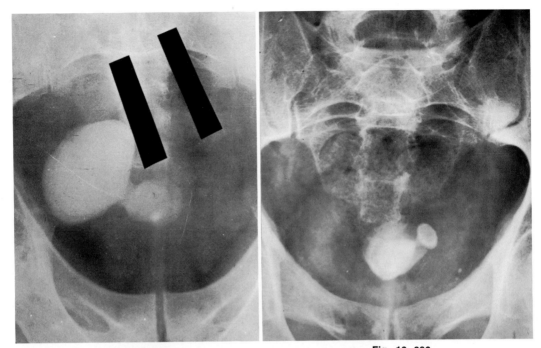

Fig. 12–235 Fig. 12–236

Figures 12–235 and **12–236.** *Plain films.* Vesical calculus, dumbbell shape, with one portion of stone in diverticulum and other free in bladder.

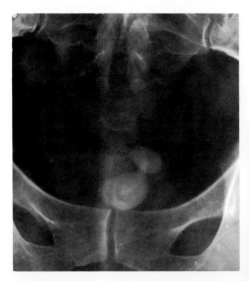

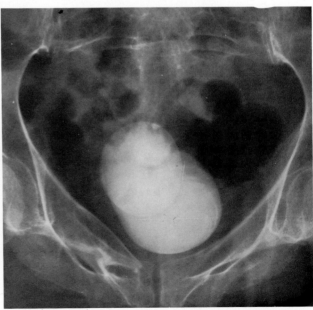

Figure 12–237. *Plain film.* Dumbbell vesical calculus at site of repair of vesicovaginal fistula. (From Cristol, D. S., and Greene, L. F.: Vesical Calculi in Women. S. Clin. North America, Aug., 1945, pp. 987–992.)

Figure 12–238. *Plain film.* Large vesical calculi in woman aged 61.

women are uncommon but do occur (Fig. 12–238). Multiple calculi situated in vesical diverticula may produce roentgenograms of unusual appearance (Figs. 12–239 and 12–240).

Differential Diagnosis From Encrusted Lesions in Bladder and Extravesical Shadows

Encrustations in the bladder caused by encrusted cystitis (Chapter 10), vesical tumor (Chapter 14), or a postradium slough may simulate true vesical calculi. Extraurinary calcification in the vesical region may simulate vesical stone and be excluded only by means of cystoscopic examination. Most such shadows are in the gen-

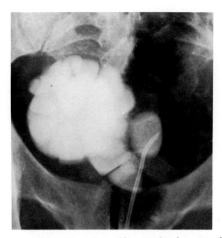

Figure 12–239. *Plain film.* **Multiple vesical calculi filling large vesical diverticulum,** which arises from right wall of bladder. There are a few stones free in bladder adjacent to diverticulum. Urethral catheter in bladder.

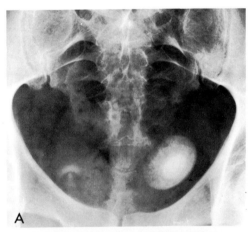

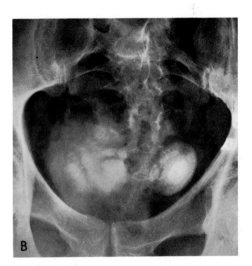

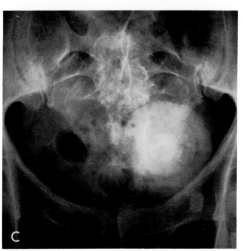

Figure 12–240. Laminated calculus in vesical diverticulum. **A,** *Plain film.* Large laminated vesical calculus overlying left half of bladder. **B,** *Excretory cystogram.* Medium partially fills right half of bladder, which is trabeculated and contains multiple cellules. Stone appears to be extravesical in this cystogram because contrast medium has not entered diverticulum. **C,** *Plain film* made 24 hours later. Residual contrast medium in large vesical diverticulum in which calculus is situated.

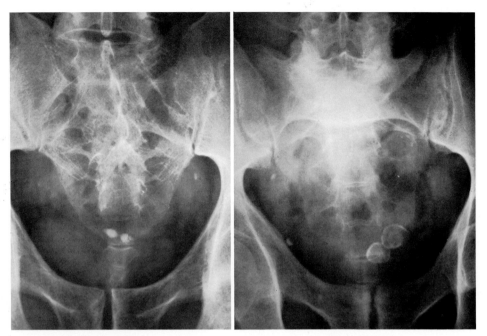

Fig. 12–241   **Fig. 12–242**

Figures 12–241 and 12–242.   Extravesical calcifications that look like vesical calculi. *Plain films.* Multiple calcific shadows over vesical region, suggesting vesical calculi. Cystoscopy showed no stones in bladder.

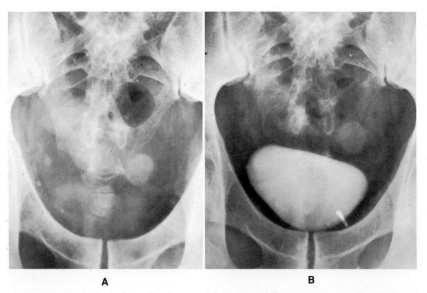

A   **B**

Figure 12–243.   Extravesical shadow (fecal material in sigmoid?) mimics vesical calculus. **A,** *Plain film.* Circular shadow over left side of bony pelvis, overlying vesical region in a man. Suggests vesical calculus. **B,** *Retrograde cystogram.* Shadow definitely excluded; is not in urinary tract.

ital organs of women, although frequently they are seen in men, in which case their accurate identification is most difficult (Figs. 12–241, 12–242, and 12–243; see also Chapter 7).

Management of Vesical Calculi

SURGICAL MANAGEMENT OF VESICAL CALCULI

Vesical calculi may be removed by cystoscopic manipulation and conventional or electrohydraulic litholapaxy. Transurethral resection of an obstructive prostate can be carried out at the same time. Occasionally, litholapaxy may be performed via the sinus tract of an indwelling suprapubic catheter. Large, hard calculi (especially when impacted in a diverticulum), endemic stones, and stones formed around solid, large foreign bodies require cystolithotomy; suprapubic prostatectomy may also be undertaken at the same time.

CHEMOLYSIS OF VESICAL CALCULI

Dissolution of sterile uric acid vesical calculi in unobstructed asymptomatic patients may be achieved by hydration, urinary alkalinization, and administration of allopurinol (see section on uric acid lithiasis) (Fig. 12–244). In patients with struvite calculi who are poor surgical risks or who refuse surgical procedures, intermittent (four to six times daily) or continuous intravesical instillation of hemiacidrin (Renacidin) or Suby and Albright's solutions G (pH 4.0) or M (pH 4.5) may achieve gratifying results (D. R. Smith, 1972). These procedures are, however, likely to fail with markedly radiopaque (hard) calculi.

PROSTATIC CALCULI

Classification of Prostatic Calculi

Prostatic calculi may be divided into three groups, namely, native, migrant, and secondary. By native is meant that the calculi were formed originally within the substance of the prostate gland. Migrant calculi are those that have formed elsewhere in the urinary tract and have become lodged in the prostatic urethra (see discussion of urethral calculi). Secondary calculi are usually formed in the prostatic fossa in association with infection, obstruction, or both. Prostatic calculi often are missed because the plain film is not centered low enough to show the prostatic region (see Chapter 7).

NATIVE PROSTATIC CALCULI

Native prostatic calculi usually are multiple and relatively small, varying from 1 to 10 mm in diameter. In occasional cases, however, the calculi are very large and numerous and may almost completely replace the substance of the prostate gland. They are rarely observed in boys and are infrequent in men less than 40 years of age. The majority occur in men aged from 50 to 65 years (Straffon and Higgins), and their incidence in benign hypertrophied prostate gland (7 per cent) is almost equal to that in prostatic carcinoma (6.3 per cent) (Cristol and Emmett).

Detailed studies by Vernon Smith (1966) indicate that prostatic calculi are not a product of secondary changes in corpora amylacea but rather are a separate entity. It is suggested that corpora amylacea are a product of normal prostatic secretion, consisting of laminated mucoprotein matrix that can become covered by apatite (minimal or no calcification in center) and form corpora calculi when trapped in the prostatic acinar complex during the normal process of aging. Prostatic calculi are formed under fundamentally similar settings, but they differ from corpora calculi in that the initial event involves massive deposition of calcium phosphate (apatite) in the central area.

MIGRANT AND SECONDARY PROSTATIC CALCULI

Migrant and secondary prostatic calculi usually are larger and fewer than native calculi.

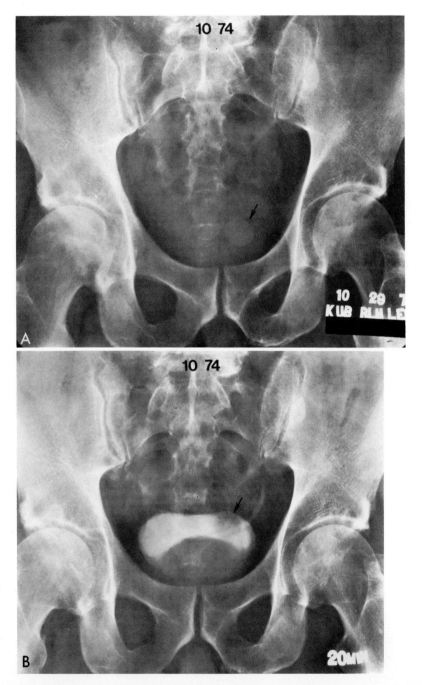

Figure 12–244.   Effect of chemolysis on uric acid bladder stone. Patient was a 71-year-old hyperuricemic asymptomatic man. Urographic studies were carried out for evaluation of hypertension. **A**, *Plain film*. Large stone of poor density left side of bladder *(arrow)*. **B**, *Excretory urogram*. Negative filling defect produced by uric acid stone *(arrow)*. Note prostatic enlargement.

Legend continued on following page

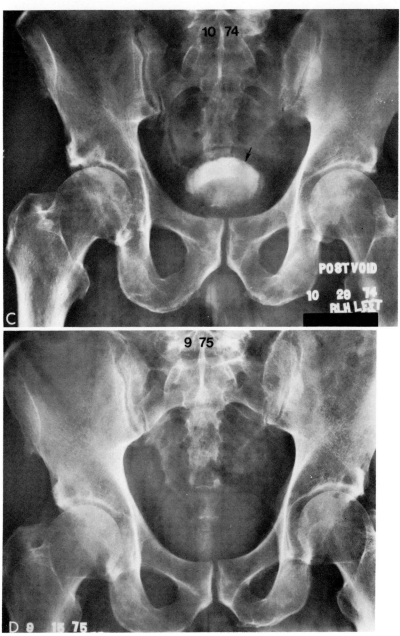

Figure 12–244. *Continued.* **C,** *Excretory urogram.* Postvoiding film shows moderate amount of residual urine. Stone is again seen as negative shadow *(arrow).* **D,** *Plain film, 11 months after treatment.* Calculus has completely dissolved and is no longer visible.

Illustration and legend continued on following page

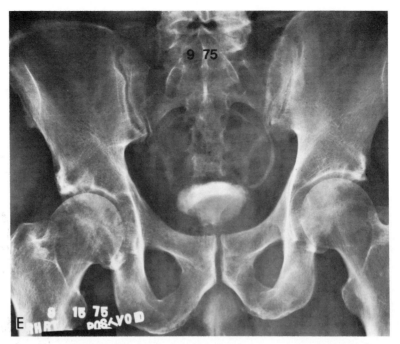

Figure 12–244. *Continued.* **E,** *Excretory urogram.* Nothing to suggest residual calculus. Note prostatic enlargement and small amount of residual urine. *Comment:* Chemolytic program consisted of hydration, urinary alkalinization, and administration of allopurinol.

They may produce sudden or intermittent interruption of the urinary stream with or without pain or hematuria. Rarely acute epididymitis may be the presenting symptom. It is not always possible to distinguish roentgenographically between native and migrant stones, so the patient's history and the results of other urologic investigation, especially cystoscopic examination, may be necessary to enable one to make a decision (Figs. 12–245 through 12–249).

mately 20 per cent of cases (Straffon and Higgins). Under these circumstances it is vital to rule out prostatic tuberculosis, which is more likely to occur in the younger age group, and, more importantly, carcinoma and infarction in the older age group. Passage of a urethroscope may produce a grating sensation, concomitant rectal palpation of the prostate against the instrument may elicit crepitation, and calculi may be observed protruding into the prostatic urethra.

Clinical Features of Prostatic Calculi

Prostatic calculi have no pathognomonic symptoms. Small ones may pass spontaneously, and terminal hematuria may be present. Rarely, a prostatic abscess may form and give rise to deep pain in the perineum and rectum that is aggravated by defecation, and to fever and constitutional symptoms.

Small calculi are usually not palpable by digital rectal examination, but large stones may be felt as hard "nodules," and crepitation may be elicited in approxi-

Roentgen Features of Prostatic Calculi

Diagnosis usually can be made on the basis of the typical appearance and location of the shadows of the calculi seen in the plain film. The shadows are situated in the region of the symphysis pubis, may be approximately 1 to 3 cm to either side (depending on the size of the gland), and may be above or below the level of the symphysis, depending on the length of the prostate, their location in the prostate, and

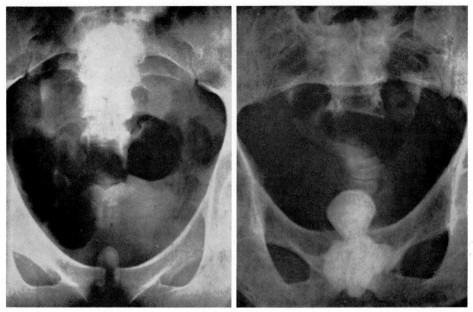

Figure 12–245. *Plain films.* **Examples of migrant prostatic calculi. A,** Stone formed in bladder and dropped into prostatic urethra. **Neurogenic bladder.** Stone was pushed into bladder with cystoscope, and litholapaxy was performed. **B,** Another case. Migrant prostatic stone. Dumbbell calculus which formed following perineal prostatectomy several years previously. Large portion of stone projected into bladder. Suprapubic removal.

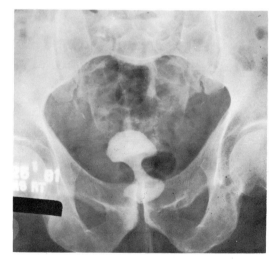

Figure 12–246. *Plain film.* **Migrant dumbbell stone in prostatic urethra and bladder** following suprapubic prostatectomy and removal of vesical calculi.

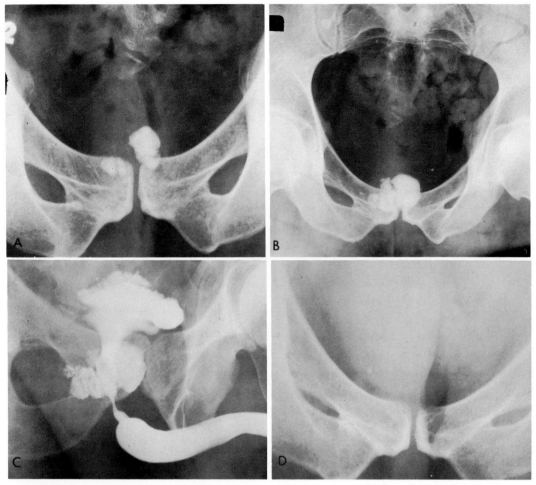

Figure 12–247. "Secondary" prostatic calculi. Cord bladder and incontinence due to myelodysplasia in a man, 24 years of age. Patient wears penile incontinence clip and has chronic pyuria. **A**, *Plain film*, April 1952. Prostatic calculi of moderate size. **B**, *Plain film*, January 1961. Considerable increase in size of calculi. **C**, *Retrograde urethrogram*, February 1961. Suggests stones have originated in old prostatic abscess cavities. **D**, *Plain film* following transurethral removal of stones. No stones are present.

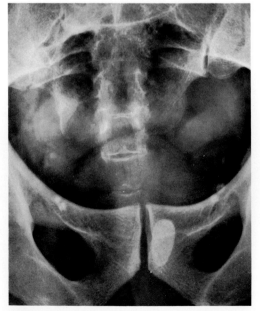

Figure 12–248. *Plain film.* **Secondary prostatic calculus** that has formed in prostatic urethra (following suprapubic prostatectomy done 1 year previously). Stone was dislodged into bladder with cystoscope, and litholapaxy was performed.

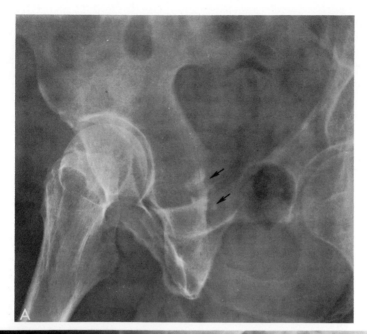

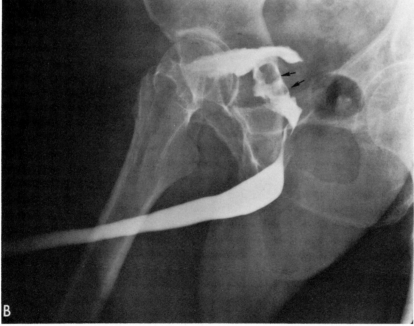

Figure 12–249. Secondary prostatic calculi. Patient had undergone transurethral prostatic resection 7 months earlier, had been shown to be infected, and presented with poor stream. **A,** *Plain film.* Calculi in region of prostate *(arrows).* **B,** *Retrograde urethrogram.* Deformity of prostatic fossa due to previous surgery. Note negative filling defects *(arrows)* caused by calculi. Stones were dislodged into bladder with cystoscope. Residual prostatic adenoma was resected, and litholapaxy was performed (calcium phosphate stones).

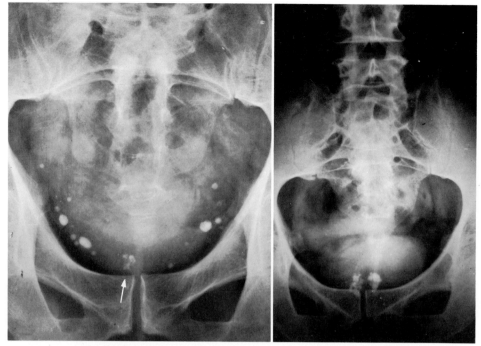

Fig. 12–250   Fig. 12–251

Figure 12–250. *Plain film.* Phleboliths on both sides of bony pelvis. Multiple minute prostatic calculi to right of midline.

Figure 12–251. *Plain film.* Multiple prostatic calculi.

the angle at which the film is exposed. When the shadows are projected a considerable distance above the symphysis, it may be difficult to decide whether they are vesical or prostatic calculi (Figs. 12–250 through 12–257; see Chapter 7).

Management of Prostatic Calculi

Asymptomatic prostatic calculi require no treatment. Many patients with so-called chronic prostatitis and prostatic calculi manifest irritative lower urinary tract symp-

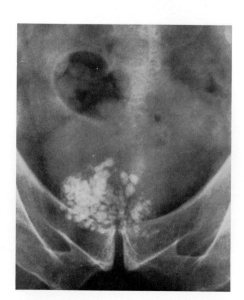

Figure 12–252. *Plain film.* Multiple prostatic calculi.

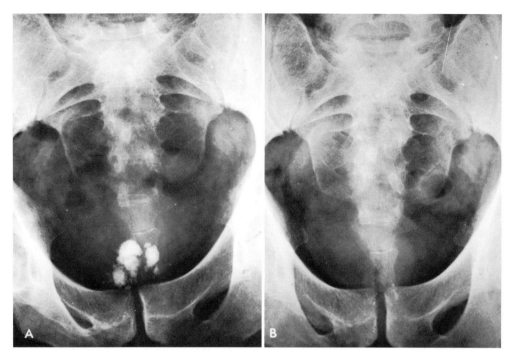

Figure 12–253. *Plain film.* **Multiple prostatic calculi removed by transurethral prostatic resection. B,** *Plain film* (postoperative). A few minute calculi remaining after transurethral removal of prostatic calculi.

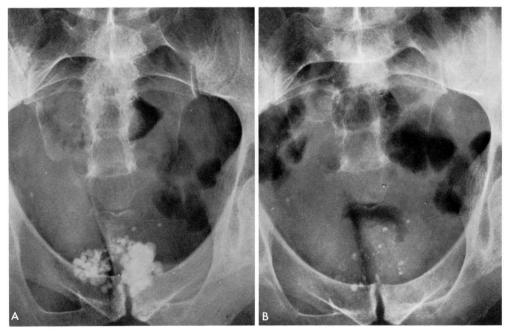

Figure 12–254. **Multiple prostatic calculi removed by transurethral prostatic resection. A,** *Plain film.* **B,** *Plain film* (postoperative). A few minute calculi remaining after transurethral removal of prostatic calculi.

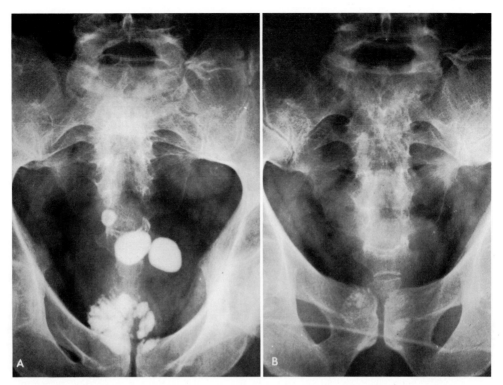

Figure 12–255. A, *Plain film.* **Multiple prostatic calculi forming almost complete replacement of prostate gland. Multiple vesical calculi.** B, *Plain film* (postoperative). A few prostatic calculi remaining after litholapaxy for vesical calculi and transurethral removal of prostatic calculi.

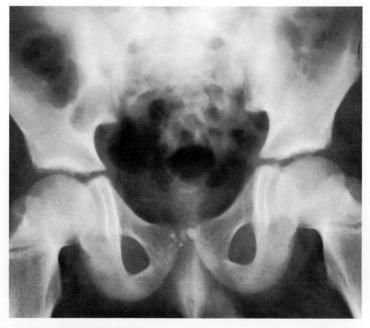

Figure 12–256. *Plain film.* **Prostatic calculi** in boy aged 11 years. (Calculi known to have been present since age 6.) (Courtesy of Dr. Robert Payne.)

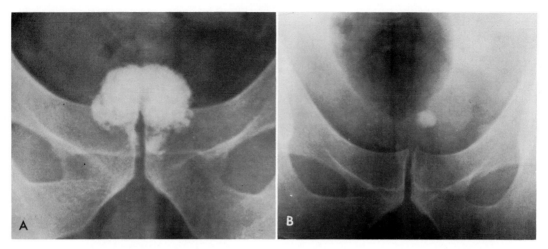

Figure 12–257. *Plain films.* **Spontaneous evacuation of prostatic calculi. A,** Extensive replacement of prostate with multiple prostatic calculi, which could be palpated easily on digital rectal examination. **B,** Seven months later. Patient had spontaneously passed large number of calculi. A few had caught in urethral meatus, requiring extraction with forceps. One large calculus and a few small calculi remain

toms. More often than not, transurethral resection of the prostate in the absence of clearly demonstrable obstruction transforms these sufferers of perineal pain into urologic cripples whose irritative symptoms and perineal pain continue relentlessly and may be further confounded by urinary incontinence. On the other hand, clearly obstructive stone-bearing prostates with or without infection require removal. Transurethral resection is usually adequate but does not guarantee the removal of all the calculi, and recurrent stone formation may ensue. Occasionally, prostatic calculi may be very large and numerous, causing extensive destruction and infection of the prostate. Retropubic adenectomy, and, rarely, total prostatectomy can be employed under these circumstances. For management of migrant prostatic urethral calculi, see the section on urethral calculi.

URETHRAL CALCULI

Urethral calculi are the least common form of urinary calculous disease in the United States. During a 25-year period, only 47 patients with urethral calculi (34 men and 13 women) were encountered at the Mayo Clinic (Paulk and associates). Urethral calculi are probably encountered most often in the Orient, where vesical calculi are common among children (Malek and Kelalis, 1975b).

Urethral calculi may be formed as a primary event within the urethra, or the stones may originate in the bladder or kidney with secondary descent into the urethra. We prefer the terms *native* for stones that form within the urethra and *migrant* for those that form within the bladder or elsewhere and subsequently drop down. The traditional use of the terms "primary" and "secondary" is misleading, because these terms are widely used in a nonanatomic, metabolic sense to signify the exact opposite. In this sense, primary stone formation results from an underlying metabolic abnormality, whereas secondary stones form as a result of pathologic deviation of normal mineralization within the urinary tract in association with infection, obstruction, or foreign bodies (Malek and Boyce, 1973).

Native urethral calculi usually form in association with chronic urinary infection, either within a urethral diverticulum or proximal to urethral obstruction (Figs. 12–258 through 12–262). Generally, these stones are composed of calcium phosphate and carbonate and do not cause acute symptoms, because they develop and grow

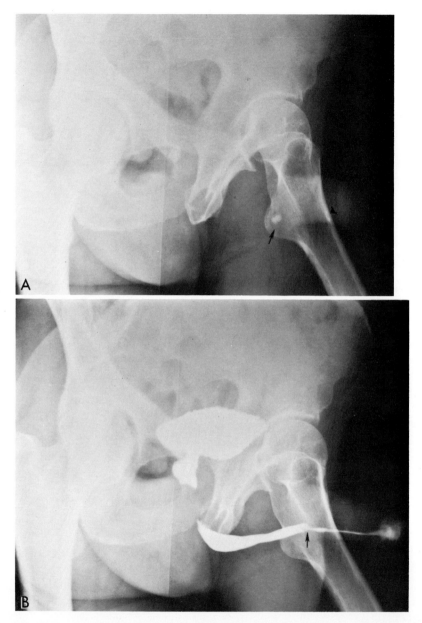

Figure 12–258. "Native" urethral stone formed proximal to urethral stricture. **A,** *Plain film.* Stone in penile urethra *(arrow).* **B,** *Retrograde urethrogram.* Long distal urethral stricture. Stone shows as faint negative filling defect *(arrow).* (From Paulk, S. C., Khan, A. U., Malek, R. S., and Greene, L. F.)

Fig. 12-259

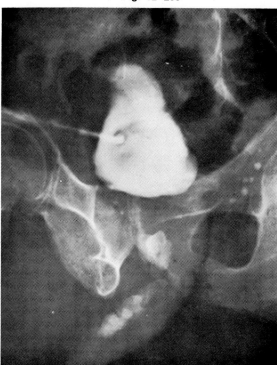

Figure 12-259. *Retrograde cystogram,* made through suprapubic tube. **Multiple urethral calculi occupying almost entire perineal urethra.** They formed as **result of urethral stricture.** (Courtesy of Dr. Gordon W. Strom.)

Figure 12-260. *Plain film.* **Large urethral calculus forming cast of scrotal and perineal fistula, associated with diverticulum, in case of long-standing urethral stricture.** At operation, scrotal fistula was opened and scrotum was divided. Fistulous tract entered large diverticulum completely filled with calculus, which was removed in one piece. Diverticulum excised. (Courtesy of Dr. Gordon W. Strom.)

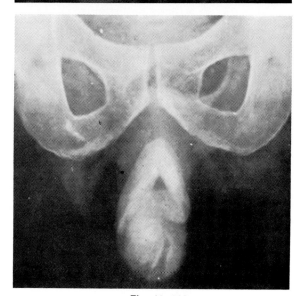

Fig. 12-260

slowly within the urethral lumen or else are sequestered within a diverticulum. On the other hand, migrant stones, having achieved sizable dimensions higher up in the urinary tract, often cause acute symptoms because of their sudden descent into and persistent or intermittent lodgement within the urethral lumen. Migrant calculi are ten times as common in men as native calculi (Figs. 12-263 and 12-264). Conversely, urethral calculi in women are practically always formed in a urethral diverticulum (native stone) (Fig. 12-265) (Paulk and associates).

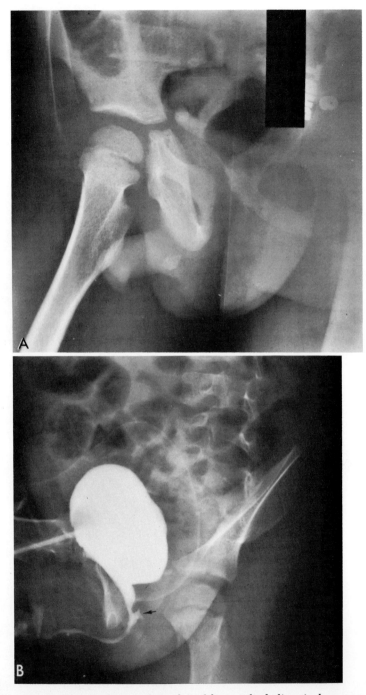

Figure 12–261.   "Native" urethral stone formed in false urethral diverticulum caused by repair of rectourethral fistula in 5-year-old boy. **A,** *Plain film.* Calculus in region of penoscrotal urethra. **B,** *Retrograde urethrogram* (after removal of calculus by external urethrotomy) shows pocket (false diverticulum) where calculus had formed *(arrow).* (From Malek, R. S., 1976.)

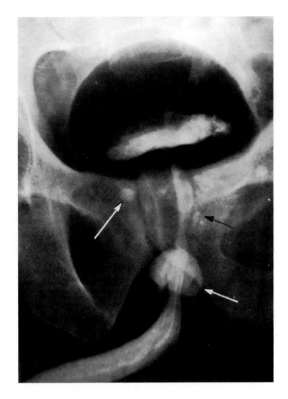

Figure 12–262. Calculi in diverticulum of bulbous urethra. **Multiple prostatic calculi.** *Urethrogram.* Two large calculi superimposed on each other, situated in diverticulum of bulbous urethra. Also multiple prostatic calculi. These stones were removed through external urethrotomy incision.

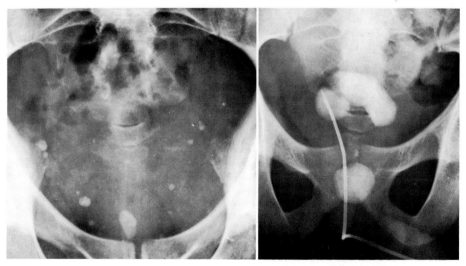

Fig. 12–263   Fig. 12–264

Figure 12–263. **Migrant prostatic calculus.** *Plain film.* Patient with **cord bladder.** Stone lodged in prostatic urethra, no doubt originating in bladder. Stone was dislodged with cystoscope and removed.

Figure 12–264. **Multiple vesical calculi. One has been passed into prostatic urethra.** *Plain film.* Patient with **neurogenic vesical dysfunction.** Multiple vesical calculi. Stone caught in prostatic urethra. This stone was dislodged into bladder with cystoscope, and litholapaxy was performed.

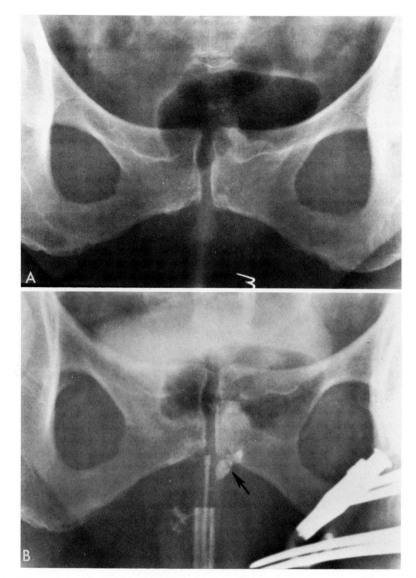

Figure 12–265. "Native" urethral calculus in a woman with urethral diverticulum. **A,** *Plain film.* Calculus is nonopaque. **B,** *Double-balloon retrograde urethrogram.* Diverticular cavity containing radiolucent calcium phosphate–carbonate stone *(arrow)* is outlined. Diverticulectomy. (From Paulk, S. C., Khan, A. U., Malek, R. S., and Greene, L. F.)

Clinical Features of Urethral Calculi

Clinical presentation is variable. Unlike Amin, in whose series from Kuwait 88.9 per cent of the patients presented with acute urinary retention, we found only one patient with acute retention. Most men in our experience present with dysuria or weak stream, whereas women usually complain of dysuria or perineal pain. All patients are likely to have lower urinary tract lesions or to have had previous prostatic surgery, and almost 50 per cent have infection (Paulk and associates).

Diagnosis of Urethral Calculi

Diagnosis was made urographically in only 42.5 per cent of our patients. The reasons for missing a majority of these calculi roentgenologically include the radiolucency of some stones, exclusion of the external genitalia from some routine excretory urograms, and inattention to areas below the symphysis pubis during interpretation of the excretory urogram, probably because of the rarity of urethral calculous disease. Retrograde urethrography is essential in suspected cases and is most helpful in delineating associated urethral disease in male patients. In women, however, retrograde urethrographic diagnosis of urethral diverticulum continues to remain a problem; only 3 of 13 diverticula in women were discovered in this manner (see Figures 12–258 through 12–265). Cystourethroscopy is essential in all patients of either sex. It confirms the diagnosis in all patients and is, additionally, therapeutic in those patients who are manageable by endoscopy.

Management of Urethral Calculi

The frequent association of urethral calculi with other urethral disease complicates its management, which in itself is fraught with danger of excessive surgical trauma to the urethra and consequently to the upper urinary tract.

In men, a calculus in the fossa navicularis may be removed with thumb forceps after meatotomy. Penile urethral calculi are usually amenable to removal *through* the lumen of the cystoscope. Attempts to milk the stone externally in either direction, to crush it in the urethra, or to extract it other than *through* the lumen of a cystoscope (as done with a stone basket or with a biopsy forceps grasping the stone and then withdrawing the whole instrument with the stone protruding from its tip) should be condemned because of trauma sustained by the urethra and the danger of subsequent stricture formation. Bulbous and posterior urethral (prostatic) calculi are encountered most often. These may be guided endoscopically into the bladder. Most can be irrigated out or removed by transurethral litholapaxy; the remaining few, together with vesical calculi, may require cystolithotomy.

Generally, open surgical procedures are required when the urethral calculus is impacted (external urethrotomy), lodged in a urethral diverticulum (diverticulectomy), or associated with transurethrally unmanageable vesical or urethral disease (cystolithotomy).

Although correction of urethral disease and treatment of urinary infection may prevent the recurrence of urethral calculi, other possible underlying etiologic factors must be carefully determined. In a majority of our patients with urethral calculi who underwent metabolic evaluation, an underlying cause was found. Indeed, a urethral stone may be the only presenting symptom of the stone-forming tendency, and the affected patient deserves a complete evaluation (Paulk and associates).

REFERENCES

Aguilo, J. J., Malek, R. S., and Hattery, R. R.: Unpublished data.

Amin, H. A.: Urethral Calculi. Brit. J. Urol. 45:192–199, 1973.

Andersen, D. A.: Historical and Geographical Differences in the Pattern of Incidence of Urinary Stones Considered in Relation to Possible Aetiological Factors. In Hodgkinson, A., and Nordin, B. E. C.: Renal Stone Research Symposium. London, J. & A. Churchill, 1969, pp. 7–31.

Arcelin: L'exploration radiologique des voies urinaries. In Encyclopédie française d'urologie. Paris, Octave Doin et Fils, 1914, vol. 2, pp. 99–184.

Arons, W. L., Christensen, W. R., and Sosman, M. C.: Nephrocalcinosis Visible by X-ray, Associated With Chronic Glomerulonephritis. Ann. Int. Med. 42:260–282 (Feb.) 1955.

Atsmon, A., de Vries, A., and Frank, M.: Uric Acid Lithiasis. Amsterdam, Elsevier Publishing Company, 1963, 251 pp.

Benendo, B., and Litwak, A.: "Milk of Calcium" in Renal Cyst. Brit. J. Radiol. 37:70–71 (Jan.) 1964.

Bennett, A. H., and Colodny, A. H.: Urinary Tract Calculi in Children. J. Urol. 109:318–320 (Feb.) 1973.

Berg, R. A., Chan, Y. S., and Goode, R.: Milk-of-Calcium Hydronephrosis. J. Urol. 107:905–907 (June) 1972.

Blacklock, N. J.: The Pattern of Urolithiasis in the Royal Navy. In Hodgkinson, A., and Nordin, B. E. C.: Renal Stone Research Symposium. London, J. & A. Churchill, 1969, pp. 33–47.

Boyce, W. H.: Radiology in the Diagnosis and Surgery of Renal Calculi. R. Clin. North Am. 3:89–102 (Apr.) 1965.

Boyce, W. H.: The Renal Tubule in the Genesis of Renal Calculi. In Schreiner, G. E.: Proceedings of the Third International Congress of Nephrology. Basel, S. Karger, 1967, vol. 2, pp. 354–363.

Boyce, W. H.: Organic Matrix of Human Urinary

Concretions. Amer. J. Med. *45*:673–683 (Nov.) 1968.

Boyce, W. H., and Elkins, I. B.: Reconstructive Renal Surgery Following Anatrophic Nephrolithotomy: Followup of 100 Consecutive Cases. Tr. Am. A. Genito-Urin. Surgeons *65*:126–131, 1973.

Boyce, W. H., Garvey, F. K., and Strawcutter, H. E.: Incidence of Urinary Calculi Among Patients in General Hospitals, 1948 to 1952. J.A.M.A. *161*:1437–1442 (Aug. 11) 1956.

Burnett, C. H., Commons, R. R., Albright, F., and Howard, J. E.: Hypercalcemia Without Hypercalcinuria or Hypophosphatemia, Calcinosis and Renal Insufficiency: A Syndrome Following Prolonged Intake of Milk and Alkali. New England J. Med. *240*:787–794 (May 19) 1949.

Butt, A. J.: Historical Survey of Etiologic Factors in Renal Lithiasis. *In* Butt, A. J.: Etiologic Factors in Renal Lithiasis. Springfield, Illinois, Charles C Thomas, Publisher, 1956, pp. 6–7.

Camiel, M. R.: Stone in the Intramural Bladder Portion of the Ureter: Urographic Observations. Radiology 78:959–962 (June) 1962.

Chutikorn, C., Valyasevi, A., and Halstead, S. B.: Studies of Bladder Stone Disease in Thailand. II. Hospital Experience: Urolithiasis at Ubol Provincial Hospital, 1956–1962. Am. J. Clin. Nutr. *20*:1320–1328 (Dec.) 1967.

Clark, P. B., and Nordin, B. E. C.: The Problem of the Calcium Stone. *In* Hodgkinson, A., and Nordin, B. E. C.: Renal Stone Research Symposium, London, J. & A. Churchill, 1969, p. 2.

Cristol, D. S., and Emmett, J. L.: Incidence of Prostatic Calculi in Association With Benign Hyperplasia or Malignant Lesions of the Prostate Gland. Proc. Mayo Clin. Staff Meet. *19*:265–267 (May 31) 1944.

de Vries, A., Kochwa, S., Lazebnik, J., Frank, M., and Djaldetti, M.: Glycinuria, A Hereditary Disorder Associated With Nephrolithiasis. Am. J. Med. *23*:408–415 (Sept.) 1957.

Dhanamitta, S., and Valyasevi, A.: Personal communication.

Drummond, K. N., Michael, A. F., Ulstrom, R. A., and Good, R. A.: The Blue Diaper Syndrome: Familial Hypercalcemia With Nephrocalcinosis and Indicanuria; a New Familial Disease, With Definition of the Metabolic Abnormality. Am. J. Med. *37*:928–948 (Dec.) 1964.

Eckstein, H. B.: Harnsteine im Kindesalter. Z Kinderchir Grenzgeb *2*:451–465 (Oct.) 1965.

Edling, N. P. G.: Further Studies of the Interureteric Ridge of the Bladder. Acta Radiol. *30*:69–75, 1948.

Engel, W. J.: Nephrocalcinosis. J.A.M.A. *145*:288–294 (Feb. 3) 1951.

Epstein, F. H.: Freedman, L. R., and Levitin, H.: Hypercalcemia, Nephrocalcinosis and Reversible Renal Insufficiency Associated With Hyperthyroidism. New England J. Med. *258*:782–785 (Apr. 17) 1958.

Esposito, W. L.: Specific Nephrocalcinosis of Chronic Glomerulonephritis. Am. J. Roentgenol. *101*:688–691 (Nov.) 1967.

Fellers, F. X., and Schwartz, R.: Etiology of the Severe Form of Idiopathic Hypercalcemia of Infancy: A Defect in Vitamin D Metabolism. New England J. Med. *259*:1050–1058 (Nov. 27) 1958.

Fetter, T. R., Zimskind, P. D., Graham, R. H., and Brodie, D. E.: Statistical Analysis of Patients With Ureteral Calculi. J.A.M.A. *186*:21–23 (Oct. 5) 1963.

Finlayson, B.: Renal Lithiasis in Review. Urol. Clin. North Am. *1*:181–212 (June) 1974.

Gelzayd, E. A., Breuer, R. I., and Kirsner, J. B.: Nephrolithiasis in Inflammatory Bowel Disease. Am. J. Dig. Dis. *13*:1027–1034 (Dec.) 1968.

Geraci, J. E., Harris, H. W., and Keith, N. M.: Bilateral Diffuse Nephrocalcinosis: Report of Two Cases. Proc. Staff Meet. Mayo Clin. *25*:305–315 (June 7) 1950.

Gutman, A. B., and Yü, T-F: Uric Acid Nephrolithiasis. Am. J. Med. *45*:756–779 (Nov.) 1968.

Henken, E. M.: "Milk of Calcium" in a Renal Cyst: Report of a Case. Radiology *84*:276–278 (Feb.) 1965.

Hinman, F., Jr.: Peripelvic Extravasation During Intravenous Urography, Evidence for an Additional Route for Backflow After Ureteral Obstruction. J. Urol. 85:385–395 (Mar.) 1961.

Hofmann, A. F., Tacker, M. M., Fromm, H., Thomas, P. J., and Smith, L. H.: Acquired Hyperoxaluria and Intestinal Disease: Evidence That Bile Acid Glycine Is Not a Precursor of Oxalate. Mayo Clin. Proc. *48*:35–42 (Jan.) 1973.

Howell, R. D.: Milk of Calcium Renal Stone. J. Urol. 82:197–199 (Aug.) 1959.

Hurxthal, L. M., and O'Sullivan, J. B.: Cushing's Syndrome: Clinical Differential Diagnosis and Complications. Ann. Intern. Med. *51*:1–16 (July) 1959.

Huth, E. J.: Nephrolithiasis and Nephrocalcinosis. *In* Black, D. A. K.: Renal Disease. Ed. 2, Oxford, Blackwell Scientific Publications, 1967, pp. 421–445.

Inada, T., Miyazaki, S., Omori, T., Nihira, H., and Hino, T.: Statistical Study on Urolithiasis in Japan. Urol. Int. 7:150–165, 1958.

Joachim, G. R., and Becker, E. L.: Spontaneous Rupture of the Kidney. Arch. Int. Med. *115*:176–183 (Feb.) 1965.

Jungmann, K.: Das Kolikurogramm (Ausscheidungsurographie während der Nierenkolik). Zentralbl. Chir. 93:426–432 (Mar. 23) 1968.

Khan, A. U., and Malek, R. S.: Spontaneous Urinary Extravasation. J. Urol. *116*:161–165 (Aug.) 1971.

Lagergren, C., and Öhrling, H.: Urinary Calculi Composed of Pure Calcium Phosphate: Roentgen Crystallographic Analysis and Its Diagnostic Value. Acta chir. Scandinav. *117*:335–341, 1959.

Lightwood, R., and Payne, W. W.: British Pediatric Association: Proceedings of the Twenty-third General Meeting. A. M. A. Arch. Dis. Child. 27:302–303 (June) 1952.

Lonsdale, K.: Human Stones. Science, *159*:1199–1207 (Mar. 15) 1968.

Malek, R. S.: Urologic Aspects of Hyperparathyroidism. Bull. N. Y. Acad. Med. *50*:576–579 (May) 1974.

Malek, R. S.: Urolithiasis. *In* Kelalis, P. P., King. L. R., and Belman, A. B.: Clinical Pediatric Urology. Philadelphia, W. B. Saunders Co., 1976, pp. 865–895.

Malek, R. S., Aguilo, J. J., and Hattery, R. R.: Radiolucent Filling Defects of the Renal Pelvis: Classifi-

REFERENCES **1367**

cation and Report of Unusual Cases. J. Urol. *114*:508–513 (Oct.) 1975.

Malek, R. S., and Boyce, W. H.: Intranephronic Calculosis: Its Significance and Relationship to Matrix in Nephrolithiasis. J. Urol. *109*:551–555 (Apr.) 1973.

Malek, R. S., and Boyce, W. H.: Observations on the Ultrastructure and Genesis of Urinary Calculi. J. Urol. *117*:336–341 (March) 1977.

Malek, R. S., and Kelalis, P. P.: Nephrocalcinosis in Infancy and Childhood. J. Urol. *114*:441–443 (Sept.) 1975a.

Malek, R. S., and Kelalis, P. P.: Pediatric Nephrolithiasis. J. Urol. *113*:545–551 (Apr.) 1975b.

Malek, R. S., and Kelalis, P. P.: Hyperparathyroidism: Its Manifestations in the Urinary Tract During Childhood. J. Urol. *115*:717–719 (June) 1976.

Malek, R. S., Moghaddam, A., Furlow, W. L., and Greene, L. F.: Symptomatic Ureteral Stumps. J. Urol. *106*:521–528 (Oct.) 1971.

Malek, R. S., Wilkiemeyer, R. M., and Boyce, W. H.: The Stone Forming Kidney: A Study of Functional Differences Between Individual Kidneys in Idiopathic Renal Lithiasis. J. Urol. *116*:11–14 (July) 1976.

Mates, J.: External Factors in the Genesis of Urolithiasis. *In* Hodgkinson, A., and Nordin, B. E. C.: Renal Stone Research Symposium. London, J & A Churchill, 1969, pp. 59–64.

Maurer, R. M., and Wildin, R. E.: Milk-of-Calcium Renal Stone: Report of a Case. Radiology 84:274–275 (Feb.) 1965.

Melnick, I., Landes, R. R., Hoffman, A. A., and Burch, J. F.: Magnesium Therapy for Recurring Calcium Oxalate Urinary Calculi. J. Urol. *105*:119–122 (Jan.) 1971.

Modlin, M.: The Aetiology of Renal Stone: A New Concept Arising from Studies on a Stone-Free Population. Ann. Roy. Coll. Surg. (Eng.) *40*:155–177 (Mar.) 1967.

Mortensen, J. D., and Emmett, J. L.: Nephrocalcinosis: A Collective and Clinicopathologic Study. J. Urol. *71*:398–406 (Apr.) 1954.

Mukai, T., and Howard, J. E.: Some Observations on the Calcification of Rachitic Cartilage by Urine: One Difference Between "Good" and "Evil" Urines, Dependent upon Content of Magnesium. Bull. Johns Hopkins Hosp. *112*:279–290, 1963.

Myers, W. P. L.: Hypercalcemia in Neoplastic Disease. Cancer 9:1135–1140 (Nov.–Dec.) 1956.

Passmore, R.: Observations on the Epidemiology of Stone in the Bladder in Thailand. Lancet *1*:638–640 (Mar. 28) 1953.

Paulk, S. C., Khan, A. U., Malek, R. S., and Greene, L. F.: Urethral Calculus. J. Urol. *116*:436–439 (Oct.) 1976.

Plimpton, C. H., and Gellhorn, A.: Hypercalcemia in Malignant Disease Without Evidence of Bone Destruction. Am. J. Med. *21*:750–759 (Nov.) 1956.

Potter, W. M., Greene, L. F., and Keating, F. R., Jr.: Vesical Calculi and Hyperparathyroidism. J. Urol. *96*:203–206 (Aug.) 1966.

Prien, E. L., and Frondel, C.: Studies in Urolithiasis. I. The Composition of Urinary Calculi. J. Urol. *57*:949–991 (June) 1947.

Pullman, R. A. W., and King, R. J.: Milk of Calcium Renal Stone. Am. J. Roentgenol. *87*:760–763 (Apr.) 1962.

Pyrah, L. N., and Hodgkinson, A.: Nephrocalcinosis. Brit. J. Urol. *32*:361–373, 1960.

Pyrah, L. N., Hodgkinson, A., and Anderson, C. K.: Primary Hyperparathyroidism. Brit. J. Surg. *53*:245–316 (Apr.) 1966.

Randall, R. E., Jr.; Strauss, M. B., and McNeely, W. F.: The Milk-Alkali Syndrome. Arch. Int. Med. *107*:163–181 (Feb.) 1961.

Richtsmeier, A. J.: The Symptoms of Hypercalcemia Associated With Sarcoidosis Masquerading as Peptic Ulcer. Ann. Int. Med. *51*:1371–1378 (Dec.) 1959.

Riesz, P. B., and Wagner, C. W., Jr.: Unusual Renal Calcification Following Acute Bilateral Renal Cortical Necrosis: A Case Report. Am. J. Roentgenol. *101*:705–707 (Nov.) 1967.

Rosenberg, M. A.: Milk of Calcium in a Renal Calyceal Diverticulum: Case Report and Review of Literature. Am. J. Roentgenol. *101*:714–718 (Nov.) 1967.

Samuels, L. D., and Smith, J. P.: Nephrocalcinosis in Children: Diagnostic Visualization by Strontium-87m Scintiscans. J. Urol. *108*:788–791 (Nov.) 1972.

Scholz, D. A., and Keating, F. R., Jr.: Milk Alkali Syndrome: Review of Eight Cases. Arch. Int. Med. 95:460–468, 1955.

Scholz, D. A., and Keating, F. R., Jr.: Renal Insufficiency, Renal Calculi and Nephrocalcinosis in Sarcoidosis: Report of Eight Cases. Am. J. Med. *21*:75–84 (July) 1956.

Seldin, D. W., and Wilson, J. D.: Renal Tubular Acidosis. *In* Stanbury, J. B., Wyngaarden, J. B., and Fredrickson, D. S.: The Metabolic Basis of Inherited Disease. Ed. 3, New York, McGraw-Hill Book Company, 1972, pp. 1548–1566.

Shaw, R. E.: Spontaneous Rupture of the Kidney. Brit. J. Surg. *45*:68–72 (July) 1957.

Smith, D. R.: Urinary Stones. *In* Smith, D. R.: General Urology. Ed. 7, Los Altos, California, Lange Medical Publications, 1972, pp. 207–227.

Smith, L. H.: Treatment of Renal Lithiasis Associated With Infection. Mod. Treat. *4*:505–514 (May) 1967.

Smith, L. H.: Nephrolithiasis: Current Concepts in Pathogenesis and Management. Postgrad. Med. *52*:165–170 (Sept.) 1972a.

Smith, L. H.: The Diagnosis and Treatment of Metabolic Stone Disease. Med. Clin. N. Amer. *56*:977–988 (July) 1972b.

Smith, L. H.: Medical Evaluation of Urolithiasis. Etiologic Aspects and Diagnostic Evaluation. Urol. Clin. North Am. *1*:241–260 (June) 1974.

Smith, L. H., Fromm, H., and Hofmann, A. F.: Acquired Hyperoxaluria, Nephrolithiasis, and Intestinal Disease: Description of a Syndrome. New England J. Med. *286*:1371–1375 (June) 1972.

Smith, L. H., Jones, J. D., and Keating, F. R., Jr.: Primary Hyperoxaluria. *In* Hodgkinson, A., and Nordin, B. E. C.: Renal Stone Research Symposium. London, J. & A. Churchill, 1969, pp. 297–307.

Smith, M. J. V.: Prostatic Corpora Amylacea. Monographs in Surg. Sciences 3:209–265 (Sept.) 1966.

Snyder, C. H.: Idiopathic Hypercalcemia of Infancy. Am. J. Dis. Child. *96*:376–380 (Sept.) 1958.

Straffon, R. A., and Higgins, C. C.: Urolithiasis. *In*

Campbell, M. F., and Harrison, J. H.: Urology. Ed. 3, Philadelphia, W. B. Saunders Company, 1970, vol. 1, pp. 687–765.

Suki, W. N., Eknoyan, G., and Martinez-Maldonado, M.: The Control of Idiopathic Hypercalciuria With Diuretics and Salt Restriction. *In* Scott, R., Jr.: Current Controversies in Urologic Management. Philadelphia, W. B. Saunders Company, 1972, pp. 345–350.

Sutor, D. J.: The Nature of Urinary Stones. *In* Finlayson, B., Hench, L. L., and Smith, L. H.: Urolithiasis: Physical Aspects. Washington, D. C., National Academy of Sciences, 1972, pp. 43–60.

Taneja, O. P.: Pathogenesis of Ureteric Reflux in Vesical Calculous Disease of Childhood: A Clinical Study. Brit. J. Urol. 47:623–629 (Dec.) 1975.

Thier, S. O., and Segal, S.: Cystinuria. *In* Stanbury, J. B., Wyngaarden, J. B., and Fredrickson, D. S.: The Metabolic Basis of Inherited Disease. Ed. 3, New York, McGraw-Hill Book Company, 1972, pp. 1504–1519.

Thomas, W. C., Jr.: Medical Aspects of Renal Calculous Disease. Treatment and Prophylaxis. Urol. Clin. North Am. 1:261–278 (June) 1974.

Thomas, W. C., Jr., Connor, T. B., and Morgan, H. G.: Some Observations on Patients With Hypercalcemia Exemplifying Problems in Differential Diagnosis, Especially in Hyperparathyroidism. J. Lab. Clin. Med. 52:11–19 (July) 1958.

Valyasevi, A., and Van Reen, R.: Pediatric Bladder Stone Disease: Current Status of Research. J. Pediatr. 72:546–553 (Apr.) 1968.

Vermooten, V.: Congenital Cystic Dilatation of the Renal Collecting Tubules: A New Disease Entity. Yale J. Biol. Med. 23:450–453 (June) 1950–1951.

Walker, W. H., Pearson, R. E., and Johnson, N. R.: Milk-of-Calcium Renal Stone: Case Report. J. Urol. 84:517–520 (Oct.) 1960.

Walls, J., Schorr, W. J., and Kerr, D. N. S.: Prolonged Oliguria With Survival in Acute Bilateral Cortical Necrosis. Br. Med. J. 4:220–222 (Oct. 26) 1968.

Wesson, M. B., and Fulmer, C. C.: Influence of Ureteral Stones on Intravenous Urograms. Am. J. Roentgenol. 28:27–33 (July) 1932.

Wilkiemeyer, R. M., Boyce, W. H., and Malek, R. S.: Validity of the Intravenous Pyelogram in Assessment of Renal Function. Surg. Gynec. Obst. 135:897–900 (Dec.) 1972.

Williams, D. I., and Eckstein, H. B.: Urinary Lithiasis. *In* Williams, D. I.: Paediatric Urology. New York, Appleton-Century-Crofts, 1968, pp. 323–339.

Williams, H. E., and Smith, L. H., Jr.: Primary Hyperoxaluria. *In* Stanbury, J. B., Wyngaarden, J. B., and Fredrickson, D. S.: The Metabolic Basis of Inherited Disease. Ed. 3, New York, McGraw-Hill Book Company, 1972, pp. 196–219.

Wilson, D. M., Smith, L. H., Segura, J. W., and Malek, R. S.: Renal Lithiasis: An Optimistic Outlook. Minn. Med. 57:368–373 (May) 1974.

Wilson, J. K. V., and Brown, W. H.: Nephrocalcinosis Associated With Sarcoidosis. Radiology 62:203–214 (Feb.) 1954.

Winsbury-White, H. P.: Stone in the Urinary Tract. St. Louis, The C. V. Mosby Company, 1954, 328 pp.

Wyngaarden, J. B.: Xanthinuria. *In* Stanbury, J. B., Wyngaarden, J. B., and Fredrickson, D. S.: The Metabolic Basis of Inherited Disease. Ed. 3, New York, McGraw-Hill Book Company, 1972, pp. 992–1002.

Yendt, E. R.: Gagné, R. J. A., and Cohanim, M.: The Effects of Thiazides in Idiopathic Hypercalciuria. Am. J. Med. Sci. 251:449–460 (Apr.) 1966.

INDEX

INDEX

Page numbers in *italics* indicate illustrations. Page numbers followed by (t) indicate tables.

Abdominal aorta, aneurysm of, 2029–2033
  ureteral obstruction and, 2205, *2206*
  vs. retroperitoneal fibrosis, 2206
Abdominal compression, in plain film, 7, 8
Abdominal muscles, congenital absence of, *734, 777–779, 1050*
Abscess, hepatic, confusing shadows from, *413*
  ischiorectal, communicating with urethra, *1852*
  of prostatic ducts, 888–889
  ovarian, ureteropyelectasis and, *2200*
  pelvic, sonography in, *2064*
  pericecal, vs. calcified tumor of appendix, *423*
  perinephric, *440*
    nephrobronchial fistula and, *851*
    psoas muscle and, *440*, 441
    renal cortical abscess and, *850, 861*
    renal displacement and, *861*
    sonographic diagnosis of, 308, *315–316*
  perirenal, 843–848, 867(t)
  perivesical, *1856*
  prostatic, 888–891
    bilharzial, *938*
    tuberculous, *918*
  psoas, *1856*
    confusing shadows from, *416*
    in renal tuberculosis, *904*
    secondary to Pott's disease, *903*
  renal, 298, 842–867
    angiographic changes in, 867(t)
    calcification in, 1488(t)
    clinical aspects of, 844–848
    cortical, *167, 854–855, 857–859*
    etiology of, 842–843   .
      in duplicated kidney, *672*
      in fused kidney, *517*
      perinephric abscess and, *850, 861*
    pathophysiology of, 843–847
    sonographic diagnosis of, 296–298, *862*
    vs. infected cyst, 296–308, *309–314*
  retroperitoneal, in Crohn's disease, *871*
  sonographic diagnosis of, 296–298, *862*
Accessory urethra, 755–761
"Acorn" deformity of vesical neck, *1103–1104*
Actinomycosis, renal, 895–898
Acute renal failure, 1865–1867. See also *Renal failure.*
Acute tubular necrosis, 297, *1876*. See also *Renal tubular necrosis.*

Acute tubular necrosis (*Continued*)
  in renal transplant, *202*
  vs. allograft rejection, 2054–2055
  vs. suppurative pyelonephritis, 296, *297*
Adenocarcinoma, 54, 140, 253–258, 439, 532, *1506*
  adrenocortical, *1717*
  in children, 1671–1673, *1674*
  incidence of, 1468(t)
  Lindau-von Hippel disease and, 1534, *1539, 1541–1542*
  mucinous, confusing shadows from, *433*
    in horseshoe kidney, *1535*
  of renal pelvis, 1572
  of seminal vesicle, 1647–1649
  renal, *1552*
    calcification in, 445, 1493, *1499–1500*
    clear cell, *1521*
    clinical considerations in, 1486–1487
    cortical, *1497*
      bilateral, *1529*
      calcification in, *1499–1500*
      vs. epithelioma of renal pelvis, *1494, 1496*
      vs. ureteropelvic obstruction, *1496*
    destruction of renal architecture by, *1503*
    differential diagnosis of, 1493–1504
    hypovascular, *1519–1520*
    in duplicated kidney, *673*
    in ectopic kidney, *607*
    in horseshoe kidney, *640, 1535*
    in lower left pole, *1507, 1508*
    in solitary kidney, *1507*
    incidence of, 1468(t)
    metastasis of, *1509, 1510, 1526*
      adrenal, *1744*
      osteolytic, *466–467*
    necrotic, *1520–1521*
    normal urogram with, 1498, *1504*
    papillary, *1521*
    renal cyst and, 1528, *1536*
    rupture of collecting system and, *1496*
    traumatic rupture of, *1786*
    tuberculosis and, *913*
    urographic diagnosis of, 1487–1498, *1499–1501*
    vena caval obstruction and, *1522–1524*
    vs. brucelloma, 895
    vs. cyst, 51, *1505*
    vs. epithelioma of renal pelvis, 1492, 1493, *1494, 1569*

i

Adenocarcinoma (*Continued*)
  renal, vs. extrarenal tumor, 1493, *1500–1503*
    vs. hematoma, 1493–1498, *1501–1503*
    vs. lobar dysmorphism, 650, *653–655*
    vs. papilloma of renal pelvis, *1492*
  retroperitoneal, *1588*
  ureteral, 1577, *1583*
    primary, *1583*
  urethral, in male, *1643*
Adenoma, adrenal, *1710*
  benign, *142*
    Cushing's disease and, *1715*
    cystic, hemorrhagic, *1735*
    primary aldosteronism with, *1747–1748*
    scintigraphic study in, *1753*
    vs. ganglioneuroma, *1736*
  adrenocortical, *1716*, 1730–1731, *1732–1735*
    calcification in, *1735*
    in adrenogenital syndrome, *1719*
    in Cushing's disease, *1718*
  benign papillary, *171*, 1469–1472, *1597*
  incidence of, 1468(t)
  nephrogenic, 1641
  of renal cortex, incidence of, 1468(t)
  renal, 1469–1472
    clinical features of, 1469–1470
    functioning, *1717*
    papillary benign, *1469*
    pathologic aspects of, 1470–1471
    roentgen features of, 1471–1472
    treatment of, 1472
    tubular benign, *1469*, 1470
Adrenal arteriography, 120–121, 1722–1746
Adrenal artery, *120*
  carcinoma of, *1731–1735*, *1737–1743*
    CT scanning in, *1751*
  excess function of, 1707–1709
  hyperplasia of, angiography in, 1735, *1744–1747*
    in Cushing's disease, *1744–1745*
    multinodular, *1746*
  tumors of, 1706–1709, *1716*
Adrenal gland(s), anatomy of, 1700
    vascular, 1723–1726
  arteriography of, 120–121, 1722–1746
  calcified, confusing shadows from, 421–422
  cysts of, *1701–1703*
    calcified, *1709*
  invasion of, by renal adenocarcinoma, *1744*
  mass lesions of, CT scanning in, 367–368
  normal, *1711*, *1722–1726*
  on CT scan, *1751*
  "pseudotumors" of, 1711–1713, *1714*
  radionuclide evaluation of, 210–212
  renal agenesis and, 574
  sonography of, 331–332, 1750, *1751*
  tumors of, *369*, 1700–1753. See also *Tumors, adrenal.*
Adrenal hematoma, *40*
Adrenal medulla, tumors of, 1704–1706
Adrenal rests, incidence of, 1468(t)
Adrenal vein sampling, for hormone assay, 122
Adrenal venography, 121–122, 1729
Adrenogenital syndrome, 1708
  adrenocortical adenoma in, *1719*
"Adult type" polycystic renal disease, 1414–1427, *1429–1432*

Agenesis, renal, 571–577
  cyst of seminal vesical and, *771*
  ectopic ureter and, *692*
  myelodysplasia with, *1095*
  urethral, *753*
  vesical, 751, *753*
Air, shadows from, 403–404
Air cystogram, 66–67
Air pyelogram, 64
Albarran, gland of, hypertrophy of, *1144*
Allergic states, contrast medium reactions and, 21–22
Alveolar carcinoma. See *Adenocarcinoma, renal.*
Amyloid, composition of, 1915
Amyloidosis, 1913–1925
  classification of, 1915
  diagnosis of, 1917–1918
  experimental, 1915
  heredofamilial, 1916–1917
  in multiple myeloma, 1916, 1959
  localized, 1916
  of renal pelvis, 1921, *1922*
  primary, 1915–1916
  radiographic findings in, 1918–1925
  renal, 1921–1925
  secondary, 1916
  ureter, 1918–1921
  vesical, 1918, *1919*
Anaerobic urinary infection, in women, 2134
Anal atresia, 791–801. See also *Ectopic anus.*
Analgesic nephropathy, *1927*, *1929*, 1930–1931, *1936*, *1939*
Anesthesia, in renal angiography, 100–101
Aneurysm(s), calcified, confusing shadows from, 409–411
  of abdominal aorta, 2029–2033
    ureteral obstruction and, 2205, *2206*
    vs. retroperitoneal fibrosis, 2206
    vs. tumor, *2030*
  of iliac artery, 2029–2033
    confusing shadows from, *409*
  of renal artery, *1897*
Angiitis, necrotizing, angiography in, 1891(t)
Angiography. See also *Arteriography* and names of specific procedures.
  in bilateral adrenocortical hyperplasia, 1735–1746
  in genitourinary tuberculosis, 918
  in renal failure, 1889–1900
  in renal trauma, 1786–1806
  in vesical tumors, 1633–1639
  renal, 94–149. See also *Renal angiography.*
Angiolipoleiomyoma, renal, *1479*
Angiomyolipoma, *130*, *141*, *1474*
  CT evaluation of, 362–363
  in children, 1673
    in tuberous sclerosis, *1675*
    vs. polycystic renal disease, *1675*
  renal, 1474–1481, *1482–1484*
  spontaneous rupture with, *1477*
  tuberous sclerosis and, *1484*
  vs. polycystic disease, *1485*
Angiomyolipomatoma, in tuberous sclerosis, *262–263*
Angiotomography, 98
Anomalies, congenital, 565–808. See also names of specific anomalies.
  arteriography in, 143
  clinical classification of, 565–566
  radionuclide evaluation of, 192
  ureteral calculi and, 1321, *1325*

Antegrade pyelography, 167–183. See also *Per-cutaneous translumbar pyelography.*
Anterior urethral valves, 1116–1119
Antihistamines, reactions and, 22–23
Anus, abnormalities of, types of, *796*
  ectopic, 791–801. See also *Ectopic anus.*
  "imperforate," 791–801. See also *Ectopic anus.*
  normal development of, *795*
Aorta, abdominal, aneurysm of. See *Aneurysm, of abdominal aorta.*
  confusing shadows from, *410–411*
  primary arteritis of, 2033–2034, *2035*
Aortography, in retroperitoneal fibrosis, 2217
  translumbar, 115–116
  complications of, 126–127
Aortoiliac vascular system, retroperitoneal fibrosis and, 2206, *2208*
Aortorenal arteriography, 106–109, *110–112,* 1992–1993
Aplasia, renal, 571–577
Appendix, tumor of, vs. pericecal abscess, *423*
Arteriography, adrenal, 120–121, 1722–1746
  in pheochromocytoma, 1726–1729
  midstream abdominal aortic, 106–109, *110–112,* 1992–1993
  renal. See *Renal arteriography.*
  triple contrast, *1636*
Arteriolar nephrosclerosis, angiography in, 142–143
Arteriovenous fistula, displacement of urinary structures by, *2033*
  following cyst aspiration, *174*
  in renal transplant, 2056–2057
  of iliac and hypogastric vessels, 2029–2033
  post-traumatic, *1797,* 1799
  renal, 2012–2018
    acquired, 2012, *2014–2018*
    congenital, 2012, *2013*
    idiopathic, 2012
  vesical, *2044*
Arteritis, primary aortic, 2033–2034, *2035*
  renal
    immunologically mediated, 2035–2036
    pheochromocytoma and, 2035
    syphilitic, 2036
Artery(ies), aberrant, ureteropelvic obstruction and, *992*
  collateral, ureteral defects and, *2042*
  femoral, confusing shadows from, *411*
  hypogastric, aneurysm of, *2032*
  iliac, aneurysm of, 2029–2033
    confusing shadows from, *408, 411*
    preureteral, 678–680
  renal. See *Renal artery.*
  ureteral, anomalous, *2052*
Artifacts, in CT scanning, 343–344
Ascites, chylous, 392
Aspiration biopsy, of renal masses, 150–167. See also *Renal mass puncture.*
Atheromatous stenosis of renal arteries, *133–134*
Atherosclerosis, hypertension and, 1993–1995
  renal arterial, *133–134*
Atresia, anal, 791–801. See also *Ectopic anus.*
Atrophy, renal. See *Kidney, atrophy of.*
Autonephrectomy, *444*
  in tuberculosis, *900–901, 903–904*

Backflow, calyciorenal, 1812–1821
  pyelointerstitial, *1814–1816*
  pyelolymphatic, 1816, *1818–1819*
  pyelorenal, 1812–1821
  pyelosinus, 1816, *1817, 1820*
  pyelotubular, 1812, *1813–1814*
Bacterial cystitis, 883
Bandages, confusing shadows from, 405
Banti's disease, *1604*
Barium, residual, confusing shadows from, *426*
Bead-chain cystourethrography, 2158–2163
"Beaded" ureter, *914,* 916
Benign prostatic hyperplasia, 1135–1145
Berman's sign, 1577
Bertin, column of, vs. renal tumor, 1493
Bilharziasis, 921–939, *940*
  genital involvement and, 927
  pathogenesis of, 922
  pathology of, 922–927
  roentgen diagnosis in, 927–939
  urinary fistulas and, *1852–1854*
  vesical carcinoma and, 926–927
  vesicoureteral reflux in, 925–926, *932*
  vs. tuberculosis, 934–936
Biopsy, renal, complications of, *1787, 1799–1800*
  sonography in, 233–235
Bladder, agenesis of, 751, *753*
  air in, *882*
  amyloidosis of, 1918, *1919*
  anatomic variations in, 546–552
  anomalies of, 736–751
    clinical classification of, 566
    renal agenesis and, 574–575
  as substitute vagina, 2198, *2199*
  bilharziasis in, 923–924, 927–928, *929, 930, 932,* 932–933
  calcification of, tuberculous, *905*
  calculi of, 1338–1349. See also *Calculi, vesical.*
  carcinoma of. See *Carcinoma, vesical.*
  cecal, 2098, *2102*
  contracture of, irradiation and, *1622*
    periureteral diverticula and, *820*
  cord, calculous disease and, *1363*
  displacement of, by arteriovenous fistula, *2033*
    by ectopic hydronephrotic kidney, *602*
    by prostatic hyperplasia, *1141–1142*
    by retroperitoneal tumor, *1550*
  diverticula of, 1129–1135. See also *Diverticula, vesical.*
  diverticulitis of colon and, *873*
  duplication of, 745–751, *752*
  dysfunction of, unrecognized myelodysplasia and, 1904–1095
  embryology of, 729–732
  encrustations of, vs. calculi, 1347–1349
  endometriosis of, 2182
  exstrophy of, 458, *459,* 736–745, *748–750*
    pseudo-, *737*
    ureterosigmoidostomy in, carcinoma in, *747–748*
    vesicorectostomy in, 2076, *2077*
    vesicoureteral reflux and, *1051*
  extravesical impressions on, *440,* 547–550, 2185, *2186–2187*
  fistulas of, 1848–1849, *1849–1851,* 2044
  foreign bodies in, *447–449,* 2197
  hernia of, 2228–2233
    transitory ("bladder ears"), 2229

Bladder (*Continued*)
  hourglass, 751
  ileal, 2098–2108, *2109–2119*
  in prostatic hyperplasia, *1138–1139*
  incomplete filling of, diagnostic errors and, *555*
  injury to, 1827–1840
  instability of (urge incontinence), 2156–2163
  leaks in, renal transplantation and, 2069–2073
  leukemic infiltration of, *1699*
  leukoplakia of, 2246–2247
  lymphatic network of, *1640*
  mucosal edema of, vs. cystitis emphysematosa, *880*
  neck of. See *Vesical neck.*
  neurofibromatosis of, *1642*
  neurogenic, 1080–1100. See also *Neurogenic bladder.*
  normal, *1626*
  "pine tree" deformity of, *2210*
  radionuclide evaluation of, 207–210
  rupture of, 1828–1834
  saddle deformity of, 550, *551*
  trabeculation of, in neurogenic bladder, 1080–1082, *1098–1099*
    in prostatic hyperplasia, *1138*
  tuberculosis and, *905*, *917*, 917
  tumors of, 1618–1641. See also *Tumor(s), vesical.*
"Bladder ears," 2229
Bladder neck. See *Vesical neck.*
Bladder wall, thickness of, estimation of, 1618–1619
Blastema, renal nodular, *1671*
Bleeding, submucosal, of renal pelvis, *1776*
Blood clot, vs. tumor of renal pelvis, *1565*
Blood vessels, aberrant, ureteral obstruction by, *682*, 683, *991–993*
  calcified, confusing shadows from, 405–411
Blue-diaper syndrome, 1263–1264
Bolus technique of nephrotomography, 57
Bonney-Marshall test, 2157
Botryoid sarcoma, clinical findings in, *1693–1697*
  of renal pelvis, *1585*
  prostatic, *1697*
  treatment of, 1698
  vaginal, *1696*
  vesical, *1693–1695*
Bowel, contrast excretion into, *16*
  retroperitoneal fibrosis in, 2206, *2208*
Bowel gas, renal sonography and, 221, *224*
Boyce-Vest vesicorectostomy, *2077*
"Brat board," *74*
Breast, carcinoma of, osteolytic metastasis from, *467*
Bronchogenic carcinoma involving kidney, *1551*
Brucellosis, of urinary tract, 891–895
Buerger's disease, 2036–2038

C sign of subcapsular extravasation, 115
"Cake" kidney, *608–609*, 615, *616*
Calcific deposits, opaque shadows from, 442–446
Calculi, 1171–1368
  branched. See *Calculi, renal, staghorn.*
  calcium phosphate, *1180*, 1181
  caliectasis and, *1217–1219*
  classification of, 1173–1176, 1177(t)
  composition, architecture, and formation of, 1172–1173
  computed tomography in, 370–372
  cystine, *1181*, *1189*

Calculi (*Continued*)
  diversion procedures and, *2108–2111*
  focal hydronephrosis and, *282–283*
  in ectopic ureter, *1325*
  in medullary sponge kidney, *1445*, *1448–1451*
  in megaloureter, *1322*
  in presacral tumor, *1614*
  in prostatic utricle, 768
  in renal pelvis, leukoplakia with, *2242–2243*
    postoperative, *2024*
  in sarcoidosis, 1261–1262
  in ureteral valve, *685*
  in ureterocele, *718*, *719*, 726
  in ureteropelvic juncture, *1199*, *1217*
  in urethral diverticulum, *2138*
  incidence of, 1171–1172
  infection and, 1279–1283
  jackstone, *1228*, *1342–1343*, *1344*
  laminated, *1181*, *1197*, *1205–1206*, *1228*
  matrix, 1181, *1182*
  nonopaque, 1201, *1202–1213*
  plain film in, 5–7, *10–11*
  poor-density, 1201, *1202–1213*
  primary, 1173
  prostatic, 83, 85, 769, *1343–1345*, 1349–1359
    confusing shadows from, 436
    migrant and secondary, 1349–1352, *1353–1355*, *1363*
    multiple, *1356–1358*, *1363*
    native, 1349
    roentgen features of, 399, *1352–1356*
    spontaneous evacuation of, *1359*
    vs. phleboliths, *1356*
  radionuclide studies in, 192, *193–194*
  renal, *371*, *442*, *443*, *991*, 1176–1285
    abscess with, *856*
    burr-like, *1228*
    calcium oxalate, *1285*
    calyceal, *401*, *442*, *1189–1190*
    clinical features of, 1176–1179
    cortical, 1230–1234, *1235*
    cystine, *1203*, *1245–1248*, *1249–1250*
    encysted, 1230–1234, *1235*
    idiopathic, 1273–1279
    in calyceal diverticula, *980*, *982*, 1230–1234, *1236–1237*
    in children, 1284–1285
    in duplex kidney, 662–666
    in ectopic kidney, 603–606
    in horseshoe kidney, *629*, *632–638*, *643*
    in malrotated kidney, 585–587
    in medullary sponge kidney, *1445*, *1448–1451*
    in multiple myeloma, *1262*
    infection and, 1279–1283
    laboratory investigation of, 1177–1179
    laminated, *1197*, *1205–1206*, *1228*
    management of, medical, 1241–1283
      surgical, 1283–1284
    "milk of calcium," *1234–1236*, *1238–1239*
    nonopaque, 1201, *1202–1213*
    of recumbency, *1219*, *1266*, 1280–1283
    pathogenesis of, 1241–1283
      enzyme disorders and, 1248–1252
      hypercalcemic states and, 1252–1265. See also *Hypercalcemia.*
      hypercorticism and, 1263, *1264*
      idiopathic, 1273–1279
      intestinal disease and, 1269–1273, *1274*

Calculi (*Continued*)
  pathogenesis of, renal tubular syndromes and,
    1241–1248
    steroid therapy and, 1263, *1264*
    uric acid lithiasis and, 1265–1269, *1270–1275*
    urosepsis and, 1279–1283
  pathologic renal changes from, 1213–1241
  poor-density, 1201, *1202–1213*
  radiographic characteristics of, 1180–1213
  radionuclide studies in, 192, *193*
  recurring, 1230, *1233–1234*
  roentgen studies of, 1179–1241
    calcific shadows and, 1183–1201
    preliminary plain film and, 1179–1180
    ureteral catheter and, 1191
    urography and, 1191–1201
  sonographic diagnosis of, 339
  staghorn, *193, 338, 400–401, 442, 669, 743, 1180,*
    1202–1203, 1222, *1229–1232*
    carcinoma of renal pelvis and, *1572*
    in bilharziasis, *931*
    infected, *1280*
  tumor with, *439*
    uric acid, *1204*
    vs. calcified renal artery, *1185*
    vs. gallstones, 412–416, *1188*
    vs. pyelectasis, *400*
    vs. tuberculous calcification, *902,* 1222, *1227*
  scrotal fistula and, *1361*
  secondary, 1173–1176, 1213–1222
  "silent", 5–6
  sonography in, 338, *339*
  struvite, *1180*
  sulfonamide, *1172*
  thyrotoxicosis and, 1263, *1265*
  transplantation and, 2069–2070
  ureteral, 442–443, *444,* 1294–1338
    clinical features of, 1294
    difficulty in visualizing on plain film, 1294–1310
    dilatation and, 1321, *1322–1324*
    diversion procedures and, *2070*
    in bilharziasis, *929–930, 936*
    in duplex kidney, 662–666
    in intramural ureter, 1323–1330
    in prostatic hyperplasia, *1312*
    in ureteral stumps, 1331, *1332*
    laminated, *1321*
    large, 1321, *1322–1324*
    management of, nonsurgical, *1336,* 1338
      surgical, 1331–1338
    migratory, *1326*
    miscellaneous types of, 1321–1331
    nonopaque, 1317–1321
    opaque, 1301–1307
    papillary necrosis and, *1943*
    poor-density, 1317–1321
    pyeloureterectasis and, *1317–1319*
    radionuclide studies in, 192, *194*
    roentgen studies of, 1294–1331
      extraurinary shadows and, *443–444,* 1294–1300
      oblique and lateral views in, 1310–1317
      obstructive nephrogram in, 1307–1310
      opaque catheter in, 1301–1307
      overlying bone and, 1294, *1295–1298*
      plain film in, 1294–1310
      transient renal nonfunction and, 1307, *1308*
      visualization problems in, 1294–1310
    rupture of renal pelvis and, *1820*
    transient renal nonfunction and, 1307, *1308*

Calculi (*Continued*)
    ureteral, transurethral manipulation of, 1331,
      1333–1335
    uric acid, *1337*
    urinary extravasation and, 1330–1331
    vs. kinks, *402*
    vs. phleboliths, 1188, 1294, *1299–1300*
    vs. renal tubular necrosis, *1876*
    vs. stricture, *1321*
    vs. tumor, *1320–1321*
    vs. vesical calculi, *1323–1324*
  urethral, 446, 1359–1365
    vs. urethritis cystica, 939
  uric acid, *1959*
  vesical, 444–446, *447–448,* 1338–1349
    burr-like, 1342–1343, *1344*
    catheter drainage and, *2075*
    clinical features of, 1340–1349
    dumbbell, *1346*
    endemic, 1338–1340
    foreign-body, 1338, *1339*
    in bilharziasis, *930*
    in diverticulum, *1134,* 1343–1347
    in duplex kidney, 668
    jackstone, 1342–1343, *1344*
    management of, 1349, *1350*
    migrant, *1363*
    poor radiopacity of, 1340–1341
    roentgenographic characteristics of, 1341–1343
    vs. encrusted bladder lesions, 1347–1349
    vs. extravesical shadows, 1347–1349
    vs. renal calculi, *606*
    vs. ureteral calculi, *1323–1324*
  vs. calcified costal cartilage, 404, *405*
  vs. phleboliths, *407*
  vs. pyelectasis, *400–401*
  vs. ureteral kinks, *402*
Calculosis, intranephronic, 1173
Caliectasis, *999*
  calculi and, *1217–1219*
  false diagnosis of, 515
Calyceal diverticula, *195,* 974–986, 1453–1455
  calculi in, 1230–1234, *1236–1237*
Calyceal tips, irregular, vs. calculi, *401*
Calyciorenal backflow, 1812–1821
Calyx. See *Renal calyx.*
Candidiasis, renal, 895–898
Carbon dioxide cystography, *1626, 1627–1630*
Carbonic anhydrase inhibition, calculous disease and,
  1245
Carcinoma, adrenocortical, 1731–1735, *1737–1743*
  CT scanning in, *1751*
  Cushing's disease and, *1737*
  Cushing's syndrome and, *1719*
  hepatic invasion by, *1742*
  simple cyst and, *1740–1741*
  alveolar. See *Adenocarcinoma, renal.*
  bronchial, metastatic, *1553*
  cervical, 2193–2195, *2196*
  extraureteral obstruction and, 1014, *1015–1016*
  hepatic, *1602*
  hypernephroid. See *Adenocarcinoma, renal.*
  in ureterosigmoidostomy, 747–748
  of renal pelvis, *170,* 284–288
    analgesic nephropathy and, *1932*
    in children, 1686, *1687*
    in horseshoe kidney, *641–642*
    metastatic renal, *1492,* 1493, *1494*
    transitional cell, *284–288*

Carcinoma (*Continued*)
  of seminal vesicles, *1647–1649*
  ovarian, *432*, 433, 2197
  pancreatic, metastatic, *1586*
    vs. retroperitoneal fibrosis, 2206
  parenchymal. See *Adenocarcinoma, renal.*
  penile, *386*
    lymphography in, 392
  prostatic, 387, 1146, 1648–1650, *1697*
    lymphography in, 391–392
    metastasis from, *466, 468–472, 474*
      castration and, 471, *474*
      vs. Paget's disease, 465–479
      vs. fluoride osteosclerosis, *473*
  renal, *155–156, 169, 198*
    calcification in, *1500*
    epithelial, vs. renal blood clots, 965
    in adult polycystic disease, *1429*
    lymphography in, 392
    metastatic, 1549–1554
      vs. endometriosis, 2184–2185
      vs. renal cyst, *264–273*
    renal cell, *155, 156, 169, 198, 362*
      arteriovenous fistula and, *2016*
      calcification in, 1498(t)
      in horseshoe kidney, *641*
      in solitary kidney, *168*
      lymphography in, 392
    splenic, vs. retroperitoneal tumor, *1604*
    squamous cell, calcification in, 1498(t)
    testicular, 337–339, *384–386*, 387–391
    transitional cell, calcification in, 1498(t)
      of renal pelvis, *284–288*
    urachal, 1632–1633, *1634*
      in children, 1689
    ureteral, nonpapillary, *1583*
      transitional cell, *1575–1576*
      in female, 2198–2199
      in male, 1643–1646
    urethral, *1645–1646*, 2198–2199
    uterine, 2195–2197, *2198*
    vaginal, 2198, *2199*
    vesical, *181, 332, 1627, 1635–1636*
      bilharziasis and, 926–927
      infiltrating, *1622–1624, 1628*
      lymphography in, 392
      transitional cell, *1575, 1637*
      vs. ureteral tumor, *1584*
    vulvular, 2198–2199
Cardiovascular disease, risks of, urography in,
    24–25
Caruncle, of female urethra, 2199
Castration, in prostatic carcinoma, 471, *474*
Catharsis, in excretory urography, 27
    in children, 38
    in plain film, 7
Catheterization, ureteral, in retrograde pyelography,
    58–61
Cecal bladder, 2098, *2102*
Central nervous system, renal arteriography and, 124
Cervix, carcinoma of, 2193–2195
Chemodectoma, vesical, *1721*
Chemotherapy, in Wilms' tumor, 1666–1667
Cholecystogram, confusing shadows from, 424
Cholesteatoma, 2240–2246. See also *Leukoplakia, of
    renal pelvis.*

Chondrosarcoma, of left ilium, *463*
Chordoma, retroperitoneal, 1610
    sacral, *463*
Choriocarcinoma, metastatic, *1551*
Chromaffinoma. See *Pheochromocytoma.*
Chromoscopy, 696–697
Chromosomal sex, 780, 781(t)
Chronic renal failure, 1867–1868. See also *Renal
    failure.*
Chylous ascites, 392
Chyluria, 2220–2228
    lymphography in, 392
    nontropical, 2220, *2223*
    tropical, 2220, *2222, 2225–2227*
Circumcaval ureter, 677–678
Clear cell adenocarcinoma. See *Adenocarcinoma.*
Clips, surgical, confusing shadows from, *428–429*
Cloaca, embryology of, 566–569, 729–730, 755,
    792–793
Coccyx, congenital defects of, 1088–1091, *1093–1096*
Colitis, granulomatous, in Crohn's disease, 872
Collateral arteries, ureteral defects and, *2042*
Collateral circulation, in renal arterial stenosis, 136,
    137
Colon, diverticulitis of, *873*
Colostomy, confusing shadows from, 405, *406*
    cutaneous sigmoid, ureterosigmoidostomy with,
      2093–2095, *2096*
Colpocystorectography, 2160–2161
Compensatory hypertrophy of kidney, 523–526,
    527–528, 578–579
Computed tomography, 339–373
    in adrenal disease, 367–368, 1711, 1721, 1750, *1751*
    in calculous disease, 370–372
    in hydronephrosis, 368–370
    in masses, 354–368
      of pelvis, bladder, and prostate, 354–360
    in renal parenchymal disease, 372
    in retroperitoneal fibrosis, 2217
    technique of, 341–354
      anatomic considerations in, 344–354
        of renal anatomy, 344–350
        of retroperitoneal anatomy, 350–354
      artifacts and, 343–344
      image interpretation and, 344
Conduit, ileal, *179*
Congenital absence of abdominal muscles, *734,*
    777–779, *1050*
Congenital aneurysm of renal artery, 2004, *2005*
Congenital anomalies. See *Anomalies, congenital.*
Congenital mesoblastic nephroma, 1669, *1671*
Congenital multicystic kidney, 1430–1435, *1436–1437*
Congenital stenosis of urethral meatus, 1122–1123,
    1124
Congenital urethral diverticulum, 1150
Congenital urethral valves, anterior, 1116, *1118–1119*
    cystic renal dysplasia with, 1435–1437
    hydronephrosis and, *2081–2082*
    in female, 1119, *1120–1122*
    in male, 1106–1116
      clinical problem in, 1107–1108
      treatment of, 1115–1116
      urographic diagnosis in, 1108–1115
Conn's syndrome (primary aldosteronism), 1708
Contraceptive devices, confusing shadows from, *430*
    infection and, 2131–2134

Contrast medium (media), 13–23
  delayed appearance of, in renovascular hypertension, 1986–1987
  dosage of, 22
  excretion mechanism of, 16–18
  extravasation of, in adenocarcinoma, *1504*
    in ureter, *1820*
  in excretory urography, in adults, 30–32
    in children, 39
  in lymphography, 379–380
  in renal angiography, 101, 124
  in retrograde pyelography, 61–62
  physical properties of, 14–16, 15(t)
  plasma concentrations of, *17–18*
  pretesting and, 22, 123
  reactions to, 18–27
    cardiovascular, 24–25
    hepatorenal syndrome and, 1871
    in renal angiography, 123–124
    in renal failure, 23
    premedication and, 123
    sensitivity testing and, 22, 123
    treatment of, 26–27
Cord bladder, calculous disease and, *1363*
"Corkscrew" ureter, *914*, 916
Corpus cavernosa, calcification of, confusing shadows from, 437
Corpus luteum cysts, ovarian, 2191–2193
Corticoid therapy, calculous disease and, 1263, *1264*
Corticosteroids, reactions and, 23
Costal cartilages, calcified, vs. renal calculi, *1183–1184*
  confusing shadows from, 404, *405*
Crescent sign of hydronephrosis, *966*
  chronic pyelonephritis and, *1851*
Crohn's disease (regional ileitis), *870–872*
Crystals, urinary, microscopic appearance of, *1179*
CT scanning, 339–373. See also *Computed tomography.*
Cushing's disease, adrenal adenoma and, *1715*
  adrenocortical carcinoma in, *1737*
  adrenocortical hyperplasia and, *1744–1745*
  radionuclide studies in, *1752*
Cushing's syndrome, 1707–1708
  adrenocortical adenoma in, *1718*
  adrenocortical carcinoma in, *1717*
  adrenocortical hyperplasia in, 1720–1721
  nonendocrine, 1709
Cutaneous sigmoid colostomy, ureterosigmoidostomy with, 2093–2095, *2096*
Cutaneous ureterostomy, 2076–2080, *2081*
  transureteroureterostomy and, 2083–2084, *2085–2087*
Cutaneous vesicostomy, 2074, *2075*
Cut-film changer, Elema-Schonanader, *96*
Cyclophosphamide cystitis, 885
Cysts, adrenal, *1701–1703*
  calcified, *1709*
  hemorrhagic, cortical adenoma and, *1735*
  corpus luteum, of ovary, 2191–2193
  deep pelvic, 765–776
    clinical classification of, 566
    vs. tumor, 1616, *1618*
  dermoid, 1608–1610
    confusing shadows from, *434*, 435
    ovarian, *434*, 435, 2191, *2192–2193*
    pelvic, *464*

Cysts (*Continued*)
  dermoid, retroperitoneal, 1608–1610
    of omentum, *945*
  echinococcus, *446*, 940–949
  hepatic, 945, *946*, *1603*
    confusing shadows from, *413*
  infected, sonography in, 298–308, *309–314*
  müllerian duct, 765, *766–767*
    vs. prostatic utricle cysts, 767
    vs. seminal vesicle cysts, 769
  of Gartner's duct, 774, *775*
  of prostatic utricle, 765–767, *769–770*
  of seminal vesicle, 768–773, *774*
  ovarian, *440*, 2191–2193
    dermoid, *434*, 435, 2191, *2192–2193*
  pancreatic, *1599–1601*
  parapelvic, *161*, *364*, *1380–1384*, *1385–1388*
    calyceal dilatation and, *976*
    racemose, *161*
  pararenal pseudo-, features of, 1370(t)
  perirenal, 1455–1463
  prostatic, 774, *775–776*
  pyelogenic, 95, 974–986, 1453–1455
    calculi in, 1230–1234, *1236–1237*
  renal, 439, 523, *525*, 1369–1466. See also *Cystic disease; Medullary cystic disease; Polycystic renal disease; Renal dysplasia.*
    adenocarcinoma in, *1536*
    arteriography in, *139*
    aspiration of, 152–162. See also *Renal mass puncture.*
      complications of, 164–167
      sonographic guidance of, 227–233
    benign, *346*, *361*, *364*
    calcification in, *445*
    carcinoma in, 1528, *1536*
    echinococcus, *446*, 940–949. See also *Renal hydatidosis.*
      vs. hepatic cyst, *946*
    fluid characteristics in, 158–162
    hydatid, *446*, 940–949. See also *Renal hydatidosis.*
    in duplex kidney, *649*, *670*, *671*
    in ectopic kidney, *606–607*
    infected, vs. renal abscess, 298–308, *309–314*
    management of, sclerosing agents in, 155–158
    "milk of calcium" stone in, *1239*
    multilocular, *162–163*, 1437–1441
      features of, 1370(t)
      hypernephroma and, *1375*
      vs. simple cyst, *1386*
      vs. Wilms' tumor, *1442*
    multiple, 1383–1384, *1387–1389*
      vs. polycystic disease, *1432*
    pyelogenic, 1453–1455
    radionuclide evaluation of, *197*
    roentgen findings in, 162–164
    simple, *157–159*, 1371–1410
      adrenocortical carcinoma and, *1740–1741*
      aspiration of, 1396–1405
      calcification in, 1498(t)
      features of, 1370(t)
      fluid assay findings in, 273(t)
      hemorrhagic, 164–165
      roentgen diagnosis of, 1372–1396
      spontaneous regression of, *1385*
      vs. tumor, *1391–1410*, *1513*

Cysts (*Continued*)
  renal, sonographic findings in, 250–253,
      254–255
    supernumerary kidney and, *570*
    trauma and, *1786*
    ureteritis cystica and, 875
    vs. carcinoma, *51*, 264–269, *270–273, 1505*
    vs. hydatidosis, 943–945
    vs. renal carbuncle, *857*
    vs. tumor, 151–152, *1387, 1390–1410*, 1504–1534,
        1505–1527
      criteria for differentiation of, 1507(t)
      CT evaluation in, 360–367
      sonographic evaluation in, 245–276. See also
          Sonography, in renal mass lesions.
  retroperitoneal, 1589–1618
    dermoid, 1608–1610
    of mesodermal origin, 1594–1606
  sacral, *464*
  spinal and pelvic, 462–464
  splenic, *1605*
  umbilical, 734, *735*
  urachal, vs. omental echinococcus cyst, *945*
  ureteral, *1578*
Cyst fluid, biochemical values of, 158–162
Cystadenoma, *171, 1469, 1471*
  renal, 1469–1472
  retroperitoneal, *1597*
Cystic disease. See also *Cyst(s), renal; Polycystic
    renal disease; Renal dysplasia.*
  classification of, 1369(t)
  features of, 1370(t)
  medullary, 1441–1453
    medullary sponge kidney, 1441–1451
    uremic, 1451–1453, *1454–1455*
      features of, 1370(t)
  sonographic diagnosis of, 243–245, *246–250*
Cystic lymphangioma, *1599*
Cystine calculi, *1203*
Cystinuria, calculous disease and, 1245–1248,
    1249–1250
Cystitis, 883–888
  bacterial, 883
  cyclophosphamide, 885
  cystica, 873–876
  emphysematosa, 878–883
  eosinophilic, 885, *886*
  glandularis, 885–888
  "honeymoon", 2134
  in women, 2131–2134
  interstitial (Hunner's ulcer), 883–885, 2142–2144
  postcoital, 2134
  radiation, *1964, 2914*, 2195
  tuberculous, 888, *917*, 2134–2135
Cystocele, 2163–2167
Cystography, air, 66–67
  pelvic pneumography and, in vesical carcinoma,
      1637–1639
  carbon dioxide, perivesical insufflation and, 1619,
      1626, 1627–1630
  common errors in interpreting, 552, *554–555*
  excretory, 65, 67, 546–552
  interureteric ridge sign in, 2163
  normal findings in, 546–552
  radionuclide, 207–210
  residual urine determination by, 67–68
  retrograde, 65–66, 546–552
  uterine pressure and, 547–550

Cystoscopy, excretory urography and, 44–45
  in ectopic ureteral orifice, 695–696
Cystostomy, suprapubic, 2074, *2075*
Cystourethrography, 70–74, 552–563
  bead-chain, 2158–2163
  expression, 71, 73
  in females, 561–563
  in males, 552–557
    in infants and children, 559–561
  retrograde, in prostatic hyperplasia, 1135–1141
    vs. voiding, *557*
  voiding, 72–76
    fluoroscopic control in, 73
    free voiding vs. voiding against resistance in, 72
    in children, 74–76
    ordinary technique of, 72
    patient position for, *66*
    simple, 71
    technique of Waterhouse in, 72–73

Dark cell carcinoma. See *Adenocarcinoma.*
Davis intubated ureterotomy, *1004*
Deep pelvic cysts, 765–776
  clinical classification of, 566
  vs. tumor, 1616, *1618*
Dehydration, for excretory urography, 27–28
  in children, 38
Delayed pyelogram, 64
Dermoid cyst(s). See *Cyst(s), dermoid.*
Detrusor instability, 2156–2163
Diabetes mellitus, glomerular disease in, 1910–1913
  renal failure in, 24
  renal papillary necrosis in, *1914*, 1931
  risks of, urography in, 24
  spermatic tract calcification in, 435, *436*, 901
  urinary tract infections in, 878, *879, 881–882*
Differentiated ganglioneuroma, in children, 1686
Diffuse nephroblastomatosis, 1671, *1673*
Diffuse proliferative glomerulonephritis, 1901–1902
Direct magnification renal angiography, 97–98
"Disk" kidney, *608–609, 613*, 615
Distal urethral stenosis, 1102–1106, 2136–2138
Diversion, urinary, 2073–2127. See also *Urinary
    diversion.*
Diverticula, calyceal, *195*, 974–986, 1453–1455
  calculi in, 1230–1234, *1236–1237*
  paraureteral, *1024*
    vesicoureteral reflux and, *1043*
  periureteral, vesical contracture and, *820*
  ureteral, 672–676
  urethral, 761–765
    calculi in, 1363–1364, *2138*
    diffuse, 762–765
    false, calculus in, *1362*
    in female, 2138–2142
    in male, *764*, 765, 1149–1150, *1151–1152*
    post-traumatic, of prostatic urethra, *764*
    saccular, 761–762
    vs. ectopic ureteral orifice, 699–700, *703*, 2177
  vesical, *208*, 1129–1135
    calculi in, *447*, 1134, 1343–1347
    multiple, *1135*
    prostatic hyperplasia and, *1136*
    tumors in, 1630–1632, *1633*
    vesicoureteral reflux and, *1044*
    vs. extravesical impression, 2185, *2186–2187*
    vs. shadows, *554*

Diverticula (*Continued*)
  vesicourachal, 733–734
  vesicoureteral reflux and, *1042–1044*
Diverticulitis, of colon, 873
Drip-infusion urography, *43–44*, 46–51, 57–58, 971, 973
  in renal insufficiency, *43*
  in urinary diversion, *44*
Dromedary hump, 518–520, *522*
Drug abuse, arteritis and, *2037*
  renal failure in, *1897*
  retroperitoneal fibrosis and, *2209*, 2212
  tubulointerstitial disease and, *1927*
Ductus deferens, normal anatomy of, *80*
Duplex kidney, associated pathologic conditions and, 654, *656*, 662–672
  cyst in, *649*, *1391*
  ectopic ureteral orifice and, *696*
  hypernephroma in, *673*
  lobar dysmorphism in, *655*
  lower-pole pelvis of, 657–662
  obstructive uropathy in, 654–657
  pseudotumor in, *650*, *653–655*
  pyeloureterectasis in, 662, *663–664*
  reflux in, 654–657
  size of, 648, *652*
  transitional cell epithelioma in, *1563*
  tuberculosis in, *670*
Dysgenesis, renal, 571–577
Dysplasia, renal, 571–577, 1427–1437. See also *Renal dysplasia.*

Echinococcus cysts, *446*, 940–949. See also *Renal hydatidosis.*
Ectopia, anal, 791–801. See also *Ectopic anus.*
  of ureteral orifice, 684–708, 2177. See also *Ectopic ureteral orifice.*
  renal, *130*, 584–591. See also *Renal ectopia.*
  ureteral, *658*, *688*, *690*, *704–705*, 727–729
Ectopic ACTH syndrome, 1709
Ectopic anus, associated anomalies and, 798–799
  at urethrovesical juncture, *798*
  at urogenital sinus, *799*, *800*
  classification of, 795–798
  embryologic explanation for, 792–793
  management of, 799–800
  perineal, *794*
  posterior urethral, *798*
  roentgen technique in, 793–794
Ectopic ureteral orifice, diagnostic methods in, 695–697
  double, 690–691
  embryogenesis of, 684–688
  familial tendency of, 700–703
  in female, 692–694, *695–696*, 697–703, 2177
  in male, 706–708, *709–712*
  obstruction vs. reflux in, 691–692
  sites of, *686*, 690
  statistical data and, 688–690
  unilateral vs. bilateral, 690, *692–694*
  unusual cases of, 697–699, 703–706
  urinary incontinence and, 692–694, *695–696*, 697–703, 2177
  vs. urethral diverticulum, 699–700, *703*, 2177
Ectopic ureterocele, *237–238*, 715, 719–726, 727–728, *1053*

Edema, of vesical mucosa, vs. cystitis emphysematosa, *880*
  ureteral, in calculous disease, 1323–1330
Ejaculatory duct(s), normal anatomy of, *80*
  prostatic calculi in, *85*
  reflux into, *79*, 87
Embryology, of cloaca, 792–793
  of genital tract, *687*, 783–784
  of kidney, 579
  of urinary tract, 566–569
Emphysema, renal, *879*
Emphysematous cystitis, 878–883
Emphysematous pyelonephritis, 853
Endemic stone disease, 1338–1340
Endometriosis, of urinary tract, 2181–2185
"End-stage" renal disease, angiographic features of, 1890(t), *1892*
Enteritis, regional, 872
Enzyme disorders, calculous disease and, 1248–1252, *1253–1255*
Eosinophilic cystitis, 885, *886*
Ependymoma, spinal erosion from, *463*
Epididymis, obstruction of, 86–87
Epididymitis, radionuclide study of, *211*
Epididymography, 85–87
Epinephrine, in renal angiography, 98–99, 138
Epispadias, 736–745
Epithelioma, in ectopic kidney, *607*
  vesical, *1620*, *1629*, *1630*
Ergot, retroperitoneal fibrosis and, 2212
Ethiodal, 379
Excretory cystogram, 65, *67*
Excretory pyelogram. See *Excretory urography.*
Excretory urography, 12–64
  as preliminary to cystoscopy, 44–45
  as test of renal function, 42–44
  basic concepts of, 12–13
  contrast media for, 13–23. See also *Contrast medium (media).*
  disadvantages of, 45
  drip-infusion technique in, *43–44*, 46–51, 57–58, 971, 973
  history of, 2–5
  hypotension and, 24–27
  in acute pyelonephritis, 810–812, *813–817*, 817
  in adrenal neoplastic disease, 1709–1722
  in adults, 27–38
    contrast medium in, 30–32
    roentgen technique in, 32–38
  in calculous disease of ureter, 1301–1307
  in cardiovascular disease, 24–25, 1984–1989
  in children, 38–42
  in diabetes, 24
  in multiple myeloma, 25–26
  in pyelectasis, 969, *973*
  in renal failure, 23, 1871–1889
    risks of, 1868–1871
  in renal trauma, 1768–1777
  in renovascular hypertension, 1984–1989
    isotope renography with, 1989–1990
  in simple renal cyst, 1372–1390
  increased risk factors in, 23–26
  minute-sequence technique in, 52–53
  normal, *191*
  radiation dose in, 45–46
  ureteral compression in, 28–30, *31–33*
    hypertensive effect of, *1872*
Exposure time, plain film and, 11, *12*
Expression cystourethrography, 71

Exstrophy, of bladder, 458, 459, 736–745, 748–750
    pseudo-, 737
    ureterosigmoidostomy in, carcinoma in, 747–748
    vesicorectostomy in, 2076, 2077
    vesicoureteral reflux and, 1051
Exstrophy-epispadias complex, 736–745
Extravasation, urinary, in calculous disease, 1330–
        1331
    isotope scan in, 2060
Eye, melanoma of, metastatic to urinary tract, 1588

Fallopian tubes, agenesis of, renal agenesis and, 575
Familial Mediterranean fever, amyloidosis in, 1917
Fanconi syndrome, in multiple myeloma, 1959
Fecal material, shadows from, 403–404
Feminizing syndrome, 1708–1709
Fetal bones, confusing shadows from, 422–423
Fetal lobulation, 347, 518, 520
    vs. chronic pyelonephritis, 839
Fibroepithelioma, ureteral, 1688
Fibrolipoma, retroperitoneal, calcified, 1600
Fibrolipomatosis, renal, 526–531
    vs. chronic pyelonephritis, 839
    vs. pelvic lipomatosis, 2233
Fibroma, benign polypoid, of renal pelvis, 1554
    renal, 1473–1474
    peripelvic, 1473
Fibromatous uterine tumors, confusing shadows
        from, 429, 432, 433
Fibromyoma, uterine, 2189–2190
Fibromyxolipoma, renal, 1472
Fibromyxosarcoma, retroperitoneal, 1593
Fibrosarcoma, renal, vs. tumor of renal pelvis, 1543
Fibrosis, of uterus, 440
    retroperitoneal, 2205–2220. See also
        Retroperitoneal fibrosis.
Filling defect(s), air bubbles and, 539
    gas shadow simulating, 539
Film, selection of, for plain film, 11–12
"Fish hook" deformity of ureter, 1142
Fistula(s), arteriovenous. See Arteriovenus fistula.
    bilharzial perineal, 937
    iatrogenic, urinary incontinence and, in women,
        2167–2175
    ileovesical, 1851
    lymphatic, 393
    lymphaticocalyceal, in chyluria, 2223–2227
    lymphaticopelvic, 1843
    nephrobronchial, 1843
        perinephric abscess with, 851
    nephrocutaneous, 1842
    perineal, calculus and, 1361
    postirradiation, 2195, 2197
    pyeloduodenal, 1846
    rectofossa navicularis, 797
    rectoperineal, in female, 797
        in male, 796
    rectourethral, 796
        postoperative calculi and, 1362
    rectovaginal, 797
        embryologic development of, 795
    rectovesical, 796
    renal, 1842–1846
    renocolic, 182–183, 1841, 1845
    renogastric, 1844–1845

Fistula(s) (Continued)
    scrotal and perineal, calculus and, 1361
    terminology of, 1840
    tuberculous, renocolic, 1845
        renogastric, 1844
    types of, in female, 797
        in male, 796
    ureteral, 1846, 1847–1848
    ureterocutaneous, 1846
    ureteroileal, 1846
    ureteroperineal, 2176
    ureterovaginal, 1858–1861
        incontinence and, 2167–2173
    urethral, 1849–1854
    urethrocavernous, 1854–1855
    urethrocutaneous, 2075
        iatrogenic, 1156
    urethroperineal, 1853
        congenital, 760, 761
    urethrorectal, 1854, 1856
    urethrovaginal, 1861
        incontinence and, 2176
    urinary, 1840–1861
        classification of, 1842
        diagnosis of, 1840–1842
    urinary-vaginal, 1854–1861
    urogenital, 791–792. See also Ectopic anus.
    vesical, 1848–1849, 1849–1851, 2044
    vesicocervical, incontinence and, 2174
    vesicocutaneous, in renal transplantation, 2072
    vesicointestinal, 1848–1849, 1849–1851
    vesicosigmoidal, 1850
    vesicourethral, iatrogenic, 1155
    vesicouterine, 2198
    vesicovaginal, 1857–1858, 1861
        postirradiation, 2197
        postoperative calculi and, 1346
Fluoride osteosclerosis, vs. prostatic carcinoma, 473
Fluoroscopy, in children, 41–42
Flushing technique of genitography, 785
Foreign bodies, confusing shadows from, 446–449
Fundus ring, 561
Fungal infection of kidney, 895–898
Fungus ball, candidal, 896

Gallbladder, confusing shadows from, 416, 424
    contrast excretion into, 16
    hydrops of, 1602
    renal malrotation and, 438
Gallstones, confusing shadows from, 410, 412–416
    renal malrotation and, 438
    vs. renal calculus, 1188
Gamma scintillation camera, 186
Ganglioneuroma, adrenal, vs. adenoma, 1736
    differentiated, in children, 1686
    retroperitoneal, 1614
Gartner's duct, cysts of, 774, 775
Gas, bowel, obscuring ureteral calculi, 1298, 1309
    rectal, vs. filling defect, 555
        vs. prostatic hyperplasia, 1140
    shadows from, 403–404, 539
Gas-producing infections of urinary tract, 878–883
Gastric fundus, fluid in, vs. adrenal tumor, 1712
Gastroenteropathy, protein-losing, lymphography in,
        392
Gender, 781

Genital system, embryologic differentiation of, 687
Genital tract, bilharziasis in, 927–928
  embryology of, 783–784
Genitalia, anomalies of, renal agenesis and, 575
  embryology of, 751–755
  external, differentiation of, 754
Genitography, in intersexual state, 784–785, 779–791
Genitourinary tract, male, normal anatomy of, 556
Gland of Albarran, hypertrophy of, 1144
Glomerulonephritis, acute, 1904, 1906
  angiography in, 142–143
  chronic, 1904–1905, 1906–1909
    angiographic features of, 1890(t), 1891(t)
    nephrocalcinosis and, 1290–1293
  diffuse proliferative, 1901–1902
  focal, 1901, 1926
  membranous, 1902–1903
  nephrocalcinosis in, 1909–1910
Glycinuria, calculous disease and, 1248
"Goblet sign" of ureteral tumor, 1577, 1579–1582
Gonadal sex, 780–781
Gout, 1265, 1956–1957
Granular cell adenocarcinoma. See Adenocarcinoma.
Granular cell carcinoma. See Adenocarcinoma.
Granuloma, plasma cell, of renal pelvis, 1556
Granulomatous prostatitis, 889–890, 891
Grawitz's tumor, 1486–1534. See also
  Adenocarcinoma.
Gynecologic problems related to urinary tract,
  2130–2204

Hamartoma, 1474–1481, 1482–1484. See also
  Angiomyolipoma.
  renal, 1475, 1476–1481, 1482–1484
    fetal, 1669
    in infant, 1670
  tuberous sclerosis and, 1484
  ureteral, secondary, 1560
  vs. polycystic disease, 1485
Heavy metal salts, confusing shadows from, 425
Heitz-Boyer diversion, 2095, 2097
Hemangioendothelioma, renal, with Lindau-von
  Hippel disease, 1542
  retroperitoneal, 1594
Hemangioma, hepatic, vs. adrenal tumor, 1713
  in children, 1689, 1691
  of renal pelvis, 1555
  renal, 1474
  ureteral, 1559, 1560
  vesical, 1641–1643
Hemangiopericytoma, retroperitoneal, 1616
Hematoma, confusing shadows from, 423
  intrarenal, 1501
  of renal pelvis, 1776
  perirenal, 1503
    following biopsy, 1787
    spontaneous, 1775
  subcapsular, 1501, 1773–1774
    calcified, 1501
  vs. adenocarcinoma, 1493–1498, 1501–1503
Hematometrocolpos, 2177–2178
Hemorrhage, in plain film, 441
Hepatomegaly, 438
Hepatorenal syndrome, 1871
Hermaphroditism, true, 785

Hernia, inguinal, vesical diverticulum and, 1131
  ureteral, 2228–2233
  vesical, 2228–2233
Hodgkin's disease, of ureter, 1587
Hodgkin's lymphoma, 358, 1545, 1548
Hormonal sex, 781
Hormone assay, adrenal vein sampling for, 122
Horseshoe kidney, 240–243, 439, 619–641
  associated anomalies and, 625–631
  duplication in, 643
  embryogenesis of, 619–620
  mucinous adenocarcinoma in, 1535
  pathologic conditions associated with, 631–642
  prostatic hypertrophy and, 628
  pyelocaliectasis in, 630
  sonographic diagnosis of, 238, 240–243
  supernumerary kidney with, 572
  trauma and, 1785
  tuberculosis in, 639–640
  urographic findings in, 620–625
  vs. bilateral malrotation without fusion, 628
  vs. fused kidney, 618
Hunner's ulcer, 883–885, 2142–2144
Hydrocalycosis, 974–986
Hydrocalyx, 974–986
  vs. tumor, 975
Hydrocele, 338
  radionuclide study of, 211
  renalis, 1370(t), 1455–1463, 2065
Hydrocolpos, 704
  vaginal atresia and, 2180
Hydrometrocolpos, 2178–2181
Hydronephrosis, 278–281, 955–974, 2067. See also
  Pyelectasis.
  arteriography in, 142, 143
  bilateral, 1038
  cervical carcinoma and, 2194–2195, 2196
  computed tomography in, 368–370
  crescent sign of, 966
  focal, secondary to calculous disease, 282–283
  in ectopic kidney, 599, 602
  in horseshoe kidney, 631, 643
  in prostatic obstruction, 1136
  in retroperitoneal fibrosis, 292
  in ureteropelvic obstruction, 290–291, 293
  intermittent, 994–999
  moderate, 289
  postradiation, 2194
  secondary calculi in, 1220–1221
  sonographic diagnosis of, 276–290, 291
  vesicoureteral reflux and, 1057
  vs. adenocarcinoma of renal cortex, 1496
Hydroureter, 693, 1577
  in prostatic obstruction, 1136
  secondary calculi in, 1221
Hydroureteronephrosis, bilateral, 1063–1064
Hydroxyproline, calculous disease and, 1340
Hyperaldosteronism, primary, adrenal adenoma in,
  1747–1749
  adrenal venography in, 1746
Hypercalcemia, calculous disease and, 1252–1265
  Cushing's syndrome and, 1263
  hypercorticism and, 1263, 1264
  hyperthyroidism and, 1263, 1265
  hypervitaminosis D and, 1262
  idiopathic infantile hypercalcemia and, 1263–1264

Hypercalcemia (*Continued*)
  calculous disease and, immobilization and, *1219,*
      1264–1265
    immobilization and, *1219,* 1264–1265
    milk-alkali syndrome and, 1262
    neoplasms and, 1262–1263
    primary hyperparathyroidism and, 1254–1261,
        1282
    sarcoidosis and, *1260,* 1261–1262
  idiopathic infantile, 1263–1264
Hypercorticism, calculous disease and, 1263, *1264*
Hypernephroid carcinoma. See *Adenocarcinoma,*
    renal.
Hypernephroma, 532, 1486–1534. See also
    Adenocarcinoma, renal.
Hyperoxaluria, 1248–1252, *1253–1255*
  acquired, 1273, *1273–1274*
Hyperparathyroidism, calculous disease and,
    1254–1261, *1282,* 2188
  primary, uterine myofibroma and, *2188*
Hypersensitivity reactions, to contrast medium,
    18–27. See also *Contrast medium (media).*
Hypertension, arterial, excretory urography in,
    34–35
  differential diagnosis of, 1891(t)
  malignant, angiographic appearance of, *1893*
  paroxysmal, on voiding, *1721*
  pheochromocytoma and, *1721,* 1726, 2035
  radiation nephritis and, 1964
  renovascular, 1979–2002
    angiographic findings in, 1891(t)
    basic concepts of, 1979–1981
    causes of, 132(t), 1993–2001
    diagnosis of, 1981–1993
    fibroplasia of renal artery and, *1877*
    iatrogenic, *2023*
    incidence of, 1981
    management of, 2001
    radionuclide evaluation in, 205, *206–207,*
        1988–1990
    renal artery occlusion and, *1878*
    trauma and, *1801–1802, 1804*
Hyperthyroidism, calculous disease and, 1263, *1265*
Hypertrophy, compensatory renal, 578–579
Hypervitaminosis D, calculous disease and, 1262
  vs. idiopathic infantile hypercalcemia, 1263–1264
Hypogastric artery, aneurysm of, *2032*
  ureteral obstruction and, *2041*
Hypoplasia, renal, 238, 240
    congenital, 577–578, *579*
      vs. chronic pyelonephritis, 839
Hypotension, urographic procedures and, 24–27

Idiopathic infantile hypercalcemia, 1263–1264
Idiopathic renal lithiasis, 1273–1279
Ileal bladder, 2098–2108, *2109–2119*
Ileal conduit, *179,* 2098–2108, *2109–2119*
Ileal loop, *179,* 2098–2108, *2109–2119*
Ileitis, regional, *870–871*
Ileocystography, *2076*
Ileocystostomy, 2074–2075, *2076*
Ileopyelostomy, 2116, *2119*
Ileostomy, urinary, 2098–2108, *2109–2119*
Ileovesical fistula, *1851*
Iliac artery, aneurysm of, 2029–2033
  confusing shadows from, *408, 411*
  preureteral, 678–680
Iliac vessel, calcification of, *1187*

Immobilization, calculous disease and, *1219,* 1264–
    1265, 1280–1283
"Imperforate" anus, 791–801. See also *Ectopic anus.*
Imperforate hymen, hematometrocolpos and,
    2177–2178
Incontinence of urine, after transurethral resection,
    1161, 1162
  in female, 2155–2176
    acquired urinary fistula and, 2167–2175
    cystocele and, 2163–2167
    ectopic ureteral orifice and, 692–694, *695–696,*
        697–703, 2177
    labial fusion and, 2177
    procidentia and, 2163–2167
  in male, postoperative, 1161, *1162*
  stress, 2156
    vs. detrusor instability, 2156–2163
  urge, 2156
    vs. stress incontinence, 2156–2163
Indigo-carmine test, 2169–2171, 2174
Infantile polycystic renal disease, 1414–1415,
    1415–1416
Infarction, renal, *1888–1889*
  in sickle hemoglobinopathy, 1944–1945
  radionuclide studies in, 205–206
  segmental, vs. pyelonephritis, 838
Infection, anaerobic, 2134
  calculous disease and, 1297–1283
  gas-producing, 878–883
  genitourinary, 909–954. See also names of specific
      diseases.
  renal papillary necrosis and, 1931
  response of collecting system to, 867–872
  sonographic diagnosis of, 290–319
  urinary, anaerobic, 2134–2135
    in women, 2131–2134
  vesicoureteral reflux and, *1047*
Inferior vena cava, adenocarcinoma obstructing,
    1522–1524
  embryogenesis of, 677, *678*
Inferior vena cavography, in renal tumors,
    1522–1524, 1532
  in Wilms' tumor, *119*
  normal, *117*
Inflammatory lesions of female pelvis, 2199–2201
Infusion urography, *43–44,* 46–51, 971, *973*
Inguinal hernia, vesical diverticulum and, *1131*
Injection granulomas, confusing shadows from, *426*
Interpapillary line, 822
Intersexuality, 779–791
  classification of, 785–790
    genitographic, 786–790
    morphologic, 785
  embryologic explanation of, 783–784
Interstitial cystitis, 883–885, 2142–2144
Interureteric ridge, cystographic visualization of,
    550–552, *553*
Interureteric ridge sign, 2163
Intestinal disease, calculous disease and, 1269–1273,
    1274
Intranephronic calculosis, 1173
Intrarectal probe, 335
Intrarenal backflow, 1812–1821
Intrarenal reflux, chronic pyelonephritis and, 819–
    821
Intrathoracic kidney, 593, *596–597*
  vs. ectopic kidney, 598
Intrauterine contraceptive device (IUD), urinary
    infection and, 2131–2134
Intravenous nephrotomography, 55–58

Intravenous pyelogram (IVP). See *Excretory urography.*
Intubated ureterotomy of Davis, *1004*
Iodized oil, confusing shadows from, *425–427*
^{131}I-orthoiodohippurate, 186–187
  in renal mass detection, 198
  plasma disappearance curve of, *189*
  radiation dose from, *187*
Irradiation, vesical contracture and, *1622*
Ischemia, renal, 1946–1953
Ischiorectal abscess, communicating with urethra, *1852*
Isolated rectal pouch, 2093–2095, *2096*
IUD, confusing shadows from, *430*
  urinary infection and, *2131–2134*

Jackstone calculi, *1228, 1342–1343, 1344*
Juvenile medullary cystic disease, 1451–1453, *1454–1455*
Juvenile nephronophthisis, 1451–1453, *1454–1455*

Kidney. See also *Renal.*
  abscess of, 842–867. See also *Abscess, perirenal; Abscess, renal.*
  agenesis of, 571–577
    ectopic ureter and, *692*
  anatomy of, 481–484, *508*
    vascular, 2002–2003
  anomalies of, clinical classification of, 565
    in form, 604–642
    in number, 569–577
    in position, 579–604
    in size, 577–579
    in structure, 642. See also *Multicystic disease.*
    vs. disease, *523*
  architecture of, destruction of by adenocarcinoma, *1503*
  ascent and rotation of, *579*
  asymmetry of, *439, 441, 510*
  atrophy of, 238, 240
    back-pressure, *1887*
    congenital, 571–577
    hydronephrotic, vs. pyelonephritis, 838–839
    iatrogenic, *2024*
    in nephrosclerosis, *1953*
    postobstructive, *1943*
    postoperative, *2023*
    renal arterial occlusion and, *2022*
    vesicoureteral reflux and, *1056*
  autonephrectomy of, in tuberculosis, *900–901, 903–904*
  bifid, adenocarcinoma in, *1491*
  bilharziasis in, 928, 933–936
  blood supply of, *2003*
  "cake", *608–609, 613*
  calcification of, 444–445, 1285–1293. See also *Nephrocalcinosis.*
    tuberculous, *444, 902–904*
  calculi of, 1176–1285. See also *Calculi, renal.*
  carcinoma of. See *Carcinoma, renal.*
  collecting system of, infection and, 867–872
  compensatory hypertrophy of, 523–526, *527–528,* 578–579
  congenital neoplasia of, 1668–1671
  cysts of, 1369–1466. See also *Cyst(s), renal.*

Kidney (*Continued*)
  damage to, from contrast medium, 124
  diffuse nephroblastomatosis of, 1671, *1673*
  "disk", *608–609, 613*
  displacement of, *352–353*
    by abdominal aortic aneurysm, *2031*
    by neoplasm, 1493, *1496–1497*
    by perinephric abscess, *861*
  duplex, 648–672. See also *Duplex kidney.*
  duplication of, *178*
    ectopic ureteral orifice with, 696–697
    horseshoe kidney with, 625–626
    pyelonephritis and, 837
    sonographic diagnosis of, 235–236, *237–238*
    tuberculous autonephrectomy in, *904*
    vesicoureteral reflux and, *1035, 1042*
  dysgenesis of, 571–577
  dysplasia of, 1427–1437. See also *Renal dysplasia.*
  ectopic. See *Renal ectopia.*
  embryology of, 566–568, 579, 584–588
  endometriosis of, 2184–2185
  "endstage" disease of, 319, 1890(t), *1895*
  enlargement of, false, *519*
    in leukemia, *1677*
  fetal lobulation of, *347,* 518, *520*
  fistulas of, 1842–1848
  foreign bodies in, *448, 1783*
  fungal infection of, 895–898
  fused, *439,* 608–619, *627.* See also *Horseshoe kidney.*
    vesicoureteral reflux and, *1046*
  horseshoe, 619–641. See also *Horseshoe kidney.*
  hydronephrosis and, 955–956, *961*
  hypoplasia of, arteriography in, *145*
    congenital, 577–578, *579*
    sonographic diagnosis of, 238, 240
    vs. chronic pyelonephritis, 839
  in renal parenchymal disease, 1886(t)
  in renovascular hypertension, 1986–1987
  infantile, 577–578, *579*
  infarct in, *1888–1889.* See also *Infarction, renal.*
  injury to, 1767–1821
    classification of, 1767–1768
    complications of, arteriography and, 1789–1802
    late sequelae of, 1807–1811
      arteriography and, 1802–1806
    roentgen diagnosis of, 1768–1806
      angiography in, 1786–1806
      excretory urography in, 1768–1777
      retrograde pyelography in, 1777–1786
    treatment of, 1811–1812
  intrathoracic, 593, 596–597
    vs. ectopic kidney, *598*
  leukemic infiltration of, *1544,* 1677–1679
  lobar dysmorphism in. See *Lobar dysmorphism.*
  L-shaped, *609, 615*
  "lump", *608–609, 613*
  malrotation of, 580, 581–584, *585–588*
    cystic disease and, *1379, 1381, 1385*
    gallbladder distention and, *438*
    in ectopic kidney, *604*
    pathologic conditions associated with, 584, *585–587*
    vs. horseshoe kidney, *628*
  mass lesions of. See *Renal mass(es).*
  medullary sponge, 1370(t), 1441–1451
  multicystic, 1430–1435, *1436–1437,* 1498(t)
    sonographic diagnosis of, 245, *249–250*

Kidney (*Continued*)
   nephrostomy drainage of, 175, *176–177*
   nodular blastema of, 1671
   nonvisualization of, ureteral calculi and, 1307, *1308*
   normal, interpapillary line in, 822
     on sonogram, 220
   "Page", post-traumatic, *1802*
   parenchyma of. See *Renal parenchyma.*
   pelvic (sacral), 239, 592–593, *594–595.* See also
     Pelvic kidney.
   pelviocalyceal system of, 484–487
   polycystic disease of, 1410–1427. See also *Polycystic*
     renal disease.
   position of, 488–492
   "pseudotumor" of, 272, *274–277,* 650, 653–655,
     835–836, 1036–1037
   ptosis of, 542–546
     in female, 2135, *2136*
     vs. ectopia, 588–589, *590*
   pyelectasis and, 955–956
   pyonephrotic, *860*
   radionuclide studies of, 185–207
   "reflux," *1029, 1031–1032*
   scarring of, 523
   separated function study in, 1990–1991
   sigmoid, *609*
   size of, hypertension and, 1984–1985
     in renal failure, 1884, *1885,* 1886(t)
     in renal papillary necrosis, 1933
   solitary. See *Solitary kidney.*
   spleen transposed with, *274–277*
   supernumerary, 569–571, *572–573*
   transplantation of, 2051–2073. See also *Renal*
     transplantation.
   tuberculosis in, 305–308, 907–914, 1940, *1942,* 2245
   tubular ectasia of, 1370(t), 1441–1451
   vesicoureteral reflux and, 1050–1059. See also
     Vesicoureteral reflux.
Kilovoltage, effect of, on plain film, 10–11
KUB, 5–11, 396–480. See also *Plain film.*

Labial fusion, urinary incontinence and, 2177
Laminated calculi, *1205–1206*
Laxative(s). See *Catharsis.*
Lead shot, confusing shadows from, *426*
Leiomyoma, of renal pelvis, *1554*
   renal, 1473
     in children, *1677*
   vesical, in children, *1689*
Leiomyosarcoma, *1542*
   of renal pelvis, *1585*
   renal, *1540*
   retroperitoneal, *1591, 1594*
   vesical, vs. deep pelvic cyst, *1618*
Leukemia, renal infiltration by, *1544, 1677*
   vesical infiltration of, *1699, 1699*
Leukoplakia, 2239–2247
   carcinoma and, *1571*
   of renal pelvis, 2240–2246
   renal tuberculosis and, *2245*
   ureteral, *2243,* 2246
Lindau-von Hippel disease, 1534, *1539, 1541–1542*
Lipoid nephrosis, histologic findings in, *1925*
Lipoma, retroperitoneal, *1595–1596*
Lipomatosis, of renal pelvis, *327–329*
   sonographic diagnosis of, 323–326

Lipomatosis (*Continued*)
   of renal sinus, 526–531, *532*
     vs. pelvic lipomatosis, 2233
   pelvic, 2233–2236, *2237–2240*
Lipomyxosarcoma, renal, *1543*
Liposarcoma, cystic, retroperitoneal, *1593*
Lipuria, vs. chyluria, 2228
Liver, carcinoma of, *1602, 1742–1743*
   confusing shadows from, 412, *413, 438*
   echinococcus cyst of, 945, *946*
   enlarged, *438*
   hemangioma of, vs. adrenal tumor, *1713*
Lobar dysmorphism, 272, *274–277,* 655, 835–836,
     1036–1037
   in duplex kidney, 650, *653–654*
   vs. tumor, 650, *653–654*
L-shaped kidney, *609,* 615
Lumbar spine, anomalies of, 459–462
Lumbar vertebrae, confusing shadows from, 404
"Lump" kidney, *608–609, 613*
Lung granuloma, calcified, vs. renal calculus,
   1186
Lymph nodes, calcified, confusing shadows from,
   418–421
   mesenteric, *1187*
   metastatic involvement of, 384–385
   normal, *381–382, 383*
Lymphangiography, in retroperitoneal fibrosis, 2217
   in vesical tumors, 1639, *1640*
Lymphangioma, cystic, *1599, 1615*
   renal, *1472*
   vesical, 1641–1643
     in children, *1691*
Lymphatic channels, cannulation of, 379
   normal, 381–383
   peripheral, locating of, 378–379
Lymphaticocalyceal fistula, in chyluria, 2223–2227
Lymphedema, 392, *393*
Lymphoblastoma, retroperitoneal, with calcification,
   1546
Lymphocele, *2066*
   in renal transplant rejection, *331*
Lymphocyst, 393
Lymphography, 377–395
   as aid to retroperitoneal node dissection, 389
   complications of, 393–394
   cordis injector for, *380*
   history and development of, 377
   in pathologic states, 383–393
     in chylous ascites, 392
     in chyluria, 392
     in idiopathic retroperitoneal fibrosis, 393
     in lymphatic fistula, 393
     in lymphedema, 392, *393*
     in malignancies, 384–392
     in protein-losing gastroenteropathy, 392
     in testicular neoplasms, *384–386,* 387–391
   indications for, 383(t)
   normal, 378, *381–383*
     of spermatic cord, 389
   technique of, 378–381
   terminology of, 377
Lymphoma, 322–326, 388
   Hodgkin's, *358*
   perirenal, *321*
   renal, malignant, 1544–1549
Lymphomyxosarcoma, retroperitoneal, *1591*
Lymphosarcoma, renal, *1546*

Lymphosarcoma (*Continued*)
  retroperitoneal, *1545, 1590, 1595*
Lysergic acid diethylamide, retroperitoneal fibrosis
  and, 2212

Makar's stricture, 933–934, *935*
Malacoplakia, 876–878
Malta fever, 891–895
Mass lesions, computed tomography in, 354–368
  in adrenal lesions, 367–368
  in pelvic, vesical, and prostatic lesions,
    354–360
  in renal lesions, 360–367
  parapelvic, *349*
  renal. See *Renal mass(es)*.
Mass puncture, 150–167. See also *Renal mass
  puncture*.
McCarthy ejaculatory duct instrument, 78
Mediterranean fever, familial, amyloidosis in, *1917*
Medullary cystic disease, 1370(t), 1441–1453,
  1454–1455
Medullary sponge kidney, 1441–1451
  calculi in, *1445, 1448–1451*
  features of, 1370(t)
  vs."adult type" polycystic disease, 1443, *1446–1447*
Medullary uremic cystic disease, 1451–1453,
  1454–1455
Megaloureter, calculi in, *1322*
Megalourethra, 762–765
Megaureter, refluxing, *1029*, 1038, 1079–1080
Melanoma, metastatic to kidney and ureter, *1588*
Meningocele, 1082–1090
Meningomyelocele, *460, 462*, 1082–1095, *1096*
  vesicoureteral reflux with, *1045*
Mesenchymal tumors, incidence of, 1468(t)
  remnants of, in female, *686*
Mesonephric duct, embryology of, 566–569
Metastasis, osteolytic vs. osteoblastic, 465–467
Methyldopa, retroperitoneal fibrosis and, 2212
Methysergide, retroperitoneal fibrosis and, *2209*, 2212
Michaelis-Gutmann bodies, 876
Middeldorpf tumors, 1610–1618
Middle aortic syndrome, 2033–2034, *2035*
Milk-alkali syndrome, calculous disease and, 1262
Minute-sequence urography, 52–53
Moniliasis, renal papillary necrosis and, *896*
Müllerian duct cysts, 765, *766–767*, 769
Multicystic kidney, 1430–1435, *1436–1437*, 1498(t)
  sonographic diagnosis of, 245, *249–250*
Multilocular cysts, *162–163*, 1437–1441
Multinodular hyperplasia of adrenal cortex, *1746*
Multiple catheter technique of genitography, 785
Multiple myeloma, 464–465, 1957–1960
  amyloidosis and, 1916
  excretory urography in, 25–26
  radiographic findings in, 1960
Multiple renal arteries, *129, 2057*
Multiple sclerosis, neurogenic bladder and, 1082
Myelodysplasia, *461*, 1082–1095
  neurologic defects in, 1091, *1092*
  unrecognized, bladder dysfunction and, 1094–1095
Myelolipoma, adrenal, *1704*
Myeloma, renal involvement and, *1549*
Myofibroma, uterine, *2188–2189*
Myxoma, of renal sinus, *1473*

Necrosis, renal papillary, 1928–1943. See also *Renal
  papillary necrosis*.
Necrotizing angiitis, 1891(t), 1899
Needle puncture, of renal masses, 150–167. See also
  Renal mass puncture.
Neonates, renal function studies in, 191
Nephritis, radiation, 1962–1965
Nephroblastomatosis, diffuse, 1671, *1673*
Nephrobronchial fistula, *851, 1843*
Nephrocalcinosis, *1240*, 1285–1293
  advanced, *1293*
  conditions associated with, 1285(t)
  cortical, *1292, 1911*
  hypercorticism and, *1263–1264*
  in glomerulonephritis, *1290–1293, 1909–1912*
  in primary hyperparathyroidism, *1256*
  in sarcoidosis, *1260, 1962*
  medullary, *1240, 1242–1244, 1286–1290*
  vs. calculi of recumbency, *1219*
  vs. medullary sponge kidney, 1444
  vs. tuberculous calcification, *903*
Nephrocutaneous fistula, *1842*
Nephrogram, 54–55
  in renal failure, 1871–1884
  obstructive, 1307–1310
Nephroma, congenital mesoblastic, 1669, *1671*
  vs. Wilms' tumor, 1664
Nephronophthisis, 1451–1453, *1454–1455*
Nephropathy, analgesic, *1929*, 1930–1931, *1939*,
    2036, *2038*, 2212
  uric acid, 1955–1957, *1958*
Nephroptosis, 542–546
  in female, 2135, *2136*
  vs. ectopia, 588–589, *590*
Nephrosclerosis, 1890(t), 1946–1953
Nephrosis, lipoid, histologic findings in, *1925*
  osmotic, 23
Nephrostomy, 2116–2125
  by percutaneous puncture, 175, *176–177*
  infected urolithiasis and, 1280, *1281*
Nephrotic syndrome, 1925–1926
  in end-stage renal disease, *1895*
  in sickle hemoglobinopathy, 1945
Nephrotomography, 55–58, 1307–1310
  in differentiation of tumor and cyst, 1504–1507,
    1505–1527
  in simple cyst, 1390–1392
Neurilemmoblastosis, 262–263, 1481–1486, *1675*
Neurilemmoma (Schwannoma), 1606, *1607, 1614*
Neuroblastoma, adrenal, *336, 1685*
  renal, in children, 1680–1686
Neurofibroma, of lumbosacral canal, *464*
  retroperitoneal, 1606
  vesical, in children, 1688–1689, *1690*
  in von Recklinghausen's disease, *1690*
Neurofibromatosis, of renal artery, 2038–2040
  vesical, *1642*
Neurogenic bladder, 1080–1100
  acquired, 1080–1082
  calculous disease and, *1363*
  congenital, 1082–1095
    trabeculation of bladder in, *1098–1099*
  renal function in, radionuclide studies in, 199–200
  trabeculation of, 1080–1082
  urethral sphincter in, 1082, *1083–1086*
  vesicoureteral reflux and, *1049*
  vs. congenital vesical neck obstruction, 1094–1095,
    1096

Nodes, enlarged, retroperitoneal, *354*
Nodular renal blastema, 1671
Nonchromaffin paraganglioma, vesical, *1721*
Nonendocrine Cushing's syndrome, 1709

Obesity, confusing shadows from, 405, *406*
Obstructive ureterectasis, 1011–1017
Oliguria, in acute renal failure, 1866
Omentum, echinococcus cyst of, *945*
Organ of Zuckerkandl, pheochromocytoma of, *1617*, 1709
Osmotic nephrosis, 23
Osteitis, condensans ilii, 457–458
    deformans, 475–479
    pubis, 453–457
Osteoarthritis, *450–451*, 452
Osteoblastic metastasis, 467–474
    vs. osteolytic, 465–467
Osteochondrofibrosarcoma, renal, *1592*
Osteochondroma, *462*
Osteolytic metastasis, vs. osteoblastic, 465–467
Osteomyelitis, of vertebrae, 453, *454*
Osteosclerosis, fluoride, vs. carcinoma of prostate, *473*
Ovarian vein, sarcoma encircling, *1594*
Ovarian vein syndrome, left, *2152*
    right, 2149–2155
Ovary, abscess of, ureteropyelectasis and, *2200*
    agenesis of, 575
    carcinoma of, *432*, *433*, 2197
    cysts of, 2191–2193
        confusing shadows from, *434*, *435*
Overexposure, in plain film, *403*

P sign of retroperitoneal extravasation, *1115*
"Page kidney," post-traumatic, *1802*
Paget's disease of bone, 475–479
Pancreas, carcinoma of, vs. retroperitoneal fibrosis, 2206
    confusing shadows from, 414, 417–418
    cyst of, *1599*
    cystadenoma of, *1600*
    normal, *345*
    pseudocyst of, *1601*
Papillary cystadenocarcinoma. See *Adenocarcinoma.*
Papillary necrosis, in diabetes mellitus, *1914*
    in renal tuberculosis, 907–909
    moniliasis and, *896*
Papillary transitional cell epithelioma of renal pelvis, *1564–1567*
Papilloma, paracervical bilharzial, *938*
    trigonal, *1621*
    vesical, *1621*
        prostatic hypertrophy and, *1620*
Papillomatosis, *1621*
    bilharzial, of ureter, *934*
Paraganglioma, vesical, 1641, *1642, 1721*
Parapelvic cysts, *161, 364, 1380–1384, 1385–1388*
    calyceal dilatation and, *976*
    racemose, *161*
Pararenal pseudocyst, 1370(t), 1455–1463, 2065
Paraureteral diverticula, *1024, 1043*
Parenchymal carcinoma. See *Adenocarcinoma.*
Patient preparation, for excretory urography, 27–28
    in children, 38

Patient preparation (*Continued*)
    for plain film, 7
    for radionuclide renal studies, 187
    for renal angiography, 100
    for renal mass puncture, 152
Pelvic inflammatory disease, in female, 2199–2201
Pelvic kidney, 239, 592–593, *594–595*
    duplication of bladder and urethra with, *752*
    reflux and, *1046*
    squamous cell carcinoma and calculus in, *1572*
    trauma and, *1786*
Pelvic lipomatosis, 2233–2236, *2237–2240*
Pelvic pneumography, in vesical carcinoma, *1637–1639*
Pelvic vasculature in female, *1637*
Pelviocalyceal system, vascular impressions on, 983–986
Pelvioileal conduit, *2117–2119*. See also *Ileal conduit.*
Pelvioileoneocystostomy, *2120, 2123*
Pelvis, sagittal section of, female, *357*
    male, *356*
Penis, carcinoma of, *386*
    lymphography in, *392*
    duplication of, *750*
Penoscrotal juncture, iatrogenic fistula of, *1156*
    stricture of, *1155, 1158–1159*
Percutaneous catheterization, vascular complications of, 125–126
Percutaneous needle aspiration, 150–167. See also *Renal mass puncture.*
Percutaneous nephrostomy, catheter for, *233*
Percutaneous noncatheter brachial method of renal angiography, 116–117
Percutaneous transaxillary catheterization, in renal angiography, 114–115
Percutaneous transfemoral catherization, in renal angiography, 101–113
Percutaneous translumbar pyelography, 167–183
    clinical application of, 179–183
    complications of, 179
    indications for, 175–179
    technique of, 167, 175
Periarteritis nodosa, *1898–1899*
Perimedial dysplasia of renal artery, 1998, *1999*
Perineal ectopic anus, *794*
Perineal fistula, calculus and, *1361*
Perineal sigmoidostomy, with ureterorectostomy, *2095, 2097*
Perineal urethrostomy, 2073
Perinephric abscess. See *Abscess, perinephric.*
Perinephric cyst, 1370(t), 1455–1463, 2065
Perirenal abscess, 843–848, 867(t)
Perirenal air, with ruptured duodenum, *854*
Perirenal cyst, 1370(t), 1455–1463, 2065
Perirenal hematoma, 1503, *1775, 1787*
Perirenal space, air in, *854*
Peristalsis, pelvic and ureteral, urogram and, 532–535, *536*
    retrograde, in duplicated ureter, 648, *649*
Periureteric venous ring, *2043*
Perivesical insufflation, in measurement of bladder wall, 1619
Pessaries, confusing shadows from, 428, *430*
Peyronie's disease, calcification of corpus cavernosa in, 437
Phenacetin, retroperitoneal fibrosis and, 2212
Phenacetin nephropathy, *1929, 1939, 2036, 2038,* 2212

Pheochromocytoma, 1701, 1704–1706
  adrenal, *1714–1715, 1727–1729*
  angiography in, 1726–1730
  calcification in, *1710*
  excision of, arteritis and, 2035
  extra-adrenal, 1720, *1730*
  hypertension and, *1721*, 1726, 2035
  metastatic, *369*
  of organ of Zuckerkandl, *1617*, 1709
  radionuclide study of, *211*
  sites of, 1720(t)
  tests for, 1705–1706
  vesical, *1721*
Phleboliths, confusing shadows from, 407
  vs. prostatic calculi, *1356*
  vs. ureteral calculus, *1188, 1294, 1299–1300*
Photographic film selection, for plain film, 11–12
"Pine tree" deformity of bladder, *2210*
"Pipestem" ureter, *914–915,* 916
Pixel, *340*
Plain film (KUB), 5–11, 396–480
  abdominal compression in, 7, 8
  exposure of, *1298*
  good quality in, importance of, 402–404
  in bilharziasis, 927–932
  in calculous disease, 1179–1180, 1294–1310
  in renal hydatidosis, 942
  in simple cyst, 1372–1374
  in skeletal lesions, 450–479
  in tuberculosis, 899–907
  method of examining, 396–399
  preliminary, 5–7, 400–402
    in children, 38–39
  shadows in, 403–449. See also *Shadows.*
  technique of, 7–11
  terminology and, 396
Pneumothorax, after renal mass puncture, *173*
Polyarteritis nodosa, *1897, 1899, 2005,* 2006–2007,
  2028–2029
Polycystic disease, of liver, *1603*
Polycystic renal disease, 1410–1427
  "adult type," 1414–1427, *1429–1432*
    features of, 1370(t)
    in children, 1414
  CT evaluation of, 363, *365*
  in duplex kidney, *671*
  infantile, 1410–1414, *1415–1416*
    features of, 1370(t)
  sonographic findings in, 243–245, *246–248*
  vs. hamartoma, *1485, 1675*
  vs. medullary sponge kidney, 1443, *1446–1447*
Polyp(s), malignant, at ureterocolic anastomosis, *2089*
  ureteral, 1555–1559, *1687, 1688*
  urethral, 1119–1122, *1123*
    in children, 1699
Positive-pressure urethrography, 70, *71*
Postarterial ureter, 678–680
Postcaval ureter, 677–678
Postcoital distress, 2134
Posterior urethral valves, 1106–1116, *1869*
Posterior urethrovesical (PUV) angle, 2158–2160
Postirradiation fistula, 2195, *2197*
Pott's disease, psoas abscess and, *903*
Pregnancy, pyelonephritis of, 2147–2149
  pyeloureterectasis in, 2144–2147
  radionuclide renal evaluation in, 206–207
  renal ectopia in, *602*
Primary aldosteronism, 1708
  radionuclide evaluation of, *212, 1752–1753*

Primary hyperoxaluria, 1248–1252, *1253–1255*
Primary hyperparathyroidism, calculous disease and,
  1254–1261, *1282*
Primary systemic sclerosis, 1953–1955
Procidentia, 2163–2167
Prostate gland, abscess of, bilharzial, *938*
    tuberculous, *918–919*
  bacterial disease of, 888–891
  benign hyperplasia of, 1135–1145
    ureteral stone and, *1312*
  bilharzial involvement of, 939
  calcification of, 436
    tuberculous, 901, *905*
  calculi in, *83, 85,* 769, *1343, 1345,* 1349–1359
  carcinoma of. See *Carcinoma, prostatic.*
  cysts of, 774, 775–776
  encrustation of, vs. vesical tumor, *1141*
  hypertrophy of, *357, 628, 1620*
  normal, *80*
    vs. enlarged, *333–335*
  tumors of, 1648–1650
    in children, 1699
Prostatectomy, incontinence and, 1161, *1162*
Prostatic ducts, abscess of, 888–889
Prostatic utricle, calculi in, *768*
  dilatation of, 765–767, *769–770*
  examination of, 87–88
  normal, *769*
Prostatitis, 888–891
  granulomatous, *889–890,* 891
  tuberculous, *919, 921*
Proteinuria, Tamm-Horsfall, *1878*
Prune belly syndrome, 777–779
  vesicourachal diverticulum in, *734*
  vesicoureteral reflux and, *1050*
Pseudocyst, pancreatic, *1601*
Pseudocyst, pararenal, 1370(t), 1455–1463, *2065*
Pseudohermaphroditism, female, 784, 785, *790*
  hydrometrocolpos and, 2178–2181
  male, 786
Pseudohydronephrosis, 1370(t), 1455–1463, *2065*
Pseudotumor, renal, 272, *274–277,* 650, *653–655,*
  835–836, 1036–1037
Psoas abscess, *1856*
  confusing shadows from, *416*
  in tuberculosis, *904*
  secondary to Pott's disease, *903*
Psoas muscle, obliteration of, in perinephric abscess,
  440, 441
Ptosis, renal, 542–546
  in female, *2136*
  vs. ectopia, 588–589, *590*
Pudendal neurectomy, in neurogenic bladder, *1088*
Purgation. See *Catharsis.*
PUV angle, 2158–2160
Pyelectasis, 955–974. See also *Hydronephrosis.*
  in duplex kidney, 662, *663–664*
  pathophysiologic renal changes in, 955–956
  radioisotope studies in, 971–974
  roentgen findings in, 956–971
  ureteropelvic obstruction and, *956,* 989–990, *994*
  vs. calculous disease, *400–401*
  vs. "flashy" renal pelvis, *497,* 498
Pyelocaliectasis. See also *Hydronephrosis.*
  advanced, 963–969
  bilateral, *987*
  in ectopic kidney, *602*
  in horseshoe kidney, *630*
Pyelocutaneous anastomosis, 2125–2127

Pyeloduodenal fistula, *1846*
Pyelogenic cyst, *195*, 974–986, 1453–1455
  calculi in, 1230–1234, *1236–1237*
Pyelography. See also *Excretory urography.*
  antegrade, 167–183. See also *Percutaneous translumbar pyelography.*
  definition of, 1
  percutaneous translumbar, 167–183. See also *Percutaneous translumbar pyelography.*
  rapid-sequence, 52–53
  retrograde, 58–64. See also *Retrograde pyelography.*
Pyelointerstitial backflow, *1814–1816*
Pyelolymphatic backflow, 1816, *1818–1819*
Pyelonephritis, acute, *294*, 809–817
    differential diagnosis in, 817
    gross pathologic appearance of, 809
    microscopic findings in, 809–810
    roentgen findings in, 810–817
    sonographic diagnosis of, 293–296
  angiographic features of, 1890(t)
  atrophic, *1887*
    chronic, *1888*
      angiographic appearance of, *1892–1894*
    renal papillary necrosis and, *1940*
  chronic, 817–839
    angiographic features of, 1890(t)
    arteriography in, *145*, 1891(t)
    Crohn's disease and, *1851*
    "end stage" of, *845–847*
    gross pathologic changes in, 818–819
    in children, 838–839
    intrarenal reflux and, 819–821
    roentgen diagnosis in, 821–837
    route of infection in, 818
    sonographic diagnosis of, 316, *317*
    vesicoureteral reflux and, 837–838
  emphysematous, *853*
  of pregnancy, 2147–2149
  suppurative, *295, 296*
    vs. transplant rejection, 295–296, *296*
  vs. tumor, *835–836*
  xanthogranulomatous, 839–842
    calcification in, 1498(t)
Pyelorenal backflow, 1812–1821
Pyelosinus backflow, 1816, *1817, 1820*
Pyelotubular backflow, 1812, *1813–1814*
Pyeloureterectasis, in duplex kidney, 662, *663–664*
  in ectopic ureter, *690*
  in pregnancy, 2144–2147
  ureteral calculi and, *1317–1319*
  vesical carcinoma and, *1622*
Pyeloureteritis, 873–876
Pyonephrosis, *318–319, 860*
  sonographic diagnosis of, 316–319
Pyuria, vs. chyluria, 2228

Radiation cystitis, *1964, 2194,* 2195
Radiation dose, in excretory urography, 45–46
  in radioisotope studies, *187*
Radiation nephritis, 1962–1965
Radiation protection, in renal angiography, 99–100
Radiation therapy, in Wilms' tumor, 1665–1666
Radioactive isotope seeds, confusing shadows from, *428*
Radioisotope(s), selection of, for renal studies, 186–187

Radionuclide studies, 185–213
  in adrenal neoplasm, *1751–1752*
  in calculous disease, 192, *193–194*
  in congenital anomalies, 192
  in horseshoe kidney, *621*
  in neurogenic bladder, 199–200
  in obstructive uropathy, 196–197, 971–974
  in pregnancy, 206–207
  in renal and perirenal abscess, 862
  in renal infarction, 205–206
  in renal mass lesions, 197–199
  in renal transplantation, 200–205, 2057–2062
  in renal trauma, 200
  in renovascular hypertension, 205, *206–207,* 1988–1989
    excretory urography with, 1989–1990
  in vesicoureteral reflux, 192–196
  of the adrenals, 210–212, *1751–1752*
  of the bladder, 207–210
  of the kidney, 185–207
    age factors in, 191
    applications of, 190–207
    equipment for, 185–186
    evaluation of, 189
    in patient screening, 190–192
    normal, *190–191*
    patient preparation for, 187
    radioisotopes in, 186–187
    scintillation camera technique in, 187–189
  of the testis, 210, *211*
  residual urine calculation in, *188*
Rapid-sequence pyelography, 52–53
Reactions, to contrast medium, 18–27
Rearing sex, 779–781
Recklinghausen's disease, 1606, *1690*
Rectofossa navicularis fistula, 797
Rectoperineal fistula, 796–797
Rectourethral fistula, 796
Rectovaginal fistula, 797
  embryologic development of, 795
Rectovesical fistula, 796
Rectum, normal development of, 795
Reductive ureteroplasty, 1079–1080
  intrarenal chronic pyelonephritis and, 819–821
Reflux, into ejaculatory duct, 79, 87
  vesicoureteral, 1017–1080. See also *Vesicoureteral reflux.*
Refluxing megaureter, 1038, 1079–1080
Regional enteritis, 872
Regional ileitis (Crohn's disease), *870–871*
Reinjection urography, 971, *973*
Renal abscess, *298,* 842–867. See also *Abscess, renal.*
Renal actinomycosis, 895–898
Renal agenesis, 571–577
  cyst of seminal vesicle and, *771*
  ectopic ureter and, *692*
  myelodysplasia and, *1095*
Renal angiography, 94–149. See also *Renal arteriography.*
  adrenal arteriography in, 120–121
  adrenal venography in, 121–122
  anesthesia in, 100–101
  applications of, 132–147
  contrast medium in, 101
  direct magnification, 97–98
  epinephrine in, 98–99, 138
  equipment for, 94–97
  general considerations in, 94

Renal angiography (*Continued*)
  hazards of, 123–127
  in acute pyelonephritis, 812, *815–816*
  in arteriolar nephrosclerosis, 142–143
  in congenital anomalies, 143
  in glomerulonephritis, 142–143
  in mass lesions, 137–142
  in renal abscess, 862–867
  in renal vascular disease, 132–136
  in tuberculosis, 918
  magnification studies in, 97–98, *113, 114*
  normal, 127–132
    arterial phase of, 127–131
    nephrographic phase of, 131–132
    venous phase of, 132
  patient preparation in, 100
  patient selection in, 1992–1993
  percutaneous noncatheter brachial method of,
    116–117
  percutaneous transaxillary catheterization in, 114–
    115
  percutaneous transfemoral catherization (Seldinger
    technique) in, 101–113
  radiation protection in, 99–100
  radiographic techniques for, 97–100
  renal venography in, 117–120
  selective renal arteriography in, 109–113
  stereoscopic, 97
  tomography in, 98
  translumbar method of, 115–116
Renal arteriography, in chronic pyelonephritis, *145*
  in differentiation of tumor and cyst, 1392–1396,
    1504–1507, *1505–1527*
  in postoperative evaluation, 143, *146–147*
  in renal transplantation, 143–145, *147*, 2052–
    2057
Renal arteriovenous fistula, 2012–2018, *2019*
Renal artery, aneurysm of, 2003–2012
    calcified, *2010*
      confusing shadows from, *409*
    classification of, 2004–2011
    congenital, 2004, *2005*
    extraparenchymal, 2007–2011
    fusiform, *2009*
      calcified, *2008*
    in systemic lupus erythematosus, *1897*
    intrarenal, 2004–2006
      atherosclerotic, 2004, *2010*
    medial dissecting, *2010*
    polyarteritis type of, *2005*, 2006–2007
    saccular, 2008–*2009*
      calcified, *2007*
    traumatic, *1798*
  anomalies of, renal agenesis and, 575, *577*
  calcified, vs. renal calculus, *1185*
  confusing shadows from, *409–410*
  emboli of, *2021*
  fibromuscular dysplasia of, *1896, 1986*, 1995–
    2001, *2007–2009*
    focal type, *135*
    hypertension and, *1877*
    intimal, *1997*, 2000–2001, *2010*
    medial, 1997–1998
    multifocal type, *134, 136*
    periarterial, *1997*, 1998–2000
    perimedial, 1998, *1999*
    tubular type, *135*
  iatrogenic dissection of, 112

Renal artery (*Continued*)
  inflammation of, drug-induced, 2036, *2038*
    immunologically mediated, 2035–2036
    pheochromocytoma and, 2035
    syphilitic, 2036
  medial dissection of, 1998, *1999*
  multiple, *129, 2057*
  neurofibromatosis of, 2038–2040
  occlusion of, *1878, 2058*
    acute, 2018–2024, *2025*
    atheromatous, *1996*
    iatrogenic, *2024*
    by transcatheter embolization, 1532–1534
  stenosis of, atherosclerotic, 1993–1995, *1997*
    collateral circulation and, 136, *137*
    hypertension and, *1985*
    in transplant rejection, *2037*, 2055–2056
    renal vein renin activity and, 1991–1992
  thrombosis of, in renal transplantation, *2056*
  traumatic lesions of, 1789–1802, 2004, *2020–2022*
Renal atrophy, hydronephrotic, vs. pyelonephritis,
    838–839
  postobstructive, *1943*
  vesicoureteral reflex and, *1061*
Renal biopsy, sonography in, 233–235
Renal blastema, nodular, 1671
Renal calyx (calyces), *508*
  anatomic variations in, abnormal, 1488, *1489–1491*
    normal, *493, 500–503, 506–516, 1488*
  calculi in, *1189–1190, 1214–1218*
  cupping of, *516*
  dilatation of, 956–961, 974–986
  elongated, abnormal, 1488, *1489–1491*
    normal, *1488*
  in adenocarcinoma, *1491–1492*
  in neoplastic disease, 1487–1493, *1566*
  in renal failure, 1884–1889
  in renovascular hypertension, 1987
  infundibulum of, vascular obstruction of, 983–986
  kidney architecture and, 483–484
  leukoplakia of, *2241*
  multiplicity of, *514*
  normal, *500–503*
  obstructive atrophic changes in, *959*
  papillary tumor of, *1569*
  peristaltic activity of, *535*
  spider-leg deformity of, 1488
  T-shaped, *514–515*
  tumors of, 1487–1493, *1566, 1569–1570*
Renal candidiasis, 895–898
Renal carbuncle, 854–855, *857–859*
  perinephric abscess and, *850, 861*
Renal cell carcinoma. See *Carcinoma, renal cell.*
Renal cortex, 483, *484*, 508
  abscess of, *167*
  necrosis of, 1965–1971
  tumors of, 1467–1554. See also *Tumors, of renal*
    cortex.
Renal dysgenesis, 571–577
Renal dysplasia, 571–577, 1427–1437
  ectopic ureter in, *708*
  features of, 1370(t)
  multicystic, 1430–1435, *1436–1437*
    sonographic diagnosis of, 245, *249–250*
Renal ectopia, *130*, 584–591
  arteriography in, *144*
  crossed, 593–604, *608–611*
    bilateral, 608

Renal ectopia (*Continued*)
  crossed, embryogenesis of, 594–595
    solitary, 600–601, *608*
      with fusion, *599, 608–614, 617–618*
        pelvic lipomatosis and, *2237*
        multicystic dysplasia and, *1437*
      without fusion, *599, 600, 608*
  embryogenesis of, 585, 588
  in pregnancy, *602*
  pathologic conditions associated with, 601–604,
    605–607
  pyelocaliectasis in, *602*
  radionuclide evaluation of, 192, *195*
  simple, 588, *589–591*
  sonography in, 236–238, *239*
  vs. intrathoracic kidney, *598*
  vs. ptosis, 542–546, 588–589
Renal failure, 1865–1900
  acute, 1865–1867, *1882*
    atrophic pyelonephritis and, *1887–1888*
    calculous disease and, *1876*
    cortical necrosis and, 1965–1971
    in alcoholism, *1880–1881*
    in multiple myeloma, 1959
    posterior urethral valves and, *1869*
    renovascular disorders and, *1877–1878*
    ureteropelvic obstruction and, *1870*
    vs. ureteral obstruction, *1874–1876*
  chronic, 1867–1868
    angiographic findings in, 1891(t)
    "end-stage," *1892*
      nephrotic syndrome and, *1895*
      sonography in, 319
  hepatorenal syndrome in, 1871
  radiographic findings in, 1868–1900
    angiography in, 1889–1900
    excretory urogram in, 1871–1889
      nephrogram in, 1871–1884
      risks of, 23, 1868–1871
  sonographic diagnosis in, *235*, 319
Renal fibrolipomatosis, 526–531, *532*
  vs. pelvic lipomatosis, 2233
Renal function, excretory urography and, 42–44
  radionuclide evaluation of, 199–200
  separated study of, 1990–1991
Renal hydatidosis, diagnosis, 942–949
    differential, 943–945
  epidemiology of, 940–941
  genitourinary infestation and, 941–942
  needle aspiration in, 945–949
  arteriography in, *145*
Renal hypoplasia, 238, 240
Renal infarction. See *Infarction, renal.*
Renal injuries, 1767–1821. See also *Kidney, injury to.*
Renal insufficiency, drip-infusion urography in, *43*
Renal ischemia, 1946–1953
Renal mass(es), angiography in, 137–142
  CT scanning in, 360–367
  radionuclide studies in, 197–199
  roentgen findings in, 162–164
  sonographic differentiation of, 245–276. See also
    Sonography, in renal mass lesions.
Renal mass puncture, 150–167
  complications of, 166(t), *172–174*
  contrast studies and, 154–155
  equipment for, 152, *153, 227–228*
  fluid aspirate characteristics in, 158–162
  hazards of, 164–167

Renal mass puncture (*Continued*)
  patient preparation for, 152
  patient selection for, 150–152
  roentgen findings and, 162–164
  sonographic guidance for, 227–233
  technique of, 152–158
Renal medulla, *508*
Renal outline mapping, by sonography, 233–235
Renal papilla(e), 483, *484*
  aberrant, 506, *507*
  necrosis of, 1928–1943. See also *Renal papillary necrosis.*
  pyelectasis and, 956–961
Renal papillary necrosis, analgesic abuse and, *1929,
    1930–1931, 1936*
  associated disease states and, 1931
  clinical course of, 1928
  differential diagnosis of, 1940–1943
  gross pathology of, 1928–1930
  infection and, 1931
  medullary, *1929*, 1934–1938
  moniliasis and, *896*
  obstructive uropathy and, 1931–1932
  papillary, 1933–1934, *1935–1938*
  pathogenesis of, 1930–1932
  radiographic findings in, 1932–1939
  sickle hemoglobinopathy and, 1932, 1944–1946
  tuberculosis and, *907–908, 1941–1942*
  urothelial tumors and, 1932
  vs. obstructive atrophy, 959
Renal parenchyma, anatomic variation in, 517–526
  atrophy of, *372*
    vesicoureteral reflux and, *1061–1062*
  calcium deposition in, 1285–1293. See also
    Nephrocalcinosis.
  fetal lobulation in, 518, *520*
  kidney architecture and, 483–484
  normal variations in, 517–526
  thickness of, 517–518, *520*
  tumors of, 1467–1554. See also *Tumors, renal corti-
    cal.*
  vascular distribution in, 2002–2003
Renal parenchymal disease, 1901–1976
  angiographic features of, 1890(t)
  computed tomography in, *372*
  general considerations in, 1901
  glomerular, 1901–1926. See also names of specific
    diseases.
    amyloidosis, 1913–1925
    in diabetes mellitus, 1910–1913
    nephrotic syndrome, 1925–1926
    radiographic findings in, 1903–1910
  radiographic appearance of, 1886(t)
  tubulointerstitial, 1926–1971. See also *Tubulo-
    interstitial disease* and names of specific
    diseases.
Renal pelvis, aberrant papillae in, 506, *507*
  ampullary, *995*
  amyloidosis of, 1921, *1922*
  anatomic variations in, 492–506
  anomalies of, clinical classification of, 566
    horseshoe kidney and, *630*
    in number, 642–672
  atypical insertion of ureter into, *495–496*
  bifid, 498–500, *502*, 646
    malrotation with, *583*
    retrograde peristalsis in, 533–534
  "branching ureter" type of, *498*

Renal pelvis (*Continued*)
  calculi in, *1192–1198, 1200–1201, 1207–1208,*
    1216, 1218
  carcinoma of, 284–288. See also *Carcinoma, of*
    renal pelvis.
  distortion of, by incomplete filling, 500, 501–503
  "drooping-flower," *659, 694*
  duplication of, *647, 652, 694, 1817, 1820.* See also
    Duplex kidney.
    comparative size of, *646–648, 650–652*
    complete, *650–651*
    incomplete, *644–646, 651, 656*
    malrotation with, 656
    terminology of, 646
  extrarenal, *495, 497*
  "flabby", *958*
    vs. pyelectasis, *497, 498*
  funnel, *995*
  hematoma in, *1776*
  intrarenal, *495*
  kidney architecture and, 483–484
  leukoplakia of, 2240–2246
  lipomatosis of, *327–329*
    sonographic diagnosis of, 323–326
  mucosal striation in, 868, *1034*
  multifid, *645*
  normal, 484–487, *497*
  oval, *496*
  overdistention of, by contrast medium, *496*
  peristalsis in, urogram and, 532–535
  pressure deformities of, *496,* 500–506
  pyelectasis and, *961–963*
  retroperitoneal fibrosis in, *2211*
  rupture of, adenocarcinoma and, 1493, *1495*
    during urography, *1821*
    ureteral calculus and, *1820*
  "spastic", in renovascular hypertension, 1987
  square, *496*
  submucosal bleeding in, *1776*
  symmetry of, in same individual, 486, *487*
  trifid, *498–500, 647, 689*
  tumors of, 1554–1589. See also *Tumors, of renal*
    pelvis.
  vascular impressions on, 500–506
Renal pyramids, 483, *484*
  pyelectasis and, *956–961*
Renal scans, 185–207. See also *Radionuclide studies.*
Renal sinus, *508*
  anatomic variations in, 526–531
  myxoma of, *1473*
Renal sinus lipomatosis, 526–531, *532,* 2233
Renal transplantation, 2051–2073
  complications of, urologic, 2064–2073
    leaks in, ureteral, 2067–2068
      ureterovesical, *2071*
      vesical, 2069–2073
    obstruction in, *203,* 2068–2069
    vascular, 2055–2056
      arteriovenous fistula, 2056–2057
  function evaluation in, 2052–2064
    arteriography in, 143–145, *147,* 2052–2057
    radioisotope scanning in, 200–205, 2057–
      2062
    sonography in, 326, *330–331,* 2062–2064
  ileal conduit diversion and, *2103*
  normal allograft in, *2053, 2061, 2062*
  rejection in, *331, 2037*
    acute, *2053–2055*
    arteriographic evaluation of, 2053–2055

Renal transplantation (*Continued*)
  rejection in, chronic, 2054, *2055*
    hyperacute, 2054
    radioisotope study of, *2059*
    vs. acute tubular necrosis, 2054–2055
    vs. suppurative pyelonephritis, 295–296, *296*
  renal papillary necrosis and, *1932*
  ureteral hernia in, *2233*
Renal tubular acidosis, calculous disease and,
  1241–1245
Renal tubular ectasia, 1441–1451
  nephrocalcinosis and, 1287
Renal tubular necrosis, *1876, 1882*
  vs. ureteral obstruction, *1874–1876*
Renal tubular syndromes, calculous disease and,
  1241–1248, *1249–1250*
Renal vein, renin activity of, 1991–1992
  thrombosis of, *1877,* 2024–2028
    arteriography in, *138*
    in adults, 2025–2026
    in infants and children, 2024–2025, *2026*
    in transplantation, 2056
  tumor and, *1522–1524,* 1528–1532
Renal venography, 117–120
Renocolic fistula, *182–183*
Renin-angiotensin-aldosterone system, 1979–1980
Renogastric fistula, *1844–1845*
Renography, isotope. See *Radionuclide techniques.*
Renovascular hypertension, 1979–2002. See also
  Hypertension, renovascular.
Residual urine, calculation of, by cystography, 67–68
  in radionuclide studies, *188*
Retrocaval ureter, 677–678, *679–682*
Retrograde cystography, 65–66
Retrograde cystourethrography, in prostatic hyper-
  plasia, 1135–1141
Retrograde ileocystography, *2076*
Retrograde peristalsis, 533–534
Retrograde pyelography, 58–64
  air-pyelogram in, 64
  delayed pyelogram in, 64
  in genitourinary tuberculosis, 917–918
  in pyelectasis, 969–971
  in renal trauma, 1777–1786
  in tuberculosis, 917–918
  ureteral catheterization in, 58–61
Retrograde urethrography, 68–70
Retroiliac ureter, 678–680
Retroperitoneal fibrosis, *180,* 292, 2205–2220
  bowel involvement by, 2206, *2208*
  clinical features of, 2205–2207
  computed tomography in, 2217
  drug-induced, *2209*
  gross and microscopic appearance of, 2207
  in renal pelvis, *2211*
  lymphography in, 393
  pathogenesis of, 2207–2212
  radionuclide studies in, *196*
  roentgen diagnosis of, 2212–2217
  treatment of, 2217–2220
Retroperitoneal xanthofibrosarcoma, *170*
Retrorectal tumors, 1610–1618
Rhabdomyosarcoma, 1691–1699. See also *Botryoid*
  sarcoma.
  in horseshoe kidney, *643*
  prostatic, 1698
  retroperitoneal, *1593*
  vesical, 1697–1698
Right ovarian vein syndrome, 2149–2155

Roll-film changer, Elema-Schonanader, 96
Roux-en-Y pelvioileoneocystostomy, 2120
RTA (renal tubular acidosis), calculous disease and,
    1241–1245

Sacral (pelvic) kidney, 592–593, 594–595. See also
    Pelvic kidney.
Sacrum, anomalies of, 459–462, 1088–1091, 1093–
    1096
    cysts of, 464
    normal, 460
Sarcoidosis, 1260, 1960–1962
    calculous disease and, 1261–1262
    nephrocalcinosis in, 1260, 1962
    pulmonary, 1961–1963
    radiographic findings in, 1960–1962, 1963
    renal, 1961
Sarcoma, botryoid, 1693–1697. See also Botryoid
    sarcoma; Rhabdomyosarcoma.
    renal, in duplicated kidney, 673
        incidence of, 1468(t)
        polypoid fungating, 1543
    vesical, 1628
Scaphoid megalourethra, 763
Schistosomiasis, 921–939, 940. See also Bilharziasis.
Schwannoma, retroperitoneal, 1606, 1607
Scintigraphy, adrenal, 1750–1753
Scintillation camera studies, 185–213. See also
    Radionuclide studies.
Scleroderma, 1953–1955
Scoliosis, 458
Scout film, 5–11, 396–480. See also Plain film.
Scrotal fistula, calculus and, 1361
Segmental ureterectasis, 1008, 1010, 1011
Seldinger needle-cannula, 102
Seldinger technique, 101–113
Selectan neutral, formula of, 4
Seminal vesicle(s), bilharzial involvement of, 939, 940
    calcification of, bilharzial, 932
        tuberculous, 906
    carcinoma of, 1647–1649
    cysts of, 768–773, 774
    ectopic ureteral orifice in, 706–708, 709–712
    normal anatomy of, 80
    tumors of, 1646–1648
Seminal vesicle tract, malignant lesions of, 85
    traumatic lesions of, 85
Seminal vesiculitis, 82–84
    tuberculous, 919
Seminal vesiculography, 76–85
Sensitivity testing, 123
Separated renal function study, 1990–1991
Septum of Bertin, 483
Sex, chromosomal, 780
    determinants of, 782(t)
    genital, external, 781
        internal, 781
    gonadal, 780–781
    hormonal, 781
    nature of, 780–784
    of rearing, 779–781
Sexual differentiation, normal, 781–783
Shadows, in gastrointestinal tract, 403–404
    intestinal gas and, 539
    nonopaque, in lower abdomen, 441, 442
        in upper abdomen, 437–441

Shadows (Continued)
    opaque, extraurinary, from adrenal glands, 421–422
        from body surfaces, bandages, and clothing,
            405, 406
        from calcified blood vessels, 405–411
        from calcified intra-abdominal structures,
            412–418
        from carcinoma of ovary, 432, 433
        from costal cartilages and lumbar vertebrae,
            404, 405
        from dermoid cysts of ovary, 434, 435
        from female pelvis and genital tract, 428–433
        from fetal bones, 422–423
        from gallstones, 410
        from male pelvis and genital tract, 435–437
        from mesenteric and retroperitoneal lymph
            nodes, 418–421
        from miscellaneous calcifications, 423
        from mucus-producing adenocarcinoma, 433
        from previous cholecystogram, 424
        from previous operative procedures, 426–427,
            429–430
        from opaque material in bowel, 424–426
        from residual medication, 424, 425, 427
        urographic identification of, 1301
    in urinary tract, 442–449
        from calcific deposits, 442–446
        from foreign bodies, 446–449
    vs. renal calculi, 1183–1201
    vs. ureteral calculi, 1294–1300
    vs. vesical calculi, 1347–1349
    vs. vesical diverticulum, 554
Sickle cell trait. See Sickle hemoglobinopathy.
Sickle hemoglobinopathy, 1944–1946, 1947–1950
    renal papillary necrosis and, 1932
Sigmoid conduit, 2095–2097, 2098–2101
Sigmoid kidney, 609, 615
Sigmoidostomy, perineal, with ureterectostomy,
    2095, 2097
    urinary, 2095–2097, 2098–2101
Simple voiding cystourethrography, 71
Sinus, abdominal draining, 1846
    suprapubic, 1841
    urachal alternating, 734–736
Skeletal system, lesions of, 450–479
Solitary kidney, carcinoma in, 168, 1507
    retrocaval ureter with, 681
    transitional cell epithelioma in, 1564
    ureterocalyceal stricture in, 974
    Wilms' tumor in, 1667
Sonography, 214–339
    abbreviation nomenclature for, 218(t)
    as guide for percutaneous aspiration, 227–233
    equipment for, 216–217, 227
    frequencies used in, 216(t)
    in adrenal diseases, 331–332, 1750, 1751
    in calculous disease, 338, 339
    in congenital anomalies, 235–245
    in cystic disease of seminal vesicle, 773
    in hydronephrosis, 276–290, 291
    in infection, 290–319
        in end-stage kidney, 319
        in infected cyst, 298–308, 309–314
        in perinephric abscess, 308, 315–316
        in pyelonephritis, acute, 293–296
            chronic, 316, 317
            suppurative, 295–296, 296
        in pyonephrosis, 316–319

Sonography (*Continued*)
in infection, in renal abscess, 296–298, *862*
in renal tuberculosis, *305–308*
in pelvic abscess, *2064*
in renal biopsy, 233–235
in renal mass lesions, 245–276, 1507–1514
in neoplasm, 253–263
in renal cyst, 250–253, *254–255*, 1507–1514
pitfalls in, 263–276
in renal outline mapping, 233–235
in renal sinus lipomatosis, 323–326
in renal transplantation, 326, *330–331*, 2062–2064
in retroperitoneal fibrosis, 2217, *2218*
in retroperitoneal neoplasia, 319–323
in vesical tumors, 1639
of bladder, 331, *332*
of normal kidneys, 216–227
of prostate, 331, *333–335*
of testis, 337–339
of ureter, 326
scanning technique in, 220–221, *222*
terminology of, 215–216
Spermatic cord, normal lymphogram of, *389*
Spermatic tract, confusing shadows from, 435, *436*
"Spider-leg" vessels, in Wilms' tumor, 1657
Spina bifida, 459–461, 1082–1095
arrested ascent of spinal cord in, *1091*
cystica, 1613
occulta, *459*
without meningocele, *1092*
Spinal cord, injury of, neurogenic bladder
secondary to, *1081–1082*
Spindle ureter, 535–537, *539*
Spine, tuberculosis of, 452–453
"Spinning top" deformity, *1103–1104*
Spiral-flap ureteropelvioplasty, *1004*
Spleen, confusing shadows from, 412, *438*
cyst of, *1605*
distortion of, by renal mass, 1487
enlargement of, vs. retroperitoneal tumor, *1604*
kidney transposed with, *274–277*
Splenic artery, confusing shadows from, *410*
Splenic impression, 518–520, *522*
Splenomegaly, *438*
Staghorn calculi. See *Calculi, renal, staghorn.*
Stereoscopic renal angiography, 97
Steroid therapy, calculous disease and, 1263, *1264*
Stoma, colonic, confusing shadow from, *406*
Stones, 1171–1368. See also *Calculi.*
Stress incontinence, 2156–2163
Stricture, third-lumbar (Makar's), 933–934, *935*
Subcapsular hematoma, 1493–1498, *1501, 1773–1774*
Subdiaphragmatic abscess, vs. perinephric, 849
Supernumerary kidney, "free," 569–571, *572–573*
Suppurative pyelonephritis, *295, 296*
Suprapubic cystostomy, 2074, *2075*
Suprapubic sinus, *1841*
Sutures, confusing shadows from, *429*
Swick, Moses, 2–5
Sympathicoblastoma, in children, 1680–1686
Systemic lupus erythematosus, aneurysm in, *1897*

Takayasu's disease, 2033–2034, *2035*
Tamm-Horsfall proteinuria, *1878*
Tampons, confusing shadows from, 428, *431*
Teratocarcinoma, *337*

Teratoma, intrarenal, *1677*
pararenal, *1609*
renal, malignant, *1676*
retroperitoneal, 1608–1610
presacral, *1613*
sacrococcygeal, 1611–1612, *1613*
Testicular torsion, 210
Testis, carcinoma of, 337–339, *384–386*, 387–391
normal, *337*
radionuclide evaluation of, 210, *211*
tumors of, 1650–1652
Thromboarteritis (Buerger's disease), 2036–2038
Thyrotoxicosis, calculous disease and, 1263, *1265*
Tomography, 53–54. See also *Nephrotomography.*
advantages of, 8–10, *34–37*
and reinjection, 35–38
computed, 339–373. See also *Computed tomography.*
"Toothpaste sign" of vesical neck contracture, *1148*
Torsion, testicular, 210
Transcatheteral embolization of renal artery, 1532–1534
Transitional cell carcinoma, of renal pelvis, 284–288
renal, *141*
ureteral, *1575–1576*
vesical, *1575*
Translumbar aortography, 115–116
vascular complications of, 126–127
Transplantation, renal. See *Renal transplantation.*
Transureteroureterostomy, 2080–2083
cutaneous ureterostomy and, 2083–2084, *2085–2087*
Trauma, to urinary system, 1767–1840. See also
names of specific organs.
Trigone, anomalies of, renal agenesis and, 574–575
cystographic visualization of, 550–552, *553*
Trueta phenomenon, 1889–1899
Tubercular cystitis, 888
Tuberculosis, cystitis and, 888, *917*, 2134–2135
genital, 84, 918–921
vesicosigmoidal fistula and, *1850*
genitourinary, 898–921
calcification in, 899–907
clinical and laboratory findings in, 898–899
pathogenesis of, 898
roentgen findings in, 899–918
plain film in, 899–907
renal angiography in, 918
retrograde pyelography in, 917–918
urography in, 907–917
vs. bilharziasis, 934–936
in duplex kidney, 670
in horseshoe kidney, 639–640
renal, *305–308*
leukoplakia and, *2245*
papillary necrosis in, *1940, 1942*
vs. tumor, *913*
renogastric fistula and, *1844–1845*
spinal, 452–453
vs. brucellosis, 891
vs. caliectasis with calculi, 1222, *1227*
Tuberous sclerosis, 1481–1486
angiomyolipoma and, 262–263, *1484, 1675*
Tubular insufflation, confusing shadows from, *431*
Tubules, uriniferous, developmental zones of, *568*
Tubulointerstitial disease, 1926–1971
drug abuse and, *1927*
in multiple myeloma, 1957–1960

Tubulointerstitial disease (*Continued*)
  in sarcoidosis, 1960–1962
  nephrosclerosis, 1946–1953
  radiation nephritis, 1962–1965
  renal cortical necrosis, 1965–1971
  renal papillary necrosis and, 1928–1943
  scleroderma, 1953–1955
  sickle hemoglobinopathy, 1944–1946, *1947–1950*
  uric acid nephropathy, 1955–1957, *1958*
Tumors, 1467–1766. See also under individual
    names, such as *Carcinoma, Sarcoma,* etc.
  adrenal, *369,* 1700–1753
    adrenogenital syndrome and, 1708
    classification of, 1700–1703
    computed tomography in, 367–368, 1711, 1721,
      1750, *1751*
    cortical, 1706–1709, *1716,* 1730–1731, *1732–1735*
      angiography in, 1730–1735
      clinical syndromes and, 1707–1709
      functioning, 1707
      in Cushing's disease, *1718*
      nonfunctioning, 1706–1707
    Cushing's syndrome and, 1707–1708
    ectopic, 1720
    feminizing syndrome and, 1708–1709
    medullary, *1682,* 1704–1706
    primary aldosteronism and, 1708
    radiographic visualization of, 1709–1750
      by arteriography, 1722–1745, *1746*
      by excretory urography, 1709–1722
      by venography, 1748, *1749–1750*
    scintigraphic evaluation of, 1750–1753
    sonographic evaluation of, 331–332, 336, 1750, *1751*
    vs. aortic aneurysm, *2030*
    vs. fluid in gastric fundus, *1712*
  calculous disease and, *439,* 1262–1263
  extrarenal, vs. adenocarcinoma, 1493, *1500–1503*
    vs. hematoma, 1493–1498, *1501–1503*
  genitourinary, in female, 2185–2199
      benign, 2185–2191
      malignant, 2193–2199
      ovarian cysts, 2191–2193
  in children, 1652–1699
    congenital, 1668–1671
    infantile, 1668–1671
  metastasized, calcification in, 1498(t)
  neovascularity of, 1657–1658
  of appendix, vs. pericecal abscess, *423*
  of renal calyx, *1569–1570*
  of renal cortex, benign, epithelial, 1469–1472
    incidence of, 1468–1469
    mesenchymal, 1472–1481
    calcification of, 1493, *1499–1500*
    malignant, epithelial, 1486–1534. See also
      Adenocarcinoma, renal.
      histogenesis of, 1486
      Lindau-von Hippel disease and, 1534, *1539,*
        1541–1542
      mesenchymal, 1534–1542
      metastatic, 1542–1554
      secondary, 1542–1554
  of renal pelvis, 1554–1589
    benign, 1554–1560
    in children, *1585,* 1686–1688
    incidence of, 1468(t)
    malignant, 1560–1589
      epithelial, 1562–1572

Tumors (*Continued*)
    of renal pelvis, malignant, incidence of, 1561(t)
      lethal potentiality of, 1561(t)
      nonepithelial, 1582–1589
    vs. adenocarcinoma, *1492*
    vs. blood clot, *1565*
    vs. fibrosarcoma, *1543*
  of seminal vesicles, 1646–1648
  pelvic, *441,* 442
  pelvic bone, 462–464
  prostatic, 1648–1650
    in children, 1699. See also *Rhabdomyosarcoma.*
  renal, calcification in, 1493, 1498(t), *1499–1500*
    classification of, 1467–1468
    cortical, 1467–1554
      benign, 1467–1486
      malignant, 1486–1554
    in children, 1652–1686
    incidence of, 1468(t)
    malignant, *140*
    metastatic, 1549–1554
      calcification in, 1498(t)
    pseudo-, 272, *274–277,* 650, *653–655,* 835–836,
      1036–1037
    solid, *354*
    sonographic findings in, 253–263
    transitional cell, *141*
    vascular obstruction by, *1521–1524*
    vascularity of, 1514–1520, *1537*
    vs. aortic aneurysm, *2030*
    vs. cyst, *1387, 1390–1410,* 1504–1534
      CT evaluation in, 360–367
      sonographic evaluation in, 245–276
    vs. hydrocalyx, *975*
    vs. lobar dysmorphism, 650, *653–654*
    vs. pyelonephritic scars, *835–836*
    vs. renal carbuncle, *857*
    vs. renal tuberculosis, *913*
  retroperitoneal, 1589–1618
    benign, 1590(t), 1594–1602
    classification of, 1589(t)
    confusing shadows from, *440*
    embryonal, 1608–1610
    incidence of, 1589, 1590(t)
    malignant, 1590(t)
    Middeldorpf, 1610–1618
    of mesodermal origin, 1589–1606
      benign, 1594–1602
      malignant, 1589–1594, *1595*
    of neurogenic origin, 1606–1608
    presacral, 1610–1618
      classification of, 1611(t)
    sonographic diagnosis of, 319–323
    vs. intra-abdominal lesions displacing kidneys
      and ureters, 1602–1605
  spinal primary, 462–464
  testicular, 1650–1652
  urachal, in children, 1689
  ureteral, benign, 1554–1560
    in children, *1688*
    nonpolypoid, 1559, *1560*
    polypoid, 1555–1559
    urographic diagnosis of, 1559–1560
    Bergman's sign in, 1577
    in children, 1686–1688
    in pelvic kidney, *607*
    incidence of, 1468(t)

Tumors (*Continued*)
  ureteral, malignant, 1560–1582
    diagnosis of, "goblet sign" in, 1577, *1579–1582*
      inaccuracy in, 1572–1576
    epithelial, 1560–1580
      multiplicity of, 1561–1562
      primary, 1572–1580
    incidence of, 1561(t)
    lethal potentiality of, 1561(t)
    nonepithelial, 1582–1589
    nonpapillary, 1577–1582, *1585*
    papillary, 1576–1577, *1578–1583*
    secondary, directly invasive, 1585–1589
      metastatic, 1586–1589
    symptoms of, 1572
    urographic diagnosis of, 1576–1582, *1583*
    vesical tumors with, *1575*
   vs. calculus, *1321*
   vs. endometriosis, *2184*
   vs. vesical carcinoma, 1584
  urethral, 1643–1646
   in children, 1699
  urothelial, analgesic nephropathy and, 1932
   in children, 1689
  uterine, fibroid, 2185–2191
    confusing shadows from, 439, *432, 433*
    extravesical pressure by, *551*
  vesical, 1618–1641
   adrenal, *1721*
   benign, 1641–1642
   calcification of, 1630, *1631*
   in children, 1688–1689. See also *Rhabdomyo-*
    sarcoma.
   lymphangiography in, 1639
   malignant, 1618–1641
    angiography in, 1633–1639
    epithelial, 1618–1639
     calcification of, 1630, *1631*
     in vesical diverticula, 1630–1632, *1633*
     nonpapillary (solid) infiltrating, 1623–1630
     papillary noninfiltrative, 1619–1623
     urachal carcinoma and, 1632–1633
    metastatic, 1639–1641
    nonepithelial. See *Rhabdomyosarcoma.*
    nonpapillary (solid) infiltrating, 1623–1630
    papillary noninfiltrative, 1619–1623
    ureteral tumors with, *1575*
   sonography in, 1639
   vs. leukoplakia, *2246*, 2246–2247
   vs. prostatic encrustation, *1141*
  Wilms'. See *Wilms' tumor.*
Two-film technique, advantages of, 8, *9*

Ulcer(s), Hunner's, 883–885, 2142–2144
Ultrasound, 214–339. See also *Sonography.*
Umbilical cyst, 734, *735*
Umbilical sinus, 734, *735*
Underexposure, in plain film, *403*
Undulant fever, 891–895
Unilateral multicystic disease, 1430–1435, *1436–1437*
Unilateral renal dysplasia, 1430–1435, *1436–1437*
Upper urinary tract, anatomy of, 481–487
Urachal sinus, alternating, 734–736
Urachus, anomalies of, 732–736
  carcinoma of, 1632–1633, *1634*
   in children, 1689

Ureter, amyloidosis of, 1918–1921
  anatomic relation of, 483
  anomalies of, clinical classification of, 566
   in number, 642–672
   in origin and termination, 684–729
   in position and form, 672–682
   renal agenesis and, 574
  "beaded," *914*, 916
  bifid, 642, *644*
  bilharzial pathology of, 924–926, 928, *929–931,*
   933–936
  blind-ending, 672, *673–675*
  branched rudimentary, 672, *673–675*
   tuberculous, *905*
  calcification of, 444
   vs. bilharziasis, 901
  calculi of, 1294–1338. See also *Calculi, ureteral.*
  caliber variations in, 535–537
  catheterization of, in retrograde pyelography, 58–61
  "corkscrew", *914*, 916
  cysts of, *1578*
  deviation of, *352–353*
   by abdominal aneurysm, *2031–2032*
   by iliac artery, *538*
   by retroperitoneal lymphadenopathy, *1548*
   in duplex kidney, *662*
   normal, 2212, *2215*
  dilatation of. See also *Ureterectasis; Ureteropyelec-*
   tasis.
   calculi in, 1321, *1322–1324*
   in infection, 867–868
   in neoplastic disease, *1577*
   venous, 2149–2155
  diverticulum of, 672–676
  duplication of, *647*, 693, *702*
   complete, 642–644, *645, 650–651*
   incomplete, 642, *644, 648, 653, 689*
    retrograde peristalsis in, 648, *649*
   sonographic diagnosis in, 235–236, *237–238*
   supernumerary kidney with, *571*
   terminology of, 646
   ureterocele in, *713*
   vesicoureteral reflux and, *1052, 1070*
  ectopic, 658, *688*
   calculi in, *1325*
   vesicoureteral reflux and, *1051–1052*
  edema of, in calculous disease, 1323–1330, *1335*
  embryology of, 568–569
  endometriosis of, 2182–2184
   vs. stricture, *2183*
  filling defects in, air bubbles and, *539*
  "fish hook", *1142*
  hernia of, 2228–2233
  high insertion of, *993, 1003*
  incomplete filling of, diagnostic errors from,
   537–538, *539, 541*
  injury to, 1822–1827
   iatrogenic, *180*, 1824–1826, *2168*
  intramural, calculi in, 1323–1330
   extravesical position of, neurologic disease with,
    1045
  kinks in, 538–542
   vs. calculi, *402*
  leaks in, in renal transplantation, 2067–2068
  leukoplakia of, *2243*, 2246
  mucosal striation in, 868, *1034*
  "notching" of, *1988*, 2041, *2042–2043*
  obstruction of, *991*. See also *Ureteropelvic juncture,*
   obstruction of.

Ureter (*Continued*)
obstruction of, abdominal aortic aneurysm and, 2205, *2206*
by aberrant vessels, *682,* 683
by arteriovenous fistula, *2033*
by cervical carcinoma, 2193, *2194*
by congenital adhesions, *1017*
by infiltrating carcinoma, *1622*
by leukemic infiltration, *1680*
by neoplasm, 1014, *1015–1016*
by ovarian cysts, *2192–2193*
by postoperative temporary edema, *1071*
by uterine fibroids, *2190*
by valves, 682–683, *684–685*
by vascular lesions, 1014–1017, 2020–2045
by vesical diverticulum, *1133*
congenital, 680–683
inflammatory, 1014
in renal transplantation, *203*
papillary necrosis and, *1943*
radioisotope study of, *2059*
retroperitoneal fibrosis and, 2205–2220. See also *Retroperitoneal fibrosis.*
vs. acute renal failure, *1874–1875.*
vs. renal tubular necrosis, *1874–1875*
orifice of. See *Ureteral orifice.*
peristalsis in, 532–535
"pipestem", *914–915,* 916
polypoid lesions of, *1555–1559,* 1687, *1688*
position of, normal, 537
postarterial, 678–680
postcaval, 677–678
replacement of, 2116–2125
retrocaval, 677–678, *679–682*
retroiliac, 678–680
"scalloping" of, *1988, 2041, 2042–2043*
sonographic evaluation of, 326
spasm of, catheterization and, 541–542
"spastic", in renovascular hypertension, 1987
spindle deformity of, 535–537, *539*
strictures of, 539–542
congenital, 680–682
in infection, 868–873
in transplantation, *2070*
long, *1004*
malignancy and, 1582
vs. calculus, *1321*
vs. endometriosis, *2193*
surgical injury to, *180,* 1824–1826, *2168*
triplication of, *647*
tuberculous changes in, 914–916
tumors of, 1554–1589. See also *Tumors, ureteral.*
valves of, congenital, 682–683, *684–685*
venous compression of, in pregnancy, 2147. See also *Ovarian vein syndrome.*
Y-type, 646, 648, *649,* 653
Ureteral artery, anomalous, *2052*
Ureteral bud, 567–568
Ureteral caliber reduction-modelage, 1079–1080
Ureteral compression, 28–30, *31, 33, 1820*
Ureteral ileus, *41*
Ureteral orifice, ectopic, 684–708. See also *Ectopic ureteral orifice.*
jet of urine from, 552, *554*
secondary obstruction of, *1012–1013*
Ureteral stumps, stone-bearing, 1331, *1332*
Ureterectasis, 1005–1017

Ureterectasis (*Continued*)
vesical diverticulum and, *1132*
Ureteritis, cystica, *935*
tuberculous, *909*
Ureterocecostomy, 2098, *2102*
Ureterocele, 708, 713–726
ectopic, 237–238, 715, 719–726, 727–728, *1053*
simple, 708, 713–715, *716–719*
Ureterocolic anastomoses, 2084–2086
Ureterocutaneous fistula, *1846*
Ureteroileal fistula, *1846*
Ureteroileoneocystostomy, 2121–2123
Ureteroileostomy, 2098–2108, *2109–2119*
Ureterointestinal anastomoses, 2098–2116, *2117–2119*
Ureterolithotomy, 1331–1338
Ureteroneocystostomy, 1066–1079
complications of, 1070–1079
results of, *1067–1069, 1073, 1075–1079*
Ureteropelvic juncture, anomalous vessel crossing, *991*
bizarre types of, *494–495*
calculi in, *1199, 1217*
hamartoma of, *1560*
obstruction of, 986–1004
aberrant blood vessels and, *991–993*
bilateral tendency of, 986
clinical features of, 999–1000
high ureteral insertion and, *993*
hydronephrosis and, *290–291,* 956, *994–999*
in infant, *293*
in infants and children, 986–987
pathogenesis of, 987–999
intermittent hydronephrosis in, 994–999
radioisotope study of, *2059*
renal failure and, *1870*
secondary calculi in, *1221–1222*
surgical considerations in, 1000–1004, *2126*
temporary diversion in, *2126*
trauma and, *1788*
urographic diagnosis of, 999–1004
vs. adenocarcinoma of renal cortex, *1496*
vs. reflux, *1028*
peristaltic narrowing of, *536*
"signet-ring" deformity of, *1688*
spasm of, catheterization and, *536*
Ureteropelvioplasty, spiral flap, *1004*
Y-V, *1003–1004*
Ureteroperineal fistula, *2176*
Ureteroplasty, 1079–1080
Ureteropyelectasis, 1005–1017
general principles in, 1005
incomplete filling in, diagnostic errors and, 1005–1008, *1009*
ovarian abscess and, *2200*
pelvic inflammatory disease and, *2200*
vesical neck contracture and, *1149*
Ureterorectostomy, 2093, *2095*
with perineal sigmoidostomy, 2095, *2097*
Ureterosigmoidostomy, 2086–2093, *2094*
carcinoma in, 747–748
cutaneous sigmoid colostomy with, 2093–2095, *2096*
gas in urinary tract and, *879*
in exstrophy of bladder, 744–745
Ureterostomy, cutaneous, 2076–2080, *2081*
transureteroureterostomy and, 2083–2084, *2085–2087*

Ureterovaginal fistula, 1858–1861, 2172–2174
  incontinence and, 2167–2173
  vesicovaginal fistula with, 1861
Ureterovesical juncture, bilharziasis and, 925–926
  obstruction of, 1011–1017
    in renal transplantation, 2068–2069
  vesicoureteral reflux and, 1039
Urethra, accessory, 755–761
  "acorn" deformity of, *1103–1104*
  anomalies of, 755–765
  anterior, 559
    congenital valves of, 1116–1119
  bilharzial involvement of, 936–939
  bulbomembranous, carcinoma of, *1645*
  calculi of, 446, 939, 1359–1365
  caliber of, vesical neck contracture and, *1102*
  carcinoma of, *1644–1646*, 2198–2199
  congenital valves in, 1106–1119. See also
    Congenital urethral valves.
  continence zone of, 2158
  distal, stenosis of, 1102–1106, 2136–2138
    voiding effect on, *1105*
  diverticulum of, 761–765
  duplication of, *750–752*, 755–761
  embryology of, 751–755
  female, carcinoma of, 2198–2199
    caruncle of, 2199
    congenital valves of, 1119, *1120–1122*
    length of, incontinence and, 2157–2158
    normal, *562*
    tumors of, *1646*
  fistulas of, 1849–1854
  foreign bodies in, *449*
  injury to, 1123–1129, 1157–1161, 1827–1840
  male, anatomic considerations in, 552–557
    normal, infants and children, 559–561
    tumors of, 1643–1646
    urographic considerations in, 557–559
  meatus of, congenital stenosis of, 1122–1123, *1124*
  megalo-, 762–765
  membranous, 559
  polyps of, 1119–1122, *1123*
    in children, 1699
  posterior, *562*
    congenital valves of, 1106–1116, *1869*
    ectopic anus at, *798*
    injury to, 1827–1840
  prostatic, 558–559
    ectopic ureteral orifice in, *707*
  rupture of, 1834–1840
  sphincter of, neurogenic bladder and, 1082, *1083–1086*
  "spinning top" deformity of, *1103–1104*
  stenosis of, in women, 1102–1106, 2136–2138
  stricture of, calculus and, *1360–1361*
    congenital, 1123–1129
    iatrogenic, 1123–1129, 1157–1161
    in adult male, 1150–1161
    in children, 1123–1129
    inflammatory, 1152–1157
    postneisserian, *1853*
    traumatic, 1129, 1157–1161
  trifurcation of, *760*
  tumors of, 1643–1646, 1699
  variations of, during cystourethrography, *1104*
Urethral continence zone, 2158
Urethral diverticulum. See *Diverticula, urethral.*

Urethral meatus, congenital stenosis of, 1122–1123, *1124*
Urethral polyps, 1119–1122, *1123*
Urethral sphincter, neurogenic bladder and, 1082, *1083–1086*
Urethral stenosis, distal, 1102–1106, 2136–2138
Urethral valves, congenital, 1106–1119. See also
  Congenital urethral valves.
Urethritis cystica, bilharzial, *939*
  vs. urethral calculi, 939
Urethrocavernous fistula, *1854–1855*
Urethrocutaneous fistula, *2075*
  retrograde, 68–70, *71*
Urethrography, 794
Urethroperineal fistula, congenital, *760, 761, 1853*
Urethroscopy, in ectopic ureteral orifice, 695–696
Urethrorectal fistula, 1854, *1856*
Urethrostomy, perineal, 2073
Urethrovaginal fistula, 1861, *2176*
Urethrovesical juncture, ectopic anus at, *798*
Urge incontinence, 2156–2163
Uric acid lithiasis, *1205*, 1265–1269, *1270–1275*
  ureteral, *1337*
Uric acid nephropathy, 1955–1957, *1958*
Urinary diversion, 2073–2127. See also names of
  specific operations.
  at bladder level, 2074–2076, *2077*
  at renal level, 2116–2127
  at ureteral level, 2076–2098, *2101–2102*
  at urethral level, 2073
  in exstrophy of bladder, 744–745
  permanent, 2073
  temporary, 2073
  ureterointestinal anastomoses in, 2098–2116, *2117–2119*
Urinary extravasation, abdominal, iatrogenic, *2168*
  isotope scan in, *2060*
Urinary ileostomy, 2098–2108, *2109–2119*
Urinary retention, in neurogenic bladder, *1087, 1089*
Urinary sigmoidostomy, 2095–2097, *2098–2101*
Urinary stasis, 955–1170. See also *Caliectasis,*
  Pyelectasis, Ureterectasis, etc.
  classification of, 955
  infected urolithiasis and, 1279–1283
  of lower urinary tract, 1080–1162
  terminology of, 955
Urinary system, injury to, 1767–1840. See also names
  of specific organs.
Urinary tract, calcification of, in tuberculosis, 899–907
  endometriosis of, 2181–2185
  gas-producing infections of, 878–883
  upper, anatomy of, 481–487
Urinary-vaginal fistulas, 1854–1861
Urine, crystals in, *1179*
  differential assay of, 1706
  residual, 67–68, *188*
Uriniferous tubules, developmental zones of, *568*
Urinoma, 1370(t), 1455–1463, *2065*
Urogenital fistula, 791–792. See also *Ectopic anus.*
Urogenital sinus, 730–732
  ectopic anus at, *799–800*
Urographic contrast medium, 13–23. See also
  Contrast medium (media).
Urography, definition of, 1–2
  drip-infusion, *43–44*, 971, *973*
  historical perspective on, 2
  in calculous disease, 1191–1201

Urography (*Continued*)
  in genitourinary bilharziasis, 932–939
  in genitourinary tuberculosis, 907–917
  in renal and perirenal abscess, 851–861
  in renal hydatidosis, 942–945
  normal, 481–564
    general considerations in, 481–487
    nephroptosis and, 542–546
    of the bladder and urethra, 546–563
    of the kidney, 488–531
    of the ureters, 532–542
  peristalsis and, 532–535
  reinjection, in pyelectasis, 971, *973*
  techniques and applications of, 1–93. See also
    names of specific techniques.
  terminology in, 1–2
Urolithiasis, 1171–1368. See also *Calculi.*
Uroselectan, formula of, *4*
Uterine myofibroma, *2188–2189*
Uterus, anomalies of, renal agenesis and, 575
  carcinoma of, 2195–2197, *2198*
  didelphys, *704–705*
  extravesical pressure of, 2185, *2186–2187*
  fibroid tumors of, 2185–2191
    confusing shadows from, 429, *432, 433*
  fibrosis of, *440*
  prolapse of, 2163–2167
Utricle, prostatic, calculi in, *768*
  dilatation of, 765–767, *769–770*
  normal, *769*
Utriculography, 87–88

Vagina, agenesis of, renal agenesis and, 575, *576*
    renal ectopia and, *595*
  aplasia of, solitary ectopic kidney and, *600*
  atresia of, hydrocolpos and, *2180*
  carcinoma of, 2198, *2199*
  duplication of, *704*
  examination of, for ectopic ureteral orifice,
    695–696
  opacification of, 2160–2161
  powder in, confusing shadows from, 428, *431*
  substitute, bladder as, 2198, *2199*
Vaginography, 794
Valves, congenital urethral, 1106–1119. See also
    Congenital urethral valves.
  ureteral, 682–683, *684*
    impacted calculus in, *685*
Vasa deferentia, calcification of, *435–436*
  in diabetes, 435, *436*, 901
  tuberculous, *905–906*
  genitourinary hydatidosis in, *943*
Vascular infundibular obstruction, 983–986
Vein, renal. See *Renal vein.*
Vena cava, adenocarcinoma obstructing, *1522–1524*
  embryogenesis of, 677, *678*
  invasion of by tumor, 1528–1532
Vena cavography, in renal tumors, *119, 1522–1524,*
    1532
  normal, *117*
Venography, adrenal, 121–122, 1748–1749, *1750*
  in retroperitoneal fibrosis, 2217
  renal, 117–120
Vertebrae, confusing shadows from, 404
  ligamentous calcification of, *450*
  osteomyelitis of, 453, *454*
Verumontanum, normal anatomy of, *80*

Vesical diverticulum, 1129–1135. See also
    Diverticula, vesical.
Vesical mucosa, edema of, vs. cystitis emphysematosa,
    880
Vesical neck, "acorn" deformity of, *1103–1104*
  contracture of, postoperative, 1146–1149
    "toothpaste sign" of, *1148*
    urethral caliber and, *1102*
  in neurogenic bladder, 1082
  obstruction of, bilharzial, 926–927, 936, *937*
    congenital, *1049, 1137*, 1100–1102
      vs. neurogenic dysfunction, 1094–1095, *1096*
    in adult male, 1135–1149
      benign prostatic hyperplasia and, 1135–1145
      postoperative, 1147–1149
      prostatic carcinoma and, 1146
  "spinning top" deformity of, *1103–1104*
  transurethral resection of, *1087, 1089*
Vesical neck elevation test, for stress incontinence,
    2157
Vesicoappendiceal fistula, *1850*
Vesicocervical fistula, *2174*
Vesicocutaneous fistula, in renal transplantation, *2072*
Vesicoenteric fistula, *1850*
Vesicointestinal fistula, 1848–1849, *1849–1851*
Vesicorectostomy, *2076, 2077*
Vesicosigmoidal fistula, *1848–1849*
Vesicostomy, cutaneous, 2074, *2075*
Vesicoureteral reflux, 995, 1017–1080
  calculous disease and, *1178*
  chronic pyelonephritis and, 837–838
  diverticula and, *1042–1044*
  duplication and, *1042*
  ectopic ureteral orifice and, 691–692
  etiology of, 1038–1050
    ureterovesical juncture and, 1039
  general considerations in, 1018
  grading of, 1019–1022, *1022–1024*
  iatrogenic, *1053–1054*
  in adults, 1059–1062
  in bilharziasis, 925–926, *932*
  in duplex kidney, 654–657
  in ectopic kidney, *614*
  management of, 1062–1080
    conservative, 1062–1066
      results of, *1065–1066*
    surgical, 1066–1080
  neurologic disease and, *1045*
  primary, 1040–1046
  prognosis in, 1050–1059
  radionuclide evaluation of, 192–196, *209*
  roentgen findings in, 1018–1038
  secondary, 1046–1050
Vesicouterine fistula, *2198*
Vesicovaginal fistula, 1857–1858
  incontinence and, 2173–2176
  postirradiation, *2197*
  ureterovaginal fistula with, 1861
Vesiculogram, abnormal, 81–85
  normal, 80–81
Vestibule, examination of, 695–696
Vitamin D, calculous disease and, 1262
von Recklinghausen's disease, 1606
Vulva, carcinoma of, 2198–2199

Waterhouse technique, 72–73
Wilms' tumor, *259–261*

Wilms' tumor (*Continued*)
  bilateral, *1665–1666*
  calcification in, 1498(t), 1653, *1655*
  in solitary kidney, *1667*
  incidence of, 1468(t)
  inferior vena cavography in, *119*
  prognosis in, 1667–1668
  pulmonary metastasis of, *1652*
  "spider leg" neovascularities in, 1657
  staging of, 1664
  treatment of, 1664–1667
    by chemotherapy, 1666–1667
    by radiation therapy, 1665–1666
      side effects of, *1668*
  vascularity of, 1657–1658, *1659–1662*
  vs. congenital mesoblastic nephroma, 1664
  vs. multilocular cyst, *1442*
  vs. pararenal pseudocyst, *1462*

Wire mesh, confusing shadows from, *429–430*
Wolffian duct, embryology of, 566–569
  remnants of, in female, *686*
Women, urologic problems of, 2130–2204

Xanthinuria, 1252, *1255*
Xanthofibrosarcoma, retroperitoneal, *170*
Xanthogranulomatous pyelonephritis, 839–842
  calcification in, 1498(t)

"Yo-yo phenomenon," 648, *649*
Y-V ureteropelvioplasty, *1003–1004*